ANNUAL REVIEW OF PHARMACOLOGY AND TOXICOLOGY

EDITORIAL COMMITTEE (1987)

ANNUAL REVIEW OF PHARMACOLOGY AND TOXICOLOGY

VOLUME 27, 1987

ROBERT GEORGE, Coeditor

University of California School of Medicine, Los Angeles

RONALD OKUN, Coeditor

University of California School of Medicine, Los Angeles

ARTHUR K. CHO, Associate Editor

University of California School of Medicine, Los Angeles

ANNUAL REVIEWS INC.   4139 EL CAMINO WAY   PO BOX 10139   PALO ALTO, CALIFORNIA 94303-0897

ANNUAL REVIEWS INC.
Palo Alto, California, USA

International Standard Serial Number: 0362–1642
International Standard Book Number: 0–8243–0427–6
Library of Congress Catalog Card Number: 61–5649

Typesetting by Kachina Typesetting Inc., Tempe, Arizona; John Olson, President
Typesetting coordinator, Jeannie Kaarle

PRINTED AND BOUND IN THE UNITED STATES OF AMERICA

Annual Review of Pharmacology and Toxicology
Volume 27, 1987

CONTENTS

vi   CONTENTS   *(Continued)*

SOME RELATED ARTICLES IN OTHER *ANNUAL REVIEWS*

From the *Annual Review of Biochemistry*, Volume 56, 1987:

Inositol Trisphosphate and Diacylglycerol: Two Interacting Second Messengers, Michael J. Berridge
Intracellular Calcium Homeostasis, Ernesto Carafoli

From the *Annual Review of Medicine*, Volume 38, 1987:

Antiarrhythmic Drug Selection, Philip J. Podrid
Mechanisms Involved in Gastric Mucosal Resistance to Injury, David Fromm
Treatment of Pulmonary Embolism, Jack Hirsh
Chronic Lead Nephropathy, Peter W. Craswell
Interferon for the Treatment of Infections, Monto Ho
Clinical Pharmacology of Benzodiazepines, Malcolm Lader
Clinical Perspectives on Neuropeptides, D. A. Lewis and F. E. Bloom
The Treatment of Infertility, Henry G. Burger and H. W. Gordon Baker

From the *Annual Review of Neuroscience*, Volume 10, 1987:

Perspectives on the Discovery of Central Monoaminergic Neurotransmission, Arvid Carlsson
Molecular Properties of the Muscarinic Acetylcholine Receptor, Neil M. Nathanson
An Integrated View of the Molecular Toxinology of Sodium Channel Gating in Excitable Cells, Gary Strichartz, Thomas Rando, and Ging Kuo Wang
Developmental Regulation of Nicotinic Acetylcholine Receptors, Stephen M. Schuetze and Lorna W. Role
Calcium Action in Synaptic Transmitter Release, George J. Augustine, Milton P. Charlton, and Stephen J Smith

From the *Annual Review of Physiology*, Volume 49, 1987:

Regulation of Intracellular pH in the Stomach, Terry E. Machen and Anthony M. Paradiso
Thyroid Hormones and Brain Development, Jean H. Dussault and Jean Ruel
Gastroenteropancreatic Peptides and the Central Nervous System, Dianne P. Figlewicz, Francoise Lacour, Alfred Sipols, Daniel Porte, Jr., and Stephen C. Woods
Functions of Angiotensin in the Central Nervous System, M. Ian Phillips
Sex Steroids and Afferent Input: Their Roles in Brain Sexual Differentiation, Carlos Beyer and Harvey H. Feder

Ann. Rev. Pharmacol. Toxicol. 1987. 27:1–21

INHIBIN

Choh Hao Li and Kristipati Ramasharma

Laboratory of Molecular Endocrinology, University of California, San Francisco, California 94143

INTRODUCTION

Mottram & Cramer (1) laid the foundations of the inhibin (IB) concept six decades ago when they observed severe morphological changes in the anterior pituitary gland of a male rat whose germinal elements in the testes had been selectively damaged by radiation. This observation led to the suggestion that the pituitary gland is in some way regulated by a testicular factor other than steroid hormones. This hypothesis was further supported by experiments involving parabiotic rats. These parabiotic pairs consisted of a normal and a castrated rat. The hyperactivity of the pituitary gland in the castrated partner was prevented by treatment with water-soluble testicular extracts (2). Subsequently, McCullagh (3) coined the name "inhibin" for this hypothetical testicular factor. The inhibin concept remained an unresolved riddle in endocrine physiology for a long time (4–7). During this time the two gonadotropins [luteinizing hormone (LH) and follicle-stimulating hormone (FSH)] were successfully isolated and characterized (8). Insensitive bioassays of FSH and LH were replaced by more specific and sensitive radioimmunoassays. Using these assays, more definite quantitative information about the hypothalamo-pituitary-gonadal axis was derived. Several lines of evidence from clinical and experimental data suggested the divergent secretions of FSH and LH. All of these studies supported unequivocally the concept of inhibin (9–11). In addition, inhibin (which was originally described in the male) has now been found in the female. Inhibinlike activity has been detected in a variety of gonadal-related fluids and extracts (12–21). Inhibin may be defined as a proteinaceous material of gonadal origin that is involved in the regulation of pituitary FSH secretion in both sexes.

1

0362-1642/87/0415-0001$02.00

BIOASSAY

Detection and quantitation methods are essential in isolation and purification of biologically important substances. These assay procedures should meet the criteria of simplicity, specificity, sensitivity, precision, and reproducibility. Unfortunately, no such assay methods are available for measuring inhibin activity; many only detect the activity. A standard reference preparation of inhibin is not available to compare the activity and potency ratios from different laboratories. Although a detailed discussion of these assays is beyond the scope of this article, we attempt to point out some common problems in these assays.

In Vivo Methods

Several in vivo methods for assaying inhibin activity have been developed and critically evaluated (21–30). Most of these methods rely on the suppression of circulating levels of FSH after the injection of inhibin-enriched preparations. In many instances the endogenous circulating levels of FSH must be elevated before a significant FSH-suppressing effect is observed.

We have used an in vivo rat system for assay of inhibin activity. Briefly, immature male rats (34-days old) are injected subcutaneously with the appropriate amounts of test sample in 0.2 ml of saline at two different time intervals [8 hours (hr) and 11 hr]. The synthetic LH-releasing hormone (LHRH) at a dose of 5 μg/rat is administered subcutaneously at 14 hr, and at 15 hr the animals are sacrificed under light ether anesthesia and blood samples are withdrawn. The serum content of FSH and LH are analyzed by specific radioimmunoassays (RIA).

Alternatively, male rats (34-days old) are bilaterally castrated under light ether anesthesia, and the test samples are immediately injected subcutaneously in appropriate amounts in 0.2 ml of saline. The second dose of the same sample is administered on day 35, and the blood samples are collected after 6 hr. The serum levels of FSH and LH are analyzed by RIA. A twofold increase of FSH and LH levels is usually observed in these immature castrated rats, as compared to those in the control animals of the same age group. The IB-containing fraction, when tested at different concentrations, suppresses FSH in a dose-dependent manner. The maximum FSH suppression in this model system ranged from 45–75%. Although the fraction specifically suppresses FSH in this model system, occasionally a small degree (20–30%) of LH suppression occurs.

The in vivo methods are usually not very sensitive, and FSH-suppressing activity varies from assay to assay. Therefore, this type of assay is not practical for routine use in screening the large number of fractions obtained during isolation procedure. Hence, a simple in vitro assay to measure inhibin activity must be developed.

In Vitro Methods

The rat anterior pituitary culture assay has been used to assay inhibin activity (31, 32). This assay procedure is reasonably sensitive and can be used routinely to screen the large number of fractions obtained during the isolation procedure. Also, it has a good index of precision and gives acceptable dose-response curves. However, this method is time consuming and requires at least 72 hr to detect significant FSH suppression after the addition of test material. Under the conditions of LHRH stimulation, it requires additional 5–8 hr to block the release of FSH. In addition, both FSH and LH levels are suppressed, and the system then becomes less specific (33–35). Hence, it is more appropriate to depend on the basal suppression of FSH secretion in the in vitro culture system.

Pituitary halves obtained from adult male rats, when incubated in vitro in an appropriate medium, respond well to synthetic LHRH and release significant amounts of FSH and LH. The pituitary tissue retains its morphological integrity under these conditions. Addition of inhibin-containing preparations markedly reduces FSH, but not LH, in this system (5). Based on this method, an in vitro mouse pituitary incubation assay has been developed (36). The immature mouse pituitary responds well to synthetic LHRH, its agonists, and its antagonists (37, 38). The amounts of FSH and LH released by the mouse pituitary into the medium are analyzed by specific radioreceptor assays, which measure the biologically active hormones. Inhibin-containing preparations from human seminal plasma, bull seminal plasma, ovine testicular extract, bovine follicular fluid, and human follicular fluid show a selective suppression of FSH secretion without a significant effect on LH secretion in this test system. A slightly modified mouse pituitary incubation system has been applied to suppress basal levels of FSH secretion using inhibin from porcine follicular fluid. The mouse pituitary gives maximal response to LHRH when tested in a cumulative experiment; similar response may be difficult to produce in a cell culture system (39–41).

Since the in vitro mouse pituitary system has been used in our laboratory to isolate α-inhibins from human seminal fluid, we describe this assay procedure here. The pituitary tissue obtained from a 20–22-day-old mouse is incubated in the Dulbecco's modified Eagle's medium containing 0.1% bovine serum albumin (BSA) at 37°C in an atmosphere of 95% O_2 and 5% CO_2. Appropriate amounts of test samples are added in 0.5 ml of the above medium, and the tissue is incubated for 1 hr, after which synthetic LHRH (3 μg/pituitary) is added and the incubation is continued for 3 hr. Thus, the total incubation period is 4 hr. In a second set of incubation assays, the mouse pituitary is challenged at different time intervals with appropriate amounts of the test material and LHRH. The medium is separated from the pituitary tissue, and levels of the mouse pituitary gonadotropins are estimated by specific radioreceptor assays. FSH radioreceptor assays are performed with bull testes preparation and ovine FSH as the ligand, whereas the LH receptor assays use rat testes homogenate and ovine LH as the ligand.

INHIBINS FROM SEMINAL FLUID

The concept of inhibin regulation of pituitary gonadotropin secretion was originally described in the male (1–3). Several attempts have been made to isolate inhibin from testes-related fluids and extracts from various species (15), as well as from human seminal plasma (42–44).

Human Inhibinlike Peptide

Ramasharma and coworkers (45, 45a) isolated and determined the structure of a peptide with inhibinlike activity from human seminal plasma. It was named inhibinlike peptide (ILP). Briefly, ILP was obtained from ethanol precipitates of sperm-free human ejaculates by a combination of procedures (44) including ion-exchange chromatography on sulphopropyl-Sephadex C-50 and DEAE-Sephadex A-25, gel filtration on Sephadex G-50, and HPLC on Waters C_{18} micro-Bondapak column. The peptide is shown to behave as a single substance in HPLC as well as in polyacrylamide gel electrophoresis at pH 4.5.

The amino acid analyses of ILP give the following composition in molar ratio: Lys_5, His_7, Arg_3, Asp_4, Ser_{1-2}, Glu_{2-3}, Gly_6, Ala_1, Val_2, Ile_1, Phe_1 (45). The primary structure of the peptide has been determined (45, 45a), as shown in Figure 1. The peptide is very basic and consists of 7 histidine, 5 lysine and 3 arginine residues, with one residue each of aspartic and glutamic acids.

Incubation of whole mouse pituitaries with ILP inhibited LHRH-induced FSH release. The inhibitory action of ILP on FSH release was dose-dependent, and it had no effect on LH release (45), as shown in Figure 2, part A. When injected into castrated male rats (34-days old), ILP inhibited the rise in circulating FSH levels, whereas no effect on LH levels was observed (Figure 2, part B). ILP has been synthesized by the solid-phase method, and the synthetic product was shown to be homogeneous in HPLC and paper electrophoresis (46). In both the in vitro mouse pituitary assay and the in vivo LHRH-induced FSH release in immature male rats, the FSH-suppressing activities of the synthetic and natural ILP are comparable (46).

Liu et al (47) employed an impure synthetic ILP to demonstrate that "synthetic 31-amino acid inhibin-like peptide lacks inhibin activity." As stated by these authors, "only 15–30% of the material (synthetic peptide) had the complete correct sequence. The remaining peptides had one or more amino acids missing, mainly the histidine residues at positions 1, 9 or 17." Any conclusions drawn from experiments using such crude peptide mixtures are meaningless.

```
                    5                      10
       H-His-Asn-Lys-Gln-Glu-Gly-Arg-Asp-His-Asp-

                    15                     20
       Lys-Ser-Lys-Gly-His-Phe-His-Arg-Val-Val-

                    25                         31
        Ile-His-His-Lys-Gly-Gly-Lys-Ala-His-Arg-Gly-OH
```

Figure 1   Amino acid sequence of ILP.

Antisera raised in rabbits to synthetic ILP afford a highly specific and sensitive RIA for the peptide (48) using a synthetic [Tyr⁴]-ILP analog as primary radioiodinated ligand. Synthetic ILP completely displaces antiserum binding of [^{125}I-Tyr⁴]-ILP with half maximal displacement at 36-fmoles ILP/tube. ILP, [Tyr⁴]-ILP and ILP-(9–31) had essentially equal potency, while ILP-(1–25), ILP-(1–23) had reduced activity. Apparently, the antiserum recognizes the COOH-terminal segment of ILP.

Human α-Inhibin-92

Using the RIA for ILP, two new peptides structurally related to ILP have been isolated and characterized from human seminal plasma (49). One consists of 52 amino acids and the other of 92 amino acids. They are designated α-IB-52 and α-IB-92, respectively. Sequence analyses show that the NH$_2$-terminal 31 amino acids of α-IB-52 are identical to those of ILP, and the COOH-terminal

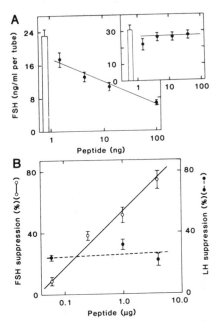

Figure 2   (*A*) Action of ILP on gonadotropin release by mouse pituitary (open bars = control values). (*B*) Effect of ILP on FSH and LH release in castrated male rats.

```
                    5                      10                      15
H-Thr-Tyr-His-Val-Asp-Ala-Asn-Asp-His-Asp-Gln-Ser-Arg-Lys-Ser-

                   20                      25                      30
Gln-Gln-Tyr-Asp-Leu-Asn-Ala-Leu-His-Lys-Thr-Thr-Lys-Ser-Gln-

                   35                      40                      45
Arg-His-Leu-Gly-Gly-Ser-Gln-Gln-Leu-Leu-His-Asn-Lys-Gln-Glu-

                   50                      55                      60
Gly-Arg-Asp-His-Asp-Lys-Ser-Lys-Gly-His-Phe-His-Arg-Val-Val-

                   65                      70                      75
Ile-His-His-Lys-Gly-Gly-Lys-Ala-His-Arg-Gly-Thr-Gln-Asn-Pro-

                   80                      85                      90
Ser-Gln-Asp-Gln-Gly-Asn-Ser-Pro-Ser-Gly-Lys-Gly-Ile-Ser-Ser-

                   92
Gln-Tyr-OH.
```

Figure 3 Amino acid sequence of α-IB-92. Residues 41–92 constitute α-IB-52, and residues 41–71 constitute ILP.

52 amino acids of α-IB-92 are identical to the structure of α-IB-52 (see Figure 3). Bioassay data (Figure 4) in mouse pituitaries in vitro shows that α-IB-52 is 3.4 times, and α-IB-92 over 40 times, more active than ILP peptide in suppressing follitropin release (49).

Lilja & Jeppsson (50) reported a basic protein in hSP with the same amino acid sequence as α-IB-52. These authors believed that the basic protein is the major degradation product of the gel-forming protein secreted by the seminal vesicles.

α-IB-92 has been synthesized by the thiocarboxyl segment strategy (51). Three segments were synthesized by the solid-phase method, purified, and characterized: [GlyS³⁴]-α-IB-92-(1–34) (I), CF₃CO-[GlyS⁶⁵]-α-IB-92-(35–

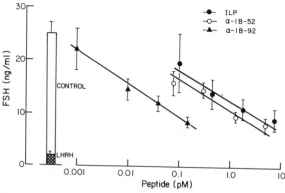

Figure 4 Effect of ILP, α-IB-52, and α-IB-92 on LHRH-induced FSH secretion by mouse pituitary; means ± SEM (n = 5).

65) (II), and Msc-α-IB-92-(66–92) (III), where Msc is 2-(methylsulfonyl)-ethyloxycarbonyl. All were reacted with citraconic anhydride followed by removal of the Msc group in III to give Ia, IIa, and IIIa, respectively. Peptide IIIa was coupled to IIa by the silver nitrate–N-hydroxysuccinimide procedure, and after removal of uncoupled segments and the trifluoroacetyl group, Ia was coupled, followed again by removal of uncoupled segments. Final deblocking to remove citraconyl groups was accomplished under exceptionally mild conditions in aqueous acetic acid. The synthetic product was identical to natural α-IB-92 in amino acid analysis, reversed-phase high-performance liquid chromatography (HPLC), gel electrophoresis, and tryptic mapping. The synthetic peptide was indistinquishable from natural α-IB-92 in a radioimmunoassay and in an in vitro mouse pituitary assay (see Table 1). In the mouse pituitary assay system, a dose of 0.001 nM of either synthetic or natural α-IB-92 causes significant inhibition of FSH release in the presence of 10 ng of LHRH.

Antiserum of high titer (1 : 40,000 final dilution) was obtained from one rabbit that had been immunized with α-IB-52 (52). It cross-reacted with ILP and α-IB-92 with equal affinity. The antiserum showed no cross-reaction to any of the known pituitary or hypothalamic peptides. Using radioiodinated α-IB-92 as the primary ligand, a specific and sensitive RIA for α-IBs has been developed with the ED_{50}, and the slope of 10 different assays (mean $\pm$ SE) ranged 2.23 $\pm$ 0.1 ng/tube and 0.57 $\pm$ 0.03, respectively (52). The minimal detectable dose was found to be 0.1 to 0.2 ng/tube. The recovery of added α-IB-92 to the blank serum at two concentrations (10 and 50 ng) was 85.5% (n = 20) in three different experiments. The intra- and interassay coefficient of variations for a pool of unidentified human serum was 9.49% and 14.0%,

Table 1 Comparison of natural (N) and synthetic (S) α-IB-92 in a mouse pituitary assay (MPA) and radioimmunoassay (RIA)

Assay	Peptide	ED_{50} (nM[a])	Slope	Relative potency
MPA	α-IB-92 (N)	0.0959 (0.075–0.12)	0.620	1
	α-IB-92(S)	0.0766 (0.052–0.112)	0.870	1.25 (0.67–2.3)
RIA	α-IB-92 (N)	0.140 (0.13–0.15)	0.640	1.0
	α-IB-92 (S)	0.128 (0.119–0.13)	0.552	1.1 (0.88–1.4)

[a]95% confidence limits in parentheses.

respectively. The pool of human serum showed a dose-dependent response. Human pituitary and hypothalamic extracts also showed a concentration-dependent response; the dose-response curve for the pituitary extract shifted to the left after fractionation on Sephadex G-100 column. The amounts of immunoreactive material (52) in human pituitary, hypothalamus, and serum, as expressed in ng per gram wet weight of tissue or ml, are estimated to be pituitary, 70.3; hypothalamus, 12.9; and serum (normal adult male), 7.2. The presence of immunoreactive α-IB-92 (12.9 ng/ml) in human follicular fluid was also shown (K. Ramasharma, unpublished data).

When the human serum sample was fractionated on a Sephadex G-100 column, the immunoreactive material eluted earlier than did the authentic α-IB-92 or α-IB-52. When α-IB-92 was mixed with blank human serum and chromatographed on the same column, the immunoreactivity again appeared in the void volume. Under identical chromatographic conditions, the immunoreactive material in the human pituitary and hypothalamic extracts was also found in the high-molecular-weight region (52).

The immunoreactive fraction obtained from gel filtration and further fractionated on sodium dodecylsulfate-polyacrylamide gel electrophoresis (SDS-PAGE) was resolved into several bands. These bands were electrophoretically transferred to nitrocellulose paper. Immunoreactive material from human pituitary extract appeared to behave as α-IB-92 and α-IB-52. The hypothalamic extract and human serum showed α-IB-92-related material (52).

A surprising finding was that pituitary and hypothalamic extracts contain immunoreactive α-IB-related peptides (52). Preliminary studies demonstrated the existence of α-IB in sheep and rat pituitary glands as examined by RIA. When these extracts were subjected to gel filtration, the immunoreactivity appeared mostly in the high-molecular-weight region. However, blotting analysis clearly indicates the presence of immunoreactive α-IB-92 and α-IB-52. The significant amounts of immunoreactivity were found in the anterior pituitary, but not in the posterior lobe. The amount of α-IB immunoreactivity found in the hypothalamus is lower than that observed in the pituitary (52).

Although the pituitary gland is the primary site of action of inhibin, several other organs such as the hypothalamus, pineal gland, and gonads have also been implicated (15). Results obtained using partially purified inhibin preparations suggested that inhibin must bind to the cell membrane before it evokes the cellular response in FSH suppression (53–55). The binding ability of α-IB-92 has been verified using human or ovine pituitary membrane preparations (56). Human pituitary membrane homogenate was prepared in 50-mM Tris-HCl buffer (pH 7.4), containing 0.3-M sucrose and 0.01% bacitracin. The binding studies were carried out using 50-mM Tris-HCl (pH 7.4) containing 0.1% BSA and 0.01% bacitracin at 4°C for 16 hr. The

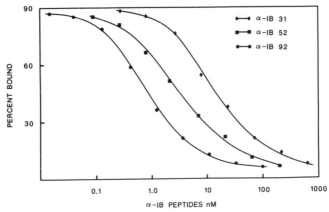

Figure 5   Competition of the binding of [^{125}I]α-IB-92 to human pituitary membrane preparation by α-IB-92, α-IB-52 and ILP (α-IB-31).

membrane-bound radioactivity was separated by Whatman filter paper (GF/B) and counted in the Beckman gamma counter. The results were computed for curve fitting in a computer.

The binding of labeled α-IB-92 to the human pituitary membrane was concentration dependent. The [^{125}I]-α-IB-92 binding to the human pituitary membrane can be displaced by the unlabeled peptide in a dose-dependent manner (Figure 5). The binding is specific, as most of the pituitary hormones and hypothalamic peptides failed to displace the bound label. α-IB-52 and ILP exhibit lesser binding affinities in displacing the label (Figure 5), compared to that of α-IB-92. These data demonstrate the existence of α-IB-92 binding sites on the human pituitary membrane.

Human β-Inhibin

Sheth et al (57) reported the isolation of a polypeptide with inhibinlike activity from human seminal plasma. This polypeptide has an amino acid content of nearly 130 residues, with serine as the NH$_2$-terminal amino acid. The amino acid sequence of the first 30 residues has also been determined (57). The polypeptide was later designated β-inhibin, and was completely sequenced (58). The primary structure of β-inhibin (shown in Figure 6) confirms the earlier data (57) on the NH$_2$-terminal sequence. It consists of 94 residues with one each of methionine and histidine, two each of arginine, leucine, phenylalanine, and tryptophan, and 5 disulfide bridges. β-Inhibin contains no alanine and is chemically distinct from α-IB-92.

One of the disulfide bridges is linked between Cys-73 and Cys-87, and the others have not been identified. Sheth and coworkers (59) further indicate that the inhibinlike activities of both β-inhibin-(1–94) and β-inhibin-(67–94) are

```
                 5                  10                 15
H-Ser-Cys-Tyr-Phe-Ile-Pro-Asn-Glu-Gly-Val-Pro-Gly-Asp-Ser-Thr-

                20                 25                 30
Arg-Lys-Cys-Met-Asp-Leu-Lys-Gly-Asn-Lys-His-Pro-Ile-Asn-Ser-

                35                 40                 45
Glu-Trp-Gln-Thr-Asp-Asn-Cys-Glu-Thr-Cys-Thr-Cys-Tyr-Glu-Glu

                50                 55                 60
Glu-Ile-Ser-Cys-Cys-Thr-Leu-Val-Ser-Thr-Pro-Val-Gly-Tyr-Asp-

                65                 70                 75
Lys-Asp-Asn-Cys-Gln-Arg-Ile-Phe-Lys-Lys-Glu-Asp-Cys-Lys-Tyr-

                80                 85                 90
Ile-Val-Val-Glu-Lys-Lys-Asp-Pro-Lys-Lys-Thr-Cys-Ser-Val-Ser-

                94
Glu-Trp-Gly-Ile-OH
```

Figure 6 Amino acid sequence of β-inhibin.

equipotent on a mole-to-mole basis. A 10-ng dose of β-inhibin inhibits FSH release in rat pituitary in vitro assay, whereas 100 ng are required for the in vivo adult male rat assay (57). Neither α-IB-92 nor β-inhibin exhibits inhibin activity in the rat pituitary culture assay.

Bovine Inhibin

A highly acidic protein with an isoelectric point of pH = 2.2 has been obtained from bovine seminal plasma (60). This protein has a molecular weight of 18,200 and a Stokes radius of 1.90 nm, and is capable of suppressing human chorionic gonadotropin (hCG)-induced uterine weight increase in immature mice. The relationship of this protein to human α-IB-92 or β-inhibin is undetermined, as no structural data are presented.

INHIBINS FROM FOLLICULAR FLUID

Porcine Follicular Inhibin

Miyamoto et al (61) were the first investigators to isolate and characterize inhibin from porcine follicle fluid using cultured cells of rat anterior pituitary for bioassay. Purification steps were performed in the presence of urea to eliminate noncovalent protein–protein interactions. The purified inhibin had a molecular weight of 32,000. It behaved as a homogeneous protein in HPLC and SDS-PAGE. The hormone suppressed specifically the secretion of FSH from the pituitary cells, with an ED_{50} value of 0.9 ng/ml medium. After reduction with β-mercaptoethanol it gave rise to two subunits with molecular weights of 20,000 and 13,000, respectively. The NH$_2$-terminal sequence of

```
     1                                                          15
H-Ser-Thr-Ala-Pro-Leu-Pro-Trp-Pro-Trp-Ser-Pro-Ala-Ala-Leu-Arg-

                                                             30
    Leu-Leu-Gln-Arg-Pro-Pro-Glu-Glu-Pro-Ala-Val-His-Ala-Asp-Cys-

                                                             45
    His-Arg-Ala-Ser-Leu-Asn-Ile-Ser-Phe-Gln-Glu-Leu-Gly-Trp-Asp-

                                                             60
    Arg-Trp-Ile-Val-His-Pro-Pro-Ser-Phe-Ile-Phe-His-Tyr-Cys-His-

                                                             75
    Gly-Gly-Cys-Gly-Leu-Pro-Thr-Leu-Pro-Asn-Leu-Pro-Leu-Ser-Val-

                                                             90
    Pro-Gly-Ala-Pro-Pro-Thr-Pro-Val-Gln-Pro-Leu-Leu-Leu-Val-Pro-

                                                            105
    Gly-Ala-Gln-Pro-Cys-Cys-Ala-Ala-Leu-Pro-Gly-Thr-Met-Arg-Ser-

                                                            120
    Leu-Arg-Val-Arg-Thr-Thr-Ser-Asp-Gly-Gly-Tyr-Ser-Phe-Lys-Tyr-

                                                        134
    Glu-Thr-Val-Pro-Asn-Leu-Leu-Thr-Gln-His-Cys-Ala-Cys-Ile-OH
```

Figure 7 Deduced amino acid sequence of pfIB-α.

the large subunit was Ser-Thr-Ala-Pro and of the other, Gly-Leu-Glu-Cys.

Subsequently, two groups of investigators (62, 63) confirmed the data of Miyamoto et al (61) in obtaining the same inhibin molecule from porcine follicular fluid. In addition, the amino acid composition (278 residues) of the hormone (62) was given as residues for the 32-kd inhibin: Asx_{21}, Thr_{14}, Ser_{18}, Gly_{23}, Gly_{24}, Ala_{22}, Val_{14}, Met_6, Ile_{10}, Leu_{28}, Tyr_{11}, Phe_{10}, His_8, Trp_4, Lys_5, Arg_{16}, Cys_{14}, Pro_{30}. The first 10 NH_2-terminal residues of the 20-kd and 13-kd subunits were, respectively, Ser-Thr-Ala-Pro-Trp-Pro-Trp-Ser and Gly-Leu-Glu-Cys-Asp-Gly-Arg-Thr-Asn-Leu. In addition, Ling et al (62) isolated two forms (A and B) of inhibin with an identical α-subunit but a slightly different β-subunit. However, both forms have similar inhibin activity.

Using the NH_2-terminal-sequence data, Mason et al (64) identified cloned complementary DNAs encoding the biosynthetic precursors of the two subunits (α and β) of porcine follicular inhibin (pfIB). From the cDNA sequences, the primary structures of pfIB-α, and pfIB-β_A or pfIB-β_B, were deduced (shown in Figures 7, 8, and 9). One glycosylation site was predicted to occur in the α-subunit. Thus the α subunit has 134 amino acids with 7 cysteine residues, and the β_B subunit has 115 amino acids with 9 cysteine residues. The authors (64) suggest that the two subunits are derived from one ancestral gene, as the alignment of half of the cysteine residues in the two subunits indicates a similar distribution and some sequence homology. When compared with the amino acid sequence of human transforming growth factor-β (TGF-β) (65), pfIB-β shows some homology (see Figure 10). Sur-

```
                                                                    1
                                                                 H-Gly-Leu-
                                    10                                          20
         Glu-Cys-Asp-Gly-Lys-Val-Asn-Ile-Cys-Cys-Lys-Lys-Gln-Phe-Phe-Val-Ser-Phe-
                                              30
         Lys-Asp-Ile-Gly-Trp-Asn-Asp-Trp-Ile-Ile-Ala-Pro-Ser-Gly-Tyr-His-Ala-Asn-
                  40                                    50
         Tyr-Cys-Glu-Gly-Glu-Cys-Pro-Ser-His-Ile-Ala-Gly-Thr-Ser-Gly-Ser-Ser-Leu-
                           60                                    70
         Ser-Phe-His-Ser-Thr-Val-Ile-Asn-His-Tyr-Arg-Met-Arg-Gly-His-Ser-Pro-Phe-
                                    80                                    90
         Ala-Asn-Leu-Lys-Ser-Cys-Cys-Val-Pro-Thr-Lys-Leu-Arg-Pro-Met-Ser-Met-Leu-
                                  100                                          110
         Tyr-Tyr-Asp-Asp-Gly-Gln-Asn-Ile-Ile-Lys-Lys-Asp-Ile-Gln-Asn-Met-Ile-Val-
                           116
         Glu-Glu-Cys-Gly-Cys-Ser-OH
```

Figure 8   Deduced amino acid sequence of pfIB-β_A.

prisingly, TGF-β has recently been shown (66) to act as an inhibitor of
FSH-induced aromatase activity in cultured rat granulosa cells.

Bovine Follicular Inhibin

Using a combination of procedures including exclusion chromatography,
HPLC, and SDS-PAGE, Robertson et al (67) isolated a protein with inhibin
activity from bovine follicular fluid collected in the presence of aprotimin and
phenylmethyl-sulphonyl fluoride. Under nonreducing conditions, the protein
gave a single band in SDS-PAGE with a molecular weight of 56,000. In the
presence of mecaptoethanol, the protein gave two bands with molecular
weight of 44,000 and 14,000 with NH$_2$-termini of Asn-Ala-Val and Tyr-Leu-

```
            1                                                          15
         H-Gly-Leu-Glu-Cys-Asp-Gly-Arg-Thr-Asn-Leu-Cys-Cys-Arg-Gln-Gln-
                                                               30
            Phe-Phe-Ile-Asp-Phe-Arg-Leu-Ile-Gly-Trp-Ser-Asp-Trp-Ile-Ile-
                                                               45
            Ala-Pro-Thr-Gly-Tyr-Tyr-Gly-Asn-Tyr-Cys-Glu-Gly-Ser-Cys-Pro-
                                                               60
            Ala-Tyr-Leu-Ala-Gly-Val-Pro-Gly-Ser-Ala-Ser-Ser-Phe-His-Thr-
                                                               75
            Ala-Val-Val-Asn-Gln-Tyr-Arg-Met-Arg-Gly-Leu-Asn-Pro-Gly-Thr-
                                                               90
            Val-Asn-Ser-Cys-Cys-Ile-Pro-Thr-Lys-Leu-Ser-Thr-Met-Ser-Met-
                                                               105
            Leu-Tyr-Phe-Asp-Asp-Glu-Tyr-Asn-Ile-Val-Lys-Arg-Asp-Val-Pro-
                                  115
            Asn-Met-Ile-Val-Glu-Glu-Cys-Gly-Cys-Ala-OH
```

Figure 9   Deduced amino acid sequence of pfIB-β_B.

```
                                                                 73
PfIB-βB   Thr-( )-Ala-Val-Val-Asn-Gln-Tyr-Arg-Met-Arg-Gly-Leu-Asn-Pro-
TGF-β     Thr-Gln-Tyr-Ser-Lys-Val-Leu-Ala-Leu-Tyr-Asn-Gln-His-Asn-Pro-
                                                                 70

                                                              88   88
          Gly-( )-Thr-Val-Asn-Ser-Cys-Cys-Ile-Pro-Thr-Lys-Leu-Ser-Thr Met-
          Gly-Ala-Ser-Ala-Ala-Pro-Cys-Cys-Val-Pro-Gln-Ala-Leu-Glu-Pro-( )-
                                                                       85

                                                            103
          Ser-Met-Leu-Tyr-Phe-Asp-Asp-Glu-Tyr-Asn-Ile-Val-Lys-Arg-Asp-
          Leu-Pro-Ile-Val-Tyr-Tyr-Val-Gly-Arg-Lys-Pro-Lys-Val-Glu-Gln-
                                                                     100

                                                    115
          Val-Pro-Asn-Met-Ile-Val-Glu-Glu-Cys-Gly-Cys-Ala-OH
          Leu-Ser-Asn-Met-Ile-Val-Arg-Ser-Cys-Lys-Cys-Ser-OH
                                                         112
```

Figure 10 Comparison of pfIB-β_B and TGF-β sequences.

Gln, respectively. Thus, bovine follicular inhibin (bfIB) is a 56-kd protein consisting of disulfide-linked 44-kd and 14-kd polypeptide chains.

Robertson et al also isolated a 31-kd form of inhibin from bovine follicular fluid (68). The 31-kd protein gave 2 bands after reduction on SDS-PAGE, with molecular weights of 20 kd and 15 kd. An antiserum to 56-kd inhibin can neutralize the bioactivity of both the 56-kd and 31-kd preparations. This ability may suggest that 31-kd inhibin is derived from the 56-kd molecule.

Independently, Fukuda et al (69) described the isolation of 32-kd inhibin from bovine follicular fluid using procedures similar to those for their work on pfIB (61). The 32-kd bfIB described by Fukuda et al (69) is apparently the same protein as the 31-kd inhibin described by Robertson et al. It consists of two polypeptide chains (20 kd and 13 kd) with NH$_2$-termini of Ser-Thr-Pro-Pro and Gly-Leu-Glu-Cys, respectively. Thus, the 31-kd bovine inhibin is very closely related to the porcine 32-kd hormone (61–63).

Monoclonal antibodies to bfIB 32-kd subunits (20 kd and 13 kd) have been prepared by Miyamoto et al (70). Using these antibodies, six different forms of inhibin with molecular weights of 120,000, 108,000, 88,000, 65,000, 55,000, and 32,000 have been identified in bovine follicular fluid. These forms are further divided into two groups: one (120 kd, 108 kd, and 88 kd) consists of three polypeptide subunits with disulfide linkages, and the other (65 kd, 55 kd, and 32 kd) consists of two subunits also with disulfide bridges. These bioactive forms of bfIB contain segments that are 20-kd and 13-kd polypeptide chains of 32-kd inhibin. The authors (70) suggest the largest form of bfIB has the structure shown in Figure 11. Restricted proteolytic processing of the largest form would give rise to different forms of bioactive inhibin.

Cloning and sequence analysis of cDNA for the 56-kd bfIB of Robertson et

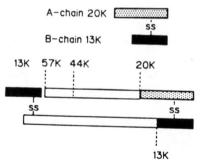

Figure 11   Proposed structure for the largest form of bfIB (From Ref. 70, Figure 4).

al (67) has been described (71). [Forage et al (71) stated that α-inhibin is "a protein of prostatic origin." In a paper by Li et al (49), the authors did not mention the origin of α-inhibin. In fact, recent data from a cytoimmunochemical technique indicate that α-inhibin-92 is located in the testis (D. T. Lau, unpublished data).] From the NH_2-terminal-sequence data of the two subunits, it is possible to obtain the oligonucleotide probe for the isolation of the cDNA of two 56-kd inhibin subunits (71). The amino acid sequence of the subunits is deduced from sequence analysis of cDNA. The α subunit (see Figure 12) consists of 300 amino acids with two potential N-glycosylation sites at Asn residues in positions 80 and 202. The β subunit consists of 116 amino acids with no sites for N-glycosylation and is identical to the porcine β_A subunit (see Figure 8). In agreement with Miyamoto et al (70), the 32-kd form of bfIB is derived by combination of 56-Kβ with a segment of the α subunit [56 Kβ-(167–300)] (71).

Human Follicular Inhibin

A comparison of chromatographic behavior of inhibin activity from human and bovine follicular fluid has been presented by van Dijk et al (72). Both inhibins are retained by immobilized lectins. The human hormone is apparently somewhat more basic (pI = 5.1–5.7) than bovine IB (pI = 4.75–5.25). Human and bovine inhibins behave similarly in various chromatographic assays.

Using porcine inhibin α, β_A and β_B cDNA as hybridization probes (64), Mason et al (73) identified cDNA clones for inhibins from human ovary mRNA. The primary structures of the subunits as deduced from the complete nucleotide sequence of cDNAs are nearly identical to their porcine equivalents. Human follicular fluid has two forms of inhibin (73) as does the porcine ovary (62, 63). These two forms have an identical α subunit but somewhat different β subunits.

```
                 1                              10
            H-His-Ala-Val-Gly-Gly-Phe-Met-Arg-Arg-Gly-Ser-Glu-
             20                              30
        Pro-Glu-Asp-Gln-Asp-Val-Ser-Gln-Ala-Ile-Leu-Phe-Pro-Ala-Ala-Gly-Ala-Ser-
                            40
        Cys-Gly-Asp-Glu-Pro-Asp-Ala-Gly-Glu-Ala-Glu-Glu-Gly-Leu-Phe-Thr-Tyr-Val-
             50                              60
        Phe-Gln-Pro-Ser-Gln-His-Thr-Arg-Ser-Arg-Gln-Val-Thr-Ser-Ala-Gln-Leu-Trp-
                 70                              80
        Phe-His-Thr-Gly-Leu-Asp-Arg-Gln-Glu-Thr-Ala-Ala-Ala-Asn-Ser-Ser-Glu-Pro-
                     90                          100
        Leu-Leu-Gly-Leu-Leu-Val-Leu-Thr-Ser-Gly-Gly-Pro-Met-Pro-Val-Pro-Met-Ser-
                        110                          120
        Leu-Gly-Gln-Ala-Pro-Pro-Arg-Trp-Ala-Val-Leu-His-Leu-Ala-Thr-Ser-Ala-Phe-
                            130
        Pro-Leu-Leu-Thr-His-Pro-Val-Leu-Ala-Leu-Leu-Leu-Arg-Cys-Pro-Leu-Cys-Ser-
             140                          150
        Cys-Ser-Thr-Arg-Pro-Glu-Ala-Thr-Pro-Phe-Leu-Val-Ala-His-Thr-Arg-Ala-Lys-
                 160                          170
        Pro-Pro-Ser-Gly-Gly-Glu-Arg-Ala-Arg-Arg-Ser-Thr-Pro-Pro-Leu-Pro-Trp-Pro-
                     180                          190
        Trp-Ser-Pro-Ala-Ala-Leu-Arg-Leu-Leu-Gln-Arg-Pro-Pro-Glu-Glu-Pro-Ala-Ala-
                         200                          210
        His-Ala-Asp-Cys-His-Arg-Ala-Ala-Leu-Asn-Ile-Ser-Phe-Gln-Glu-Leu-Gly-Trp-
                             220
        Asp-Arg-Trp-Ile-Val-His-Pro-Pro-Ser-Phe-Ile-Phe-Tyr-Tyr-Cys-His-Gly-Gly-
             230                          240
        Cys-Gly-Leu-Ser-Pro-Pro-Gln-Asp-Leu-Pro-Leu-Pro-Val-Pro-Gly-Val-Pro-Pro-
                 250                          260
        Thr-Pro-Val-Gln-Pro-Leu-Ser-Leu-Val-Pro-Gly-Ala-Gln-Pro-Cys-Cys-Ala-Ala-
                     270                          280
        Leu-Pro-Gly-Thr-Met-Arg-Pro-Leu-His-Val-Arg-Thr-Thr-Ser-Asp-Gly-Gly-Tyr-
                     290                          300
        Ser-Phe-Lys-Tyr-Glu-Met-Val-Pro-Asn-Leu-Leu-Thr-Gln-His-Cys-Ala-Cys-Ile-OH
```

Figure 12   Deduced amino acid sequence of α chain of 56-kd bfIB.

CONCLUDING REMARKS

Feedback effects of gonadal steroids, as well as LHRH, on secretion of gonadotropins from the pituitary gland have been firmly established (74). After inhibin was observed nearly 60 years ago (1–3), inhibins have now been isolated and characterized from human seminal plasma and porcine or bovine follicular fluid. Figure 13 summarizes the present knowledge on the control FSH release from the pituitary. Whether a separate molecule from the hypothalamus also controls FSH secretion remains to be investigated.

Inhibins from human seminal plasma (hSP) are more simple peptides; they

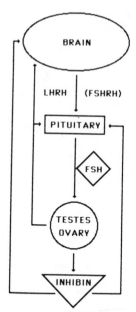

Figure 13   Diagram indicating the control of FSH secretion.

are active in vivo and in vitro assay systems in the presence of LHRH but not active in cultured pituitary cells (45, 49, 57–59). On the other hand, follicular inhibins, consisting of two subunits of glycoproteins with disulfide bridges, are active in pituitary cells in culture, but no data on them are available from in vivo bioassay systems (61–64, 67–71, 73). α-IB-92 from hSF is present in human serum, pituitary, hypothalamic (52), and follicular fluid (K. Ramasharma, unpublished data). In addition, specific binding sites in human and ovine pituitary membranes have been demonstrated (56).

The pituitary site of inhibin action is well documented in several in vivo and in vitro model systems (75). The female inhibin requires at least 72 hr to reduce FSH secretion in an in vitro pituitary cell culture system. On the other hand, male inhibin requires a relatively short time, but requires LHRH. These differential effects of inhibin in suppressing FSH raise the possibility that two types of modulating agents may be present in the gonad.

The hypothalamus was suggested as an additional site of action of inhibin (76). Endogenous LHRH levels in hypothalamic tissue were effectively reduced when incubated in vitro in the presence of seminal plasma inhibin preparations (15). On the contrary, de Greef et al (77) reported suppression of circulating FSH levels without changes in LHRH levels in the portal blood. If these results are correct, they probably indicate the existence of a separate FSH-releasing hormone (FSHRH) (78). The exact nature of these interactions between inhibin and LHRH or FSHRH remains to be established. Furthermore, certain inhibin preparations affect the gonadal function by directly inhibiting the synthesis of DNA in the testis (79). Such local regulatory mechanisms are important for paracrine control of germ-cell development and follicular maturation.

The mechanism of action of inhibin remains unexplored. How inhibin modulates the intracellular events and effects differential secretions of FSH and LH is not clear. As indicated earlier, the anterior pituitary cultures must be exposed to inhibin-containing preparations for 72 hr for a significant FSH suppression to occur. Considering this time lag one could suggest that inhibin is somehow involved in the blockade of one of the molecular events (transcriptional or translational) leading to the biosynthesis of FSH molecules. The nature of the interplay of LHRH, steroid hormones, and inhibin (see Figure 13) in suppressing the release of FSH without affecting LH release remains unexplained. Whether cyclic nucleotides, particularly cyclic GMP, are involved in mediating the action of inhibin should be investigated.

The physiological role of inhibin is to convey the feedback signal(s) to the pituitary gland regarding the peripheral concentrations of FSH and subsequently to modulate FSH-dependent events in the testes, as well as in the ovary. The precise role of FSH in the adult male in regulating spermatogenesis is not completely resolved (80). However, if the rate of sperm production is a function of circulating levels of FSH, then inhibin could convey these quantitative signals to the pituitary gland. Preliminary data available indicate that reduction of inhibin activity occurs concomitantly to a reduction in the activity of germinal elements (81–84). On the other hand, if the immature male rats are treated with bfIB preparation, the development of spermatogenesis is delayed (85). Administration of hSP inhibin preparation to immature rats resulted in a reduction of ^{3}H-thymidine incorporation into testicular DNA (79, 86). These experimental results support a predominant role for inhibin in prepubertal males rather than in the adult male.

In the female, there is a good correlation of circulating levels of FSH and ovarian function. Inhibin might play a physiologically important role in those situations where there is a divergent secretion of LH and FSH (87–89). Studies in monkeys suggest that inhibin plays an important role in the follicular development (90). However, it is not possible to ascertain the quantitative contribution of inhibin in the follicular development.

As pointed out earlier, much of the supporting evidence for the inhibin concept comes from clinical and pathological situations associated with primary disorders of spermatogenesis. Inhibin might be a marker to determine the etiology of puberty and menopause. Circulating levels of inhibin might be a good index for assessing the functional status of granulosa cells in the ovary (15, 16). It has also been suggested that inhibin might be a potential contraception agent (5). Inhibin can certainly help in understanding the hypotha-lamo-pituitary-gonadal axis in the complex biological phenomena of mamma-lian reproduction.

ACKNOWLEDGEMENTS

We thank Donald Yamashiro for critical reading of this review. The work of the authors was supported in part by grants from the National Institutes of Health (AM-6097 and GM-2907) and the Hormone Research Foundation.

Literature Cited

1. Mottram, J. C., Cramer, W. 1923. Report on the general effects of exposure to radium on metabolism and tumour growth in the rat and the special effects on testis and pituitary. *J. Exp. Physiol.* 13:209–29
2. Martins, T., Rocha, A. 1931. Regulation of the hypophysis by the testicle and some problems of sexual dynamics. *Encodrinology* 15:421–34
3. McCullagh, D. R. 1932. Dual endocrine activity of testes. *Science N.Y.* 76:19–20
4. Setchell, B. P., Davies, R. V., Main, S. J. 1977. Inhibin. In *The Testis,* ed. A. D. Johnson, W. R. Gomes, 4:189–238. New York: Academic
5. Davies, R. V., Main, S. J., Setchell, B. P. 1976. Inhibin: evidence for its existence, methods of bioassay and nature of active material. *Int. J. Androl.* 2:102–13 (Suppl.)
6. Main, S. J., Davies, R. V., Setchell, B. P. 1979. The evidence that inhibin must exist. *J. Reprod. Fert.* 26:3–14 (Suppl.)
7. Franchimont, P., Chari, S., Hazee-Hagelstein, M. T., Debouche, M. L., Duraiswami, S. 1977. Evidence for the existence of inhibin. In *The Testis in Normal and Infertile Men,* ed. P. Toren, H. R. Nankin, pp. 253–70. New York: Raven
8. Sairam, M. R., Papkoff, H. 1974. Chemistry of pituitary gonadotrophins. *Handb. Physiol. Endocrinol.* 4:111–31
9. Franchimont, P. 1972. Human gonadotropin secretion. *J. Royal. Coll. Physicians (London)* 6:283–98
10. Franchimont, P., Chari, S., Demoulin, A. 1975. Hypothalamo-pituitary-testis interaction. *J. Reprod. Fertil.* 44:335–350
11. Setchell, B. P., Sirinathsinghji, D. J. 1972. Antigonadotropic activity in rete testis fluid, a possible inhibin. *J. Endocrinol.* 53:lx–lxl
12. Setchell, B. P., Main, S. J. 1974.

Bibliography (with review) on inhibin. *Biol. Reprod.* 24:245–59
13. Baker, H. W. G., Bremmer, W. J., Burger, H. G., de Kretser, D. M., Dulmanis, A., et al. 1976. Testicular control of follicle-stimulating hormone secretion. *Recent Prog. Hormone Res.* 32:429–69
14. de Jong, F. H., Sharpe, R. M. 1976. Evidence for inhibin-like activity in bovine follicular fluid. *Nature* 263:71–72
15. Franchimont, P., Proyard, V. J., Hazee-Hagelstein, M. T., Renard, H., Demoulin, A., et al. 1979. Inhibin from concept to reality. *Vitam. Horm.* 37: 243–302
16. de Jong, F. H. 1979. Inhibin fact or artifact. *Mol. Cell. Endocrinol.* 13:1–10
17. Hafez, E. S. E. 1980. Male and female inhibin. *Arch. Androl.* 5:131–58
18. de Jong, F. H., Sander, H. J., Ultee-van Gessel, A. M., van der Molen, H. J. 1985. Specific regulation of the secretion of follicle stimulating hormone from the pituitary gland: The inhibin concept. *Front. Horm. Res.* 14:53–69
19. Channing, C. P., Gordon, W. L., Liu, W. K., Ward, D. N. 1985. Physiology and biochemistry of ovarian inhibin. *Proc. Soc. Exp. Biol. Med.* 178:339–61
19a. de Jong, F. H., Robertson, D. M. 1985. Inhibin: update on action and purification. *Mol. Cell. Endocrinol.* 42: 95–103
19b. Sheth, A. R., Arbatti, N. J. 1985. Inhibin—An updated review. *Indian J. Exp. Biology* 23:475–94
20. Sairam, M. R., Raj, H. G. M. 1981. Progress in the isolation of inhibin-like activity(ies) from different sources: A 1981 report. *Int. J. Androl.* 5:205–9 (Suppl.)
21. Hudson, B., Baker, H. W. G., Eddie, L. W., Higginson, R. E., Burger, H. G., et al. 1979. Bioassays for inhibin: a

critical review. *J. Reprod. Fertil.* 26: 17–29 (Suppl.)

22. Lee, V. W. K., Pearce, P. T., de Kretser, D. M. 1977. The assessment of rodent models in evaluating the capacity of testis extracts to suppress FSH levels. See Ref. 7, pp. 293–306

23. de Jong, F. H., Welschen, R., Hermans, W. P., Smith, S. D., van der Molen, H. J. 1978. Effect of testicular and ovarian inhibin-like activity using in vitro and in vivo systems. *Int. J. Androl* 2:115–24 (Suppl.)

24. de Jong, F. H., Welschen, R., Hermans, W. P., Smith, S. D., van der Molen, H. J. 1979. Effect of factors from ovarian follicular fluid and Sertoli cell culture medium on in vivo and in vitro release of pituitary gonadotropins in the rat: an evaluation of systems for the assay of inhibin. *J. Reprod. Fertil.* 26:47–59 (Suppl.)

25. Baker, H. W. G., Eddie, L. W., Higgenson, R. E., Hudson, B., Keogh, E. J., Niall, H. D. 1981. Assay of inhibin. In *Intragonadal Regulation of Reproduction*, ed. P. Franchimont, C. P. Channing, pp. 193–228. New York: Academic

26. Nandini, S. G., Lipner, H., Moudgal, N. R. 1976. A model for studying inhibin. *Endocrinology*. 98:1460–65

27. Chari, S., Duraiswami, S., Franchimont, P. 1976. A convenient and rapid bioassay for inhibin. *Horm. Res.* 7:129–37

28. Ramasharma, K., Murthy, H. M. S., Moudgal, N. R. 1979. A rapid bioassay for measuring inhibin activity. *Biol. Reprod.* 20:831–35

29. Schwartz, N. B., Channing, C. P. 1977. Evidence for ovarian inhibin: suppression in the secondary rise of FSH levels in proestrous rats by injection of porcine follicular fluid. *Proc. Natl. Acad. Sci. USA* 74:5721–24

30. Lorengen, J. R., Channing, C. P., Schwartz, N. B. 1976. Partial characterization of FSH suppressing activity (folliculostatin) in porcine follicular fluid using the metoestrous rat as an in vivo bioassay model. *Biol. Reprod.* 19:635–40

31. Scott, R. S., Burger, H. G., Quigg, H. 1980. A simple and rapid in vitro bioassay for inhibin. *Endocrinology* 107:1536–42

32. de Jong, F. H., Smith, S. D., van der Molen, H. J. 1979. Bioassay of inhibin-like activity using pituitary cells in vitro. *J. Endocrinol.* 80:91–102

33. Robertson, D. M., Au, C. L., de Kretser, D. M. 1982. The use of 51Cr. for

assessing cytotoxicity in an in vitro bioassay for inhibin. *Mol. Cell. Endocrinol.* 26:119–27

34. Steinberger, A. 1983. In vitro model for study of testicular inhibin. In *Male Reproduction and Fertility*, ed. A. Negro-Vilar, pp. 183–92. New York: Raven

35. de Jong, F. H., Jansen, E. H. J. M., Steinbergen, J., van Dijk, S., van der Molen, H. J. 1983. Assay and purification of inhibin. In *Role of Peptides and Proteins in Control of Reproduction*, ed. S. M. McCann, D. M. Dhindsa, pp. 257–73. New York: Elsevier

36. Ramasharma, K., Sairam, M. R., Ranganathan, M. R. 1981. Effect of inhibin-like factors on gonadotropin release by the mouse pituitary in vitro. *Acta. Endocrinol.* 98:496–505

37. Kato, K., Ramasharma, K., Sairam, M. R. 1982. Enhanced sensitivity of immature mouse pituitary for gonadotropin release. The rapid effects of synthetic LH-RH analogs (agonists and antagonists) on FSH and LH release in vitro. *Abstr. Endocrine Soc., 64th Ann. Meet.*, p. 285

38. Kato, K., Sairam, M. R. 1983. The rapid effects of luteinizing hormone releasing hormone agonists and antagonists on the mouse pituitary in vitro. *Life Sci.* 32:263–70

39. Kato, K., Sairam, M. R., Ramasharma, K. 1983. Effect of porcine follicular fluid preparations on gonadotropin secretion by the mouse pituitary gland in vitro. *J. Endocrinol.* 96:73–84

40. Sairam, M. R., Kato, K., Manjunath, P., Ramasharma, K. 1984. Isolation and characterization of a protein with inhibin-like activity from pig follicular fluid. In *Gonadal Proteins and Peptides and Biological Significance*, ed. M. R. Sairam, L. E. Atkinson, pp. 65–84. Singapore: World Sci.

41. Ramasharma, K. 1984. *Studies on the non-steroidal regulation of pituitary gonadotropin in the male*. PhD thesis. McGill Univ., Montreal, p. 160

42. Franchimont, P., Demoulin, A., Verstraelen-Proyard, J., Hazee-Hagelstein, M. T., Tunbridge, W. M. G. 1979. Identification in human seminal fluid of an inhibin-like factor which selectively regulates FSH secretion. *J. Reprod. Fert.* 26:123–33. Suppl.

43. Thakur, A. N., Vaze, A. Y., Dattatreyamurthy, B., Arbathi, N. J., Sheth, A. R. 1978. Isolation and characterization of inhibin from human seminal plasma. *Ind. J. Exp. Biol.* 16:854–56

44. Ramasharma, K., Sairam, M. R. 1982.

Isolation and characterization of inhibin from human seminal plasma. *Ann. N.Y. Acad. Sci.* 38:307–28

45. Ramasharma, K., Sairam, M. R., Seidah, N. G., Chretien, M., Manjunath, P., et al. 1984. Isolation, structure and synthesis of human seminal plasma peptide with inhibin-like activity. *Science* 223:1199–202

45a. Seidah, N. G., Ramasharma, K., Sairam, M. R., Chretien, M. 1984. Partial amino acid sequence of a human seminal plasma peptide with inhibin-like activity. *FEBS Lett.* 167:98–102

46. Yamashiro, D., Li, C. H., Ramasharma, K., Sairam, M. R. 1984. Synthesis and biological activity of human inhibin-like peptide (1–31). *Proc. Natl. Acad. Sci. USA* 81:5399–402

47. Liu, L., Book, J., Merrian, G. R., Barnes, K. M., Sherins, R. J., et al. 1985. Evidence that synthetic 31-amino acid inhibin-like peptide lacks inhibin activity. *Endocrine Res.* 11(3–4):191–97

48. Hammonds, R. G. Jr., Li, C. H., Yamashiro, D., Cabrera, C. M., Westphal, M. 1985. Radioimmunoassay for an inhibin-like peptide from human seminal plasma. *J. Immunoassay* 6(4):363–69

49. Li, C. H., Hammonds, R. G. Jr., Ramasharma, K., Chung, D. 1985. Human seminal alpha inhibins: Isolation, characterization and structure. *Proc. Natl. Acad. Sci. USA* 82:4041–44

50. Lilja, H., Jeppsson, O. J. 1985. Amino acid sequence of the predominant basic protein in human seminal plasma. *FEBS Lett.* 182:181–84

51. Blake, J., Yamashiro, D., Ramasharma, K., Li, C. H. 1986. Chemical synthesis of α-inhibin-92 by the thiocarboxyl segment coupling method. *Int. J. Peptide Protein Res.* 28: In press

52. Ramasharma, K., Li, C. H. 1986. Human seminal α-inhibins: Detection in human pituitary, hypothalamus, and serum by immunoreactivity. *Proc. Natl. Acad. Sci. USA* 83:3484–86

53. Sairam, M. R., Ranganathan, M. R., Ramasharma, K. 1981. Binding of an inhibin-like protein from bull seminal plasma to ovine pituitary membranes. *Mol. Cell. Endocrinol.* 22:251–64

54. Steinberger, A., Seethalakshmi, L., Kessler, M., Steinberger, E. 1982. Binding of 3H Sertoli cell factor to rat anterior pituitary *in vitro. Endocrinology* 111:696–98

55. Ramasharma, K. 1983. Binding of 125-labeled human seminal plasma inhibin to human pituitary membranes. *Abstr. En-*

docrine Soc. 65th Ann. Meet., p. 109

56. Ramasharma, K., Li, C. H. 1986. Seminal plasma α-inhibin: Binding to ovine and human pituitary membranes. *Abstr. Endocrine Soc. 68th Ann. Meet.*, p. 255

57. Sheth, A. R., Arabatti, N., Carlquist, M., Jornvall, H. 1984. Characterization of a polypeptide from human seminal plasma with inhibin-like activity. *FEBS Lett.* 165:11–15

58. Seidah, N. G., Arbatti, N. J., Rochemont, A. R., Sheth, A. R., Chretien, M. 1985. Complete amino acid sequence of human seminal plasma β-inhibin. *FEBS Lett.* 175:349–55

59. Arbatti, N. J., Seidah, N. G., Rochemont, J., Escher, E., Sairam, M. R., Sheth, A. R., Chretien, M. 1985. β_2-Inhibin contains the active core of human seminal plasma β-inhibin: synthesis and bioactivity. *FEBS Lett.* 181:57–63

60. Mohapatra, S. K., Duraiswami, S., Chari, S. 1985. On the identity of bovine seminal plasma inhibin. *Mol. Cell. Endocrinol.* 41:187–96

61. Miyamoto, K., Hasegawa, Y., Fukuda, M., Nomura, M., Igarashi, M., et al. 1985. Isolation of porcine follicular fluid inhibin of 32 K daltons. *Biochem. Biophys. Res. Commun.* 239:396–403

62. Ling, N., Ying, S. Y., Ueno, N., Esch, F., Denoroy, L., Guillemin, R. 1985. Isolation and partial characterization of a Mr 32,000 protein with inhibin activity from follicular fluid. *Proc. Natl. Acad. Sci. USA* 82:7217–21

63. Rivier, J., Spiess, J., McClintook, R., Vaughan, J., Vale, W. 1985. Purification and partial characterization of inhibin from porcine follicular fluid. *Biochem. Biophys. Res. Commun.* 133:120–27

64. Mason, A. J., Hayflick, J. S., Ling, N., Esch, F., Ueno, N., et al. 1985. Complementary DNA sequences of ovarian follicular fluid inhibin show precursor structure and homology with transforming growth factor β. *Nature* 318:659–63

65. Dryneck, R., Jarrett, J. A., Chen, E. Y., Eaton, D. H., Ball, J. R., et al. 1985. Human TGFβ complementary DNA sequence and expression in normal and transformed cells. *Nature* 316:701–5

66. Ying, S. Y., Becker, A., Ling, N., Ueno, N., Guillemin, R. 1986. Inhibin and TGFβ have opposite modulating effects on the FSH-induced aromatase activity of cultured rat granulosa cells. *Biochem. Biophys. Res. Commun.* 136:969–75

67. Robertson, D. M., Foulds, L. M., Leversh, L., Morgan, F. J., Hean, M.

T. W., et al. 1985. Isolation of inhibin from bovine follicular fluid. *Biochem. Biophys. Res. Commun.* 126:220–26
68. Robertson, D. M., de Vos, F. L., Foulds, L. M., McLachlan, R. I., Burger, H. G., et al. 1986. Isolation of a 31 kDa form of inhibin from bovine follicular fluid. *Mol. Cell. Endocrinol.* 44: 271–77
69. Fukuda, M., Miyamoto, K., Hasegawa, Y., Nomura, M., Igarashi, M., et al. 1986. Isolation of bovine follicular fluid inhibin of about 32 kDa. *Mol. Cell. Endocrinol.* 44:55–60
70. Miyamoto, K., Hasegawa, Y., Fukuda, M., Igarashi, M. 1986. Demonstration of high molecular weight forms of inhibin in bovine follicular fluid (bFF) by using monoclonal antibodies to bFF 32K inhibin. 1986. *Biochem. Biophys. Res. Commun.* 136:1103–9
71. Forage, R. G., Ring, J. M., Brown, R. W., McInerney, B. V., Cobon, G. S., et al. 1986. Cloning and sequence analysis of cDNA species coding for the two subunits of inhibin from bovine follicular fluid. *Proc. Natl. Acad. Sci. USA* 83: 3091–95
72. van Dijk, S., Steenbergen, C., de Jong, F. H., van der Molen, H. J. 1985. Comparison between inhibin from human and bovine ovarian follicular fluid using fast protein liquid chromatography. *Mol. Cell. Endocrinol.* 42:245–51
73. Mason, A. J., Niall, H. D., Seeburg, P. H. 1986. Structure of two human ovarian inhibins. *Biochem. Biophys. Res. Commun.* 135:957–64
74. McCann, S. M. 1974. Regulation of secretion of FSH and LH. In *Handbook of Physiology*, Sect. 7, part 2, ed. E. Knobil, W. H. Sawyer, 4:489–517
75. Franchimont, P., Lecomte-Yerna, M. J., Henderson, K., Verhoeven, G., Hazee-Hagelstein, M. T., et al. 1983. Inhibin mechanism of pituitary action and regulation of secretion. See Ref. 35, pp. 237–55
76. Lumpkin, M., Negro-Villar, A., Franchimont, P., McCann, S. M. 1983. Evidence for a hypothalamic site of action of inhibin to suppress FSH release. *Endocrinology* 108:1101–4
77. de Greef, W. J., de Jong, F. H., de Konig, J., Steenbergen, J., van der Vaart, P. D. 1983. Studies on the mechanism of the selective suppression of plasma levels of follicle-stimulating hormone in the female rat after administration of steroid-free bovine follicular fluid. *J. Endocrinol.* 97:327–38
78. McCann, S. M. 1983. Luteinizing hormone-releasing hormone past, present and future. See Ref. 34, pp. 111–26

79. Demoulin, A., Hustin, J., Lambotte, R., Franchimont, P. 1981. Effect of inhibin on testicular function. See Ref. 25, pp. 327–42
80. Means, A. R., Dedman, J. R., Tash, J. S., Tindall, D. J., Sickle, M. V., Welsh, M. J. 1980. Regulation of the testis Sertoli cell by follicle stimulating hormone. *Ann. Rev. Physiol.* 42:59–70
81. Franchimont, P., Chari, S., Schellen, A. M. C. M., Demoulin, A. 1975. Relationship between gonadotropins, spermatogenesis and seminal plasma. *J. Steroid. Biochem.* 6:1037–41
82. Scott, R. S., Burger, H. G. 1980. Inhibin is absent from azoospermic semen of infertile men. *Nature* 285:246–47
83. Scott, R. S., Burger, H. G. 1981. An inverse relationship exists between seminal plasma inhibin and FSH in men. *J. Clin. Endocrinol. Metab.* 52:796–803
84. Steinberger, A., Seethalakshmi, L., Kessler, M., Steinberger, E. 1983. Physiology of Sertoli cell factor (inhibin). In *Recent Advances in Male Reproduction: Molecular Basis and Clinical Implication*, ed. R. D'Agata, M. B. Lipsett, P. Polosa, H. T. van der Molen, pp. 79–89, New York: Raven
85. Hermans, W. P., van Leeuwen, E. C. M., Debets, M. H. M., de Jong, F. H. 1980. Involvement of follicle-stimulating hormone concentrations in prepubertal and adult male and female rats. *J. Endocrinol.* 86:79–92
86. Franchimont, P., Croze, F., Demoulin, A., Bolonge, R., Hustin, J. 1981. Effect of inhibin on rat testicular deoxyribonucleic acid (DNA) synthesis in vivo and in vitro. *Acta Endocrinol.* 98:312–20
87. Schwartz, N. B. 1981. Role of ovarian inhibin (follicullostin) in regulating FSH secretion in the female rat. In *Intraovarian Control Mechanisms*, ed. C. P. Channing, S. J. Segal, pp. 25–36. New York: Plenum
88. Schwartz, N. B. 1983. Selective control of FSH secretion. See Ref. 35, pp. 193–214
89. Channing, C. P., Anderson, L. D., Hoover, D., Kolena, L., Osteen, K., et al. 1982. The role of non-steroidal regulators in control of oocyte and follicular maturation. *Recent Prog. Horm. Res.* 38:1037–408
90. Channing, C. P., Anderson, L. D., Hoover, D. J., Gagliano, P., Hodgen, G. D. 1981. Inhibitory effects of porcine follicular fluid on monkey serum FSH levels and follicular maturation. *Biol. Reprod.* 21:867–72

Ann. Rev. Pharmacol. Toxicol. 1987. 27:23–49

MOLECULAR AND CELLULAR BASIS OF CHEMICALLY INDUCED IMMUNOTOXICITY[1]

Michael I. Luster and James A. Blank

Systemic Toxicology Branch, National Institute of Environmental Health Sciences, P. O. Box 12333, Research Triangle Park, North Carolina 27709

Jack H. Dean

Chemical Industry Institute of Toxicology, Department of Cell Biology, P. O. Box 12137, Research Triangle Park, North Carolina 27709

INTRODUCTION

Immunotoxicology is the study of adverse effects on the immune system resulting from occupational, inadvertent, or therapeutic exposure to drugs, environmental chemicals, and, in some instances, biological materials. For the purpose of this chapter, we refer to these substances collectively as "xenobiotics." Immunotoxicity is subdivided into three main research areas: (*a*) studies of altered immunological events associated with exposure of humans and animals to xenobiotics, including altered host resistance to infectious disease; (*b*) studies of allergy and autoimmunity resulting from xenobiotic exposure; and (*c*) implementation of analytical immunological methods into toxicology research. This chapter focuses only on chemical-induced immunomodulation and describes several classes of immunotoxic xenobiotics, emphasizing cellular and molecular targets.

Laboratory studies, conducted primarily in rodents, have provided evidence that the immune system is very sensitive to chemical injury (reviewed in 1–6). This sensitivity is probably due as much to the general properties of a xenobiotic (e.g. reactivity with macromolecules) as to the complex nature of the immune system, which encompasses antigen recognition and processing;

---

[1]The US Government has the right to retain a nonexclusive, royalty-free license in and to any copyright covering this paper.

cellular interactions involving cooperation, regulation, and amplification; cell activation, proliferation, and differentiation; and mediator production. Since these cellular events are also involved in embryogenesis, many immunosuppressive xenobiotics are also teratogenic. The immunological effects associated with exposure to xenobiotics are often accompanied by increased susceptibility to challenge with infectious agents or tumor cells. In several instances, effects similar to those observed in rodents have been reported in humans through therapeutic, inadvertent, or occupational exposure to xenobiotics exemplifying certain characteristics of secondary immunodeficiency disease. These effects include altered immune responses in: Michigan residents and farmers exposed to polybrominated biphenyls (PBB) through the consumption of contaminated livestock and dairy products (7, 8, 8a); Chinese and Japanese exposed to polychlorinated biphenyls (PCBs) and dibenzofurans through contaminated rice oil used in cooking (8a, 9); residents of Missouri chronically exposed to dioxin from a mobile home park (10); Spanish residents exhibiting "toxic oil syndrome" following ingestion of isothiocyanate-derived imidazolidinethione adulterated rapeseed oil (11); factory workers with aplastic anemia and leukemia occupationally exposed to benzene (12); and patients with suppressed natural killer (NK) cell activity (13) and cell-mediated immunity (CMI) (14) receiving conventional diethylstilbestrol therapy for prostatic cancer. Infectious disease and neoplasia have been a recurring consequence of chronic immunosuppression or aberrant lymphoid cell differentiation in several of these cohorts. For example, the frequency of neoplasia among Michigan PBB-cohort members exhibiting immune dysfunction is approximately 15-fold greater than that observed in the control Wisconsin farmer cohort (J. G. Bekesi, unpublished observations). These examples and our current knowledge about the pathogenesis of disease support the possibility that xenobiotic-induced damage to the immune system may be associated with a wide spectrum of diverse pathologic conditions, some of which may only become detectable after a long latency. However, whether exposure to xenobiotics present in the environment influences immunocompetence of the general population under normal circumstances is still not known.

PHARMACOLOGY OF THE IMMUNE SYSTEM

Despite the increasing list of immunosuppressive chemical xenobiotics described, researchers have made little effort to delineate the cellular and molecular events of these chemicals. These efforts have probably been hampered by the fact that much of the technology to evaluate immunosuppression, at least at the molecular level, has only recently been developed. Further, many immunotoxicants have multiple effects on immune function, making it difficult to construct the actual sequence of events or determine the specificity of these cellular–chemical interactions. Chemical immunosuppressants, like immunotherapeutic agents, may vary from those that demonstrate high specificity (i.e. targeting a subpopulation of lymphocytes by interacting with specific proteins), intermediate specificity (i.e. altering specific biochemical or cellular events that are shared by several cell types), or little specificity (i.e. general antiproliferative or cytolytic activity). Immunosuppressive xenobiotics, due to their random reactivity (e.g., sulfhydryl or nucleophilic binding), might be expected to demonstrate little specificity for immune components, although in many instances xenobiotics have been shown to target specific subpopulations and molecular sites. While it is not our intent to review the organization and function of the immune system, an understanding of the biochemical and physiological processes that occur during the development of immunocompetent cells is necessary to understand how xenobiotics can influence these events. The following is a brief overview of recent developments in our understanding of macrophage and lymphocyte maturation events.

Macrophages

Mononuclear phagocytes (MPs) or macrophages originate from granulocyte–macrophage progenitor cells in the bone marrow, where they mature into promonocytes and monocytes. Monocytes are transported via the blood to organs and tissues, where they develop into macrophages. The macrophages of the body include histiocytes, Kupffer cells, alveolar macrophages, free and fixed macrophages in lymphoid tissue, and macrophages associated with serous membranes. Bloodborne monocytes and local replication can replenish these macrophage compartments with new cells. The recruitment of monocytes from the blood is greatly enhanced and local macrophage multiplication is increased in sites of inflammation (reviewed in 15). MPs provide a major defense against mechanical injuries as well as those produced by chemicals or biological toxins, infectious agents, and neoplastically transformed cells. Dysfunction of MPs can lead to indirect tissue damage through altered host resistance to infectious agents and to neoplastically transformed cells. Additionally, direct tissue injury by the MPs or their cellular products (e.g. autoimmune diseases) can occur. Environmental agents, especially fibers, particulates, and gases (reviewed in 16), and to some extent lipophilic compounds (reviewed in 17–18), can alter MP function.

Studies from several laboratories have demonstrated that murine macrophages develop in stages (19, 20) and that the stages of development can be identified by quantifying the expression of biological and chemical markers. Some of the more commonly used markers for maturation and differentiation include secretion of reactive oxygen intermediates such as H_2O_2 (18) and quantitation of ectoenzyme levels (21). In brief, these stages are defined by the inductive signals that must be applied to induce full activation (Figure 1, Section 1). Immature MPs, when taken from sites of inflammation (i.e. responsive macrophages), express a variety of functions including increased phagocytic capacity, increased spreading and adherence to glass or plastic surfaces, secretion of neutral proteases, increased production of acid hydrolases, depressed levels of 5'-nucleotidase, and an increased capacity to generate O_2 (15). Responsive macrophages are closely akin to inflammatory macrophages, as they display the markers of increased spreading, increased phagocytosis, and increased secretion of plasminogen activator (22). Inflammatory macrophages can, in turn, be activated to kill tumor cells and facultative intracellular parasites by exposure to lymphokine and/or endotoxin. Primed macrophages also display these markers, and in addition bind neoplastic targets selectively (23). Fully activated or cytotoxic macrophages, which share the properties of the primed macrophages, kill neoplastic or virally infected targets and spontaneously secrete cytolytic protease (22, 23).

Gery et al (24) detected a factor that promotes murine thymocyte proliferation in culture supernatants produced by MPs, which was subsequently termed interleukin 1 (IL-1). Stimulants that induce IL-1 synthesis by MPs act on the plasma membrane and include lipopolysaccharide (LPS), phorbol myristic acetate (PMA), immune complexes, IFN-γ, and activated T cells (reviewed in 25). Conversely, there are a number of immunosuppressive agents including corticosteroids and prostaglandins that inhibit the production and/or release of IL-1 by macrophages. IL-1 has multiple effects on cells involved in inflammation and immune responses. Subcutaneous injection of IL-1 leads to margination of neutrophils and maximal extravascular infiltration of polymorphonuclear leukocytes (PMN). IL-1 is a chemotactic attractant and activator of PMNs, causing increased glucose metabolism, reduction of nitroblue tetrazolium, and release of lysosomal enzymes (reviewed in 25). In lymphocytes, IL-1 is not required for entry from G_0 to G_{1a} of the cell cycle, but once having entered G_{1a}, T cells respond to IL-1 by proceeding through G_{1b} to S phase. These events involve the intermediate formation of IL-2 and DNA synthesis.

B Cells

B cells originate from hematopoietic stem cells. Precursor B cells differ from immunocompetent B cells in lacking receptors for antigen on their membrane. Maturation of immunocompetent B cells into antibody-producing cells or plasma cells is divided into three stages, which include activation, proliferation, and differentiation (Figure 1, Section 2) (reviewed in 26, 27). Substantial effort has focused on early activation events that occur following antigen binding. In B cells, membrane-associated immunoglobulins serve as receptors for specific antigens. Like many agonists, including hormones, neurotransmitters and other biologically active substances, antigen binding and subsequent immunoglobulin cross-linking mediates transmembrane signaling (28). This event leads to increased phospholipid metabolism, specifically phospholipase C–catalyzed hydrolysis of phosphatidylinositol to inositol triphosphate (IP_3) and 1,2-diacylglycerol (DAG). IP_3 liberates Ca^{2+} from intracellular stores, and DAG activates protein kinase C (28). Formation of these products is associated with protein phosphorylation events and in B cells has been associated with autophosphorylation products, activation of tyrosine-protein-kinase activity, and phosphorylation of guanyl cyclase.

Progression of B cells from G_0 to G_{1a} of the cell cycle is characterized by increased expression of a Class II restricted antigen (Ia) on the surface membrane and cell enlargement. Activated cells rapidly progress into G_{1b} characterized by increased RNA synthesis and responsiveness to specific growth factors. Most of the growth-promoting factors are provided by T helper cells and include B cell–stimulatory factor (BSF or BCGF I), B cell–growth factor II (BCGF II), and, in certain instances, IL-2 (reviewed in 27). The macrophage product, IL-1, also contains growth-promoting activity for B cells. Entry into S phase of the cell cycle is accompanied by responsiveness to several differentiation signals collectively referred to as B cell–differentiation factors (BCDFs). These factors signal the cells to produce and secrete IgM antibody. The differentiation factors are also involved in the isotypic switching of antibody classes (e.g. IgM to IgG antibody-producing cells).

T Cells

Like B cells, T cell precursors originate from hematopoietic tissue (reviewed in 29). Subsequently, T cells enter the thymus and, under the influence of the thymic microenvironment, differentiate into a heterogeneous population with characteristic cell surface antigens and distinct functional properties (Figure 1, Section 3). These surface antigens are referred to as Lyt in mice and OKT in humans. The T subpopulations include T helper, T suppressor, and cytotoxic T cells (CTLs). The former two subpopulations are involved in regulation, whereas the latter is responsible for effector functions. As with transmembrane signaling events in B cells, cross-linking of the antigen receptor on T cells (T3) or mitogenic substances such as phytohemagglutinin or concanavalin A stimulate the breakdown of phosphatidylinositol, giving rise to IP_3 and DAG (30). T helper cells, in addition to antigen, require corecognition of a class II molecule present on the antigen-presenting cell and stimulation by the macrophage product, IL-1, to form lymphoblasts. Following activation, T helper cells produce IL-2, a growth factor that induces DNA synthesis in CTLs that have been activated by antigen to express receptors for

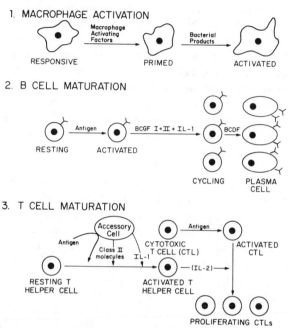

Figure 1 Macrophage and lymphocyte maturation. (*1*) Responsive macrophages are targeted by macrophage-activating factors (e.g. IFNγ), resulting in primed cells. Primed macrophages subsequently respond to bacterial products (e.g. endotoxin, muramyl dipeptide) to become fully activated. (*2*) Resting B cells are activated via antigen cross-linking. Activated B cells proliferate in response to growth-promoting factors and subsequently develop into plasma cells with the aid of differentiation factors. Other than IL-1, these growth-promoting and differentiating factors are derived from T helper cells. (*3*) T helper cells are activated by the combined action of antigens, class II molecules, and IL-1 via accessory cells. Activated T helper cells produce IL-2, which acts as a growth promoter in antigen-activated cytotoxic T cells. These processes can be negatively influenced by T suppressor cell activity. (Adapted from 15, 26, 27, 29.)

IL-2 (reviewed in 31). These cycling cells represent the effector populations responsible for lymphokine production that mediate various aspects of CMI.

IMMUNOTOXIC XENOBIOTICS

Immunotoxicology has only begun to be concerned with the consequences of chemical exposure on specific subcellular events. The following sections describe the effects of several important classes of xenobiotics on immune function. We focus the discussions on alterations in patterns of leukocyte maturation induced by these compounds.

Polycyclic Aromatic Hydrocarbons

Polycyclic aromatic hydrocarbons (PCAs) represent a class of chemicals that are ubiquitous in the environment and consist of carbon and hydrogen atoms arranged in three or more fused benzene rings (reviewed in 32). PCAs arise in the environment from energy production with fossil fuel, motor vehicle exhaust, and refuse burning. Humans are exposed to the various PCAs by breathing polluted air, eating and drinking contaminated food and water, and by tobacco smoke. The level of benzo[a]pyrene (BaP) emitted into the air in the United States is estimated at 894 tons per year.

Many natural and synthetic PCAs are carcinogenic. Interestingly, many carcinogenic PCAs have been shown to be immunosuppressive, whereas their noncarcinogenic analogs have no immunosuppressive effect (33–35). Table 1 lists several studies in which PCAs have been shown to alter humoral immunity, CMI, and/or host resistance (36–39). In addition to suppressing the antibody response to SRBC, BaP and 7,12-dimethylbenzanthracene (DMBA) (carcinogenic PCAs) also suppress antibody responses to T-independent antigens such as trinitrophenyl (TNP)-carrier conjugates including TNP-LPS and TNP-Ficoll (33, 35, 39). The TNP-Ficoll antigen is more dependent on macrophage and T lymphocyte accessory function than is the TNP-LPS antigen. Although not conclusive, data using TNP-LPS and TNP-Ficoll antigens suggest that DMBA and BaP or their metabolites can directly effect B lymphocyte maturation. Recent studies have also implicated that decreased IL-1 production may also be involved in inhibition of antibody synthesis by BaP (40). CTL activity is depressed after in vivo or in vitro DMBA exposure (36, 41). Addition of T helper cells or exogenous IL-2, but not IL-1, to CTL cultures of DMBA-exposed lymphocytes restores CTL function (38). Since T helper cells are the primary source of IL-2, and CTL function was not restored by IL-1, DMBA also appears to alter T helper cell function following in vivo or in vitro exposure.

The mechanism (or mechanisms) by which PCAs produce immunosuppression is not fully understood. To produce their carcinogenic effect, PCAs are believed to require metabolic activation to reactive species capable of forming DNA, RNA, and/or protein adducts (42). Hepatic PCA metabolism is not necessary for immunosuppression, since addition of DMBA or BaP to lymphocyte cultures results in suppression (41, 43). However, PCA metabolism may follow several alternative routes, since lymphocytes and monocytes possess inducible cytochrome P-450 activity capable of generating reactive PCA metabolites (44, 45). Although not demonstrated in lymphocytes, BaP and DMBA can also be oxidized to reactive species by prostaglandin synthetase (46). Another pathway for metabolism of methylated PCAs involves formation of methylene carbonium ions, which are capable of forming DNA

Table 1 Summary of immunologic effects by PCAs in the mouse[a]

PCA	HI	CMI	Host Resistance	Reference
BaP	+	+	–	33, 34, 39
BeP	–	–	ND	33, 34
Anthracene	–	ND	ND	33
BA	+	ND	ND	35, 37
DBA	+	ND	ND	35, 37
3-MC	+	+	+	37, 38, 45
DMBA	+	+	+	33, 39, 41

[a]Abbreviations: (+) = Suppressive; (–) = No Effect; ND = Not Determined; BaP = Benzo(a)pyrene; BeP = Benzo(e)pyrene; BA = Benzanthracene; DBA = Dibenzanthracene; 3-MC = 3-methylcholonthrene; DMBA = 7,12-dimethylbenzanthracene.

adducts (47). Although reactive PCA metabolites are responsible for altering cellular activity, PCA-induced immunotoxicity is also dependent upon the presence of the *Ah* receptor (45, 48).

Polyhalogenated Aromatic Hydrocarbons

Polyhalogenated aromatic hydrocarbons (PHAs) represent a diverse class of compounds that have received considerable attention because of their toxicity in experimental animals, possible risk of carcinogenicity in the human population, and potential widespread environmental exposure (reviewed in 49). PHAs most likely to be of a potential human health risk include selected congeners of polychlorinated biphenyls (PCBs), polybrominated biphenyls (PBBs), polychlorinated dibenzofurans (PCDFs), and polychlorinated dibenzo-p-dioxins (PCDDs). The prototype for this class of compounds is 2,3,7,8-tetrachlorodibenzo-*p*-dioxin (TCDD), a contaminant in the synthesis of the herbicide 2,4,5-trichlorophenoxyacetic acid. Numerous studies have shown that administration of toxic PHAs to laboratory animals, and in particular TCDD, causes lymphoid atrophy, immunosuppression, and alterations in host resistance to challenge with infectious agents or transplantable tumor cells (reviewed in 50–52). In fact, thymic atrophy, immunosuppression, and bone-marrow alterations are dominant characteristics of TCDD toxicity that occur in almost all species examined. The relevance of these animal studies has been fostered by clinical observations of immune alterations in individuals inadvertently exposed to various PHAs (7–10).

The specific immunological effects of TCDD and possibly other PHAs in rodents depend, to a great extent, on the age of the animals when the chemical is administered. Perinatal exposure to TCDD (i.e. during thymic organogenesis) is primarily characterized by suppression of CMI, which is not readily apparent following adult exposure (53–55). This immunological profile shares many features characteristic of neonatal thymectomy (56). Altered differentiation of intrathymic precursor cells, as occurs following neonatal thymectomy, has not been evaluated following perinatal TCDD exposure. However, T cells from treated mice demonstrate altered homing patterns (57), a feature characteristic of undifferentiated T cells. Furthermore, in vitro studies using a thymocyte and thymic epithelial cell coculture system have recently shown that TCDD inhibits the ability of thymic epithelial cells to provide the stimuli needed to induce T cell differentiation (58). Recent studies demonstrating that subchronic TCDD exposure inhibits the generation of CTLs also lend support to the premise that the thymic epithelial cell is a target tissue (59). This suggestion was indirectly evidenced by the use of murine bone-marrow chimeras, which have shown that inhibition of CTLs is due to the *Ah* genotype of the host and not of the grafted stem cell.

In contrast to subchronic or perinatal exposure, acute exposure of adult rodents to PHAs has its major effect on rapidly proliferating cell populations including hematopoietic stem cells (60, 61) and B lymphocytes, the latter manifested as suppressed antibody responses (e.g. 62–65). Unlike CMI, TCDD inhibits hematopoiesis (61) and B cell function (63, 66) by directly inhibiting maturation of the target cell.

Myelotoxicity, thymic atrophy, and immunosuppression by TCDD and PCBs appear to be associated with stereospecific binding to the *Ah* receptor present in lymphoid tissue and lymphoid cells (61, 62, 64–67). This association has been shown in genetic studies using *Ah*-responsive and -nonresponsive mouse strains, including mouse strains congenic at the *Ah* locus, where the immunotoxic effects of TCDD segregate with the *Ah* genotype. This association has also been supported in structure-activity studies where the binding affinity of various PHAs to the *Ah* receptor consistently correlated with its potency to induce immunosuppression. Furthermore, *Ah* receptors have been found in bone-marrow cells (61), lymphocytes (67), and thymic epithelial cells (58), which all are target tissues for PHA immunotoxicity.

Although immunotoxicity of PHAs is associated with binding to the *Ah* receptor, the mechanisms responsible following interaction of the receptor-ligand complex with the *Ah* locus are unknown. In fact, additional loci may be involved, since certain tissue-specific responses, such as epidermal hyperplasia in hairless mice, appear to be regulated by at least two genetic loci, *Ah* and *hr* (reviewed in 68). No consistent findings show that TCDD acts via cellular depletion mechanisms or by inducing qualitative and/or quantitative changes in regulatory products. In epidermal cell lines, TCDD alters normal patterns of proliferation and/or differentiation (reviewed in 68). Likewise, it has been proposed that TCDD induces similar maturational effects in thymic epithelial cells (58) and lymphocytes (66). For example, evidence suggests that

TCDD causes terminal differentiation of thymic epithelial cells, which results in loss of their ability to support thymocyte maturation (58). This altered pattern of differentiation may occur as a result of loss of high affinity epidermal growth factor receptors as occurs in keratinocytes treated with TCDD (69). Studies have shown qualitative and quantitative changes in phosphorylated proteins from purified B cells treated with TCDD (G. C. Clark & M. I. Luster, in preparation). Those proteins with altered phosphorylation patterns are associated with growth promoting activity in B cells. Thus, existing data indicate that TCDD immunotoxicity results from altered patterns of cell proliferation and differentiation in distinct lymphoid targets.

Heavy Metals

Metals may adversely affect the immune system and alter host resistance to infectious agents (reviewed in 4, 6, 70). Although many metals are known to alter immune function, we focus primarily on the effects of the most potent members of this group, which includes mercury (Hg), lead (Pb), and cadmium (Cd). Other heavy metals, such as platinum and gold, are of recent immunological interest. Platinum complexes, used as antineoplastic drugs, have been reported to suppress humoral immunity, lymphocyte proliferation, macrophage chemotaxis, and to induce allergic reactions (71). Gold salts, used pharmacologically as immunomodulators in rheumatoid arthritis (72), can cause nephrotoxicity in some patients that may involve an immunopathologic etiology. Gold injections cause renal disease with the involvement of immunoglobulin complexes and complement in rats, and autologous immune complex nephritis in guinea pigs (73). Gold is also capable of inducing allergic reactions and modulating lymphocyte activation.

Most reviewers have concluded that although heavy metals are immunosuppressive, under certain conditions they may be immunostimulatory (4, 70). Variables implicated in these opposite effects are dose concentration, route and duration of exposure, and strain and species differences. The most consistent effect on immune function in experimental animals following heavy metal exposure is increased susceptibility to infectious agents (74–83; Table 2). For example, increased mortality to *Listeria monocytogenes* was observed in CBA/J mice following subchronic lead exposure (78). Although lead significantly altered host resistance in these studies, it did not inhibit CMI or humoral-mediated immunity (HMI). Altered resistance to bacterial and viral infections produced by heavy metals demonstrates significant strain and species variability; in most murine studies antibody production and T cell activities are not suppressed. However, lead has been reported to inhibit phagocytosis, antigen processing, and other accessory functions in macrophages from several mouse strains (84–86).

Table 2   Summary of studies on heavy-metal effects on host resistance[a]

Host	Metal	Pathogen	Reference
Mouse	Hg	Encephalomyocarditis (EMC) virus	74
Rabbits	Hg	Pseudorabies virus	75
Mouse (SW)	Pb	*Salmonella typhimurium*	76
Rat (CR)	Pb	*Escherichia coli* and *Staphylococcus*	77
Mouse (CBA/J)	Pb	*Listeria monocytogenes*	78
Mouse (CD-1)	Pb	EMC virus	79
Mouse (S)	Pb	*Staphylococcus; Listeria monocytogenes; Candida*	80
Mouse (S)	PB	Langat virus	81, 82
Mouse (B6C3F1)	Cd	Herpes simplex virus	83

[a]Modified from Ref. 70.

The mechanism responsible for the alterations in host resistance by heavy metal exposure is unknown. Lead synergizes with endotoxin causing altered products and activities of reticuloendothelial cells, such as lipid peroxidation, superoxide anion generation, glutathiones, and glutathione-associated enzymes in mice (87), which could account for altered bactericidal and viricidal activity. In addition, although cytotoxic doses were employed (88), in vitro exposure to mercury and lead inhibits macrophage oxidative metabolism.

Mercury, lead, and cadmium reduce antibody production in some animals, but do not consistently produce this effect in all species studied (reviewed in 70). Even in the animals suppressed by heavy metals, it cannot be assumed that the defect is with the B cell. Blakley & Archer (86) have suggested that the ability of lead to inhibit humoral immunity is due to the inhibition of macrophage accessory functions. The effect of metal exposure on CMI is less well characterized. In a comprehensive study in Sprague-Dawley rats, chronic low-level pre- and postnatal exposure to lead suppressed several cell-mediated parameters, including delayed hypersensitivity and lymphoproliferative responses (89). Gaworski & Sharma (90) also noted that splenic lymphocytes from mice exposed to lead had significantly depressed proliferative responses to T and B cell mitogens. In contrast, several laboratories have reported that lead exposure does not suppress T cell proliferation (78, 82, 86). These differences are not easily reconciled, since the lead dosages and exposure periods employed do not easily account for the differences observed.

The mechanism of metal-induced injury to lymphoid cells is complex. Lead, like many metals, is a sulfhydryl alkylating agent with a high affinity for subcellular sulfhydryl groups. The immunomodulatory effects of lead on immune cells may involve an association with cellular thiols, since several studies have indicated that membrane and intracellular thiols are important in lymphocyte activation, proliferation, and differentiation. Furthermore, the inhibitory effects of lead can be reversed by the addition of exogenous thiol reagents (86).

Although many aspects of metal-induced immunopathology still need clarification, heavy metals have known influences on autoimmunity. The most common observation has been mercury-induced glomerulonephritis in Brown-Norway rats (91) or Wistar rats (92). Mercury injections induce polyclonal activation of B cells and enhance antibody synthesis to several antigens including single-stranded DNA. The precise mechanism of heavy metal–induced autoimmunity is unclear. Metal may directly modulate lymphocyte activation (e.g. enhance B cell or T suppressor cell activity), which could lead to autoimmunity (91). Since mercury and lead biochemically and biophysically alter erythrocytes, they may modify the antigenicity of erythrocytes, which results in an autoimmune hemolytic phenomena.

Organometals (Methylmercury and Organotins)

Methylmercury is readily absorbed through the intestine and passes the blood-brain and placental barriers where it can cause neuropathological changes in humans (Minamata disease). In rodents, methylmercury decreases resistance to infectious agents (reviewed in 4) and chemically induced tumors (93). Subchronic low-level methylmercury exposure in rodents causes atrophy of the thymic cortex and splenic follicles with concomitant suppression of immune functions (94–96). These observations complement Takeuchi's observation (97) of lymphoid and hemopoietic hypoplasia in the spleens of patients with Minamata disease.

Organotin compounds, used primarily as heat stabilizers, catalytic agents, and antimicrobial compounds, are also immunosuppressive in laboratory animals. Both di-n-octyltindichloride (DOTC) and di-n-butyltindichloride (DBTC) selectively depress thymic weights as well as T lymphocyte function in rats, without causing nonlymphoid toxicity (98–100). A cellular depletion mechanism is probably responsible for suppression, since decreased T cell–mitogen responsiveness in rats correlates with decreased numbers of lymphocytes with T cell surface markers (reviewed in 101). Suppression of humoral immunity by dialkyltins may be at the level of T cell regulation rather than directly affecting B cells, since T helper cell numbers are also decreased. Immune function is not impaired in mice and guinea pigs fed dialkyltins; this finding correlates with the absence of lymphoid tissue atrophy observed in these species (reviewed in 101). No species specificity is apparent following in vitro treatment; DOTC or DBTC cultured with rat, mice, or human thymocytes causes decreases in cell survival, mitogen responsiveness, and E-rosette formation (98). Organotins may interfere with T cell replication by interacting with plasma membrane sulfhydryl groups essential for amino acid transport and/or inhibiting glucose metabolism via alteration of pyruvate and α-ketoglutarate dehydrogenase activity (99).

Aromatic Amines

Benzidine (4,4-diaminobiphenyl), employed industrially in the synthesis of dyes as well as analytic reagents in various laboratory tests, is a urinary bladder carcinogen in humans (102). In rodents, benzidine causes hepatomas, mammary tumors, and, to a lesser extent, lymphoreticular neoplasms, primarily lymphomas (103). Because considerable evidence indicates that the immune response to chemically induced tumors may modulate tumor growth and/or progression, it follows that an increased incidence of neoplastic disease may occur by chemical carcinogens that also suppress immune functions. In mice, suppression of CMI occurs at dose levels of benzidine that are tumorigenic (104). In addition, benzidine exposure decreases host resistance to challenge by transplantable tumor cells or *Listeria* (104). Relevant to these observations in mice, an unconfirmed study showed a relationship between immunosuppression and neoplasia in workers engaged in the manufacture of benzidine (105). In this four-year study, only workers who were identified as having suppressed CMI (based on skin tests) demonstrated precancerous conditions and subsequent neoplasms.

The mechanisms responsible for immunosuppression by benzidine may not be the same as those responsible for its carcinogenicity. The addition of benzidine in vitro to mitogen-activated lymphocytes mimics the suppression of lymphocyte responsiveness observed following in vivo exposure. In vitro studies suggest that alterations in metabolites of the arachidonic acid–lipoxygenase pathway by benzidine (benzidine can serve as a co-oxidative substrate for hydroperoxidase) are responsible for inhibiting lymphocyte activation (104).

Estrogenic Xenobiotics

Although sex steroids such as estradiol and testosterone are not xenobiotics, they possess immunomodulatory properties (reviewed in 106). Likewise, a number of xenobiotics demonstrate both estrogenic activity (107), as determined by the rat uterine bioassay, and immunotoxicity. These include DDT, chlordecone, the mycotoxin zearalenone and its derivative zearalenol (a commercial anabolic agent), Δ^9-tetrahydrocannabinol (Δ^9-THC), and diethylstilbestrol (DES); the latter is the most potent estrogen in the series (reviewed in 108). However, other than DES, and to some extent Δ^9-THC, the immunotoxicity of these xenobiotics has not been extensively studied, and any relationship between estrogenic activity and immunotoxicity remains to be determined. The immunological effects of DES, particularly following adult exposure, are similar to those induced by 17-β-estradiol (109, 110) and following subchronic adult exposure in mice include thymic atrophy, myelotoxicity, stimulation of the reticuloendothelial system (RES), suppression of CMI, and reduction of NK cell activity (reviewed in 108, 111). Suppression of antibody synthesis in mice by DES also occurs, but is probably due either to increased antigen sequestering by macrophages or to depletion of T helper cell function and does not have a direct effect on B cells (112). Mice exposed perinatally to DES also demonstrate marked suppression (113–115). However, although immunosuppression appears to be reversible following adult exposure, the effects following perinatal exposure are persistent and may be under a different mechanism. Unlike mice, rats are resistant to immunosuppression by DES (J. Vos, personal communication).

Clinical observations and animal studies suggest that multiple mechanisms may be responsible for DES immunosuppression. Membrane-reactive estrogen metabolites (e.g. quinone intermediates) can react with the leukocyte cell membrane and modulate cell-surface interactions (116). Estrogens can also influence production of immunoregulatory factors produced by the thymic epithelium (109, 117, 118). This latter effect may be mediated by specific estrogen receptors present in thymic epithelial cells, since suppression can be blocked by steroid hormone receptor antagonists such as tamoxiphen. This putative thymic factor has not, as yet, been characterized, and any relationship with known thymic peptides remains to be determined. However, a recent report indicated that injection of estrogen reduced circulating plasma levels of thymosin $\alpha 1$ (119). Evidence also indicates that DES alters macrophage activation and T cell regulatory functions, which may also contribute to immunotoxicity. A relationship has been established between increased phagocytic activity of the RES and the amount of antigen ultimately available to the spleen, suggesting that depressed antibody responses result from altered antigen distribution or increased sequestering (reviewed in 108). Estrogens have also been reported to increase T suppressor cell activity in spleen cells of pregnant mice (120), decrease the number of T helper cells (111), and inhibit IL-2 synthesis (121). The biochemical mechanisms responsible for these effects have not been examined.

Pesticides

Several classes of insecticides have been examined for immunotoxicity, including organochlorines and organophosphates. Increasing evidence suggests that certain organochlorine pesticides, including DDT (122–124), captain (125, 126), and the chlorinated cyclodiene, chlordane (127, 128), modulate immune function. Immunosuppression by chlordane, however, may require in utero exposure (129). Due to their rapid metabolism by carboxyesterases to nontoxic metabolites, the toxicity of most organophosphate pesticides is relatively low. However, during their manufacture and storage, contaminants are formed that inhibit carboxyesterase activity. One of these contaminants, O,O,S-trimethylphosphorothioate (OOS-TMP), found in malathion, fenitrothion, and acephate, acts as a cholinergic agent at high dose levels and is immunotoxic at lower dose levels where other toxic manifestations are not observed (130–132). In mice, exposure to OOS-TMP, but not malathion, causes lymphocytopenia, thymic atrophy, suppression of antibody synthesis, and decreased generation of CTLs. However, neither lymphoproliferative responses, nor IL-2 synthesis are affected (130, 131). Methylparathion also suppresses immune function (123) and increases susceptibility to infection with *Salmonella typhimurium* (133). The immunological profile observed appears to be associated with altered macrophage activation. Macrophages treated with OOS-TMP demonstrate characteristics of inflammatory cells (low percentages of Ia antigen, increased IL-1 production, and decreased antigen binding capacity). The subcellular mechanisms for OOS-TMP immunosuppression have not been studied, however suppression does not appear to be related to altered cholinesterase activity, since O,S,S-trimethyl phosphorodithioate, a structural analog of OOS-TMP, inhibits cholinesterase activity without altering immune function (131, 132).

Benzene

Occupational exposure to benzene has frequently produced myelotoxicity expressed as leukopenia, pancytopenia, lymphocytopenia, granulocytopenia, thrombocytopenia, anemia, and bone-marrow hypoplasia (reviewed in 12). In occupational exposure a strong correlation was noted between the most frequently cited symptom, lymphocytopenia, and abnormal immunologic parameters. Benzene exposure in rabbits, rats, and mice has resulted in anemia, bone-marrow hypoplasia, and dose-related lymphocytopenia (12, 134). Benzene-induced myelotoxicity has been correlated with the appearance of benzene metabolites in the bone marrow (135), and the current evidence supports the concept that benzene toxicity is caused by one or more metabolites of benzene (136, 137).

Some investigators have stressed the importance of polyhydroxylated derivatives of benzene and their semiquinones (reviewed in 138). These studies have shown that in vitro hydroquinone and/or para-benzoquinone inhibits microtubule polymerization (139), T and B lymphocyte activation (140), and lectin-stimulated lymphocyte agglutination in rat spleen preparations (141). Since lectin-induced lymphocyte mitogenesis, cell agglutination, and capping are processes dependent upon microtubule integrity, it has been suggested that polyhydroxy metabolites of benzene (e.g. p-benzoquinone) inhibit PHA-induced lymphocyte blastogenesis and agglutination via this mechanism (reviewed in 138). The effects of benzene metabolites on microtubule assembly in vitro suggest reactivity with the two sulfhydryl groups at the GTP-binding site. However, administration of these compounds to animals does not result in typical effects of benzene toxicity, such as leucopenia, anemia, thrombocytopenia, and, eventually, aplastic anemia. Engelsberg & Snyder (142) have administered the major metabolites of benzene to mice and, using the ^{59}Fe uptake technique, failed to observe decreases in red cell production. Although these compounds are highly reactive and have profound effects when using in vitro systems, their reactivity may limit their ability to reach lymphoid tissue in biological systems. Goldstein et al (143) have suggested that ring-opening products may play a role in benzene toxicity. Thus, the toxic metabolites of benzene responsible for immunotoxicity and bone marrow suppression have yet to be identified.

Studies in rabbits exposed to benzene have described increased susceptibility to tuberculosis and pneumonia and reduced antibody response to bacterial antigens (reviewed in 12). Alterations in host resistance appear to correlate with altered immune function, since subcutaneous administration of benzene to C57BL6 mice inhibited both antibody production and lymphocyte activation (140). Alterations of immune parameters and host resistance that occur in experimental animals following benzene exposure are consistent with severe benzene toxicity in humans, which is often characterized by an acute, overwhelming infection. Evaluation of a large number of workers exposed to benzene revealed depressed levels of serum complement, IgG, and IgA, but not IgM (144, 145). Thus, benzene appears to be an immunotoxicant for humans, although the magnitude of this effect and the exposure threshold for immunotoxicity remain to be established.

Fungal Products

Several groups of mycotoxins, including ochratoxin, trichothecenes, and aflatoxin, are immunotoxic in laboratory animals. Ochratoxins are a series of 3,4-dihydro-3-methyl isocoumarin derivatives produced by several species of fungi belonging to the *Aspergillus* and *Penicillium* genera (146). Human exposure to ochratoxin A (OA) occurs through ingestion of contaminated cereal grains or contaminated animal tissue (reviewed in 147). OA can suppress antibody responses to both T-dependent (148, 149) and T-independent antigens (150) in mice. Administration of the 4-hydroxy metabolite of OA suppressed antibody secretion to the same extent as the parent compound, suggesting that a metabolite formed by liver microsomes in the presence of NADPH is responsible for OA immunosuppression (149). While the mechanism of immunosuppression and toxicity is unknown, Haubeck et al (148) demonstrated that coadministration of phenylalanine prevents OA-induced immunotoxicity. This same protective effect has been shown for OA inhibition of protein synthesis and growth of hepatoma cells in culture (151). With previous experiments demonstrating that phenylalanine inhibits OA toxicity (152), Haubeck et al suggest that increasing the enzyme substrate, phenylalanine, can reduce the inhibitory effect on the enzyme system and prevent OA-induced immunosuppression (148).

T$_2$ toxin, one of the most potent trichothecenes, has been linked to cases of alimentary toxic leukopenia in the USSR (153). Immunotoxicological effects of the trichothecenes include decreased antibody responses (154), decreased lymphoproliferation to T and B lymphocyte mitogens (155, 156), increased skin-graft survival time (154), and inhibition of macrophage activation (157). T$_2$ toxin inhibits protein synthesis in various eukaryotic cells (158), including alveolar macrophages and lymphocytes (157, 159). The inhibitory effect on protein synthesis is believed to be the primary cause for cellular toxicity.

Aflatoxin B$_1$ (AFB-1) is one of the most acutely toxic aflatoxins known, as it is both a hepatotoxin and a hepatocarcinogen (160, 161). AFB-1 also directly inhibits B and T lymphoproliferative responses in vitro. This effect is markedly enhanced when lymphocytes and AFB-1 are preincubated with hepatocytes (162), suggesting a need for metabolism. Antibody production is only inhibited when AFB-1 is preincubated with hepatocytes (162). Metabolites of AFB-1 have been shown to alkylate DNA. This akylation could account for the need of hepatocyte preincubation (163). The direct inhibitory effect of AFB-1 on lymphoproliferation could be attributed to its ability to act as an antimitotic agent (164).

Dimethylnitrosamine

Dimethylnitrosamine (DMN) has been shown to be carcinogenic and toxic in a variety of animal species (165) and is a suspected carcinogen in humans (166). Metabolic activation of DMN results in a metabolite that alkylates nucleic acids (167). DMN is also immunotoxic in mice, suppressing HMI and CMI (168, 169) and increasing susceptibility to tumor cell challenge (170); however, it also has an additional stimulatory effect on bone-marrow monocyte progenitors (168). DMN suppresses the antibody response to both T-dependent and T-independent antigens in vivo, but has no effect in vitro. Likewise, DMN does not alter mitogen-induced lymphoproliferative responses in vitro, suggesting metabolism may be needed to produce immunosuppression. Inclusion of rat hepatocytes in cell cultures to generate DMN metabolites did not produce suppression, which suggests extrahepatic DMN metabolism or an indirect in vivo effect (162). Examination of antibody production in vitro, using combinations of spleen cells from treated and untreated mice, indicates that suppression is due to altered B lymphocyte function (171).

Pulmonary Irritants

Human exposure to asbestos is associated with pulmonary diseases including fibrosis, asbestosis, and mesothelioma (reviewed in 172). Immunological impairments, such as decreased delayed-type hypersensitivity responses, reduced numbers of circulating T cells, and depressed T cell proliferation are associated with the pulmonary abestosis (reviewed in 173). In addition to suppression of CMI, increased levels of serum immunoglobulins and auto-antibodies have been observed in asbestosis patients (174). NK cell activity is also decreased in asbestotic individuals (175, 176). Altered alveolar mac-rophage activity plays a significant role in asbestos-induced immunological dysfunction. Asbestos particles reaching the alveoli are phagocytized by macrophages, resulting in cell lysis and release of lysosomal enzymes, in-flammatory products, and the previously ingested asbestos fibers (177). A cytotoxic effect on alveolar and splenic macrophages has also been demon-strated in vitro (178). While macrophages appear to be the most likely target within the lung, data also suggests that asbestos may directly affect T cell function, which may account for immune dysfunction by asbestos (179). The temporal relationship of these immune alterations to the onset of asbestosis and neoplasia remains to be clarified.

Beryllium was utilized in the fluorescent lamp industry and is currently used in the construction of lightweight metal alloys. Exposure to beryllium can result in dermatitis, acute pneumonitis, and chronic pulmonary granulo-matosis or berylliosis (reviewed in 180). While most cases of acute pneumo-nitis are thought to originate from chemical irritation, berylliosis and some acute pneumonitis involve delayed hypersensitivity responses (181, 182). The antigen producing this hypersensitivity reaction is presumed to be a be-ryllium–protein complex (183). Sensitivity to beryllium may have a genetic basis, since it is transmitted as a non-sex-linked dominant trait in guinea pigs (184). Exposure of lymphocytes from sensitized subjects to beryllium con-jugates results in increased lymphocyte transformation (185) and production of macrophage migration inhibition factor (186). Alveolar macrophages phagocytize beryllium and release lysosomal enzymes (187, 188). The pathogenesis of berylliosis and its relationship to immunological changes are not fully defined.

Silica is encountered in many occupational settings including sandblasting and mining. Acute or chronic exposure to silica dust can result in silicosis, a condition characterized by pulmonary fibrosis. Several immunological changes are associated with silicosis, including increased serum im-munoglobulin levels, autoantibodies, and an increased incidence of auto-immune disease (189, 190). Increased tumor immunity has also been reported and may be attributed to elevated numbers of macrophages at the pulmonary lesion (191). In contrast to humoral immunity, depression of CMI, as evi-denced by prolonged skin graft rejection and decreased resistance to viral mycotic or mycobacterial infections, has been reported (192, 193). Silica can be cytotoxic to macrophages in vitro (194) and can induce their activation (195). A soluble fibrogenic factor, which stimulates hydroxyproline and DNA synthesis in fibroblasts, is produced by macrophages activated by silica (196).

This interaction between activated macrophages and fibroblasts has been suggested to play a role in the pathogenesis of silicosis (reviewed in 197).

CONCLUSION

The immune system is highly complex; in it maturation is subject to orderly control by endogenous (lymphokines, cytokines) and exogenous (bacterial products) mediators. These mediators possess activation, growth-promotion, and/or differentiation properties, and are under the influence of potent, but not well-understood, regulators. A large number of xenobiotics adversely affect the immune system (based on observations in rodents and limited studies in humans inadvertently exposed) through disruption of cell-maturation processes. Considering the widespread distribution and stability of some of these agents in the environment, our concern is that current knowledge on the adverse health effects in humans may represent only the "tip of the iceberg" and that xenobiotic exposure may play a greater role than heretofore suspected in disease causation. Likewise, exposure to immunoalterative xenobiotics might represent additional risk to individuals with already fragile immune systems (e.g. those weakened by malnutrition, infancy, and old age). Due to obvious limitations in human clinical studies, an understanding of these risks depends to a great extent upon the clarification of cellular and molecular events underlying xenobiotic-induced immune alterations in experimental animals.

ACKNOWLEDGMENTS

The authors appreciate the assistance of Mrs. Louise Oyster and Mrs. Dori Germolec for assisting in the preparation of this chapter. We also thank Drs. G. Rosenthal, M. P. Ackerman, and J. Collins for their comments.

Literature Cited

1. Dean, J. H., Luster, M. I., Munson, A. E., Amos, H. A., eds. 1985. *Immunotoxicology and Immunopharmacology.* New York: Raven. 511pp.
2. Gibson, G. G., Hubbard, R., Parko, D. V., eds. 1983. *Immunotoxicology.* New York/London: Academic. 505 pp.
3. Mullen, P. W., ed. 1984. *Immunotoxicology: A Current Perspective of Principles and Practice.* Berlin/Heidelberg/New York/Tokyo: Springer-Verlag. 161 pp.
4. Koller, L. 1980. Immunotoxicology of heavy metals. *Int. J. Immunopharmacol.* 2:269–79
5. Vos, J. G. 1977. Immune suppression as related to toxicology. *CRC Crit. Rev. Toxicol.* 5:67–101

6. Dean, J. H., Luster, M. I., Boorman, G. A. 1982. Immunotoxicology. In *Immunology-Toxicology*, ed. P. Sirois, pp. 349–97. New York: Elsevier North Holland
7. Bekesi, J. G., Holland, J. F., Anderson, H. A., Fischbein, A. S., Rom, W., et al. 1978. Lymphocyte function of Michigan dairy farmers exposed to polybrominated biphenyls. *Science* 199: 1207–9
8. Bekesi, J. G., Roboz, J., Fischbein, A., Roboz, J. F., Solomon, S., Greaves, J. 1985. Immunological, biochemical and clinical consequences of exposure to polybrominated biophenyls. See Ref. 1, pp. 393–406
8a. Kimbrough, R. D. 1987. Human health

effects of polychlorinated biphenyls (PCBs) and polybrominated biphenyls (PBBs). *Ann. Rev. Pharmacol. Toxicol.* 27:87–111

9. Chang, K. J., Hsieh, K. H., Lee, T. P., Tung, T. C. 1982. Immunologic evaluation of patients with polychlorinated biphenyl poisoning: Determination of phagocytic Fc and complement receptors. *Environ. Res.* 28:329–34

10. Hoffman, R. E., Stehr-Green, P. A., Webb, K. B., Evans, G., Knutsen, A. P., et al. 1986. Health effects of long-term exposure to 2,3,7,8-tetrachlorodibenzo-*p*-dioxin. *J. Am. Med. Assoc.* 255:2037–38

11. Kammuller, M. E., Penninks, A. H., Seinen, W. 1984. Spanish toxic oil syndrome is a chemically induced GVHD-like epidemic. *Lancet* 1:1174–75

12. International Agency for Research on Cancer. 1982. Evaluation of the carcinogenic risk of chemical to humans: Some industrial chemicals and dyestuffs. *IARC Monogr.* 29:93–148

13. Kalland, T., Haukass, S. A. 1981. Effect of treatment with diethylstilbestrol-polyestradiol phosphate or estramustine phosphate (Estracyt®) on natural killer cell activity in patients with prostatic cancer. *Invest. Urol.* 18:437–41

14. Albin, R. J., Bruns, G. R., Guinan, P., Bush, I. M. 1974. Effect of diethylstilbestrol diphosphate on lymphocytic blastogenesis. *J. Endocrinol.* 62:681–82

15. Adams, D. O., Hamilton, T. A. 1984. The cell biology of macrophage activation. *Ann. Rev. Immunol.* 2:283–87

16. Gardner, D. E. 1984. Alterations in macrophage function by environmental chemicals. *Environ. Health Perspect.* 55:343–58

17. Loose, L. D., Silkworth, J. B., Charbonneau, T., Blumenstock, F. 1981. Environmental chemical-induced macrophage dysfunction. *Environ. Health Perspect.* 39:79–91

18. Dean, J. H., Adams, D. O. 1985. The effect of environmental agents on cells of the mononuclear phagocyte system. In *The Reticuloendothelial System,* Vol. 8, ed. J. W. Hadden, A. Szentivanyi, pp. 389–409. New York: Plenum

19. Cohn, Z. A. 1978. The activation of mononuclear phagocytes: Fact, fancy, and future. *J. Immunol.* 121:813–14

20. Meltzer, M. S. 1981. Tumor cytotoxicity by lymphokine-activated macrophages: Development of macrophage tumoricidal activity requires a sequence of reactions. *Lymphokines* 3:319–29

21. Morahan, P. S., Edelson, P. J., Gass, K. 1980. Changes in macrophage ectoenzymes associated with anti-tumor activity. *J. Immunol.* 125:1312–23

22. Johnson, W. J., Marino, P. A., Schreiber, R. D., Adams, D. O. 1983. Sequential activation of murine mononuclear phagocytes for tumor cytolysis: Differential expression of markers by macrophages in the several stages of development. *J. Immunol.* 131:1038–46

23. Adams, D. O., Marino, P. 1984. Activation of mononuclear phagocytes for destruction of tumor cells as a model for study of macrophage development. In *Contemporary Hematology-Oncology,* Vol. 3, ed. A. S. Gordon, R. Silber, J. LoBue, pp. 69–136. New York: Plenum

24. Gery, I., Gershon, R. K., Waksman, B. H. 1972. Potentiation of the T-lymphocyte response to mitogens. *J. Exp. Med.* 136:128–42

25. Oppenheim, J. J., Kovacs, E. J., Matsushima, K., Durum, S. K. 1986. There is more than one interleukin 1. *Immunol. Today* 7:45–56

26. Klaus, G. G. B., Hawrylowicz, C. M. 1984. Cell-cycle control in lymphocyte stimulation. *Immunol. Today* 5:15–19

27. Howard, M., Paul, W. E. 1983. Regulation of B-cell growth and differentiation by soluble factors. *Ann. Rev. Immunol.* 1:307–33

28. Coggeshall, K. M., Cambier, J. C. 1984. B cell activation. VIII. Membrane immunoglobulins transduce signals via activation of phosphatidylinositol hydrolysis. *J. Immunol.* 133:3383–88

29. Habu, S., Okumura, K. 1984. Cell surface antigen marking the stages of murine T cell ontogeny and its functional subsets. *Immunol. Rev.* 82:118–39

30. Imoden, J. B., Stobo, J. D. 1985. Transmembrane signalling by the T cell antigen receptor: Perturbation of the T_3-antigen receptor complex generates inositol phosphates and releases calcium ions from intracellular stores. *J. Exp. Med.* 161:446–56

31. Robb, R. J. 1984. Interleukin 2: The molecule and its function. *Immunol. Today* 5:203–11

32. Zedeck, M. S. 1980. Polycyclic aromatic hydrocarbons, a review. *J. Environ. Pathol. Toxicol.* 3:537–67

33. Stjernsward, J. 1966. Effect of noncarcinogenic and carcinogenic hydrocarbons on antibody-forming cells measured at the cellular level. *J. Natl. Cancer Inst.* 36:1189–95

34. Dean, J. H., Luster, M. I., Boorman, G.

A., Lauer, L. D., Luebke, R. W., Lawson, L. D. 1983. Immune suppression following exposure of mice to the carcinogen benzo(a)pyrene but not the noncarcinogenic benzo(e)pyrene. *Clin. Exp. Immunol.* 52:199–206

35. White, K. L. Jr., Lysy, H. H., Holsapple, M. P. 1985. Immunosuppression by polycyclic aromatic hydrocarbons: A structure-activity relationship in $B_6C_3F_1$ and DBA/2 mice. *Immunopharmacol.* 9:155–64

36. Wojdani, A., Alfred, L. J. 1984. Alterations in cell-mediated immune functions induced in mouse splenic lymphocytes by polycyclic aromatic hydrocarbons. *Cancer Res.* 44:942–45

37. Malmgren, R. A., Bennison, B. E., McKinley, T. W. Jr. 1952. Reduced antibody titers in mice treated with carcinogen and cancer chemotherapeutic agents. *Proc. Soc. Exp. Biol. Med.* 72:484–88

38. Lubet, R. A., Brunda, M. J., Taramelli, D., Dansie, D., Nebert, D., Kouri, R. E. 1984. Induction of immunotoxicity by polycyclic hydrocarbons: Role of the *Ah* locus. *Arch. Toxicol.* 56:18–24

39. Ward, E. C., Murray, M. J., Lauer, L. D., House, R. V., Irons, R., Dean, J. H. 1984. Immunosuppression following 7,12-dimethylbenz(a)anthracene exposure in $B_6C_3F_1$ mice. Effects on humoral immunity and host resistance. *Toxicol. Appl. Pharmacol.* 75:299–308

40. Lyte, M., Bick, P. H. 1986. Modulation of interleukin-1 production by macrophages following benzo(a)pyrene exposure. *Int. J. Immunopharmacol.* 8:377–81

41. Dean, J. H., Ward, E. C., Murray, M. J., Lauer, L. D., House, R. V., et al. 1986. Immunosuppression following 7,12-dimethylbenz(a)anthracene exposure in $B_6C_3F_1$ mice—II. Altered cell-mediated immunity and tumor resistance. *Int. J. Immunopharmacol.* 8:189–98

42. Miller, E. C., Miller, J. A. 1966. Mechanisms of chemical carcinogenesis: nature of proximate carcinogens and interactions with macromolecules. *Pharmacol. Rev.* 18:805–38

43. White, K. L. Jr., Holsapple, M. P. 1984. Direct suppression of *in vitro* antibody production by mouse spleen cells by the carcinogen benzo(a)pyrene but not by the noncarcinogenic congener benzo(e)pyrene. *Cancer Res.* 44:3388–93

44. Whitlock, J. D. Jr., Cooper, H. L., Gelboin, H. V. 1972. Aryl hydrocarbon (benzopyrene) hydroxylase is stimulated in human lymphocytes by mitogens and benz(a)anthracene. *Science* 177:618–19

45. Alfred, L. J., Wojdani, A. 1983. Effects of methylcholanthrene and benzanthracene on blastogenesis and aryl hydrocarbon hydroxylase induction in splenic lymphocytes from three inbred strains of mice. *Int. J. Immunopharmacol.* 5:123–29

46. Marnett, L. J., Reed, G. A., Johnson, J. T. 1977. Prostaglandin synthetase dependent benz(a)pyrene oxidation: Products of the oxidation and inhibition of their formation by antioxidants. *Biochem. Biophys. Res. Commun.* 79:569–71

47. Watabe, T., Ishizuka, T., Isobe, M., Ozawa, N. 1982. 7-hydroxymethyl sulfate ester as an active metabolite of 7,12-dimethylbenz(a)anthracene. *Science* 215:403–4

48. Frank, D. M., Yamashita, T. S., Blumer, J. L. 1982. Genetic differences in methylcholanthrene-mediated suppression of cutaneous delayed hypersensitivity in mice. *Toxicol. Appl. Pharmacol.* 64:31–41

49. Kimbrough, R. D., ed. 1980. *Halogenated Biphenyls, Terphenyls, Naphthalenes, Dibenzodioxins and Related Products.* New York: Elsevier North Holland Biomed. 406 pp.

50. Vos, J. G., Faith, R. E., Luster, M. I. 1980. Immune alterations. See Ref. 49, pp. 241–66

51. Silkworth, J., Vecchi, A. 1985. Role of the Ah receptor in halogenated aromatic hydrocarbon immunotoxicity. See Ref. 1, pp. 263–75

52. Thomas, P., Faith, R. 1985. Adult and perinatal immunotoxicity induced by halogenated aromatic hydrocarbons. See Ref. 1, pp. 305–13

53. Vos, J. G., Moore, J. A. 1974. Suppression of cellular immunity in rats and mice by maternal treatment with 2,3,7,8-tetrachlorodibenzo-p-dioxin. *Int. Arch. Allergy Appl. Immunol.* 47:777–89

54. Faith, R. E., Luster, M. I., Moore, J. A. 1978. Chemical separation of helper cell function and delayed hypersensitivity responses. *Cell. Immunol.* 40:275–84

55. Luster, M. I., Boorman, G. A., Dean, J. H., Harris, M. W., Luebke, R. W., et al. 1980. Examination of bone marrow immunologic parameters and host susceptibility following pre- and postnatal exposure to 2,3,7,8-tetrachlorodibenzo-p-dioxin. *Int. J. Immunopharmacol.* 2:301–10

56. Stutman, O. 1978. Intrathymic and ex-

trathymic T cell maturation. *Immunol. Rev.* 42:138–84

57. Faith, R. E., Luster, M. I. 1979. Investigations on the effects of 2,3,7,8-tetrachlorodibenzo-p-dioxin (TCDD) on parameters of various immune functions. *Ann. N.Y. Acad. Sci.* 320:564–71

58. Greenlee, W. F., Dold, K. M., Irons, R. D., Osborne, R. 1985. Evidence for direct action of 2,3,7,8-tetrachlorodibenzo-p-dioxin (TCDD) on thymic epithelium. *Toxicol. Appl. Pharmacol.* 19:112–20

59. Clark, D., Sweeney, G., Safe, S., Hancock, E., Kilburn, D., Gualdie, J. 1983. Cellular and genetic basis for suppression of cytotoxic T cell generation by halogenated aromatic hydrocarbons. *Immunopharmacol.* 6:143–53

60. Beran, M., Brandt, I., Slaninc, P. 1983. Distribution and effect of some polychlorinated biphenyls in the hemopoietic tissues. *J. Toxicol. Environ. Health* 12:521–32

61. Luster, M. I., Hong, L. H., Tucker, A. N., Clark, G., Greenlee, W. F., Boorman, G. A. 1985. Acute myelotoxic response in mice induced *in vivo* and *in vitro* by 2,3,7,8-tetrachlorodibenzo-p-dioxin. *Toxicol. Appl. Pharmacol.* 81:156–65

62. Kerkvliet, N., Brauner, J. 1984. Humoral immune suppression by contaminants of technical grade pentachlorophenol with special reference to 1,2,3,4,6,7,8-heptachlorodibenzo-p-dioxin. *J. Leuk. Biol.* 36:392

63. Holsapple, M., McNerney, P., Barnes, D., White, K. 1985. Suppression of humoral antibody production by exposure to 1,2,3,6,7,8-hexachlorodibenzo-p-dioxin. *J. Pharmacol. Exp. Ther.* 231:518–26

64. Silkworth, J. B., Antrim, L., Grabstein, E. M. 1984. Correlations between polychlorinated biphenyl immunotoxicity, the aromatic hydrocarbon locus, and liver microsomal enzyme induction in C57B1/6 and DBA/2 mice. *Toxicol. Appl. Pharmacol.* 75:156–65

65. Vecchi, A., Sironi, M., Canegrati, M. A., Recchia, M., Garattini, S. 1983. Immunosuppressive effects of 2,3,7,8-tetrachlorodibenzo-p-dioxin in strains of mice with different susceptibility to induction of aryl hydrocarbon hydroxylase. *Toxicol. Appl. Pharmacol.* 68:434–41

66. Tucker, A. N., Vore, S. J., Luster, M. I. 1986. Suppression of B cell differentiation by 2,3,7,8-tetrachlorodibenzo-p-dioxin. *Mol. Pharmacol.* 29:372–77

67. Carlstedt-Duke, J., Kurl, R., Poellinger, L., Gillner, M., Hansson, L.-A., et al. 1982. The detection and function of the cytosolic receptor for 2,3,7,8-tetrachlorodibenzo-p-dioxin (TCDD) and related carcinogens. In *Chlorinated Dioxins and Related Compounds: Impact on the Environment,* ed. O. Hutzinger, pp. 355–65. New York: Pergamon

68. Poland, A., Knutson, J. C. 1982. 2,3,7,8 - Tetrachlorodibenzo - p - dioxin and related halogenated aromatic hydrocarbons: Examination of the mechanism of toxicity. *Ann. Rev. Pharmacol. Toxicol.* 22:517–54

69. Hudson, L. G., Toscano, W. A., Greenlee, W. F. 1985. Regulation of epidermal growth factor binding in human keratinocyte cell line by 2,3,7,8-tetrachlorodibenzo-p-dioxin. *Toxicol. Appl. Pharmacol.* 77:251–59

70. Lawrence, D. A. 1985. Immunotoxicity of heavy metals. See Ref. 1, 341–53

71. von Hoff, D. D., Slavik, M., Muggia, F. M. 1976. Allergic reactions to cis platinum. *Lancet* 1:90–93

72. Harth, M. 1981. Modulation of immune responses of gold salts. *Agents Actions* 8:465–76

73. Ueda, S., Wakashim, Y., Takei, I., Mori, T., Iesato, K., et al. 1980. Autologous immune complex nephritis in gold injected guinea pigs. *Nippon Jinzo Gakkai Shi* 22:1221–1230

74. Gainer, J. H. 1977. Effects of heavy metals and of deficiency of zinc on mortality rates in mice infected with encephalomyocarditis virus. *Am. J. Vet. Res.* 38:869–72

75. Koller, L. D. 1973. Immunosuppression produced by lead, cadmium and mercury. *Am. J. Vet. Res.* 34:1457–58

76. Hemphill, F. E., Kaeberle, M. L., Buck, W. B. 1971. Lead suppression of mouse resistance to *Salmonella typhimurium*. *Science* 172:1031–32

77. Cook, J. A., Hoffman, E. O., Di Luzio, N. R. 1975. Influence of lead and cadmium on the susceptibility of rats to bacterial challenge (39117). *Proc. Soc. Exp. Biol. Med.* 150:741–47

78. Lawrence, D. A. 1981. *In vivo* and *in vitro* effects of leadx on humoral and cell-mediated immunity. *Infect. Immun.* 31:136–43

79. Gainer, J. H. 1974. Lead aggravates viral disease and represses the antiviral activity in interferon inducers. *Environ. Health Perspect.* 7:113–19

80. Salaki, J., Louria, D. B., Thind, I. S. 1975. Influence of lead intoxication on

experimental infections. *Clin. Res.* 23: 417A

81. Thind, I. S., Kahn, M. Y. 1978. Potentiation of the neurovirulence of langat virus infection by lead intoxication in mice. *Exp. Mol. Pathol.* 29:342–47

82. Koller, L. D., Roan, J. G., Kerkvliet, N. I. 1979. Mitogen stimulation of lymphocytes in CBA mice exposed to lead and cadmium. *Environ. Res.* 19:177–88

83. Thomas, P. T., Ratajczak, H. V., Aranyi, C., Gibbons, R., Fenters, J. D. 1986. Evaluation of host resistance and immune function in cadmium-exposed mice. *Toxicol. Appl. Pharmacol.* 80: 446–56

84. Koller, L. D., Roan, J. G. 1977. Effects of lead and cadmium on mouse peritoneal macrophages. *J. Reticuloendothel. Soc.* 21:7–12

85. Kerkvliet, N. I., Baecher-Steppan, L. 1982. Immunotoxicity studies on lead: Effects of exposure on tumor growth and cell-mediated tumor immunity after syngeneic or allogeneic stimulation. *Immunopharmacol.* 4:213–24

86. Blakley, B. R., Archer, D. L. 1981. The effect of lead acetate on the immune response in mice. *Toxicol. Appl. Pharmacol.* 61:18–26

87. Sakaguchi, O., Abe, H., Sakaguchi, S., Hsu, C. C. 1982. Effect of lead acetate on superoxide anion generation and its scavengers in mice given endotoxin. *Microbiol. Immunol.* 26:767–78

88. Castranova, V., Bowman, L., Reasor, M. J., Miles, P. R. 1980. Effects of heavy metal ions on selected oxidative metabolic processes in rat alveolar macrophages. *Toxicol. Appl. Pharmacol.* 53:14–23

89. Faith, R. E., Luster, M. I., Kimmel, C. A. 1979. Effect of chronic developmental lead exposure on cell-mediated immune functions. *Clin. Exp. Immunol.* 35:413–20

90. Gaworski, C. L., Sharma, R. P. 1978. The effects of heavy metals on [³H]thymidine uptake in lymphocytes. *Toxicol. Appl. Pharmacol.* 46:305–13

91. Druet, P., Teychenne, P., Mandet, C., Bascou, C., Druet, E. 1981. Immune-type glomerulonephritis induced in the Brown-Norway rat with mercury-containing pharmaceutical products. *Nephron* 28:145–48

92. Makker, S. P., Aikawa, M. 1979. Mesangial glomerulonephropathy with desposition of IgG, IgM and C3 induced by mercuric chloride. *Lab. Invest.* 41:45–50

93. Neilan, B. A., Taddeini, L., McJitton, C. E., Hankwerger, B. S. 1980. Decreased T-cell function in mice exposed to chronic low levels of lead. *Clin. Exp. Immunol.* 39:746–49

94. Blakely, B. R., Sisodia, C. S., Mukkur, T. K. 1980. The effect of methylmercury, tetraethyl lead, and sodium arsenite on the humoral immune response in mice. *Toxicol. Appl. Pharmacol.* 52: 245–54

95. Hirokawa, K., Hayashi, Y. 1980. Acute methylmercury intoxication in mice. *Acta Pathol. Jpn.* 30:23–32

96. Ohi, G., Fukunda, M., Seta, H., Yagyu, H. 1976. Methylmercury on humoral immune responses in mice under conditions simulated to practical situations. *Bull. Environ. Contam. Toxicol.* 15:175–90

97. Takeuchi, T. 1968. Pathology of minamata disease. In *Minamata Disease*, ed. Study Group of Minamata Disease. Japan: Kumamoto Univ. Publ.

98. Seinen, W., Vos, J. G., Brands, R., Hooykaas, H. 1979. Lymphocytotoxicity and immunosuppression by organotin compounds. Suppression of graft-versus-host reactivity, blast transformaion and E-rosette formation by di-n-butlytin-dichloride and di-n-octyltindichloride. *Immunopharmacol.* 1:343–55

99. Penninks, A. H., Verschuren, P. M., Seinen, W. 1983. Di-n-butyltindichloride uncouples oxidative phosphorylation in rat liver mitochondria. *Toxicol. Appl. Pharmacol.* 70:115–20

100. Miller, K., Scott, M. P. 1985. Immunological consequences of dioctyltin dichloride (DOTC)-induced thymic injury. *Toxicol. Appl. Pharmacol.* 78: 395–403

101. Vos, J. G., Krajnc, E. I., Wester, P. W. 1985. Immunotoxicity of Bis(tri-n-butyltin) oxide. See Ref. 1, pp. 327–40

102. Haley, T. J. 1975. Benzidine revisited: A review of the literature and problems associated with the use of benzidine and its congeners. *Clin. Toxicol.* 8:13–42

103. Vesselinovitch, S. D., Rao, K. V. N., Mihailovich, N. 1975. Factors modulating benzidine carcinogenicity bioassay. *Cancer Res.* 35:2814–19

104. Luster, M. I., Tucker, A. N., Hayes, H. T., Pung, O. J., Burka, T., et al. 1985. Immunosuppressive effects of benzidine in mice: Evidence of alterations in arachidonic acid metabolism. *J. Immunol.* 135:2754–61

105. Gorodilova, V. V., Mandrik, E. V.

1978. The use of some immunological reaction for studying the immune response in persons presenting a high oncological risk. *Sov. Med.* 8:50–53

106. Ahlquist, J. 1976. Endocrine influences on lymphatic organs, immune responses, inflammation and autoimmunity. *Acta Endocrinol.* 83:1–136

107. Katzenellenbogen, J. A., Katzenellenbogen, B. S., Tatee, T., Robertson, D. W., Landvatter, S. W. 1980. The chemistry of estrogens and antiestrogens: Relationships between structure, receptor binding and biological activity. In *Estrogens in the Environment,* ed. J. A. McLachlan, pp. 33–51. Amsterdam: Elsevier North Holland

108. Luster, M. I., Pfeifer, R. W., Tucker, A. N. 1985. Influence of sex hormones on immunoregulation with specific reference to natural and synthetic estrogens. In *Endocrine Toxicology,* ed. J. A. McLachlin, K. Korach, J. Thomas, pp. 67–83. New York: Raven

109. Luster, M. I., Hayes, H. T., Korach, K., Tucker, A. N., Dean, J. H., et al. 1984. Estrogen immunosuppression is regulated through estrogenic responses in the thymus. *J. Immunol.* 133:110–16

110. Pung, O. J., Luster, M. I., Hayes, H. T., Rader, J. 1984. Influence of steroidal and nonsteroidal sex hormones on host resistance in the mouse: Increased susceptibility to *Listeria monocytogenes* following exposure to estrogenic hormones. *Infect. Immun.* 46:301–7

111. Kalland, T. 1982. Long-term effects on the immune system of an early life exposure to diethylstilbestrol. In *Environmental Factors in Human Growth and Development, Banbury Report 11,* pp. 217–42. Cold Spring Harbor, NY: Cold Spring Harbor Lab.

112. Sljivic, V. S., Warr, G. W. 1973. Oestrogens and immunity. *Period. Biol.* 75:231–45

113. Ways, S. C., Blair, P. B., Bern, H. A., Staskawicz, M. O. 1980. Immune responsiveness of adult mice exposed neonatally to diethylstilbestrol, steroid hormones or vitamin A. *J. Environ. Pathol. Toxicol.* 3:207–20

114. Kalland, T., Strand, O., Forsberg, J. G. 1979. Long-term effects of neonatal estrogen treatment of mitogen responsiveness of mouse spleen lymphocytes. *J. Natl. Cancer Inst.* 63:413–19

115. Luster, M. I., Faith, R. E., McLachlan, J. A., Clark, G. C. 1979. Effect of *in utero* exposure to diethylstilbestrol on the immune response in mice. *Toxicol. Appl. Pharmacol.* 47:287–93

116. Pfeifer, R. W., Patterson, R. M. 1985. Modulation of lymphokine-induced macrophage activation by estrogen metabolites. *J. Immunopharmacol.* 7:247–63

117. Grossman, C. J., Sholiton, L. J., Nathen, P. 1979. Rat thymic estrogen receptor. I. Preparation, location and physiochemical properties. *J. Steroid Biochem.* 11:1233–40

118. Stimson, W. H., Hunter, I. C. 1980. Oestrogen-induced immunoregulation mediated through the thymus. *J. Clin. Lab. Immunol.* 4:27–34

119. Allen, L. S., McClure, J. E., Goldstein, A. L., Barkley, M. S., Michael, S. D. 1984. Estrogen and thymic hormone interactions in the female mouse. *J. Reprod. Immunol.* 6:25–37

120. Suzuki, K., Tomasi, T. B. 1979. Immune response during pregnancy. Evidence of suppressor cells for splenic antibody response. *J. Exp. Med.* 150:898–908

121. Henriksen, O., Frey, J. R. 1982. Control of expression of interleukin-2 activity. *Cell. Immunol.* 73:106–14

122. Glick, B. 1974. Antibody-mediated immunity in the presence of mirex and DDT. *Poultry Sci.* 53:1476–85

123. Street, J. C., Sharma, R. P. 1975. Alteration of induced cellular and humoral immune responses by pesticides and chemicals of environmental concern. Quantitative studies of immunosuppression by DDT, aroclor 1254, carbaryl, carbofuran, and methylparathion. *Toxicol. Appl. Pharmacol.* 32:587–602

124. Kaminski, N. E., Wells, D. S., Dauterman, W. C., Roberts, J. F., Guthrie, F. E. 1986. Macrophage uptake of a lipoprotein-sequestered toxicant: A potential route of immunotoxicity. *Toxicol. Appl. Pharmacol.* 82:474–80

125. Vos, J. G., Krajnc, E. I. 1983. Immunotoxicology of pesticides. In *Developments in the Science and Practice of Toxicology,* ed. A. W. Hayes, R. C. Schnell, T. S. Miya, pp. 229–39. New York: Elsevier

126. Lafarge-Frayssinet, C., Decloitre, F. 1982. Modulatory effect of the pesticide captan on the immune response in rats and mice. *J. Immunopharmacol.* 4:43–52

127. Spyker-Cranmer, J. M., Barnett, J., Avery, D. L., Cranmer, M. F. 1982. Immunoteratology of chlordane: Cell-mediated and humoral immune responses in adult mice exposed *in utero. Toxicol. Appl. Pharmacol.* 62:402–8

128. Beggs, M., Menna, J. H., Barnett, J. B. 1985. Effects of chlordane on influenza Type A virus and herpes simplex Type 1 virus replication *in vitro*. *J. Toxicol. Environ. Health* 16:173–88

129. Johnson, K. W., Holsapple, M. P., Munson, A. E. 1986. An immunotoxicological evaluation of γ-chlordane. *Fund. Appl. Toxicol.* 6:317–326

130. Rodgers, K. E., Imamura, T., Devens, B. H. 1985. Effects of subchronic treatment with O,O,S-trimethyl phosphorothioate on cellular and humoral immune response systems. *Toxicol. Appl. Pharmacol.* 81:310–18

131. Rodgers, K. E., Imamura, T., Devens, B. H. 1985. Investigations into the mechanism of immunosuppression caused by acute treatment with O,O,S-trimethyl phosphorothioate. I. Characterization of the immune cell population affected. *Immunopharmacol.* 10:171–80

132. Devens, B. H., Grayson, M. H., Imamura, T., Rodgers, K. E. 1985. O,O,S-trimethyl phosphorothioate effects on immunocompetence. *Pestic. Biochem. Physiol.* 24:251–59

133. Fan, A., Street, J. C., Nelson, R. M. 1978. Immune suppression in mice administered methyl parathion and carbofuran by diet. *Toxicol. Appl. Pharmacol.* 45:235–42

134. Snyder, C. A., Goldstein, B. D., Sellakumar, A., Bromberg, I., Laskin, S., Albert, R. E. 1980. The inhalation toxicology of benzene: Incidence of hematopoietic neoplasms and hematotoxicity in AKR/J and C57BL/6J mice. *Toxicol. Appl. Pharmacol.* 54:323–31

135. Greenlee, W. F., Gross, E. A., Irons, R. D. 1981. Relationship between benzene toxicity and the dispostion of ^{14}C-labeled benzene metabolites in the rat. *Chem. Biol. Interactions* 33:285–99

136. Snyder, R., Longacre, S. L., Witmer, C. M., Kocsis, J. J., Andrews, L. S., Lee, E. W. 1981. Biochemical toxicology of benzene. In *Reviews in Biochemical Toxicology*, ed. E. Hodgson, J. R. Bend, R. M. Philpot, pp. 123–153. New York: Elsevier North-Holland

137. Irons, R. D., Neptun, D. A., Pfeifer, R. W. 1981. Sulfhydryl-dependent inhibition of lymphocyte growth and microtubule assembly by quinone metabolites of benzene. *J. Reticuloendothel. Soc.* 30: 359–72

138. Pfeifer, R. W., Irons, R. D. 1985. Mechanisms of sulfhydryl-dependent immunotoxicity. See Ref. 1, pp. 255–62

139. Irons, R. D., Neptun, D. A. 1980. Effects of the principal hydroxymetabolites of benzene on microtubule polymerization. *Arch. Toxicol.* 45:297–305

140. Wierda, D., Irons, R. D., Greenlee, W. F. 1981. Immunotoxicity in C57BL/6 mice exposed to benzene and Aroclor 1254. *Toxicol. Appl. Pharmacol.* 60: 410–17

141. Pfeifer, R. W., Irons, R. D. 1981. Inhibition of lectin-stimulated lymphocyte agglutination and mitogenesis by hydroquinone: Reactivity with intracellular sulfhydryl groups. *Exp. Mol. Pathol.* 35:189–98

142. Engelsberg, B., Synder, R. 1982. Effects of benzene and other chemicals on 72 hr ^{59}Fe utilization in Swiss albino mice. *Toxicologist* 2:121 (Abstr.)

143. Goldstein, B. D., Witz, G., Javid, J., Amoruso, M. A., Rossman, T., Wolder, B. 1982. Muconaldehyde, a potential toxic intermediate of benzene metabolism. In *Biological Reactive Intermediates. II. Chemical Mechanisms and Biological Effects*, ed. D. V. Parke, J. J. Kocsis, Jollow, G. G. Gibson, C. M. Witmer, pp. 331–40, New York: Plenum

144. Smolik, R., Grzybek-Hryncewicz, K., Lange, A., Zatonski, W. 1973. Serum complement level in workers exposed to benzene, toluene and xylene. *Int. Arch. Arbeitsmed.* 31:243–47

145. Lange, A., Smolik, R., Zatonski, W., Szymanska, J. 1973. Serum immunoglobulin levels in workers exposed to benzene, toluene and xylene. *Int. Arch. Arbeitsmed.* 31:37–44

146. Steyn, P. S. 1971. Ochratoxin and other dihydroisocoumarins. In *Microbiol Toxins*, Vol. 6, *Fungal Toxins*, ed. A. Ciegler, S. Kadis, S. J. Ajl, pp. 179–205. New York: Academic

147. Shotwell, O. L., Hesseltine, C. W., Goulder, M. L. 1969. Ochratoxin A: Occurance as natural contaminant of a corn sample. *Appl. Microbiol.* 17:765–66

148. Haubeck, H. D., Lorkowski, G., Kolsch, E., Roschenthaler, R. 1981. Immunosuppression by Ochratoxin A and its prevention by phenylalanine. *Appl. Environ. Microbiol.* 41:1040–42

149. Creppy, E., Stormer, F., Roschenthaler, R., Dirheimer, G. 1983. Effects of two metabolites of Ochratoxin A, (4R)-4-hydroochratoxin A and Ochratoxin α, on immune response in mice. *Infect. Immun.* 39:1015–18

150. Prior, M. G., Sisodia, C. S. 1982. The effects of Ochratoxin A on the immune response of Swiss mice. *Can. J. Comp. Med.* 46:91–96

151. Creppy, E. E., Lugnier, A., Roschenthaler, R., Dirheimer, G. 1979. *In vitro* inhibition of yeast phenylalanine tRNA synthetase by Ochratoxin A. *Chem. Biol. Interactions* 24:257–61

152. Creppy, E. E., Schlegel, M., Roschenthaler, R., Dirheimer, G. 1980. Phenylalanine prevents acute poisoning by Ochratoxin A in mice. *Toxicol. Lett.* 6:77–80

153. Joffe, A. 1978. *Fusarium poae* and *F. sporotrichoides* as principle causal agents of alimentary toxic aleukia. In *Mycotoxic Fungi, Mycotoxins, Mycotoxicosis*, Vol. 3, ed. T. Wylie, L. Morehouse, pp. 21–27. New York: Dekker

154. Rosenstein, Y., Lafarge-Frayssinet, C., Lespinats, F., Loissillier, F., Lafont, P., Frayssinet, C. 1979. Immunosuppressive activity of *Fusarium* toxins. Effects on antibody synthesis and skin grafts of crude extracts, T_2-toxin and diacetoxyscirpenal. *Immunology* 36:111–17

155. Forsell, J. H., Kateley, J. R., Yoshizawa, T., Pestka, J. J. 1985. Inhibition of mitogen-induced blastogenesis in human lymphocytes by T-2 toxin and its metabolites. *Appl. Environ. Microbiol.* 49:1523–26

156. Lafarge-Frayssinet, C., Lespinats, F., Lafont, P., Loisillier, F., Mousset, S., et al. 1979. Immunosuppressive effects of fusarium extracts and trichothecenes: Blastogenic response of murine splenic and thymic cells to mitogens (40439). *Proc. Soc. Exp. Biol. Med.* 160:302–11

157. Gerberick, G. F., Sorenson, W. G., Lewis, D. M. 1984. The effects of T-2 toxin on alveolar macrophage function *in vitro*. *Environ. Res.* 33:246–60

158. Smith, K. E., Conan, M., Cundliffe, F. R. 1975. Inhibition of the initiation level of eukaryotic protein synthesis by T-2 toxin. *FEBS. Lett.* 50:8–12

159. Rosenstein, Y., Lafarge-Frayssinet, C. 1983. Inhibitory effect of Fusarium T_2-toxin on lymphoid DNA and protein synthesis. *Toxicol. Appl. Pharmacol.* 70:283–88

160. Wogan, G. N., Newberne, P. M. 1967. Dose-response characteristics of aflatoxin B, carcinogenesis in the rat. *Cancer Res.* 27:2370–2376

161. Newberne, P. M., Butler, W. H. 1969. Acute and chronic effects of aflatoxin on the liver of domestic and laboratory animals: A review. *Cancer Res.* 29:236–250

162. Yang, K. H., Kim, B. S., Munson, A. E., Holsapple, M. P. 1986. Immunosuppression induced by chemicals receiving metabolic activation in mixed cultures of rat hepatocytes and murine splenocytes. *Toxicol. Appl. Pharmacol.* 83:420–429

163. Gurtoo, H. C., Dave, C. V. 1975. *In vitro* metabolic conversion of aflatoxins and benz(a)pyrene to nucleic acid–binding microsomes. *Cancer Res.* 35:382–89

164. Metcalfe, S. A., Neal, G. E. 1983. Some studies on the relationship between the cytotoxicity of aflatoxin B_1 to rat hepatocytes and metabolism of the toxin. *Carcinogenesis* 4:1013–19

165. Magee, P. N., Barnes, J. M. 1967. Carcinogenic nitroso compounds. *Adv. Cancer Res.* 10:163–246

166. Craddock, V. M. 1983. Nitrosamines and human cancer: Proof of an association? *Nature* 306:638

167. Gol-Winkler, R., Govtier, R. 1977. DNA synthesis inhibition by dimethylnitrosamine in regenerating rat liver. *Eur. J. Cancer* 13:1081–87

168. Holsapple, M. P., Tucker, A. T., McNerney, P. J., White, K. L. Jr. 1984. Effects of *N*-nitrosodimethylamine on humoral immunity. *J. Pharmacol. Exp. Ther.* 229:493–500

169. Holsapple, M. P., Bick, P. H., Duke, S. S. 1985. Effects of *N*-nitrosodimethylamine on cell-mediated immunity. *J. Leuk. Biol.* 37:367–81

170. Duke, S. S., Schook, L. B., Holsapple, M. P. 1985. Effects of N-nitrosodimethylamine on tumor susceptibility. *J. Leuk. Biol.* 37:383–94

171. Johnson, K. W., Munson, A. E., Holsapple, M. P. 1986. The B lymphocyte as a target for dimethylnitrosamine-induced immunosuppression. *Toxicologist* 6:16–21

172. Liddell, D., Miller, K. 1983. Individual susceptibility to inhaled particles—A methodological essay. *Scand. J. Work. Environ. Health* 9:1–8

173. Miller, K., Brown, R. C. 1985. The immune system and asbestos-associated disease. See Ref. 1, pp. 429–40

174. Lange, A. 1980. An epidemiological survey of immunological abnormalities in asbestos workers. *Environ. Res.* 22:176–80

175. Kubota, M., Kagamimori, S., Yokoyama, K., Okada, A. 1985. Reduced killer cell activity of lymphocytes

from patients with asbestosis. *Br. J. Ind. Med.* 42:276–80

176. Ginns, L. C., Ryo, J. H., Rogol, P. R., Sprince, N. L., Oliver, L. C., Larsson, C. L. 1985. Natural killer cell activity in cigarette smokers and asbestos workers. *Am. Rev. Respir. Dis.* 131:831–34

177. Miller, K., Weintraub, Z., Kagan, E. 1979. Manifestations of cellular immunity in the rat after prolonged asbestos inhalation. I. Physical interactions between alveolar macrophages and splenic lymphocytes. *J. Immunol.* 123:1029–38

178. Yeager, H. Jr., Russo, D. A., Yonez, M., Gerardi, D., Nolon, P., et al. 1983. Cytotoxicity of a short-fiber chrysotile asbestos for human alveolar macrophages: Preliminary observations. *Environ. Res.* 30:224–32

179. Bozelka, B. E., Gaumer, H. R., Nordberg, J., Salvaggio, J. E. 1983. Asbestos-induced alterations of human lymphoid cell mitogenic responses. *Environ. Res.* 30:281–90

180. Reeves, A. L., Preuss, O. P. 1985. The immunotoxicity of beryllium. See Ref. 1, pp. 441–55

181. Epstein, W. L. 1967. Granulomatous hypersensitivity. *Prog. Allergy* 2:36–88

182. Chiappino, G., Cirla, A. M., Vigliani, E. 1969. Delayed-type hypersensitivity reaction to beryllium compounds. *Arch. Pathol.* 87:131–40

183. Krivanek, N. D., Reeves, A. L. 1972. The effect of chemical forms of beryllium on the production of the immunologic response. *Am. Ind. Hyg. Assoc. J.* 33:45–52

184. Polak, L., Barnes, J. M., Turk, J. L. 1968. The genetic control of contact sensitivity to inorganic metal compounds in guinea pigs. *Immunology* 14:707–11

185. Hanifen, J. M., Epstein, W. L., Cline, M. J. 1970. *In vitro* studies of granulomatous hypersensitivity to beryllium. *J. Invest. Dermatol.* 55:284–88

186. Henderson, W. R., Fukuyoma, K., Epstein, W. L., Spitler, L. E. 1972. *In vitro* demonstration of delayed hypersensitivity in patients with berylliosis. *J. Invest. Dermatol.* 58:5–8

187. Kang, K. Y., Salvaggio, J. 1976. Effect of asbestos and beryllium compounds on the alveolar macrophages. *Med. J. Osaka Univ.* 27:47–58

188. Hart, B. A., Pittman, D. G. 1980. The uptake of beryllium by the alveolar macrophage. *J. Reticuloendothel. Soc.* 27:49–58

189. Doll, N. J., Stankus, R. P., Goldback, S., Salvaggio, J. E. 1981. Immune complexes and autoantibodies in silicosis. *J. Allergy Clin. Immunol.* 68:281–85

190. Jones, R. N., Turner-Warwick, M., Ziskind, M., Weill, H. 1976. High prevalence of anti-nuclear antibodies in sandblasters silicosis. *Am. Rev. Respir. Dis.* 113:393–95

191. Pernis, B. 1966. Immunological reactions and pulmonary dust disease. *Ann. Occup. Hyg.* 9:49–56

192. Miller, S. D., Zarkower, A. 1974. Alterations of murine immunologic responses after silica dust inhalation. *J. Immunol.* 113:1533–43

193. Schuyler, M., Ziskind, M., Salvaggio, J. 1977. Cell-mediated immunity in silicosis. *Am. Rev. Respir. Dis.* 116:147–53

194. Allison, A. C., Harrington, J. S., Birbeck, M. 1966. An examination of the cytotoxic effects of silica on macrophages. *J. Exp. Med.* 124:141–54

195. Stankus, R. P., Salvaggio, J. E. 1981. Bronchopulmonary humoral and cellular enhancement in experimental silicosis. *J. Reticuloendothel. Soc.* 29:153–61

196. Burrell, R., Anderson, M. 1973. The induction of fibrogenesis by silica-tested alveolar macrophages. *Environ. Res.* 6:389–94

197. Stankus, R. P., Salvaggio, J. E. 1985. The immunology of experimental silicosis. See Ref. 1, pp. 423–28

Ann. Rev. Pharmacol. Toxicol. 1987. 27:51–70

COTRANSMISSION

Graeme Campbell

Department of Zoology, University of Melbourne, Parkville, Victoria 3052, Australia

INTRODUCTION

Research in the last ten years has shown that individual neurons can contain two or more biologically active compounds, each a potential or proven transmitter substance. The discovery of such coexistence suggests that single neurons may simultaneously release more than one transmitter and that cotransmission may occur. This review describes evidence that cotransmission is a physiological process in vertebrates. It focuses on selected examples from the peripheral nervous system because proof of a transmitter role for one substance, let alone two, still requires that the transmission be both experimentally accessible and neurologically simple. The broader implications of the findings are then discussed.

It is appropriate to begin with two definitions: (*a*) *Transmitter substance:* Potter et al (1) use the simple definition that a transmitter is any substance, excluding trophic substances[1], released by a neuron to control its target cells. The definition may be the only one broad enough to include the clever theory (2) that K^+ ions, released from noradrenergic axons in the recovery phase of the axonal action potential, increase extracellular K^+ concentration and directly depolarize muscle membranes. In this way they produce the apparently nonadrenergic component of excitatory transmission to the vas deferens. As a transmitter, K^+ ions would have no synthesis, no storage vesicles, no breakdown mechanism, no postsynaptic receptors, nor any of the other accretions found in more complex definitions. But K^+ is indeed a transmitter, at least at one invertebrate synapse (3). (*b*) *Cotransmission:* This will be taken as the action of two transmitters, simultaneously released from the same neuron, on

---

[1]Trophic substances may be taken to affect the expression of the genome of a target cell, whereas transmitters act on the already expressed genome. There is every chance that some substances are both transmitters and trophic substances.

0362-1642/87/0415-0051$02.00

a single target cell. The definition is narrow but, as described in "Discussion," broader definitions become meaningless.

BACKGROUND

Elliott (4) put forward the concept of chemical neurotransmission in 1905; in 1921 Loewi (5) provided the first direct evidence for its reality. By 1933, Dale (6) was able to propose that two basic chemical transmission processes, cholinergic and adrenergic, mediate nearly all peripheral transmissions in vertebrates. The evidence seemed clear that a substance, whether acetylcholine (ACh), norepinephrine (NE), or something else, was responsible for each transmission. For lack of evidence to the contrary, the concept that a nerve releases "a substance" came to mean "a single substance." The generally unstated belief that one neuron acts via one transmitter substance dominated ideas of transmission into the 1970s. The single-transmitter concept is not "Dale's principle" (7), which was, in essence, that a single neuron probably releases similar substances at all of its synapses (1).

The first serious attack on the single-transmitter concept came from Burn & Rand (8, 9) in the late 1950s. They noted that many drugs that act on cholinergic systems also affect adrenergic transmission. They proposed that when a noradrenergic axon is activated it releases ACh, which re-acts on that axon to trigger the further release of NE. Although the Burn–Rand theory did not survive rigorous inspection (10), it started cracks in the belief in solitary transmitters.

Almost as soon as histochemical techniques for demonstrating transmitter substances became available, evidence was produced that two chemically unrelated, biologically active substances could be colocalized in one neuronal type. In the sympathetic noradrenergic innervation of the pineal gland, NE and serotonin could be colocalized, not just to the same group of nerve fibers (11) but also to the same intraneuronal storage vesicle (12). However, this example may be dismissed as a local phenomenon: the serotonin is not synthesized in the neurons but is taken up into them from an extracellular pool of serotonin leaking out of pinealocytes (13). Once inside the neuron, serotonin parasitizes NE storage vesicles, from which both amines can be released by nerve stimulation (14). In this case, serotonin can be regarded as a false transmitter, and the neuron must still be regarded as adrenergic.

The next steps towards acceptance of cotransmission came from studies of identifiable giant neurons in molluscs. In brief, it was shown that one neuron can synthesize and store two potential transmitters (15, 16) and that a single cell can produce synaptic depolarizations in a target cell, mediated jointly by two transmitters, in this case ACh and serotonin (17). The validity of the experiments is still disputed (18, 19), but these studies paved the way for the first, but still the clearest, example of cotransmission by a vertebrate neuron.

EXAMPLES

Sympathetic Neurons in Culture: NE-ACh

The clearest possible evidence of cotransmission was obtained from studies of sympathetic neurons grown in culture. The studies have been reviewed (e.g. 20–23), and primary references are not used in this summary.

When sympathetic postganglionic neurons are grown by themselves in culture, without non-neural cells or cell factors, they have the biochemical and structural characteristics of noradrenergic neurons. But when cultured with certain non-neural cells or in medium in which such cells have grown, the neurons develop cholinergic characteristics. During the change from noradrenergic to cholinergic function, the neurons show dual function and sustain a NE-ACh cotransmission. This cotransmission has been shown unequivocally in experiments in which a single neuron is allowed to grow on and to innervate a small cluster of heart myocytes. In these microcultures, the muscle acts not only as a bioassay of the transmitter (or transmitters) released from the neuron but also as the initiator of the conversion from noradrenergic to cholinergic function.

Stimulation of a neuron in an adrenergic form, as seen after brief culture, causes depolarization of the myocytes and acceleration of spontaneous firing, effects blocked by β-adrenoceptor antagonists. Electron microscopic study of such neurons loaded with 5-hydroxydopamine shows that 70–80% of the small synaptic vesicles in nerve varicosities have an electron-dense core, i.e. they are small granular vesicles, typical of noradrenergic axons. Neurons of cholinergic form are found in older cultures. When stimulated, they cause hyperpolarization and inhibit spontaneous firing of myocytes, effects blocked by atropine; the small synaptic vesicles contain no granular core (small, clear vesicles).

Most of the cultured neurons have mixed noradrenergic and cholinergic properties: stimulation commonly causes inhibition followed by excitation of myocytes, blocked by atropine and β-adrenoceptor antagonists respectively; the neurons contain a mixture of small clear and small granular vesicles, but there are fewer granular vesicles than in purely noradrenergic forms. In one single case, serial physiological studies were made on one neuron over a 45-day period, during which time the neuron changed from noradrenergic to dual-function to cholinergic.

The results leave no doubt that a single neuron can show NE-ACh cotransmission, at least as an interim state during development in vitro.

NE-ACh cotransmission might indeed occur as a temporary state during in vivo development of the sympathetic neurons innervating rat eccrine sweat glands (24), but there is little evidence that it occurs in any adult mammalian neuron (cf. 20). However, the definitive sympathetic postganglionic innervation of splenic muscle in the codfish *Gadus* may show such a cotransmission: the response to nerve stimulation is jointly mediated by NE and ACh (25), and both components of the response are eliminated by adrenergic neuron blockade or by treatment with 6-hydroxydopamine (25–27).

Some of the cultured neurons show another dual transmission involving either NE or ACh together with a different cardioinhibitory substance. The third substance appears to be adenosine or a related purine-based compound (23). To date, no neuron transmitting via all three compounds has been found, but there is no obvious reason why that should not happen.

Frog Sympathetic Ganglia: ACh-LHRH

The sympathetic chains of the bullfrog *(Rana catesbeiana)* contain a peptide that has luteinizing hormone–releasing hormone (LHRH)-like immunoreactivity (IR) (28). The LHRH-like material resembles authentic LHRH chromatographically (28), but is not identical to it (29). The peptide is released from the sympathetic chains in a Ca^{2+}-dependent manner by both high K^+ concentrations (28) and electrical stimulation of preganglionic nerves (30). The LHRH-IR has been localized to synaptic boutons on ganglion cells (30, 31). Both the immunoreactive boutons and the assayable LHRH-IR are largely lost after preganglionic denervation (30, 31).

The most posterior (ninth and tenth) ganglia of the sympathetic chains contain postganglionic neurons innervated in two different ways (see 32): B cells are innervated by rapidly conducting axons arising from the anterior sympathetic outflow; smaller C cells are innervated by slowly conducting axons arising from the spinal nerves 7 and 8. Stimulation of preganglionic fibers in the anterior chain produces, in B cells only, both fast and slow cholinergic excitatory postsynaptic potentials (epsp) mediated by nicotinic and muscarinic receptors, respectively. Stimulation of preganglionic fibers in spinal nerves 7 and 8 elicits a fast nicotinic epsp and a slow muscarinic inhibitory potential (ipsp) in C cells only. But, in addition, repeated stimulation of spinal nerves 7 and 8 produces, in both B and C cells, a noncholinergic depolarization lasting for several minutes, the late slow epsp (LSepsp) (33, 34).

Electrophysiological evidence shows that the LSepsp is mediated by the LHRH-like substance (30, 35). Ejection of authentic LHRH from a micropipette near a ganglion cell causes a prolonged depolarization and changes in membrane conductance, similar to the events of the LSepsp in both extent and time course. The LHRH-induced depolarization and the LSepsp are similarly affected by applied shifts of neuronal membrane potential (see also 36). Certain LHRH analogs, for example [D-pGlu^1,D-Phe^2,D-Trp^{3,6}]-LHRH, antagonize both the LSepsp and the LHRH-induced depolarization without affecting ACh-mediated transmission.

It appears that the LHRH-like material is in fact released from cholinergic preganglionic nerves. First, LHRH-like immunoreactivity is found in more than 90% of identified preganglionic terminals on C cells (30, 37) so it seems that there must be at least some overlap between the cholinergic and the LHRH-positive fiber populations. Second, as the strength of preganglionic stimulation is gradually increased, the cholinergic epsp shows up to five abrupt increments in height. Each increment represents the recruitment of another cholinergic fiber. With each recruitment, the LSepsp also increases in amplitude (37). Either each cholinergic fiber is matched by a peptidergic fiber with exactly the same threshold, or, more likely, each fiber is both cholinergic and peptidergic.

Curiously, although both B and C cells show the LSepsp, the B cells are remote from the LHRH-positive boutons, found predominantly on C cells (30). It seems that both the ACh and the peptide released from the terminals can reach C cells, but that only the peptide can survive diffusion over many micrometers to the B cells.

The peptidergic transmission may be physiological or an artifact of stimulation. The LSepsp can cause a discharge of postganglionic action potentials but it is normally subliminal (30, 33). But even a sub-threshold depolarization should make the nicotinic cholinergic transmission more effective (38). On the other hand, the LSepsp is not produced by a single stimulus and is best seen after periods of stimulation at 5–10 Hz (30), which may be greater than the (unknown) frequency of preganglionic action potentials in vivo.

Toad Cardiac Innervation: ACh-SOM

The postganglionic parasympathetic neurons innervating the heart of amphibians lie in the interatrial septum (see 39). The neurons innervate all cardiac chambers, including the single ventricle (40), and are the archetype of cholinergic neurons (5). In the toad *Bufo marinus,* the neurons appear to show cotransmission to heart muscle via ACh and somatostatin (SOM) (41).

All of the neurons on the toad interatrial septum contain SOM-like-IR. SOM-IR varicose nerve fibers lie on cardiac muscle throughout the heart. SOM applied to in vitro preparations acts slowly to inhibit the pacemaker and reduce the force of beat of driven atria, but is without effect on the ventricle. The negative chronotropic and inotropic effects of applied SOM are strongly tachyphylactic.

Vagal stimulation slows the spontaneously beating toad heart; it also inhibits the force of beat of driven atria and ventricles. Stimulation at 1 Hz can stop the spontaneously beating heart within 2 beats and can rapidly suppress detectable beating of driven atria, effects that are abolished by muscarinic antagonists. But when stimuli are applied at 3 Hz or more, the effects on the pacemaker and on atrial force of beat are not abolished even by high concentrations of hyoscine. (Effects on the ventricle are abolished by hyoscine.) The responses surviving muscarinic blockade are slow to develop, and resemble the response to SOM. Similar responses, in this case to postganglionic nerve stimulation, are seen when the cholinergic transmission is inhibited by treatment with hemicholinium-3 (42).

Induction of tachyphylaxis to SOM specifically inhibits the nonmuscarinic vagal effects. Conversely, when vagal transmission is "fatigued" by repeated bursts of stimulation the response to SOM is suppressed, as if by a tachyphylaxis induced by stimulation. The simplest explanation of the results is that the vagal postganglionic neurons inhibit the pacemaker and atrial muscle by releasing SOM.

Since the cholinergic postganglionic neurons lie in the heart, and since all of the intracardiac neurons contain SOM-IR, it follows that all of the cholinergic postganglionic neurons contain SOM. The evidence does not prove that any one neuron can release both ACh and SOM, but that mechanism seems most likely.

It is not clear whether the SOM mechanism is used in the normal physiology of the animal. The frequencies of stimulation needed to produce SOM-mediated transmission, although quite low, may exceed vagal firing rates occurring in the intact toad.

Cholinergic Postganglionic Neurons: ACh-VIP

Vasoactive intestinal peptide (VIP) is a 28–amino acid peptide that is widely distributed in peripheral and central neurons (see 43). It relaxes many smooth muscles and may be a transmitter substance in its own right in, for example, the gut. Lundberg and his colleagues (44–46) have concluded that certain postganglionic neurons in both parasympathetic and sympathetic pathways, mediating vasodilation in exocrine glands (e.g. nasal, salivary, pancreatic, and sweat glands), act by the corelease of ACh and VIP.

The case for ACh-VIP cotransmission to blood vessels in exocrine glands is best documented for the parasympathetic vasodilator innervation of cat salivary glands. There is good evidence that the dilator response is mediated in part by ACh. Nerve stimulation causes ACh release (47). Atropine, which prevents the vasodilation caused by ACh (48), reduces the response to low-frequency nerve stimulation (49) and indeed abolishes the dilation elicited by a single stimulus (50). But the innervation also appears to act in part via VIP. The vasculature is provided with VIP-IR axons (see 51), and nerve stimulation, especially with higher frequencies, causes VIP release (44, 47,

51–54). Atropine does not antagonize the response to VIP (44, 48, 52) or to high-frequency stimulation (49, 55). Finally, infusion of VIP antiserum reduces the dilator response to stimulation (44, 56).

It might be argued that the VIP-mediated response seen after atropine is artifactual, since atropine markedly increases the release of VIP on nerve stimulation (53, 57), presumably by preventing a muscarinic presynaptic inhibition. However, the reduction of the normal response by VIP immunoblockade shows that a VIP transmission occurs even while cholinergic transmission is functional.

Until recently when antibodies for choline acetyltransferase became available, there was no reliable histochemical marker for cholinergic neurons. Lundberg and his colleagues (58) used acetylcholinesterase as a marker, while aware that the enzyme is not restricted to cholinergic neurons. They found that many peripheral neurons in the cat contain VIP-IR, but are not obviously reactive for acetylcholinesterase. But the neurons innervating exocrine glands are both VIP-IR and acetylcholinesterase-positive (44, 45, 58). For example, the cat sphenopalatine ganglion contains the cholinergic neurons innervating the nasal mucosa (59); since 98.5% of the neurons contain VIP-IR (60), ACh and VIP neurons almost certainly overlap. However, another study (61) showed that sphenopalatine neurons are normally either VIP-IR or rich in acetylcholinesterase; only after treatment with colchicine do all neurons contain both markers. The results seem to show that the neurons innervating exocrine glands are able to express both ACh and VIP, but the possibility remains that some specialize in VIP, whereas others produce mainly ACh. Apart from that evidence, the possibility that the neurons show ACh-VIP cotransmission remains a good working hypothesis.

The vasodilator cotransmission may in fact involve three transmitters. Immunoreactivity to another vasodilator polypeptide, PHI-27 (62), is also released from the submandibular gland by parasympathetic stimulation (57). The PHI-like material detected may have been identical to or homologous with a very similar peptide, PHM-27, which is part of the VIP precursor molecule synthesized in human neuroblastoma cells (63). Thus, both of the released peptides may arise from the one precursor molecule.

ACh-VIP-PHI vasodilator cotransmission probably occurs in vivo. Natural firing rates of the parasympathetic vasomotor nerves are unknown, but may resemble the firing rate in the secretomotor fibers. The fastest reflex salivation seen in dogs can be matched by parasympathetic stimulation at 4–8 Hz (64). The average firing rate of secretory nerve fibers in rabbit, recorded directly during a reflex salivation, ranged as high as $20 \ s^{-1}$, and bursts of much higher frequency can be seen in the records (65). These firing rates exceed the rates of stimulation needed to produce both ACh- and VIP-mediated responses (49, 56).

Adrenergic Postganglionic Neurons: NE-NPY

Several biologically active peptides have been localized to noradrenergic sympathetic neurons, using double or sequential labeling with antibodies to the peptide and to a synthetic enzyme for NE (see 66, 67). For example, substance P-IR is found in many neurons of the rat superior cervical ganglion (68). Enkephalin-IR is also found in some neurons of this ganglion in the rat (69), but not the cat (70). SOM-IR occurs in some neurons in paravertebral ganglia of guinea pigs (71), but there are fewer in the rat (69) and apparently none in the cat (67, 70). Finally, a large subpopulation of noradrenergic neurons contains pancreatic polypeptide-like-IR in all mammals studied. Although there are several 36-amino acid peptides in the pancreatic polypeptide family, the material in noradrenergic neurons is probably neuropeptide Y (NPY) (see 72), and is referred to as such here. In this last case, there is some evidence for a NE-peptide cotransmission.

NPY-IR is found in a large proportion of sympathetic noradrenergic neurons (73–77). In the cat, for example, between 25% and 75% of the neurons in various para- and prevertebral ganglia contain NPY-IR (75). Some NE-NPY neurons in cattle also contain enkephalin-IR (78).

NPY-IR is found in apparently all noradrenergic neurons innervating mammalian blood vessels (73, 76, 77, 79–82) and in the adrenergic neurons innervating amphibian blood vessels (83). Certain nonvascular muscles also receive NE-NPY fibers, e.g. the heart (73, 75, 84, 85), the vas deferens (75, 86), and tracheobronchial muscle (75). However, the noradrenergic innervation of other nonvascular effectors, at least in some species, lacks NPY: iris (73); nictitating membrane (75); exocrine parenchyma of salivary glands (73, 76); myenteric and submucous ganglia of the intestine (80). The adrenergic innervation of the amphibian heart also lacks NPY (83).

The NPY-IR in noradrenergic nerve fibers can be depleted by treatment with the adrenergic neurotoxin 6-hydroxydopamine (73, 74, 76, 80, 82). Stimulation of vascular sympathetic nerves releases NPY, and the release is prevented by adrenergic neuron blockade (87, 88). Thus NPY appears to be both stored in and released from noradrenergic nerves, raising the possibility of NE-NPY cotransmission. In fact, NE and NPY have been argued to be vasoconstrictor cotransmitters to salivary gland vasculature (89), pial blood vessels (90, 91), and the spleen (78, 87, 88, 92). The latter case is particularly strong.

In the cat spleen (88), stimulation of the splenic nerve normally releases both NE and NPY. When the sympathetic innervation is intact, reserpinization depletes the splenic content of both NE and NPY: the neurogenic release of both NE and NPY is reduced, as are the splenic contractile and vasoconstrictor responses to nerve stimulation. But much of the action of reserpine on NPY seems to involve sympathetic nerve activity (93). Thus, reserpine has little effect on NPY levels after preganglionic nerve section, although it depletes NE as usual. In the reserpinized, decentralized spleen, nerve stimulation does not release NE, but the release of NPY is greater than normal, and the nerve-mediated contraction and constriction are strong. These responses are mimicked by applied NPY: they are barely affected by adrenoceptor blockade, but are still abolished by adrenergic neuron blockade. Reserpinization of the pig spleen (94), even with the sympathetic innervation intact, reduces neurogenic NE release. However, NPY release is greater than normal: nerve stimulation now causes a marked vasoconstriction that is resistant to adrenoceptor blockade and is mimicked by NPY. Therefore, in both cat and pig spleen, NPY released from adrenergic nerves seems to be a significant vasoconstrictor transmitter, at least when the release of NE has been reduced. However there is little evidence that NPY is a transmitter when NE release is normal. In fact, the above findings suggest that released NE normally suppresses NPY release. Experiments with, for example, specific antagonists of NPY are needed to establish that there is a simultaneous release of both NPY and NE in physiologically significant amounts, i.e. that cotransmission occurs.

DISCUSSION

Coexistence, Corelease, and Cotransmission

In the excitement of novel research, imprecise terminology is often used, sometimes at the expense of clarity in experimental design. It is worth examining the three terms that head this section.

The term *coexistence* presents little semantic problem. Substances are found to coexist by means of anatomically based studies of tissues or cells, so that the colocalization is always referred to an anatomical unit, e.g. a neuron or a synaptic vesicle. It seems obvious that coexistence is a necessary, but not sufficient, condition for cotransmission. For example, the cultured sympathetic neurons described above form functional synaptic connections to themselves ("autapses"). Transmission at autapses seems to be wholly cholinergic, even in neurons that have NE-ACh cotransmission to heart cells (23). While NE and ACh probably coexist at the autapse, NE has no apparent effect on the neurons, and there is no cotransmission. Incidentally, virtually every active amine or peptide localized to a neuron is released by nerve stimulation in one preparation or another: therefore, when these substances are colocalized they are probably also coreleased.

Corelease has an apparently simple meaning: the release of two or more transmitter substances together from one neuron. However, the word lacks precision: it is arbitrary how closely related in space and time the releases must be before corelease occurs. For example, the release of two transmitters by exocytosis from one synaptic vesicle is clearly corelease. But if a neuron, in defiance of the authentic "Dale's principle," released one transmitter from its dendrites and another from remote axon terminals, it would not constitute a meaningful corelease. The anatomical "unit of corelease" must lie between these extremes, but it can be defined only pragmatically. For instance, the NE-ACh cultured sympathetic neurons contain both small, granular vesicles, and small, clear synaptic vesicles, which may represent discrete stores of NE and ACh, respectively. If so, the smallest possible anatomical unit that could sustain NE-ACh corelease is a single varicosity, in which the two types of vesicle are mixed (23). But the minimal unit of corelease might prove to be much larger, e.g. several varicosities. In short, since the maximal anatomical unit for corelease cannot be defined absolutely, the word is only vaguely helpful. The critical limit in time for corelease is easier to define because that corelease clearly implies that substances emerge from a neuron in response to the same event, e.g. an action potential. From what is known of the transmitter-releasing effects of action potentials, the time window delimiting corelease might be as short as a few milliseconds, but it might be found to be much longer.

Corelease is a necessary, but not a sufficient, condition for cotransmission. In the ventricle of the toad heart, for example, SOM is probably released with ACh from vagal postganglionic neurons, but it has no known action on the muscle (41). In spite of the corelease, there is an apparently pure cholinergic transmission, not cotransmission.

Cotransmission could be defined from the point of view of either the releasing neuron or the target cell. It is used, confusingly, in both senses in the literature. The definition used here is expressed in terms of the target, for the following reasons. A chemically transmitting neuron is a device for converting an input into a release of substances. What is released is, in a sense, irrelevant to the neuron; the process of release probably reflects a single action, e.g. an entry of Ca^{2+}, regardless of how simple or complex the mixture of substances released and whether all of the substances released are transmitters. It is only when a target is defined, even if the target is the neuron itself, that the source and the nature of what is released become important. For example, it has been proposed that noradrenergic axons in the vas deferens corelease NE and NPY, the NE to act on the muscle and the NPY to act back on the axon, inhibiting further release (74, 95, 96). Such a transmission would clearly show a duality, but, in its effect, it would not differ from two completely separate transmission processes. It seems that, if cotransmission has any unique physiological significance, it would be that two or more coreleased transmitters act on the same target cell, so that the net result of transmission incorporates interactive effects of the transmitters. Again using the vas deferens as an example, researchers have proposed that neurogenic excitation is mediated in part by adenosine triphosphate and in part by NE (see 97–99). Since the whole response is antagonized by, for example, destruction of the noradrenergic innervation with 6-hydroxydopamine (100), it seems that the NE and adenosine triphosphate must be coreleased from noradrenergic nerves. In this case, where both substances act on the muscle, the conditions for cotransmission would be met.

The definition of cotransmission from the point of view of the target cell leads to conclusions that are, at first sight, strange. For example, the amphibian preganglionic ACh-LHRH neurons cotransmit to sympathetic C cells, but at the same time these terminals are not cotransmitting to B cells, which are affected only by the peptide (30).

Cotransmission as a Physiological Process

Cotransmission, as defined above, clearly does occur in experimental situations. The first two examples considered, NE-ACh neurons in culture and amphibian ACh-LHRH neurons, are the only vertebrate cases that show convincingly that one neuron can transmit to a single target cell via at least two transmitters. With regard to mammalian ACh-VIP neurons and amphibian ACh-SOM neurons, there is no direct evidence that any one neuron acts via both substances, but cotransmission is a reasonable hypothesis. The final example, that of NE-NPY neurons, was chosen to represent the many other instances of coexistence of active substances in neurons (101, 102), for which the rudiments of a case for cotransmission are available.

There is virtually no evidence that cotransmission occurs during normal behavior. In most of the postulated instances of cotransmission, the transmitters each produce obvious effects such as contraction, secretion, or altered membrane potential. In these straightforward systems, pharmacological dissection in vivo should be able to eliminate the possibility that only one of the cotransmitters is normally used. However, no reports of appropriate experiments have been found. For example, it seems that nobody has determined whether atropine does or does not abolish the vasodilation that presumably occurs during salivation in response to feeding; without such evidence it remains possible that the parasympathetic ACh-VIP cotransmission to the vasculature of salivary glands is an experimental artifact.

With that proviso in mind, the scope for cotransmission as a physiological process seems to be enormous. On one hand, many substances are now recognized as potential transmitters. Added to the classical amine and amino acid transmitters are the active peptides, more than a dozen of which have been identified in neurons (e.g. 66). There are also unexpected additions to the list of potential transmitters. For example, the corelease of dopamine-β-hydroxylase and NE (103) seems to be an accidental consequence of the sequestration of the enzyme within NE storage vesicles. But extracellularly applied dopamine-β-hydroxylase can affect cells, e.g. it can restore NE effects on desensitized pinealocyte β-adrenoceptors (104), and it might conceivably be a transmitter.

On the other hand, conceptions of what is meant by an "effect" of a transmitter substance are expanding. Koketsu (105) distinguished four types of synaptic actions of transmitters on target cells: (a) changing membrane potential or conductance, i.e. typical synaptic transmission; (b) changing the amplitude or time course of action potentials; (c) changing the amount of transmitter released, i.e. presynaptic modulation; and (d) changing the sensitivity of receptors for some other transmitter. This last type of effect, which might be called receptor modulation, is quite novel. In some cases, a potential transmitter has been shown to affect the availability or affinity of receptors for another compound, e.g. opiates and nicotinic receptors on adrenal medullary cells (106) and NPY and α_2-adrenoceptors in rat brain (107). In others, the efficacy of receptor occupation is changed, e.g. adenosine triphosphate and nicotinic receptors on frog skeletal muscle (108).

In each of the chosen examples of receptor modulation there is some evidence that both transmitter substances involved coexist in neurons in the organ. If cotransmission occurs, the "modulatory" transmitter might have the sole function of regulating the effect of the "major" transmitter, and have no effect at all if released alone. Indeed, evidence suggesting cotransmission by a major and a modulatory substance is already available. The salivation caused by parasympathetic stimulation in cats is fully blocked by atropine (55), and transmission has been regarded as simply cholinergic. However, treatment with VIP antiserum reduces the secretory response, suggesting partial mediation by VIP (56), but VIP by itself does not cause secretion (44, 52). It emerges that VIP increases the secretory response to ACh (48), perhaps by increasing the affinity of muscarinic receptors for ACh (109). Thus, it seems that the role of VIP in the salivatory ACh-VIP cotransmission is to promote transmission by ACh.

Until recently the complexity of nervous systems has seemed to derive from extensive, precisely located synaptic connections between neurons. Synaptic transmission has seemed relatively simple and susceptible to only a few integrative processes, e.g. spatial or temporal summation, facilitation, and fatigue. The existence of many possible transmitters and of many possible modes of action would necessitate a complex nervous system, even if each neuron released only one transmitter. But the occurrence of corelease means that one neuron may affect several different targets or, in the special case of cotransmission, a single target via a number of substances. This occurrence suggests a new order of complexity in the function of the nervous system, with interactions occurring between transmitters at both pre- and post-synaptic sites. One should not, however, be overwhelmed by the potential for complexity. Dale (6) knew of only a few peripheral transmissions that he could not readily class as adrenergic or cholinergic. Even now, many transmissions still seem to be explicable in terms of one transmitter.

The rather simple appearance of many peripheral transmissions in spite of the potential for complexity raises several possibilities. First, substances coreleased with a major transmitter might often be receptor modulators, acting in ways not easily detectable unless reliable antagonists for the individual cotransmitters are available. Second, routine experimental protocols may be inadequate to detect cotransmission. For example, we tend to look for short-term effects of transmitters. But peptides can have actions lasting for an hour or more (e.g. 110). Yet, stimulus intervals in most experiments are 10 min or less, during which time the effects of a long-acting substance would be essentially constant. In hindsight, the only overt sign left by long-acting cotransmitters in many experiments might be the changes in response that usually occur over the first few stimulus repetitions at the beginning of an experiment, i.e. those that we tend to dismiss as "equilibration" of the preparation. Finally, transmissions seeming simple may indeed involve only one transmitter: active substances coreleased with a major transmitter might not play any role in transmission, either because the concentrations achieved are too low or because responsive targets are not present.

Can Neuronal Types Still be Recognized?

When it seemed that neurons acted via single transmitters, only three types of peripheral motor neuron were distinguished on functional grounds. Dale (6) recognized adrenergic and cholinergic nerves fifty years ago. In the 1960s, nonadrenergic, noncholinergic inhibitory neurons in the gut, lung, and some other tissues were recognized as a third type, acting perhaps via adenosine triphosphate or VIP (see 111, 112). Evidence for further distinct types is less secure. For example, the gut contains excitatory motor nerves that seem to act via substance P, but it remains possible that the substance P is in fact released as a cotransmitter from cholinergic nerves (113).

The many examples of colocalization show that, at the least, the previous neuronal types can be subdivided. A subdivision of noradrenergic neurons into four types, based on the peptides colocalized in them, has been discussed (66, 67). Similarly, the cholinergic (i.e. choline acetyltransferase-IR) neurons of the submucous plexus in guinea pig ileum can be divided into three subtypes: ACh-substance P; ACh-NPY-SOM-cholecystokinin; and ACh without known peptides (114). But, in principle, there is no reason why, for example, SOM neurons should not be subdivided, e.g. SOM-ACh (toad vagus, guinea-pig ileum) and SOM-NE (guinea-pig sympathetic). The associations of active substances in neurons might even be chaotic, so that neurons would be more realistically classified in a multidimensional array that acknowledges no major transmitters. It even appears that neurons can express incomplete transmitter mechanisms. For example, the definitive adult ACh-VIP sympathetic neurons innervating rat eccrine sweat glands, having appeared in the neonate as noradrenergic, no longer synthesize detectable NE, yet they still express a presumably functionless catecholamine uptake (24). Half of the neurons in the guinea pig paracervical ganglion show neither tyrosine hydroxylase-IR nor detectable NE, but they express dopamine-β-hydroxylase-IR (J. L. Morris & I. L. Gibbins, personal communication), which, if biochemically active, would similarly have no obvious function.

However, the disposition of active substances is probably not merely chaotic. For example, some evidence points toward preferred groupings of "transmitters." Cultured rat sympathetic neurons can express SOM, substance P, choline acetyltransferase, and tyrosine hydroxylase. The conditions of culture can affect these expressions independently, but most circumstances favoring SOM expression also promote tyrosine hydroxylase, whereas substance P and choline acetyltransferase also are often regulated together (115). Furthermore, some of the neuronal subtypes that can be distinguished by colocalization of transmitters seem to be "natural" groups, related to a particular function. The noradrenergic innervation of the guinea pig ileum shows a detailed allocation of different neuronal subtypes to specific targets: NE-NPY fibers innervate blood vessels; NE-SOM fibers innervate muscle layers, submucous ganglia, and mucosa; NE fibers without known peptide complement innervate myenteric ganglia and share the innervation of mucosa (116). So a chemically defined neuronal type can in some circumstances be related to a specific target for innervation. The most likely reason for this specificity is that the innervated target determines at least part of the transmitter complement (21, 117, 118).

The existence of natural groupings of transmitters is supported by comparisons of homologous neurons between species. For example, the parasympathetic vasodilator innervation of salivary glands operates by ACh-VIP cotransmission in cat (45), dog (119), and rat (120, 121), but in rabbit it seems to be cholinergic with no other cotransmitter (122, 123). When cardiac vagal postganglionic neurons are compared between amphibians, ACh-SOM cotransmission is found in *Bufo* (41) and the unrelated clawed toad *Xenopus* (G. Campbell, unpublished observation). But in several other genera *(Neobatrachus, Limnodynastes, Litoria)* the neurons lack SOM-IR, the heart is unresponsive to SOM, and vagal transmission is fully blocked by muscarinic antagonists (G. Campbell, unpublished observation), as it is in *Rana* (124). If it is the influence of the target organ that dominates the range of substances expressed in the innervation, these two examples might be read as follows: (*a*) in each case, the target organ always permits, or perhaps causes, the expression of ACh in this part of its innervation; (*b*) in each organ, the neurons can express only certain other substances, e.g. VIP but not SOM in the salivary gland, SOM but not VIP in the amphibian heart; and (c) such coexpression with ACh is not obligatory. In terms of evolution, it may be that each target has repeatedly, in the course of history, fostered the expression of the particular colocalized substance, but that the substance has been cemented into place in the cellular machinery only when a function for it has been found, in this case as a cotransmitter.

In closing, it is interesting that the "stable" transmitter in these last examples, ACh, provided support for the earlier classification of neurons into three types, adrenergic, cholinergic, and something else inhibitory. There may yet be truth in the older classification, but it would have to be a subtler truth than was thought even ten years ago.

SUMMARY

Cotransmission, defined here as the control of a single target cell by two or more substances released from one neuron in response to the same neuronal event, does occur in experimental situations. It has not been shown to occur in the normal operation of an animal, but the likelihood that it does is great.

There are many examples of potential transmitters coexisting in one neuron, suggesting that cotransmission might be widespread in the peripheral nervous system. But many transmissions still seem to be mediated by a single transmitter. In such cases, coreleased substances might act on other targets or modulate the receptors for the main transmitter. But the possibility also exists that some colocalized "transmitters" have no function in transmission.

It is increasingly difficult to retain a simple classification of neuronal types based on transmitter substances. However, there are indications that some combinations of colocalized substances are "preferred" and that certain combinations typify the innervation of a particular target tissue.

ACKNOWLEDGMENTS

For their helpful discussions and comments on this review, I am grateful to Colin Anderson, John Donald, Barbara Evans, Ian Gibbins, David Hirst, Judy Morris, Peregrine Osborne, and Jamie O'Shea. Many thanks to Lyn Ramsay and Fiona Jackson for their secretarial help.

Literature Cited

1. Potter, D. D., Furshpan, E. J., Landis, S. C. 1981. Multiple-transmitter status and "Dale's principle". Neurosci. Comment. 1:1–9
2. von Euler, U. S., Hedqvist, P. 1975. A tentative transmission mechanism for the twitch elicited in the guinea-pig vas deferens by field stimulation. Med. Hypotheses 1:214–16
3. Yarom, Y., Spira, M. E. 1982. Extracellular potassium ions mediate specific neuronal interaction. Science 216:80–82
4. Elliott, T. R. 1905. The action of adrenalin. J. Physiol. 32:401–67
5. Loewi, O. 1921. Über humorale Übertragbarkeit der Herznervenwirkung. I. Pfluegers Arch. 189:239–42

6. Dale, H. H. 1933. Nomenclature of nerve fibres in the autonomic system and their effects. *J. Physiol.* 80:10–11P

7. Dale, H. H. 1935. Pharmacology and nerve endings. *Proc. R. Soc. Med.* 28:319–32

8. Burn, J. H., Rand, M. J. 1959. Sympathetic postganglionic mechanisms. *Nature* 184:163–65

9. Burn, J. H., Rand, M. J. 1965. Acetylcholine in adrenergic transmission. *Ann. Rev. Pharmacol.* 5:163–82

10. Ferry, C. B. 1966. Cholinergic link hypothesis in adrenergic neuroeffector transmission. *Physiol. Rev.* 46:420–56

11. Owman, C. 1964. Sympathetic nerves probably storing two types of monoamines in the rat pineal gland. *Int. J. Neuropharmacol.* 2:105–12

12. Jaim-Etcheverry, G., Zieher, L. M. 1968. Cytochemistry of 5-hydroxytryptamine at the electron microscope level. II. Localization in the autonomic nerves of rat pineal gland. *Z. Zellforsch. Mikr. Anat.* 86:393–400

13. Jaim-Etcheverry, G., Zieher, L. M. 1982. Co-existence of monoamines in peripheral adrenergic neurones. See Ref. 101, pp. 189–206

14. Jaim-Etcheverry, G., Zieher, L. M. 1980. Stimulation-depletion of serotonin and noradrenaline from vesicles of sympathetic nerves in the pineal gland of the rat. *Cell Tissue Res.* 207:13–20

15. Kerkut, G. A., Sedden, C. B., Walker, R. J. 1967. Uptake of dopa and 5-hydroxytryptophan by monoamine-forming neurones in the brain of *Helix aspersa*. *Comp. Biochem. Physiol.* 23:159–62

16. Brownstein, M. J., Saavedra, J. M., Axelrod, J., Zeman, G. H., Carpenter, D. O. 1974. Coexistence of several putative neurotransmitters in single identified neurons of *Aplysia*. *Proc. Natl. Acad. Sci. USA* 71:4662–65

17. Cottrell, G. A. 1977. Identified amine-containing neurones and their synaptic connexions. *Neuroscience* 2:1–18

18. Osborne, N. N. 1979. Is Dale's principle valid? *Trends Neurosci.* 2:73–75

19. Osborne, N. N. 1982. Co-existence of neurotransmitter substances in a specifically identified invertebrate neurone. See Ref. 101, pp. 207–22

20. Burnstock, G. 1978. Do some sympathetic neurons synthesize and release both noradrenaline and acetylcholine? *Prog. Neurobiol.* 11:205–22

21. Patterson, P. H. 1978. Environmental determination of autonomic neurotransmitter function. *Ann. Rev. Neurosci.* 1:1–17

22. Potter, D. D., Landis, S. C., Furshpan, E. J. 1981. Adrenergic-cholinergic dual function in cultured sympathetic neurons of the rat. In *Development of the Autonomic Nervous System*, *Ciba Found. Symp.*, 83:123–38. London: Pitman

23. Furshpan, E. J., Potter, D. D., Landis, S. C. 1982. On the transmitter repertoire of sympathetic neurons in culture. *Harvey Lect.* 76:149–91

24. Landis, S. C., Keefe, D. 1983. Evidence for neurotransmitter plasticity in vivo: developmental changes in properties of cholinergic sympathetic neurons. *Dev. Biol.* 98:349–72

25. Nilsson, S., Grove, D. J. 1974. Adrenergic and cholinergic innervation of the spleen of the cod *Gadus morhua*. *Eur. J. Pharmacol.* 28:135–43

26. Holmgren, S., Nilsson, S. 1976. Effects of denervation, 6-hydroxydopamine and reserpine on the cholinergic and adrenergic responses of the spleen of the cod, *Gadus morhua*. *Eur. J. Pharmacol.* 39:53–59

27. Winberg, M., Holmgren, S., Nilsson, S. 1981. Effects of denervation and 6-hydroxydopamine on the activity of choline acetyltransferase in the spleen of the cod, *Gadus morhua*. *Comp. Biochem. Physiol.* 69C:141–44

28. Jan, Y. N., Jan, L. Y., Kuffler, S. W. 1979. A peptide as a possible transmitter in sympathetic ganglia of the frog. *Proc. Natl. Acad. Sci. USA* 76:1501–5

29. Eiden, L. E., Eskay, R. L. 1980. Characterization of LRF-like immunoreactivity in the frog sympathetic ganglia: non-identity with LRF decapeptide. *Neuropeptides* 1:29–37

30. Jan, L. Y., Jan, Y. N. 1982. Peptidergic transmission in sympathetic ganglia of the frog. *J. Physiol.* 327:219–46

31. Jan, L. Y., Jan, Y. N., Brownfield, M. S. 1980. Peptidergic transmitters in synaptic boutons of sympathetic ganglia. *Nature* 288:380–82

32. Dodd, J., Horn, J. P. 1983. A reclassification of B and C neurons in the ninth and tenth paravertebral sympathetic ganglia of the bullfrog. *J. Physiol.* 334:255–69

33. Nishi, S., Koketsu, K. 1968. Early and late after discharges of amphibian sympathetic ganglion cells. *J. Neurophysiol.* 31:109–21

34. Libet, B., Chichibu, S., Tosaka, T. 1968. Slow synaptic responses and excitability in sympathetic ganglia of the bullfrog. *J. Neurophysiol.* 31:383–95

35. Kuffler, S. W. 1980. Slow synaptic responses in autonomic ganglia and the

pursuit of a peptidergic transmitter. *J. Exp. Biol.* 89:257–86
36. Kuffler, S. W., Sejnowski, T. J. 1983. Peptidergic and muscarinic excitation at amphibian sympathetic synapses. *J. Physiol.* 341:257–78
37. Jan, Y. N., Jan, L. Y. 1981. Coexistence and co-release of acetylcholine and the LHRH-like peptide from the same preganglionic fibers in frog sympathetic ganglia. *Neurosci. Abstr.* 7: 603
38. Schulman, J. A., Weight, F. F. 1976. Synaptic transmission: long-lasting potentiation by a postsynaptic mechanism. *Science* 194:1437–39
39. McMahan, U. J., Kuffler, S. W. 1971. Visual identification of synaptic boutons on living ganglion cells and of varicosities in postganglionic axons in the heart of the frog. *Proc. R. Soc. London Ser. B* 177:485–508
40. Gaskell, W. H. 1882. On the rhythm of the heart of the frog, and on the nature of the action of the vagus nerve. *Philos. Trans. R. Soc. London* 173:893–1033
41. Campbell, G., Gibbins, I. L., Morris, J. L., Furness, J. B., Costa, M., et al. 1982. Somatostatin is contained in and released from cholinergic nerves in the heart of the toad *Bufo marinus*. *Neuroscience* 7:2013–23
42. Campbell, G., Jackson, F. 1985. Independent co-release of acetylcholine and somatostatin from cardiac vagal neurones in toad. *Neurosci. Lett.* 60:47–50
43. Said, S. I., ed. 1982. *Vasoactive Intestinal Peptide.* New York: Raven
44. Lundberg, J. M., Änggård, A., Fahrenkrug, J., Hökfelt, T., Mutt, V. 1980. Vasoactive intestinal polypeptide in cholinergic neurons of exocrine glands: functional significance of co-existing transmitters for vasodilatation and secretion. *Proc. Natl. Acad. Sci. USA* 77:1651–55
45. Lundberg, J. M. 1981. Evidence for coexistence of vasoactive intestinal polypeptide (VIP) and acetylcholine in neurons of cat exocrine glands. Morphological, biochemical and functional studies. *Acta Physiol. Scand. Suppl.* 496:1–57
46. Lundberg, J. M., Änggård, A., Fahrenkrug, J., Johansson, O., Hökfelt, T. 1982. Vasoactive intestinal polypeptide in cholinergic neurons of exocrine glands. See Ref. 43, pp. 373–89
47. Lundberg, J. M., Änggård, A., Fahrenkrug, J., Lundgren, G., Holmstedt, B. 1982. Corelease of VIP and acetylcholine in relation to blood flow and

salivary secretion in cat submandibular salivary gland. *Acta Physiol. Scand.* 115:525–28
48. Lundberg, J. M., Änggård, A., Fahrenkrug, J. 1982. Complementary role of vasoactive intestinal polypeptide (VIP) and acetylcholine for cat submandibular gland blood flow and secretion. III. Effects of local infusions. *Acta Physiol. Scand.* 114:329–37
49. Darke, A. C., Smaje, L. H. 1972. Dependence of functional vasodilatation in the cat submaxillary gland upon stimulation frequency. *J. Physiol.* 226:191–203
50. Emmelin, N., Garrett, J. R., Ohlin, P. 1968. Neural control of salivary myoepithelial cells. *J. Physiol.* 196:381–96
51. Uddman, R., Fahrenkrug, J., Malm, L., Alumets, J., Håkanson, R., et al. 1980. Neuronal VIP in salivary glands: distribution and release. *Acta Physiol. Scand.* 110:31–38
52. Bloom, S. R., Edwards, A. V. 1980. Vasoactive intestinal polypeptide in relation to atropine resistant vasodilation in the submaxillary gland of the cat. *J. Physiol.* 300:41–53
53. Lundberg, J. M., Änggård, A., Fahrenkrug, J. 1981. Complementary role of vasoactive intestinal polypeptide (VIP) and acetylcholine for cat submandibular gland blood flow and secretion. I. VIP release. *Acta Physiol. Scand.* 113:317–27
54. Andersson, P. O., Bloom, S. R., Edwards, A. V., Järhult, J. 1982. Effects of stimulation of the chorda tympani in bursts on submaxillary responses in the cat. *J. Physiol.* 322:469–83
55. Heidenhain, R. 1872. Über die Wirkung einiger Gifte auf die Nerven der Glandula submaxillaris. *Pfluegers Arch.* 5:309–18
56. Lundberg, J. M., Änggård, A., Fahrenkrug, J. 1981. Complementary role of vasoactive intestinal polypeptide (VIP) and acetylcholine for cat submandibular gland blood flow and secretion. II. Effects of cholinergic antagonists and VIP antiserum. *Acta Physiol. Scand.* 113:329–36
57. Lundberg, J. M., Fahrenkrug, J., Larsson, O., Änggård, A. 1984. Corelease of vasoactive intestinal polypeptide and peptide histidine isoleucine in relation to atropine-resistant vasodilatation in cat submandibular salivary gland. *Neurosci. Lett.* 52:37–42
58. Lundberg, J. M., Hökfelt, T., Schultzberg, M., Uvnäs-Wallensten, K., Kohler, C., et al. 1979. Occurrence of vasoactive intestinal polypeptide (VIP)-

like immunoreactivity in certain cholinergic neurons of the cat: evidence from combined immunohistochemistry and acetylcholinesterase staining. *Neuroscience* 4:1539–59

59. Eccles, R., Wilson, H. 1973. The parasympathetic secretory nerves of the nose of the cat. *J. Physiol.* 230:213–23

60. Lundberg, J. M., Änggård, A., Emson, P., Fahrenkrug, J., Hökfelt, T. 1981. Vasoactive intestinal polypeptide and cholinergic mechanisms in cat nasal mucosa: studies on choline acetyltransferase and release of vasoactive intestinal polypeptide. *Proc. Natl. Acad. Sci. USA* 78:5255–59

61. Håkanson, R., Sundler, F., Uddman, R. 1982. Distribution and topography of peripheral VIP nerve fibers: functional implications. See Ref. 43, pp. 121–44

62. Tatemoto, K., Mutt, V. 1981. Isolation and characterization of the intestinal peptide porcine PHI (PHI-27), a new member of the glucagon-secretin family. *Proc. Natl. Acad. Sci. USA* 78:6603–7

63. Itoh, W., Obata, K., Yanaihara, N., Okamoto, H. 1983. Human preprovasoactive intestinal polypeptide (VIP) contains the coding sequence for a novel PHI-27-like peptide, PHM-27. *Nature* 304:547–49

64. Emmelin, N., Holmberg, J. 1967. Impulse frequency in secretory nerves of salivary glands. *J. Physiol.* 191:205–14

65. Kawamura, Y., Matsuo, R., Yamamoto, T. 1982. Analysis of reflex responses in preganglionic parasympathetic fibres innervating submandibular glands of rabbits. *J. Physiol.* 322:241–55

66. Hökfelt, T., Lundberg, J. M., Skirboll, L., Johansson, O., Schultzberg, M., et al. 1982. Coexistence of classical transmitters and peptides in neurones. See Ref. 101, pp. 77–125

67. Lundberg, J. M., Hökfelt, T., Änggård, A., Terenius, L., Elde, R., et al. 1982. Organizational principles in the peripheral sympathetic nervous system: subdivision of coexisting peptides (somatostatin-, avian pancreatic polypeptide- and vasoactive intestinal polypeptide-like immunoreactive materials). *Proc. Natl. Acad. Sci. USA* 79:1303–7

68. Kessler, J. A., Adler, J. E., Bohn, M. C., Black, I. B. 1981. Substance P in principal sympathetic neurons: regulation by impulse activity. *Science* 214:335–36

69. Schultzberg, M., Hökfelt, T., Terenius, L., Elfvin, L. G., Lundberg, J. M., et al. 1979. Enkephalin-immunoreactive nerve fibres and cell bodies in sympa-

thetic ganglia of the guinea-pig and rat. *Neuroscience* 4:249–70

70. Lundberg, J. M., Hökfelt, T., Änggård, A., Uvnäs-Wallensten, K., Brimijoin, S., et al. 1980. Peripheral peptide neurons: distribution, axonal transport and some aspects on possible function. In *Neural Peptides and Neuronal Communication*, ed. E. Costa, M. Trabucchi, pp. 25–36. New York: Raven

71. Hökfelt, T., Elfvin, L. G., Elde, R., Schultzberg, M., Goldstein, M. 1977. Occurrence of somatostatin-like immunoreactivity in some peripheral sympathetic noradrenergic neurons. *Proc. Natl. Acad. Sci. USA* 74:3587–91

72. Emson, P. C., DeQuidt, M. E. 1984. NPY—a new member of the pancreatic polypeptide family. *Trends Neurosci.* 7:31–35

73. Lundberg, J. M., Hökfelt, T., Änggård, A., Kimmel, J., Goldstein, M., et al. 1980. Coexistence of an avian pancreatic polypeptide (APP) immunoreactive substance and catecholamines in some peripheral and central neurones. *Acta Physiol. Scand.* 110:107–9

74. Lundberg, J. M., Terenius, L., Hökfelt, T., Martling, C. R., Mutt, V., et al. 1982. Neuropeptide Y (NPY)-like immunoreactivity in peripheral noradrenergic neurons and effects of NPY on sympathetic function. *Acta Physiol. Scand.* 116:477–80

75. Lundberg, J. M., Terenius, L., Hökfelt, T., Goldstein, M. 1983. High levels of neuropeptide Y in peripheral noradrenergic neurons in various mammals including man. *Neurosci. Lett.* 42:167–72

76. Olschowka, J. A., Jacobowitz, D. M. 1983. The coexistence and release of bovine pancreatic polypeptide-like immunoreactivity from noradrenergic superior cervical ganglia neurons. *Peptides* 4:231–38

77. Ekblad, E., Edvinsson, L., Wahlestedt, C., Uddman, R., Håkanson, R., et al. 1984. Neuropeptide Y co-exists and cooperates with noradrenaline in perivascular nerve fibers. *Regulatory Peptides* 8:225–35

78. Fried, G., Terenius, L., Brodin, E., Efendic, S., Dockray, G., et al. 1986. Neuropeptide Y, enkephalin and noradrenaline coexist in sympathetic neurons innervating the bovine spleen. Biochemical and histochemical evidence. *Cell Tissue Res.* 243:495–508

79. Uddman, R., Edvinsson, L., Håkanson, R., Owman, C., Sundler, F. 1982. Immunohistochemical demonstration of

APP (Avian pancreatic polypeptide)-immunoreactive nerve fibers around cerebral blood vessels. *Brain Res. Bull.* 9:715–18

80. Furness, J. B., Costa, M., Emson, P. C., Håkanson, R., Moghimzadeh, E., et al. 1983. Distribution, pathways and reactions to drug treatment of nerves with neuropeptide Y- and pancreatic polypeptide-like immunoreactivity in the guinea-pig digestive tract. *Cell Tissue Res.* 234:71–92

81. Uddman, R., Ekblad, E., Edvinsson, L., Håkanson, R., Sundler, F. 1985. Neuropeptide Y-like immunoreactivity in perivascular nerve fibres of the guinea-pig. *Regulatory Peptides* 10: 243–57

82. Morris, J. L., Murphy, R., Furness, J. B., Costa, M. 1986. Partial depletion of neuropeptide Y from noradrenergic perivascular and cardiac axons by 6-hydroxydopamine and reserpine. *Regulatory Peptides* 13:147–62

83. Morris, J. L., Gibbins, I. L., Campbell, G., Murphy, R., Furness, J. B., et al. 1986. Innervation of the large arteries and heart of the toad *(Bufo marinus)* by adrenergic and peptide-containing neurons. *Cell Tissue Res.* 243:171–84

84. Gu, J., Adrian, T. E., Tatemoto, K., Polak, J. M., Allen, J. M., et al. 1983. Neuropeptide tyrosine (NPY)—a major cardiac neuropeptide. *Lancet* 1983: 1008–10

85. Sternini, C., Brecha, N. 1985. Distribution and colocalization of neuropeptide Y-like immunoreactivity in the guinea-pig heart. *Cell Tissue Res.* 241:93–102

86. Stjernquist, M., Emson, P., Owman, C., Sjöberg, N. O., Sundler, F., et al. 1983. Neuropeptide Y in the female reproductive tract of the rat. Distribution of nerve fibres and motor effects. *Neurosci. Lett.* 39:279–84

87. Lundberg, J. M., Änggård, A., Theodorsson-Norheim, E., Pernow, J. 1984. Guanethidine-sensitive release of neuropeptide Y-like immunoreactivity in the cat spleen by sympathetic nerve stimulation. *Neurosci. Lett.* 52:175–80

88. Lundberg, J. M., Fried, G., Pernow, J., Theodorsson-Norheim, E., Änggård, A. 1986. NPY—a mediator of reserpine-resistant, non-adrenergic vasoconstriction in cat spleen after preganglionic denervation. *Acta Physiol. Scand.* 126: 151–52

89. Lundberg, J. M., Tatemoto, K. 1982. Pancreatic polypeptide family (APP, BPP, NPY and PYY) in relation to sympathetic vasoconstriction resistant to α-adrenocoptor blockade. *Acta Physiol. Scand.* 116:393–402

90. Auer, L. M., Edvinsson, L., Johansson, B. B. 1983. Effect of sympathetic nerve stimulation and adrenoceptor blockade on pial arterial and venous calibre and on intracranial pressure in the cat. *Acta Physiol. Scand.* 119:213–17

91. Edvinsson, L., Emson, P., McCulloch, J., Tatemoto, K., Uddman, R. 1984. Neuropeptide Y: immunohistochemical localization to and effect upon feline pial arteries and veins in vitro and in situ. *Acta Physiol. Scand.* 122:155–63

92. Lundberg, J. M., Änggård, A., Pernow, J., Hökfelt, T. 1985. Neuropeptide Y-, substance P- and VIP-like immunoreactive nerves in cat spleen in relation to autonomic volume and vascular control. *Cell Tissue Res.* 239:9–18

93. Lundberg, J. M., Saria, A., Franco-Cereceda, A., Theodorsson-Norheim, E. 1985. Mechanisms underlying changes in the contents of neuropeptide Y in cardiovascular nerves and adrenal gland induced by sympatholytic drugs. *Acta Physiol. Scand.* 124:603–11

94. Lundberg, J. M., Rudehill, A., Sollevi, A., Theodorsson-Norheim, E., Hamberger, B. 1986. Frequency- and reserpine-dependent chemical coding of sympathetic transmission: differential release of noradrenaline and neuropeptide Y from pig spleen. *Neurosci. Lett.* 63:96–100

95. Allen, J. M., Adrian, T. E., Tatemoto, K., Polak, J. M., Hughes, J., et al. 1982. Two novel related peptides, neuropeptide Y (NPY) and peptide YY (PYY) inhibit the contraction of the electrically stimulated mouse vas deferens. *Neuropeptides* 3:71–77

96. Lundberg, J. M., Stjärne, L. 1984. Neuropeptide Y (NPY) depresses the secretion of ³H-noradrenaline and the contractile response evoked by field stimulation in rat vas deferens. *Acta Physiol. Scand.* 120:477–79

97. Sneddon, P., Westfall, D. P. 1984. Pharmacological evidence that adenosine triphosphate and noradrenaline are cotransmitters in guinea-pig vas deferens. *J. Physiol.* 347:561–80

98. Sneddon, P., Burnstock, G. 1984. Inhibition of excitatory junction potentials in guinea-pig vas deferens by α,β-methylene ATP: further evidence of ATP and noradrenaline as co-transmitters. *Eur. J. Pharmacol.* 100:85–90

99. Stjärne, L., Åstrand, P. 1984. Discrete events measure single quanta of adenosine 5'-triphosphate secreted from sym-

pathetic nerves of guinea-pig and mouse vas deferens. *Neuroscience* 13:21–28

100. Fedan, J. S., Hogaboom, G. K., O'Donnell, J. P., Colby, J., Westfall, D. P. 1981. Contribution by purines to the neurogenic response of the vas deferens of the guinea-pig. *Eur. J. Pharmacol.* 69:41–53

101. Cuello, A. C., ed. 1982. *Co-transmission*. London: Macmillan

102. Osborne, N. N., ed. 1983. *Dale's Principle and Communication Between Neurones*. Oxford: Pergamon

103. Weinshilboum, R. M., Thoa, N. B., Johnson, D. G., Kopin, I. J., Axelrod, J. 1971. Proportional release of norepinephrine and dopamine-β-hydroxylase from sympathetic nerves. *Science* 1349–51

104. Thomas, J. A., Sakai, K. K., Holck, M. I., Marks, B. H. 1980. Dopamine-β-hydroxylase: a modulator of beta adrenergic receptor activity. *Res. Commun. Chem. Pathol. Pharmacol.* 29:3–13

105. Koketsu, K. 1984. Modulation of receptor sensitivity and action potentials by transmitters in vertebrates neurons. *Jpn. J. Physiol.* 34:945–60

106. Kumakura, K., Karoum, F., Guidotti, A., Costa, E. 1980. Modulation of nicotinic receptors by opiate receptor agonists in cultured adrenal chromaffin cells. *Nature* 283:489–92

107. Agnati, D. F., Fuxe, K., Benfenati, F., Battistini, N., Härfstrand, A., et al. 1983. Neuropeptide Y in vitro selectively increases the number of α_2-adrenergic binding sites in membranes of the medulla oblongata of the rat. *Acta Physiol. Scand.* 118:293–95

108. Akasu, T., Hirai, K., Koketsu, K. 1981. Increases of acetylcholine-receptor sensitivity by adenosine triphosphate: a novel action of ATP on ACh-sensitivity. *Br. J. Pharmacol.* 74:505–7

109. Lundberg, J. M., Hedlund, B., Bartfai, T. 1982. Vasoactive intestinal polypeptide enhances muscarinic ligand binding in cat submandibular salivary gland. *Nature* 295:147–49

110. Potter, E. K. 1985. Prolonged non-adrenergic inhibition of cardiac vagal action following sympathetic stimulation. Neuromodulation by NPY? *Neurosci. Lett.* 54:117–21

111. Burnstock, G. 1972. Purinergic nerves. *Pharmacol. Rev.* 21:247–324

112. Campbell, G., Gibbins, I. L. 1979. Non-adrenergic, non-cholinergic transmission in the autonomic nervous system: purinergic nerves. In *Trends in Autonomic Pharmacology*, ed. S. Kalsner, 1:102–49. Baltimore: Urban & Schwarzenberg

113. Barthó, L., Holzer, P. 1985. Search for a physiological role of substance P in gastrointestinal motility. *Neuroscience* 16:1–32

114. Furness, J. B., Costa, M., Keast, J. R. 1984. Choline acetyltransferase– and peptide-immunoreactivity of submucous neurons in the small intestine of the guinea-pig. *Cell Tissue Res.* 237:329–36

115. Kessler, J. A. 1985. Differential regulation of peptide and catecholamine characters in cultured sympathetic neurons. *Neuroscience* 15:827–39

116. Costa, M., Furness, J. B. 1984. Somatostatin is present in a sub-population of noradrenergic nerve fibres supplying the intestine. *Neuroscience* 13:911–19

117. Kessler, J. A. 1984. Environmental co-regulation of substance P, somatostatin and neurotransmitter synthesizing enzymes in cultured sympathetic neurons. *Brain. Res.* 321:155–59

118. Kessler, J. A., Adler, J., Jonakait, G. M., Black, I. B. 1984. Target organ regulation of substance P in sympathetic neurons in culture. *Dev. Biol.* 102:417–25

119. Shimizu, T., Taira, N. 1979. Assessment of the effects of vasoactive intestinal peptide (VIP) on blood flow through and salivation of the dog salivary gland in comparison with those of secretin, glucagon and acetylcholine. *Br. J. Pharmacol.* 65:683–88

120. Thulin, A. 1976. Blood flow changes in the submaxillary gland of the rat on parasympathetic and sympathetic nerve stimulation. *Acta Physiol. Scand.* 97:104–9

121. Bloom, S. R., Bryant, M. G., Polak, J. M., van Noorden, S., Wharton, J. 1979. Vasoactive intestinal peptide-like immunoreactivity in salivary glands of the rat. *J. Physiol.* 289:23P

122. Morley, J., Schachter, M., Smaje, L. H. 1966. Vasodilatation in the submaxillary gland of the rabbit. *J. Physiol.* 187:595–602

123. Edvinsson, L., Fahrenkrug, J., Hanko, J., Owman, C., Sundler, F., et al. 1980. VIP (vasoactive intestinal peptide)-containing nerves of intracranial arteries in mammals. *Cell Tissue Res.* 208:135–42

124. Hartzell, H. C. 1979. Adenosine receptors in frog sinus venosus: slow inhibitory potentials produced by adenine compounds and acetylcholine. *J. Physiol.* 293:23–49

Ann. Rev. Pharmacol. Toxicol. 1987. 27:71–86

THE PROMISE OF PHARMACOEPIDEMIOLOGY

Brian L. Strom

Clinical Epidemiology Unit, Section of General Medicine, Departments of Medicine and Pharmacology, University of Pennsylvania School of Medicine, Philadelphia, Pennsylvania 19104

INTRODUCTION

Since the 1930s a series of tragic adverse drug reactions (ADRs) has placed progressively more attention on the new field of pharmacoepidemiology. The stimulus for the 1938 Food and Drug Act was the marketing of elixir of sulfanilamide dissolved in diethylene glycol, which resulted in the death of over 100 children. The resulting public outcry led to stricter requirements for drug safety (1). In the early 1960s the world experienced the notorious "thalidomide disaster." Mothers who ingested this mild hypnotic (available mostly in Europe) during the first trimester of their pregnancy had an increased risk of delivering a child with phocomelia, i.e. one missing one or more limbs or parts of limbs (2). Fortunately the drug had not yet been marketed in the United States. The resulting Kefauver–Harris Amendment to the Food, Drug, and Cosmetic Act strengthened the requirements for testing of safety and added a new premarketing requirement for proof of efficacy. In the late 1960s and early 1970s Japan experienced an epidemic of subacute myelo-optic-neuropathy (SMON), later attributed to an antimicrobial drug used for prophylaxis and treatment of traveler's diarrhea—clioquinol (3). During the 1970s practolol was recognized as responsible for an oculomucocutaneous syndrome, but only after one million patient-years of worldwide use (4). In the 1980s ticrynafen, benoxaprofen, and zomepirac were all removed from the US market because of serious ADRs, including death.

As these and other problems developed, the potential of pharmacoepidemiology for addressing them became more clear. For years,

71

0362-1642/87/0415-0071$02.00

epidemiologists had been developing and refining the techniques necessary to do research on large populations of people. The application of these techniques to the study of the effects of drugs already marketed promised to prove or disprove the many accusations about ADRs. Pharmacoepidemiology can not prevent ADRs, but it can detect them earlier, minimizing their adverse impact. Another important, although often ignored, function of pharmacoepidemiology is that it can document drug safety.

In this paper we review the current status of pharmacoepidemiology, and discuss some of its future prospects and potential problems. Most of the past work in the field applied the techniques of analytic epidemiology to studies of ADRs. We review these techniques, discuss the special methodological problem that differentiates pharmacoepidemiology from other fields of epidemiology, i.e. the large sample size required, and then describe some of the approaches investigators have taken to address this problem. We next review some opportunities for the field that require further investigation, as well as problems that have prevented its further development. Finally, we conclude with some speculation about where the field may go in the future.

BASIC PRINCIPLES OF EPIDEMIOLOGICAL STUDY DESIGN

Epidemiology is the study of the distribution and determinants of diseases in populations. It began with the study of epidemics (infectious diseases in large numbers of people). More recently, it has expanded to include the study of chronic diseases. In the process, it has developed precise and rigorous methodologies for the study of diseases in large numbers of people. Use of these methodologies for the study of drug use and drug effects is the science of pharmacoepidemiology.

Table 1 presents a list of the major epidemiological research designs available. Associations demonstrated by designs at the top of the table are more likely to be causal than those at the bottom of the table. We discuss each in turn, from the least to the most convincing.

A *case report* is simply a report of a single patient with an exposure and an illness, e.g. a report of an oral contraceptive user suffering from a myocardial infarction. This report serves to generate hypotheses for more rigorous study with other techniques; it does not establish whether the patient is typical either of those with that exposure or of those with that illness.

A *case series* is a report of a series of patients who share either a common exposure, e.g. oral contraceptives, or a common illness, e.g. myocardial infarction. Although those patients are presumably typical of those with that exposure or with that illness, respectively, one cannot conclude from a case

Table 1   Study designs used in epidemiology

1. Randomized clinical trials
2. Prospective cohort studies
3. Retrospective cohort studies
4. Case-control studies
5. Case series
6. Case reports

series that their characteristics are unique to that exposure or illness without a concurrent control group.

Analyses of secular trends compare trends in a purported cause to trends in a purported effect, e.g. a coincident rise in oral contraceptive use and myocardial infarction rates (5). Although parallel trends provide evidence for a causal association, this technique cannot separate the causal factor from the many factors whose trends are also likely to occur, e.g. changes in smoking habits.

Case-control and cohort studies both include concurrent control groups (see Figure 1). *Cohort studies* select patients on the basis of the presence or absence of an exposure and then look for subsequent disease, e.g. they might compare oral contraceptive users to nonusers and look for a difference in myocardial infarction rates (6). Cohort studies are generally used to calculate the relative risk of developing a disease, i.e. the ratio of the incidence of disease in the study group to that in the control group. A relative risk greater than 1.0 means the study subjects are more likely to develop the disease than the control subjects, or that the exposure appears to cause the disease. A relative risk of less than 1.0 means the study subjects are less likely to develop the disease than the control subjects, or that the exposure appears to prevent the disease. A relative risk of 1.0 means there is no association between the exposure and the disease.

Case-control studies select patients on the basis of the presence or absence of a disease and then look for antecedent exposures, e.g. they might compare patients suffering from myocardial infarctions to normal controls and look at the relative rates of antecedent oral contraceptive use (7). Although both case-control studies and cohort studies suffer from many of the same limitations, including difficulty in the control of extraneous factors (e.g. family history), the choice of a control group is more difficult for a case-control study than for a cohort study. Many investigators, therefore, consider case-control studies less definitive than cohort studies. Case-control studies are generally used to calculate odds ratios, estimates of relative risks.

Finally, an *experimental study,* or randomized clinical trial, is one in which

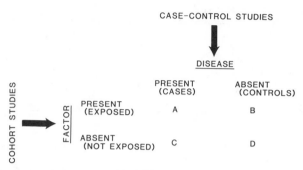

Figure 1   A cohort study compares patients with an exposure to patients without an exposure or with a different exposure, looking for differences in disease incidence. A case-control study compares patients with a disease to patients without a disease, looking for differences in drug exposure.

subjects are randomly assigned to alternative exposures and differences in outcome are observed. For example, women might be randomly assigned to either oral contraceptives or IUD's and the resulting myocardial infarction rates would be determined. The experimental design is by far the most powerful, but as the example demonstrates, it can create logistical and ethical difficulties.

NUMBERS—THE SPECIAL METHODOLOGICAL PROBLEM

Most drugs are studied in 500 to 3000 subjects prior to being marketed (8). This regulation is enforced, even if drug efficacy can be proven in 20 or 30 patients, to ensure the reliability of detecting adverse effects that occur at least once in 100 exposed patients. Therefore, most postmarketing case series, cohort studies, or randomized clinical trials need to include at least 10,000 subjects in order to add sufficient sensitivity to be worth attempting. This requirement obviously raises considerable logistical problems in designing and conducting such studies. Before we explore past solutions to these problems, however, we illustrate how sample size calculations are made for epidemiological studies. We separately present the approach one would use for: (*a*) a case series, (*b*) a cohort study or randomized clinical trial, and (*c*) a case-control study.

In a case series in pharmacoepidemiology, one generally investigates whether a disease occurs more frequently than some predetermined incidence in exposed patients. Most often the predetermined incidence is zero, and the researcher looks for any occurrences of a rare illness. To establish drug safety, a study must include a sufficient number of subjects to detect the elevated incidence, if it exists. More precisely, one needs to examine the upper limit of the 95% confidence interval for an observed frequency of zero. In most case series, researchers assume a Poisson distribution (i.e. that the frequency of the event is vanishingly small) and use that to calculate confidence intervals. (See Ref. 9 for published tables.) A helpful guide is the "rule of threes," which states that if no event of a certain kind in a population of size X is observed, a 95% certainty exists that this event occurs no more than 3 ÷ X (10). For example, if 500 drug-exposed subjects are studied prior to marketing of a particular drug, and no reactions are observed, then a 95% certainty exists that any unobserved medical event occurs in fewer than 3 in 500 subjects, or that it has an incidence less than 6 in 1000. A postmarketing study of 10,000 subjects could exclude events that occur in more than 3 in 10,000, or 1 in 3333, subjects.

More frequently pharmacoepidemiologists study more common diseases to determine if any of them has a higher incidence in patients taking a study drug than in control patients. This research requires a cohort study, comparing a drug-exposed study group to a control group. To calculate the required sample size, one must specify four variables (11, 12): (a) the α, or type I error that is tolerable, i.e. the probability of declaring there is an association when in fact one doesn't exist, conventionally set at 0.05; (b) the β, or type II error, that is tolerable, i.e. the probability of declaring there is no association when in fact one exists, conventionally set at 0.1 or 0.2; (c) the smallest relative risk one wants to be able to detect; and (d) the incidence of the outcome in the control population. Table 2 presents the sample sizes needed for each of the two study groups in a cohort study for various incidence rates in the control group and for possible values of relative risk one might want to be able to detect, assuming an α of 0.05 (two tailed) and a β of 0.2. For example, if one wants to detect a doubling of risk (a relative risk of 2.0) of a disease with an

Table 2 Sample sizes for cohort studies[a]

Relative risk	Incidence of outcome in control group					
	1/50,000	1/10,000	1/5,000	1/1,000	1/500	1/100
2.0	1,177,645	235,500	117,732	23,518	11,741	2,319
2.5	610,627	122,108	61,043	12,191	6,084	1,199
3.0	392,544	78,496	39,240	7,835	3,909	769
5.0	147,201	29,432	14,711	2,935	1,463	285
7.5	78,969	15,788	7,890	1,572	782	151
10.0	53,304	10,656	5,324	1,060	527	100

[a]Calculations are based upon a two-tailed alpha of 0.05, a beta of 0.2, and 1 control subject per expoed subject. Calculated using the formulas presented in Ref. 11 and 12.

incidence in the control group of 1 in a 100, a cohort study would require 2319 subjects in each study group. If this disease occurred in only 1 in a 1000 subjects in the control group, then 23,518 subjects would be needed in each group. If one wanted to detect only a relative risk of 5.0, then the corresponding sample sizes would be 285 and 2935, respectively.

To calculate sample sizes for a case-control study, one similarly needs to specify four variables: (a) α, (b) β, (c) the smallest relative risk you want to be able to detect, and (d) the prevalence of the drug exposure in the undiseased control group (11, 12). Table 3 presents data similar to those in Table 2, but for a case-control study. As the prevalence of exposure in the control group and/or the relative risk one wishes to detect increases, the sample size needed generally decreases. Importantly, a case-control study often requires fewer subjects than a cohort study, since the prevalence of a drug exposure of interest is often more common than the incidence of a disease of interest.

CURRENTLY AVAILABLE SYSTEMS

Traditionally, postmarketing studies of drug effects have been performed by physicians voluntarily reporting ADRs in the medical literature, to pharmaceutical companies, or to governmental agencies. This approach has the disadvantages of case reports listed above. However, it is inexpensive, it is useful for generating hypotheses about ADRs, and it is currently the only feasible method of detecting very rare ADRs. In the United States, pharmaceutical manufacturers who receive reports of ADRs are obligated to report in turn to the FDA. The FDA's spontaneous reporting system receives over 11,000 adverse drug reports annually from physicians and pharmaceutical companies: 80% of these reports come from pharmaceutical companies (13).

Table 3 Sample sizes for case-control studies[a]

Relative risk	Prevalence of drug exposure in control group					
	1/1000	1/100	5/100	10/100	25/100	50/100
2.0	23,596	2,398	516	283	152	137
2.5	12,239	1,247	272	151	85	81
3.0	7,870	804	177	100	58	58
5.0	2,954	305	70	41	27	31
7.5	1,587	165	39	24	17	22
10.0	1,072	113	28	18	14	19

[a]Calculations are based upon a two-tailed alpha of 0.05, a beta of 0.2, and 1 control subject per diseased subject. Calculated using the formulas presented in Ref. 11 and 12.

When compared to three uncontrolled case series, the FDA's spontaneous reporting system identified most of the same information (14). In Great Britain, the comparable system involves physicians' identifying potential ADRs and then completing and submitting a yellow business reply card. This yellow card system identified the increased risks of thromboembolism from oral contraceptives, hepatitis from methyldopa, jaundice from halothane, and extrapyramidal side effects from metoclopramide (15, 16). Importantly, however, it did not detect the practolol-induced oculomucocutaneous syndrome (4). Other countries have similar programs, and the World Health Organization collects and combines this information from multiple countries. Also, case reports in the medical literature continue to be an important source for suspected ADRs, although these ADRs are frequently not confirmed on subsequent study (17), and in one review of the literature only 19% of the reports had all of the necessary information (18). A checklist of data that should be included in any published case report has been developed (19).

In response to the practolol problem, Dr. William Inman, who had run the yellow card system, recently developed the innovative "Prescription Event Monitoring" system in Great Britain (20). Copies of all prescriptions for drugs of interest are obtained from the Prescription Pricing Authority and used to identify patients who had received the drug of interest. Questionnaires are then sent to the prescribers, requesting information regarding all medical events following drug exposure. The frequency of these diagnoses is compared to that in a control group of patients exposed to a similar drug, or to the same patients before or after cessation of their exposure. Preliminary experience with this system suggests that it will be useful.

Hospital-based cohort studies of short-term expected and unexpected ADRs in hospitalized patients have been conducted by the Boston Collaborative Drug Surveillance Program (BCDSP) (21, 22). These studies have provided important information about relatively common short-term ADRs. However, this system cannot be used to study medium- or long-term drug effects, to study drugs used primarily in outpatients, to study uncommon drugs or diseases, or to study new drugs, as data collection has largely ceased.

The Boston University Drug Epidemiology Unit has extended the hospital-based approach of the BCDSP, by collecting lifetime drug-exposure histories and performing hospital-based case-control studies (23). This program has provided much high-quality information on relatively uncommon ADRs. This system can only study hospitalized patients and is thus limited to illnesses that result in inpatient care. In addition, it can be used only for case-control studies and therefore cannot be used to calculate the incidence of diseases. Also, the manner in which the drug history is collected makes this system potentially subject to recall and interviewer biases.

Finally, ad hoc case-control and cohort studies may be performed if special circumstances make the described systems inadequate. The advantages of studies designed to address the question at hand are that the research methodology, patient population, and clinical setting can be tailored to fit the needs of the study question. The disadvantages are that these studies are much more expensive to perform and often will take longer to complete than would the use of an existing system. As an example, large-scale "cohort" studies conducted ad hoc by pharmaceutical companies have been conducted. Typically, a company's sales force is asked to recruit 2000 cooperative physicians, each of whom is then asked to report on the experience of five patients who received the drug (24). This approach is extremely expensive, generally well over a million dollars (25), and is open to biased reporting because of the mechanism of recruitment. Most importantly, though, is that such studies generally lack control groups, making the judgement about whether or not a medical event is likely to be due to a drug arbitrary and the detection of new ADRs unlikely. Certainly a control group could be added, but this addition would double the cost.

As an attempt to reduce the cost of pharmacoepidemiology studies, a recent trend has been to take advantage of billing databases. The BCDSP has used data from the Group Health Cooperative of Puget Sound. This HMO serves 300,000 patients and has computerized drug and hospital-discharge information. Both case-control and cohort studies can be performed using these data. While many useful studies have been carried out using this resource (26), outpatient diagnoses are not computerized and relatively uncommon drugs and illnesses cannot be studied because of the limited size of the database.

Northern and Southern California Kaiser Permanentes each have one to two million patients enrolled in their Health Maintenance Organization. Drug information and diagnostic data, both inpatient and outpatient, are linked in the same record. However, retrieval requires medical-record review; only discharge diagnoses are computerized, although Southern California Kaiser is computerizing its drug data, which will greatly increase its potential utility for pharmacoepidemiology studies. Both case-control and cohort studies can be performed on this system. Its advantages include high-quality data and a working, middle-class, and middle-age population. Its disadvantages are that it is not completely computerized, it has a limited formulary and only moderate sample size, and data cannot be collected directly from patients.

The Commission on Professional and Hospital Activities' Professional Activities Survey represents another data source, containing data on 35–40% of hospital discharges in the United States (27). While this system has great potential to find cases for case-control studies, the process of determining prior exposure requires obtaining consent from many individual hospitals, then individual physicians, and then patients, with resulting logistical difficulties and low participation rates.

The Saskatchewan Health Plan has 10 years of billing data on one million residents of that province in Canada. This system is just beginning to be used for pharmacoepidemiology studies, but appears to hold great promise because it is population-based and has a relatively representative and stable population. Both cohort and case-control studies can be performed. This system suffers from a limited formulary; limited outpatient diagnosis information, since these diagnoses use only 3 of the available 5 digits of the diagnosis codes; limited inpatient diagnosis data, which include only 4 of the available 5 digits of the diagnosis codes; the fact that physician reimbursement is dependent on the diagnosis, which might bias these data; and its moderate sample size. Inasmuch as it has not been organized or used for pharmacoepidemiology studies, further evaluation awaits additional experience.

Over the past ten years, the Food and Drug Administration has funded the development and testing of Medicaid billing data for pharmacoepidemiology studies. The Computerized On-Line Medicaid Pharmaceutical Analysis and Surveillance System (COMPASS) is composed of over six million patients from ten U.S. states. Case-control and cohort studies can be performed. The advantages of this system are that it is population based, very large, and relatively inexpensive to use. The principal disadvantage is that the validity of the diagnosis data has been questioned (28). We recently reviewed this issue in detail and concluded that the data are sufficiently valid to be useful for pharmacoepidemiology studies (29). Care must be taken, however, to ensure that all potential confounding factors of interest are available on the system and that diagnoses under study are chosen carefully, since the validity of the diagnosis data is still an issue.

OPPORTUNITIES

To date, most research in pharmacoepidemiology has focused on the study of drug effects, particularly adverse effects. As of the end of phase III clinical testing, considerable gaps remain in our information about drug effects. Areas needing further development include identification and quantitation of less common adverse effects, even serious ones; identification and quantitation of delayed adverse effects; evaluation of the efficacy and toxicity of drugs in types of patients usually excluded from premarketing testing, e.g. children, the elderly, and pregnant women; evaluation of the efficacy and toxicity of drugs used in patients with other illnesses and/or ingesting other drugs; evaluation of the efficacy and toxicity of drugs relative to the other drugs used for the same purpose; and evaluation of efficacy and toxicity for indications other than those initially tested. In this section of the paper, we review the opportunities for pharmacoepidemiological research, including both work underway and promising areas for future research.

Studies of drug effects can be divided into four categories, each with different implications for research. In the first category, research is directed toward discovering unanticipated adverse effects of drugs. This type of research can be done with an experimental study, but is better addressed with a cohort study that focuses on the drug; a case-control study (if searching for drug causes of a certain disease); or voluntary case reports. The opposite of this research is, in fact, an overlooked but extremely important role for pharmacoepidemiology—documenting drug safety by searching for unanticipated adverse effects and not finding any. Documenting safety is particularly important in light of recent drug withdrawals in response to reports of serious adverse effects that could not at the time be quantitated, e.g. zomepirac (30), and in light of the considerable litigation resulting from adverse drug effects (31).

The second set of questions relates to adverse effects of drugs that have been or could have been anticipated, either because of the pharmacology of the drug, preclinical results of animal testing, or premarketing clinical testing. The major research question to be addressed for this category is quantitative: how often does this adverse effect occur? This kind of investigation can be made with an experimental study, a cohort study, or even a case series, but not with a case-control study, as one needs an identifiable denominator. An example is the study conducted of first-dose syncope from prazosin. This adverse effect was known prior to U.S. marketing from both the prior experience in Europe and premarketing clinical testing. However, the former suggested an incidence rate of 1% and the latter, an incidence rate of 0.1%. A "Phase IV cohort study," actually a case series, was conducted by the manufacturer in response to a request by FDA. This study measured the incidence of first-dose syncope more precisely, recruiting 10,000 patients through prescribing physicians, via sales representatives. The result confirmed the premarketing suggestion of a 0.1% incidence, and was thought to be lower than that found in Europe because the latter led to marketing of a lower dosage form of the product and a recommendation to give the first dose at bedtime (25).

The third set of questions concerns unanticipated beneficial effects of drugs. An example is the beneficial effect of aspirin, given for treatment of rheumatoid arthritis, in preventing myocardial infarction (32). This result is a side effect, even if beneficial. Similar to that with unanticipated harmful effects, researchers in this area seek to discover these beneficial effects. Study design alternatives for both categories are also similar.

Finally, the fourth set of questions about drug effects concerns anticipated beneficial effects of drugs. This research determines whether a drug works as expected. Although drug efficacy needs to be established prior to marketing, multiple questions of efficacy remain after the drug is marketed (33).

These questions include the efficacy of the drug in the face of variations in drug regimen, e.g. dose per unit time, distribution of dose over time, and duration; variations in characteristics of the indication, e.g. severity, subcategories of the illness, and changes in the indication over time; and variations in characteristics of the patient being treated, e.g. age, sex, race, genetics, geographic location, diet, nutritional status, compliance, other illnesses, and use of other drugs, including tobacco and alcohol. Other questions of efficacy remaining at the time of marketing include the efficacy of the drug when used for indications other than those initially evaluated and the efficacy of the drug relative to other drugs used for the same purpose. In general, studies of drug efficacy require randomized clinical trials. However, recent work indicates that clinical trials are not always needed (34), and that the exceptions occur more often than one might have anticipated (35). This field is a new one in pharmacoepidemiology, which deserves more attention in the future.

To a large degree, the field of pharmacoepidemiology began with descriptive studies of how physicians use drugs and determinants of good prescribers vs bad prescribers (36). Subsequently, studies of drug utilization were considered more important for marketing purposes than for academic purposes, and commercial firms have done most such work recently. These firms sell their data to industry to support its marketing efforts. A number of these firms have been very generous, however, in supplying these data, without charge, to investigators as well, in support of academic research efforts (33, 35). Even more recently, there has been a resurgence of interest in academic studies of drug utilization, especially international studies (37). With the development of computerized databases, as described above, such studies are likely to increase in frequency.

A relatively undeveloped field in pharmacoepidemiology is the study of drug interactions. Only a few nonexperimental studies of drug interactions have been done (38). These studies require techniques similar to those described above for the study of other drug effects. For example, one could perform a cohort study comparing patients receiving aminophylline and digoxin to those receiving only aminophylline or only digoxin, and look for differences in the frequency of various outcomes.

A new and rapidly growing field in pharmacoepidemiology applies the principles of health economics to the study of the implications of drug use (39). As society has become more concerned with the costs of medical care, investigators have begun to conduct a series of cost-benefit or cost-effectiveness analyses, examining the financial implications of drug use. These implications involve much more than the costs of the drugs but include the costs of drug administration, the costs of adverse drug reactions, decreases in costs because of other treatments that are not used, etc. This work was markedly advanced by Smith Kline and French, who used it to support its marketing effort for cimetidine, by funding a series of studies that compared the costs of the drug to the savings from reduced peptic ulcer surgery (40). Cost-effectiveness studies of other drugs have followed, and many more are underway.

Another field of clinical epidemiology not yet applied much to the study of drug effects is the field of clinical decision making. Investigators are beginning to examine more rigorously how physicians make clinical decisions (41). Although the field of clinical decision making has been applied frequently to the evaluation of diagnostic tests, it has only rarely been applied to therapeutic decisions. Better understanding of prescribers' decision making could be useful, among other things, in understanding their choices about whether or not to treat. A better understanding of this process might provide a clearer understanding of when therapy is indicated, which is the major obstacle in expanding the use of nonexperimental study designs to address questions of drug efficacy (34).

Drug utilization review (DUR) has been performed for years. However, DUR programs generally focus exclusively on abuse or overuse of drugs, or they focus on the use of costly drugs in an attempt to reduce expenditures on drugs. More recently a new approach to DUR has been developed. This approach focuses on preventing the adverse effects resulting from inappropriate, excessive, or therapeutically incompatible drug use, thus reducing costs by preventing adverse effects from drugs (42). Other similar programs are needed, the efficacy of which must be evaluated rigorously.

Finally, the federal government has recently eased the process by which generically equivalent drugs can be approved for marketing, after expiration of the patent on the original product. Now, generically equivalent drugs can be approved after a single study in a small number of normal subjects, documenting roughly equivalent bioavailability (43). Whether or not generically equivalent drugs are in fact therapeutically equivalent has been controversial for years (44). In response to these new regulatory changes, and recent expirations of the patents of a number of products, an unusual number of generic drug products have recently been marketed (45). Studies are needed to evaluate whether these new drug products are in fact therapeutically equivalent to the trade-name predecessors.

PROBLEMS

The field of pharmacoepidemiology is also facing a number of methodological and logistical problems. Methodologically, the first problem is that no effective and reliable technique has yet been developed to study rare effects of infrequently used drugs. The sample sizes needed have been impossible to attain. Second, it remains difficult to study delayed drug effects in a reliable and efficient manner. None of the available databases have been in existence long enough for this, and even once they are, attrition from each database will probably make this type of study impractical. The only useful technique now available is the use of ad hoc case-control studies, but determining whether drug exposures occurred years previously is obviously difficult.

The third major methodological problem that remains to be addressed is how to screen for adverse drug effects. To date, virtually all adverse drug effects have first been noted as case reports, reported to the medical literature, the manufacturer, or a regulatory body. Most of the databases and the Drug Epidemiology Unit's case-control surveillance have the ability to screen for drug effects, looking for associations between drug exposures and disease occurrence. However, the number of statistical tests involved in such a screen guarantees false positive findings. If an α level of 0.05 is used, 1 out of 20 tests will be positive, purely by chance. Yet, if a smaller α is used, the screen will be insensitive. This problem has led to a reluctance to conduct such screens.

The field of pharmacoepidemiology also has two major logistical problems: funding and manpower. Obvious sources of funding for such research are the FDA, the pharmaceutical industry, and NIH. However, the FDA's budget for extramural research is extremely small, and is used only to address questions of particular regulatory importance. Although this budget for pharmacoepidemiology research was recently increased significantly, even more recently, in response to the first Gramm–Rudman budget cut of 4.3%, the budget for extramural research was reduced by 40%.

The pharmaceutical industry continues to support such work, but its needs are very short term and defined, so it does not represent a feasible source of either long-term salary support for investigators or support for studies of clinical importance that are not of marketing or regulatory importance.

Finally, NIH is organized by organ system. Any set of pharmacoepidemiology studies generally crosses organ systems, making NIH funding awkward. Although the Pharmacological Sciences Program of the National Institute of General Medical Sciences provided pivotal support of the Boston Collaborative Drug Surveillance Program at its initiation, it currently supports only basic research. It was in response to this and other problems that the Joint Commission on Prescription Drug Use, an interdisciplinary commission charged to study the opportunities and problems of pharmacoepidemiology, suggested in 1980 the formation of an independently funded, academically based Center for Drug Surveillance (25). However, such a Center has not been founded.

The other logistical problem is manpower. There are currently very few investigators in the field, and few obvious ways of training new individuals.

First, fellowship programs in Clinical Pharmacology generally do not have faculty with epidemiologic expertise. Second, Master of Public Health programs generally do not have faculty with clinical pharmacology expertise. Third, most of the current investigators in the field are not affiliated with active training programs. Obviously, the funding problems described above make recruiting new individuals into the field even more difficult. As some of the pioneers in the field approach retirement age, this problem will become more acute. The Burroughs Wellcome Foundation has established a Burroughs Wellcome Scholar Award in Pharmacoepidemiology, with the hope of attracting people into the field. Its success remains to be evaluated.

THE FUTURE

Pharmacoepidemiology is a unique new field, bridging clinical pharmacology and clinical epidemiology. There is a tremendous need for a large expansion of research in pharmacoepidemiology, both more research of the type now underway and new types of research. However, there are significant methodological and logistical obstacles that need to be overcome. If all goes well, the future is likely to see a huge expansion of the field, with an increased use of databases; more emphasis on drug safety and drug efficacy, in addition to the current emphasis on drug toxicity; and more emphasis on the financial implications of drug use. The promise of pharmacoepidemiology appears great. Time will tell whether it will be fulfilled.

ACKNOWLEDGMENTS

Supported in part by grant number FD-U-000079 from the Food and Drug Administration. The author is grateful to Dianne Greer and Susan Jordhamo for secretarial assistance.

Literature Cited

1. Temin, P. 1980. *Taking Your Medicine: Drug Regulation in the United States.* Cambridge: Harvard Univ. Press
2. Lenz, W. 1964. Malformations caused by drugs in pregnancy. *Am. J. Dis. Child.* 112:99–106
3. Kono, R. 1980. Trends and lessons of SMON research. In *Drug-Induced Sufferings,* ed. T. Soda, pp. 11–19. Princeton, NJ: Excerpta Med.
4. Nicholls, J. T. 1977. The practolol syndrome—a retrospective analysis. *Med. Pharm. Forum: Post-mark. Surveillance Adverse React. New Med.* 7:4–11
5. Beral, V. 1976. Cardiovascular disease, mortality trends and oral-contraceptive use in young women. *Lancet* 2:1047–52
6. Royal College of General Practitioners. 1974. *Oral Contraceptives and Health.* London: Pitman
7. Shapiro, S., Slone, D., Rosenberg, L., Kaufman, D. W., Stolley, P. D., et al. 1979. Oral contraceptive use in relation to myocardial infarction. *Lancet* 1:743–46
8. Strom, B. L., Melmon, K. L. 1979. Can post-marketing surveillance help to effect optimal drug therapy? *J. Am. Med. Assoc.* 242:2420–23
9. Haenszel, W., Loveland, D., Sirken, M. G. 1962. Lung cancer mortality as related to residence and smoking history. *J. Natl. Cancer Inst.* 28:947–1001

10. Lilienfeld, A. M., Lilienfeld, D. E. 1980. *Foundations of Epidemiology*, pp. 336–38. New York: Oxford Univ. Press. 2nd ed.
11. Stolley, P. D., Strom, B. L. 1986. Sample size calculations for clinical pharmacology studies. *Clin. Pharmacol. Ther.* 39:489–90
12. Schlesselman, J. J. 1974. Sample size requirements in cohort and case-control studies of disease. *Am. J. Epidemiol.* 99:381–84
13. Jones, J. K. 1980. FDA's spontaneous reaction reports data: use in postmarketing surveillance. *Clin. Pharmacol. Ther.* 27:262
14. Rossi, A. C., Knapp, D. E., Anello, C., O'Neill, R. T., Graham, C. F., et al. 1983. Discovery of adverse drug reactions: A comparison of selected phase 4 studies with spontaneous reporting methods. *J. Am. Med. Assoc.* 249:2226–28
15. Inman, W. H. 1970. Monitoring of adverse reactions to drugs in the United Kingdom. *Proc. R. Soc. Med.* 63:1302–4
16. Turner, P. 1984. Food and drugs: why different approaches to their safety? *Lancet* 1:1116
17. Lauper, R. D. 1980. The medical literature as an adverse drug reaction early warning system. See Ref. 25, pp. 1–18
18. Venulet, J., Blattner, R., von Bulow, J., Berneker, G. C. 1982. How good are articles on adverse drug reactions? *Br. Med. J.* 284:252–54
19. Soffer, A. 1984. The practitioner's role in detection of adverse drug reactions. *Chest* 86:808–9
20. Inman, W. H. W. 1984. Prescription-event monitoring. *Acta Med. Scand. Suppl.* 683:119–26
21. Cohen, M. R. 1974. A compilation of abstracts and an index of articles published by the Boston Collaborative Drug Surveillance Program. *Hosp. Pharm.* 9:437–48
22. Miller, R. R., Greenblatt, D. J. 1976. *Drug Effects in Hospitalized Patients.* New York: Wiley
23. Slone, D., Shapiro, S., Miettinen, O. S. 1977. Case-control surveillance of serious illnesses attributable to ambulatory drug use. In *Epidemiological Evaluation of Drugs*, ed. F. Colombo, S. Shapiro, D. Slone, G. Tognoni, pp. 59–70. Massachusetts: PSG
24. Gifford, L. M., Aeugle, M. E., Myerson, R. M., Tannenbaum, P. J. 1980. Cimetidine postmarket outpatient surveillance program. Interim report on phase I. *J. Am. Med. Assoc.* 243:1532–35
25. *Fin. Rep. Joint Comm. Prescr. Drug Use.* 1980. Washington, D.C.: Joint Comm. Prescr. Drug Use. 153 pp.
26. Jick, H., Madsen, S., Nudelman, P. M., Perera, D. R., Stergachis, A. 1984. Postmarketing follow-up at Group Health Cooperative of Puget Sound. *Pharmacotherapy* 4:99–100
27. Jick, H. 1979. The Commission on Professional and Hospital Activities—professional activity study. *Am. J. Epidemiol.* 109:625–27
28. Lessler, J. L., Harris, B. S. H. 1984. *Medicaid Data as a Source for Post-Marketing Surveillance Information: Final Report.* Research Triangle Park, NC: Res. Triangle Inst.
29. Strom, B. L., Carson, J. L., Morse, M. L., Leroy, A. A. 1985. The computerized on-line medicaid pharmaceutical analysis and surveillance system: A new resource for post-marketing drug surveillance. *Clin. Pharmacol. Ther.* 38:359–64
30. Strom, B. L., Carson, J. L., Morse, M. L., West, S. L. 1984. Anaphylactoid reactions from zomepirac and other nonsteroidal anti-inflammatory drugs. *Clin. Res.* 229A
31. Sheffield, L. J., Batagol, R. 1985. The creation of therapeutic orphans—or, what have we learnt from the Debendox fiasco? *Med. J. Aust.* 143:143–47
32. Boston Collaborative Drug Surveillance Group. 1974. Regular aspirin intake and acute myocardial infarction. *Br. Med. J.* 1:440–43
33. Strom, B. L., Miettinen, O. S., Melmon, K. L. 1985. Post-marketing studies of drug efficacy: why? *Am. J. Med.* 78:479–80
34. Strom, B. L., Miettinen, O. S., Melmon, K. L. 1983. Postmarketing studies of drug efficacy: when must they be randomized? *Clin. Pharmacol. Ther.* 34:1–7
35. Strom, B. L., Melmon, K. L., Miettinen, O. S. 1984. Post-marketing studies of drug efficacy: how? *Am. J. Med.* 77:703–8
36. Stolley, P. D., Becker, M. H., Lasagna, L., McEvilla, J. D., Sloane, L. M. 1972. The relationship between physician characteristics and prescribing appropriateness. *Med. Care* 10:17–28
37. Griffiths, K., McDevitt, D. G., Andrew, M., Baksaas, I., Lunde, P. K., et al. 1985. Validation of observed differences in the utilization of antihypertensive and antidiabetic drugs in

Northern Ireland, Norway, and Sweden. *Eur. J. Clin. Pharmacol.* 29:1–8

38. Slone, D., Shapiro, S. 1974. Identification of drug interactions from clinical epidemiological data. In *Drug Interactions,* ed. P. L. Morselli, S. Garattini, S. N. Cohen, pp. 375–82. New York: Raven

39. Eisenberg, J. M. 1984. New drugs and clinical economics: analysis of cost-effectiveness analysis in the assessment of pharmaceutical innovations. *Rev. Infect. Dis.* 6:S905–8. (Suppl. 4)

40. Bloom, B. S., ed. 1982. *Cost-Benefit and Cost-Effectiveness Analysis in Policymaking: Cimetidine as a Model.* New York: Biomed. Inf. Corp.

41. Weinstein, M. L., Fineberg, H. V. 1980. *Clinical Decision Analysis.* Philadelphia: Saunders

42. Morse, M. L., Leroy, A. A., Gaylord, T. A., Kellenberger, T. 1982. Reducing drug therapy-induced hospitalization: impact of drug utilization review. *Drug Inf.* 16:199–202

43. Mattison, N. 1986. Pharmaceutical innovation and generic drug competition in the USA: effects of the Drug Price Competition and Patent Term Restoration Act of 1984. *Pharm. Med.* 1:177–85

44. Strom, B. L., Stolley, P. D., Brown, T. C. 1974. Antisubstitution law controversy—a solution? *Ann. Intern. Med.* 81:254–58

45. Generic drugs. 1986. *Med. Lett.* 28:1–2

Ann. Rev. Pharmacol. Toxicol. 1987. 27:87–111

HUMAN HEALTH EFFECTS OF POLYCHLORINATED BIPHENYLS (PCBs) AND POLYBROMINATED BIPHENYLS (PBBs)[1]

Renate D. Kimbrough

Center for Environmental Health, Centers for Disease Control, Public Health Service, US Department of Health and Human Services, Atlanta, Georgia 30333

INTRODUCTION

Polychlorinated biphenyls (PCBs) are chemical compounds with the empirical formula $C_{12}H_{10-n}Cl_n$, with n = 1–10. They are a mixture of chlorinated biphenyl congeners. Theoretically, 209 such congeners are possible, but at least 20 congeners have never been identified in commercial products. In addition, PCBs may contain polychlorinated dibenzofurans and chlorinated quaterphenyls as impurities. PCBs were discovered before the turn of the century, and the useful industrial properties of mixtures obtained by chlorination of biphenyl were recognized early. In 1966 the discovery of PCBs in environmental samples (1) spurred renewed interest in the analysis and toxicity of these compounds.

In recent years many industrial nations have taken steps to control the flow of PCBs into the environment. PCBs and PCB-containing formulations are restricted (an exception is sometimes made for mono- and dichloro-PCB) for most uses, except for categories such as closed-system electrical equipment and hydraulic fluids in mining equipment.

Commercial production of PCBs began in the United States in the late 1920s. In 1971, Monsanto Chemical Company voluntarily stopped open-ended uses of PCBs, and subsequently only the lower chlorinated biphenyls

---

[1]The US Government has the right to retain a nonexclusive, royalty-free license in and to any copyright covering this paper.

87

were produced (Aroclor 1242 and 1016). In 1977 the company ceased production entirely (2). Many PCBs manufactured in the past (3) are still in use in old transformers, but even this use is decreasing. The estimated cumulative production and consumption of PCBs in the United States in the period 1930–1975 (in millions of pounds) was as follows: total production, 1400; imports, 3; domestic sales, 1253; exports, 150.

PCBs are inert chemicals that are fairly resistant to degradation. Because of their stability and lipophilicity, they have accumulated in the environment and in organisms. They have been identified in indoor air (4) at concentrations of 0.1 $\mu g/m^3$ (5), in fish (6, 7) and other food products, and in sediments from lakes and rivers (8, 9). PCBs have also been identified at varying concentrations in soil (0.01 mg/kg–100 mg/kg) (10). They do not occur naturally. Thus, their presence in the environment is linked with human activities, and concentrations are higher in urban and heavily industrialized areas than in rural and remote areas. However, trace amounts are also found in remote areas, since the air may transport such chemicals over large distances.

Although PCBs are no longer used commercially in the United States because of their persistence, they are still present in our environment. A number of transformers and capacitors that contain PCBs, however, are still in use. Results of laboratory experiments showed that pyrolysis of PCBs at temperatures of 200–600°C could result in the formation of significant amounts of the more toxic polychlorinated dibenzofurans (PCDFs) (11).

In February 1981, an electrical fire occurred in a New York State office building in Binghamton, N.Y. The fire, which originated in a switch gear in the basement, caused the bushings to crack on a nearby transformer. About 180 gallons of PCB dielectric fluid Pyralon (65% Aroclor 1254, 35% chlorinated benzenes and trace additives) were lost. A fine layer of oily soot covered many of the internal surfaces of the 18 floors of the building. Analysis of a soot sample showed that it contained various isomers of chlorinated dibenzofurans, 2,3,7,8-tetrachlorodibenzodioxin, other chlorinated dibenzodioxins, and chlorinated biphenylenes. Some of these chemicals are much more toxic than the PCBs. Because of these findings the Binghamton state office building was closed, and workers wearing respirators and protective clothing began an extensive cleanup of the building. The cleanup operations lasted four years, and the cost has been enormous (12). Since then several other transformer fires have occurred. These fires have not resulted in as much contamination as the one in Binghamton, partly because the transformers in the other fires were usually located in a separate vault (13).

The problems with polybrominated biphenyls (PBBs), which are also a mixture of chemicals, have been quite different. In 1970 a chemical company in Michigan manufactured polybrominated biphenyls as flame retardants. The same company also produced magnesium oxide, a chemical commonly mixed into feed for livestock. The flame retardant was called Firemaster and the magnesium oxide, Nutrimaster. In 1973 some bags of Firemaster were accidentally sold as Nutrimaster and mixed into animal feed. This resulted in widespread contamination in the state of Michigan (14). Since 1974 PBBs have not been produced in the United States. At the time of the exposure little was known about the toxic effects of PBBs. Ten years after the Michigan residents were exposed, no clinical illness has been causally linked to PBB exposure in this group, although chloracne was apparently noted in some workers who manufactured PBB.

HUMAN EXPOSURE

Because PCBs are ubiquitous and very persistent in the environment, humans have been and will continue to be exposed to them, particularly in industrialized countries. PCBs may be inhaled in small amounts through the air or ingested through food. In the United States today, people are primarily exposed to PCBs by consuming fish from contaminated waters (9). In the past, some farm families were exposed to PCBs from dairy products; these PCBs originated from coating material used in the inside of silos (15). In addition, workers who repair transformers and workers who handle toxic wastes may also be exposed (16).

The PCB products that were manufactured by Monsanto in the United States had the trade name "Aroclor." The particular kind of Aroclor is identified by a four-digit number. The first two digits refer to the 12 carbon atoms, and the second two refer to the percent, by weight, of chlorine in the mixture. Thus, Aroclor 1254 contains about 54% chlorine, and Aroclor 1260, about 60% chlorine.

The composition of this mixture of chemicals, with different properties, changes once it gets into the environment and into organisms. Some components of the mixture are more easily degraded in the environment than others. As a result the PCBs identified in the environment resemble Aroclor 1254 but are not identical to it. Similarly, the PCB mixtures found in humans usually resemble Aroclor 1254 if exposure occurred primarily through the environment. A different composition of the PCBs may be found in serum or adipose tissue samples from occupationally exposed workers. For instance, if the workers are primarily exposed to Aroclor 1016 or Aroclor 1242, which contain much less of the more highly chlorinated homologs, then their gas-chromatographic patterns resemble a combination of Aroclor 1016 or 1242 and Aroclor 1254. For this reason Smith et al (17), in evaluating occupational exposure, divided PCBs into high and low chlorinated biphenyls. The gas-chromatographic pattern of the PCB mixture present in humans can be used to determine whether the exposure occurred primarily through occupation or through the environment, or, in the case of occupational situations, whether most of the exposure was recent or occurred many years ago.

Although 93% of the US population eats fish, the average annual per capita consumption is small: 15 lbs. per year (6, 7). If PCBs are to be quantitated in fish, the edible portion rather than the whole fish must be examined. Because of their lipophilicity, PCBs are preferentially stored in the hepatopancreas of the fish, giving erroneously high levels if the whole fish is analyzed. Similarly, levels in cooked fish are lower (6).

Generally, PBBs are not found in the environment because they have had less commercial use than PCBs. PBB contamination is essentially restricted to Michigan's lower peninsula. Most persons who lived in Michigan during the 1973–1974 period have low-level PBB body burdens (18). The greatest degree of contamination occurred mainly in areas with contaminated farms; this segment of the population still has appreciable body burdens (19).

Since PBBs and PCBs are lipophilic, they are preferentially stored in adipose tissue. They are also present, to a smaller extent, in serum and other organs and in human milk. The concentration of these materials in different organs depends upon the lipid content of such organs, with the exception of the brain where the concentration is lower than the lipid content would indicate. PCBs and PBBs pass the placenta and are primarily excreted through bile and milk. In addition to lipid content, the ratios between adipose tissue, blood, and vital organs are influenced by exposure level, sex, age, length of exposure, and also by whether exposure is current. At very low concentrations an analytical imprecision influences the ratios much more than at higher concentrations (19). Since human milk is relatively easy to obtain, it has been used to monitor human exposure. Jensen (20) recently summarized results of such monitoring studies. Average levels of PCBs below 2 ppm (mg/kg) in milk fat have normally been found, although women living in heavily industrialized urban areas may have higher levels. The fat concentration in human milk averages 2.6–4.5% (21). At 2% fat, 1 liter (l) of milk would contain 0.04 mg or 40 μg if the PCBs were present in milk fat at a concentration of 1 ppm. If an infant weighed 5 kg and imbibed 750 ml of milk per day, it would take in about 6 μg/kg, a dose that exceeds the 1.5 μg/kg dose calculated as acceptable by Cordle et al (6). At 1% milk fat this dose would be reduced to 3 μg/kg. As the infant gains weight, the dose on a kilogram body weight basis will be reduced to some extent, however; milk is the sole food source for only about six months. After the first week, the daily milk intake is estimated to be 150 ml/kg body weight per day. This consumption gradually falls after two months and declines to 120 ml/kg body weight at four-to-six months. Finally, the amount of PCBs and other halogenated organic chemicals declines with time. However, at low concentrations this may not be obvious because of continued exposure of the mother and the variability of the analytical results. In addition to PCBs, human milk contains trace amounts of many other persistent chemicals. Whether the infant's consumption of such chemicals has any adverse health effects is not known.

Most persons, particularly in industrialized countries, have had some exposure to polychlorinated biphenyls even if they do not eat fish. The concentrations at which such exposure presents a risk are not clear. Recently, Cordle et al (6, 7) calculated the dose of PCBs to people consuming fish from Lake Michigan. They concluded that persons eating Lake Michigan fish ingested an average of 46.5 mg of PCBs per year; this amount ranged from 14.17 to 114.31 mg/year/person. The calculated mean daily dose received by the exposed group was 1.7 μg/kg/day and ranged from 0.09 to 3.94 μg/kg/day. Thus, the average sports fisherman consuming contaminated fish would receive a total PCB dose equal to 200 mg in about 4.3 years. No adverse health effects or groups of symptoms clearly related to PCB exposure could be identified in this exposed group. The presence of PCBs in the exposed persons has not caused any observable adverse health effects similar to those observed in the Yusho population (see below). However, this finding does not exclude the possibility that the effects are too subtle for detection or that they require long-term observation.

Similarly, in Michigan an analysis of 1,075 human milk samples showed that all contained PCB residues and that the residues ranged from trace amounts to 5 ppm (mg/kg) based on fat level. The public health significance of PCB residues in human breast milk and their effects on breast-fed infants are unclear. Since there are no human data on which to base public health policy, risk predictions for PCBs have been based on results from animal studies, particularly the positive bioassay studies. Reviewing these data, Cordle et al (6, 7) concluded that a 2-ppm (mg/kg) tolerance for PCB in fish be established, since a 1-ppm (mg/kg) tolerance does not greatly reduce the estimated risk.

As previously mentioned, some of the isomers of the PCBs and PBBs are much more easily degraded or metabolized. Because they can be metabolized, they are more easily excreted. Others may be retained in the body for long periods; in general, the PBBs appear to be more persistent in human tissues than the PCBs (19, 22).

POLYCHLORINATED BIPHENYLS

Background

When PCBs were first used industrially some workers developed chloracne. Results of early animal studies seemed to suggest that PCBs might have some toxic effects on the liver. Beyond that observation no information was available. Because PCBs were so inert chemically, they were not considered to cause a great deal of toxicity. In 1968 a poisoning outbreak occurred in Japan (23) that affected over 1,000 persons. These individuals had purchased rice oil, in large drums, from a single source and had used this rice oil for cooking. Chloracne was one of the leading signs in those who became ill. It was soon discovered that PCBs had been used as a heat-exchange fluid in the factory where the rice oil originated. PCBs had leaked out of the columns in which they were contained into the rice oil when the rice oil was heated. Since the disease was caused by ingesting contaminated rice oil, it was called Yusho (rice-oil disease). When the outbreak first occurred, its association with exposure to PCBs was not clear. At that time the capabilities for measuring these types of chemicals in tissues and body fluids were limited, particularly in Japan. Therefore, early in the investigation total chlorine, rather than PCBs, was measured. Retrospectively determining the precise dose these patients received is difficult. Whether the consumed oil was uniformly contaminated is also not clear. However, a relationship between the amount of rice oil ingested and some symptoms could be established (24). Because of this poisoning outbreak and other environmental problems, animal studies were started in Japan, in the United States, and in other countries to elucidate the toxic effects of PCBs. These data are summarized in several detailed reviews (16, 25, 26).

Animal Studies

This article addresses primarily the human health effects of PCBs and PBBs. Therefore we highlight only recent results from animal studies that might give a better understanding of implemented public health policies and potential human health effects. One of the difficulties in using animal data to predict human health effects for PCBs and related compounds is that animal species vary greatly in their responses. Further, many of the animal studies use relatively high doses. Therefore, determining how such animal studies relate to the human situation is difficult. Some animal species, such as the subhuman primates, the guinea pig, and the mink, are much more sensitive to the toxic effects of PCBs than the rat or the mouse; also the types of toxic effects and morphological changes in the organs of different species vary.

Most animal studies conducted during the 1970s used mixtures of PCBs. In general, PCBs were found to affect reproduction and the immune response, and to cause liver tumors in rodents (16). When different mixtures of PCBs were studied, however, the results were inconsistent. For instance, the mixture Aroclor 1254 affects reproduction in rats at much lower doses than does Aroclor 1260 (27).

More recently some of the isomers of the PCB mixture were found to be much more toxic than others (28–32). The more toxic isomers constitute only a very small portion of the mixture, particularly those with less chlorine by weight, such as Aroclor 1242 or Aroclor 1016. Recently, Schaeffer et al (33) found that a German PCB mixture—Clophen A-30, with an average composition of 1% monochlorobiphenyl, 20.7% dichlorobiphenyl, 57.4% trichlorobiphenyl, 17.3% tetrachlorobiphenyl, 1.8% pentachlorobiphenyl, 1.0% hexachlorobiphenyl, 0.6% heptachlorobiphenyl, and 0.1% octachlorobiphenyl—produced a 3% incidence of hepatocellular carcinoma, whereas Clophen A-60 produced a 61% incidence of hepatocellular carcinoma in Wistar rats. The incidence of the disease in the controls was 2%. The Clophen A-60 had an average composition of 0.2% monochlorobiphenyl, 1.1% dichlorobiphenyl, 2.2% trichlorobiphenyl, 3.1% tetrachlorobiphenyl, 19.8% pentachlorobiphenyl, 43.2% hexachlorobiphenyl, 25.3% heptachlorobiphenyl, 4.7% octachlorobiphenyl, and 0.3% nonachlorobiphenyl. Similarly, Norback & Weltman (34) and Kimbrough et al (35) were able to produce hepatocellular carcinomas in rats with Aroclor 1260, the more highly chlorinated Monsanto product.

When Aroclor 1254 was fed to rats, fewer liver tumors developed in exposed rats (36); however, the incidence of gastric intestinal metaplasia and adenocarcinoma of the stomach increased (37, 38). Whether PCB fractions without hexachlorobiphenyls, heptachlorobiphenyls, and octachlorobiphenyls produce hepatocellular carcinomas in rodents should be explored.

Particularly in the United States, mixtures such as Aroclor 1242, 1254, and 1016 were used more than Aroclor 1260. Because of these differences in potency, the PCBs in heavily contaminated areas of our environment should be characterized according to their isomeric composition. For instance, whether the PCBs in Lake Michigan are of the same composition as those found in New Bedford Harbor, Massachusetts, is not clear.

Aside from tumor formation, PCBs cause a variety of other biological effects, such as the induction of enzymes (39). In some species they may cause atrophy of the thymus, intrahepatic bile duct hyperplasia, hyperplasia of the epithelial lining of the urinary bladder, atrophy of the sebaceous glands, and hyperkeratosis of the ducts (40). Some isomers are fetotoxic, and some produce metaplasia of the sebaceous glands, nailbeds, ameloblasts, thymus corpuscles, and gastric mucosa (28, 41). Subhuman primates, mink, and guinea pigs are particularly sensitive to the toxic effects of PCBs; other species, such as the rat, the mouse, and the dog, can tolerate much higher doses. From empirical observations, humans also appear to be less sensitive to the toxic effects of PCBs. The ability to store these chemicals in adipose tissue may be protective. Generally, the subhuman primates and mink have less adipose tissue than humans. Animals with greater ability to store vitamin A on a quantitative basis, such as the hamster and the rat, are somewhat less susceptible to the toxic effects of these types of compounds (42). The mechanism by which these types of chemicals affect hepatic retinoids is not clear. Apparently, the duration of the reduction of hepatic retinoids does not correlate with the induced aryl hydrocarbon hydroxylase (AHH) activity (43).

Body Burdens

Many investigators have reported PCBs in human tissues (44, 45). In the United States, according to data from the Centers for Disease Control (CDC), mean PCB serum levels are about 5–7 ng/ml (pbb), although some patients may have higher serum levels without any documented unusual exposure. These data were also summarized by Kreiss (46). Levels in adipose tissue and in human milk fat are 100–200 times as high, since PCBs are highly lipid soluble (20). Mes et al (47) reported that PCB levels in adipose tissue of accident victims ranged from 0.9–9.4 mg/kg.

Sahl et al (48) surveyed PCB blood levels in 738 pre-employed and 1,058 currently employed workers of a utility company. The median blood level before employment was 4 mg/l and the range, 1–37 mg/l. These levels were quite similar to those in the currently employed group.

Patients who died of cancer in Denmark had somewhat higher levels of PCBs in their adipose tissue (49). Since terminal cancer patients have usually lost a great deal of weight, bioconcentration may have occurred. Similarly, in patients with highly impaired liver function, tissue concentrations of xenobiotics may be slightly higher than those in healthy persons. However, levels remained higher if parameters such as weight, height, occupation, and residence were considered (50), whereas levels of PCBs in breast fat tissue from patients with breast cancer were similar to those of controls (51).

Furthermore, Lawton et al (52) demonstrated that random errors and interlaboratory variations in procedure and methods of data reporting can influence serum and adipose PCB levels. Unless an interlaboratory quality-control system is set up, measured levels between laboratories are not necessarily comparable. For instance, Lawton et al (52) found that the results of repeated analyses on serum samples of known composition showed the 95% prediction interval for an individual measurement to be about ± 42%. This interval depends on the method of extraction, the procedure used, and the means of quantitation.

Summary of Human Epidemiology Studies

Recently, investigators studied the predominantly black population of Triana, a small rural town in the southern United States (53). This population was excessively exposed to DDT residues by consuming contaminated fish. The residents also had PCB body burdens. Fish consumption correlated positively with PCB blood levels; no other source of PCB exposure could be established. These researchers noted that PCB serum levels increased with age and that levels were lower in females of each age group. Similar findings were made for DDT residues. The serum cholesterol level was positively associated with the log PCB level, independent of age, sex, fish consumption, body-mass index, and alcohol consumption. Rates of borderline and definite hypertension for study participants were 30% higher than those expected on the basis of national rates (54). Log PCB serum values contributed significantly to explaining the variability of log systolic and diastolic blood pressure in multiple regression analysis (55). Median total cholesterol levels of individuals in the United States increase with age from about 150 to 160 mg/dl at age 20 to over 200 mg/dl at age 50. PCBs in blood are influenced by serum lipid content, and populations with inherently lower total serum cholesterol levels appear to have a different PCB serum to adipose tissue ratio. The age-associated increase in blood PCB levels could be related to the long half-life of some PCB isomers that are preferentially retained in mammals (29); as long as exposure continues, a true steady state between intake and excretion is never reached. Other variables affecting body burdens may be differences in metabolism with age. In the Triana studies, the blood levels of total DDT residues also increased with age, and others have made similar observations (56, 57). Lawton et al (58) studied workers who had been exposed to electrical-grade Aroclor 1016, 1242, and/or 1254; the study covered the period from before the workers were exposed to two years after PCB exposure ceased. Serum levels for the lower chlorinated PCBs in 1977 ranged from 57–2270 ppb and in 1979, from 12–392 ppb; for the higher chlorinated PCBs serum levels ranged from 6–142 ppb in 1977 and from 4–108 ppb in 1979. These findings again illustrate the preferential excretion of lower chlorinated PCB. Lawton et al (58) also found that cholesterol levels correlated with log serum PCBs. Similar associations with log serum PCBs were found for log gamma glutamyl transpeptidase (GGTP) and, in some cases, for log alanine aminotransferase. When the PCB concentrations were expressed as levels in serum lipids, all the associations between serum lipids or enzymes and log serum PCBs disappeared except for those between log GGTP and log PCBs. Similarly, Chase et al (59) found no significant correlation between either serum triglycerides or aminotransferases and the PCB levels in adipose tissue. How age and length of exposure affect these parameters is not adequately explained in the article. Finally, Akagi & Okumura (60) were not able to confirm a positive association between PCB blood levels and elevated blood pressure in Yusho patients.

Thus, as Brown (61) has suggested, the positive association between PCB serum levels and elevated triglycerides and serum cholesterol can be explained by the increased solubility of PCB in serum with higher lipid content.

In several cross-sectional studies of exposed workers, only minor abnormalities not necessarily related to PCB exposure have been detected

(62–66). In cross-sectional studies, however, the ability to evaluate chronic health effects is limited. In several studies, a positive association between results of one liver function test—the test for γ-glutamyltranspeptidase—and PCB blood levels has been found. Kimbrough (67) has summarized earlier studies on the health effects of PCBs observed in workers.

In 1930 and 1940, chloracne, a disfiguring skin disease, was reported among workers exposed to PCBs. One of the clinical features of chloracne is the chloracne cyst, which is skin colored and measures from 1–10 mm in diameter, with a central opening. The other dominant lesion is the comedo. The skin lesions may only involve the face, but many also extend to other parts of the body. Microscopic examination of human skin biopsies from chloracne cases shows markedly dilated hair follicles filled with keratin. The sebaceous glands involute partially or completely. The epithelial cells lining the hair follicles and the adjacent surface epithelium proliferate, and acanthosis is present. In old lesions, the epithelial lining of the greatly dilated hair follicles becomes atrophic.

Jones & Alden (68) examined 17 of 23 workers engaged in the production of PCBs. The workers had chloracne involving the face, genitalia, trunk, and extremities. Before the outbreak of chloracne in the plant, the electrical property of the PCBs had fallen below specifications, and the color had deepened. In the report, symptoms of illness were extensively described for the first worker who was diagnosed as having chloracne. This worker complained of lassitude, loss of appetite, and loss of libido. Over the years, other cases of chloracne following exposure to PCBs have been reported. Most of these involved exposure to vapors that developed when PCBs were heated (69).

At times, the skin rashes that developed in workers were accompanied by pruritus. Some workers also complained of burning of the eyes, nose, and throat; dry throat; nausea; and dizziness. Meigs et al (70) reported chloracne in workers who had been exposed to PCB vapors for 5–14 months. The concentration of PCBs in the workers' breathing zone was 0.1 mg/m^3. Evidence of slight liver injury was also present. Ouw et al (71) found air levels in a capacitor plant that ranged from 0.32–1.44 mg/m^3 Aroclor 1242 (PCB). Here workers complained of burning eyes, face, and skin in general, and persistent body odor. One worker suffered from chloracne, five complained of eczematous rashes, and a few had abnormal liver function tests. These workers had a mean PCB blood level of about 400 ppb (μg/kg). In most studies of workers with chloracne, evidence of liver injury was also found; in one study, workers who did not have chloracne were found to have abnormal liver function (69).

PCBs also affect the liver by inducing mixed-function oxidases. Alvares et al (72) determined that in five workers occupationally exposed to Aroclor 1016—a PCB mixture primarily composed of dichlorobiphenyls, trichlorobiphenyls, tetrachlorobiphenyls, and pentachlorobiphenyls—plasma antipyrine half-life was significantly lower than that in matched controls, suggesting the induction of mixed-function oxidases in the liver. These workers had been exposed to Aroclor 1016 for at least two years and had no obvious symptoms of PCB poisoning.

Other health effects are eye and upper respiratory irritation. Warshaw et al (65) studied a group of 326 workers in a capacitor plant with a mean employment of more than 15 years and mean employee ages of 41.1 years for males and 47.3 years for females. Work-related eye or upper respiratory irritation was reported by 48% of the workers, and 10% had experienced tightness in the chest. Spirometric studies were conducted on 309 workers; 66 of them were dropped from the study because they had been exposed to talc, textile dust, or asbestos. Thus, 243 men were available for analysis. In males, there were about twice as many smokers and exsmokers as nonsmokers. In females, the proportion of nonsmokers was higher. Thirty-four of the workers (14%) had a reduced vital capacity, and 27 of these demonstrated a restrictive pattern of impairment. Because of additional variables such as smoking and asbestos exposure, these findings are difficult to interpret.

Taylor et al (73), in an attempt to determine whether the fetus would be affected in capacitor workers, examined pregnancy outcome and birth weight, and found that the gestation period was reduced by one week. The infants weighed slightly less than the controls; this finding could be explained by the reduced gestation period. Smoking and alcohol consumption were not controlled, however; furthermore, whether the socioeconomic status of this group of women was similar to that of the control group is not clear. Thus, until other studies confirm these findings, they should be viewed with caution.

In several papers Jacobson and his associates reported behavioral changes and a reduced gestation period in association with higher fish intake or higher intake of PCBs (9, 74–76). Furthermore, Jacobson et al (74) reported that intrauterine PCB exposure may have a delayed effect on central nervous system functioning. Since genetic makeup, the mother's lifestyle, and acute illness also affect these parameters, these findings are difficult to interpret. Furthermore, many other chemicals are also excreted in human milk (20). Rogan & Gladen (77), for instance, found that mothers with high levels of DDE [1,1'-(2,2-dichloroethenylidene)-bis-4-chlorobenzene] in their milk tended to wean their infants earlier, as they did not thrive. Apparently, PCB levels in milk were higher in older women, women who drank alcohol regularly, and primiparas (78).

Whether high levels of DDE affect lactation is not clear. In animals, DDT homologs, but not specifically DDE, have been shown to have estrogenic effects (79). Before these findings can be clarified, additional studies must be done.

No conclusive evidence thus far reported shows that occupational exposure to PCBs causes an increased incidence of cancer. Bahn et al (80) reported results of a preliminary study of a group of 51 research and development employees and 41 refinery plant employees at a New Jersey petrochemical facility. Between 1949 and 1957 these workers had been exposed to Aroclor 1254. Three melanomas and two carcinomas of the pancreas were found. This incidence was significantly higher than expected. Exposure to other chemicals also occurred, however, and the cohort was small.

Brown & Jones (81) conducted a retrospective mortality study of 2,567 workers in two capacitor plants. The relatively few deaths (163) severely limited the statistical power of the study, and the average follow-up was only 15 years, whereas latency periods of 20–30 years are not uncommon for cancer. Over 50% of the sample had exposure to PCBs for two years or less. Deaths from liver cancer, cirrhosis of the liver, and rectal cancer were slightly higher than expected, but not significantly for both sites combined. The observed increase for cancer of the rectum was statistically significant among females at one of the plants. In a follow up study (82) no additional cancers of the rectum were noted, and the standardized mortality ratio (SMR) dropped from 336 to 211. However, two additional cancers of the liver and biliary tract were observed, bringing the total of these tumors to five as reported on the death certificates. However, a review of the medical records raises questions about at least one of these tumors.

Bertazzi et al (83) reviewed the mortality of 290 males and 1,020 females who had worked for six months or more in capacitor production. Males had a statistically significant increased number of deaths from all neoplasms. When deaths were analyzed by organ system, deaths from neoplasms of the digestive system, the peritoneum, and the lymphatic and hematopoietic tissues were higher. Among females, all causes of deaths were significantly elevated. The actual numbers in this study, however, were small.

Yusho and Yucheng

Two outbreaks of poisoning have been reported that followed the ingestion of rice oil contaminated with polychlorinated dibenzofurans, biphenyls, and quaterphenyls (PCQs). The first outbreak occurred in Japan in the summer of 1968 and the second outbreak, in Taiwan in 1979. Ironically, the outbreak in Taiwan repeated what had occurred 10 years earlier in Japan. Many studies of these two outbreaks have been published in Japanese or Chinese. In 1984 some of the information in these reports was published in English in the

American Journal of Industrial Medicine 5:1–153; the information is also summarized in volumes 59 and 60 of *Environmental Health Perspectives*.

In Japan and Taiwan the disease was first recognized because chloracne developed in the affected patients (84). In Japan, members of all of the affected households had purchased rice oil from a specific company, and the toxic rice oil produced or shipped on February 5 and 6 of 1968 contained large amounts of Kanechlor 400, a brand of PCB with a chlorine content of 48%. At the time of the outbreak, no analytical methods specific for PCBs were available in Japan; the concentration of Kanechlor 400 in the oil was therefore estimated from the organic chlorine content to be 2,000–3,000 ppm. Kanechlor 400 had been used for heating the rice oil in a metal container at over 200°C, at a reduced pressure of 3–44 mm Hg, to remove odorous material from it. Kanechlor (K) must have leaked from the heating pipe into the processed oil, but the actual mechanism of the contamination has apparently not been determined. The reanalysis of the K-rice oil, once the methods were developed, showed that some of the oil samples contained 1,000 ppm (mg/kg) PCB. This concentration was much lower than had originally been estimated. Therefore, other chlorine-containing compounds were assumed to be in the oil, and additional samples were analyzed. The oil was found to contain an average of 5-ppm polychlorinated dibenzofurans (85). According to Buser et al (86), the Yusho oil contained more than 40 polychlorinated dibenzofuran isomers, including the highly toxic 2,3,7,8-tetrachlorodibenzofuran (TCDF) and 2,3,4,7,8-pentachlorodibenzofuran (PCDF). In addition, the oil contained PCQs at a concentration of 866 ppm (87, 88).

According to estimates made by Kuratsune (89), the total amount of PCB, PCDF, and PCQs consumed by the patients was, on the average, 633 mg of PCB, 3.4 mg of PCDF, and 596 mg of PCQ. This calculates to roughly 157 μg/kg body weight/d. PCB, 0.9 μg/kg body weight/d. PCDF, and 148 μg/kg body weight/d. PCQ. At this dose the length of the latent period between exposure and onset of clinical illness was roughly 71 days, with a range from 20 to 190 days. Some of the oil the patients consumed may have contained higher or lower levels because in such situations contamination is usually not uniform. Furthermore, the patients consumed different amounts of contaminated rice oil. The severity of symptoms was positively associated with the amount of contaminated rice oil consumed (24).

Early in the outbreak the patients had chloracne, dark-brown pigmentation of the nails, itching, pigmentation of the skin, swelling of the limbs, pigmented mucous membranes, eye discharge, hyperemic conjunctivae, jaundice, swelling of the upper eyelids, a feeling of weakness, numbness of the limbs, and fever. Over 1,000 people were affected. Thirty-six babies showed fetal PCB syndrome, which consists primarily of a dark-brown pigmentation of the skin (Cola babies). The cutaneous pigmentation was caused by an increase in melanin pigment in the epidermis (90). The mucous membranes were also pigmented. In all cases, the pigmentation disappeared by the time the babies were between two and five months old. In affected infants, the face was edematous, and spotty calcifications were noticed in the parietal and occipital areas of the skull. In a few of the infants, the teeth had erupted at birth. Subsequently, the adult patients with clinical disease complained of having to expectorate a great deal and, on auscultation, wheezing was noted; however, on examination, there was no evidence of bronchial asthma or pulmonary emphysema. In many of these patients, the respiratory symptoms have persisted, and the patients have chronically infected airways. In the early 1970s, some changes were noted in the patients' serum immunoglobulin levels, but the levels returned to normal. Over time the severity and the extent of the skin lesions improved considerably in the exposed population. Fifteen years after the accident, only a very few patients had extensive chloracne (91).

About five years after the outbreak of Yusho, tissue and body fluids of Yusho patients were analyzed for various congeners of PCB and PCDF. At this time, the PCB levels in adipose tissue were 1.9 ± 1.4 ppm (mg/kg). In the liver they were 0.08 ± 0.06 ppm and in blood, 6.7 ± 5.3 ppb (μg/kg); thus, they were not very different from levels in the general population in Japan. On the other hand, the isomeric distribution for the PCBs in the Yusho patients varied from that in the control population in the same area (92). About 40 PCDF congeners were identified in the rice oil that the Yusho patients ingested. Only some PCDF congeners were retained in the body for a long time; they included 2,3,6,8-TCDF, 2,3,7,8-TCDF, 1,2,4,7,8-PCDF, 2,3,4,7,8-PCDF, and 1,2,3,4,7,8-hexachlorinated dibenzofurans. Since these congeners do not have free adjacent carbon atoms, they are not as easily metabolized and excreted. More of the 2,3,4,7,8-PCDF than the other isomers was retained in the patients' tissues. In the five patients studied, the concentration of this isomer ranged from 6.9 ppb (μg/kg) in a specimen obtained in 1969 to 0.1 ppb (μg/kg) in a specimen collected in 1977. Measurable concentrations of TCDFs were only detected in the earlier years. Although not the most toxic isomer, the 2,3,4,7,8-PCDF caused mixed-function oxidase induction at a dose of 1 μg/kg in rats, and atrophy of the thymus, suggesting toxicity at a very low dosage level. Thus, the clinical manifestations observed in these patients were primarily caused by the PCDFs, specifically by the more toxic isomers.

In the Yucheng episode, it was never determined with certainty how the rice oil was contaminated (93). In 1979 a school for blind persons informed a local health bureau in Taichung County that a strange disease characterized by an acnelike skin eruption had been occurring frequently among students and staff since the end of March. At the same time, 85 of 150 workers in a nearby plastic shoe factory had the same symptoms. Later that year, this outbreak was also reported to a local health bureau. Victims in both outbreaks had consumed the same brand of cooking rice oil, which had been manufactured by the same company and which had been purchased in the same store. For this reason the rice oil was the prime suspect in the outbreak. In additional reports of outbreaks in other companies and in the general population, all victims had consumed the same type of C-rice oil.

Finally, because the disease resembled the Yusho disease in Japan, samples of C-rice oil and patients' blood were analyzed in Japan and were found to contain either a Kanechlor-400 or a Kanechlor-500 mixture at concentrations as high as 65 and 108 ppm (mg/kg), respectively. Over 2,000 patients were finally identified as having been poisoned by contaminated rice oil. Oil samples collected from other outbreaks contained PCBs at concentrations of 31–300 ppm (mg/kg). Retrospective studies determined that the period of PCB intake ranged from 3 to 9 months. The average total intake for each person varied from 0.77 to 1.8 mg of PCB. Within the first year of the outbreak, the blood levels of PCB in 13 patients ranged from 3 ppb to 1,156 ppb. Most of the patients had blood levels between 11 and 150 ppb (μg/kg). The symptoms observed in these patients were quite similar to those already described for the patients in the 1968 Yusho outbreak in Japan.

The rice oil was not only contaminated with PCBs but also with PCDFs and polychlorinated quaterphenyls. It contained the same major components of PCDFs observed in the rice oil in Japan—namely, 2,3,4,6,7-PCDF and 2,3,4,7,8-PCDF. Relatively high concentrations of 2,3,4,5,3',4'-hexachlorobiphenyl were found in the blood and adipose tissue of the Yucheng patients. This particular PCB isomer is biologically quite active, and the concentration of 2,3,4,3'4'-pentachlorobiphenyl was also elevated in these patients. Furthermore, as in the Yusho patients, the concentration of 2,3,7,8-TCDF was comparatively low (92). Chen et al (94) analyzed additional samples of the oil, blood, and adipose tissue of the Yucheng patients. These investigators identified several TCDF and PCDF isomers. Apparently, 2,3,7,8-TCDF was only a minor component in the oil; the major component was 2,3,4,8-TCDF. One of the major furans in the toxic oil was 2,3,4,7,8-PCDF.

The concentrations of the PCDFs in different oil samples ranged from 0.21 to 1.68 ppm. Polychlorinated quaterphenyls were present in concentrations ranging from 25 to 53 ppm (mg/kg). Overall, the concentrations of PCDFs and PCQs were lower in these oil samples than in the oil samples that had caused the Yusho outbreak. Whether these oil samples were representative is not really known. The 3,4,3'4'-tetrachlorobiphenyl was also identified in the oil that caused Yucheng disease in Taiwan. This isomer is considered to be the most toxic PCB isomer present in commercial PCB preparations (95); it was present at a concentration of about 1%. Most other commercial PCB preparations, such as the Aroclors, in the United States have not been shown to contain this particular isomer.

In addition to the epidemiological studies, some disease-specific investigations were also conducted. The blood pressure of the Yucheng and Yusho patients was not affected (60). Although some of the patients in the Yusho cohort have died of cancer (90), the number has been small; because the latency period may be long, the population should be followed for a longer period to determine whether the cancer incidence will increase.

Although PCBs and related compounds are known to affect reproduction in animals, and although they affected some fetuses and neonates in the Yusho and Yucheng episodes, the information on reproduction and fetal toxicity in general is very limited. In one such study, Hara (96) examined women working in a capacitor plant who also nursed their infants and who themselves had mild chloracne and erythema of the skin. The human milk of some of these women contained, on a whole milk basis, PCB levels that ranged from below 50 ppb (μg/kg) to about 400 ppb (μg/kg). Forty children of these mothers were followed for a five-year period. Some children were found to have "decayed" nails, gingival pigmentation, mottled enamel, and dental caries. No relationships between these changes or symptoms to PCB blood levels, however, were observed. The general population in the United States and other countries also has body burdens of PCBs, PCDFs, and polychlorinated dibenzodioxins (97, 98). However, these background concentrations—particularly for the biologically active isomers—are far lower than they were in the Yusho and Yucheng patients, even several years after exposure.

Chang et al (99) examined the delayed immune response in 30 Yucheng patients and compared their responses with those of 50 controls. The mean age of patients in both groups was about 14 years. The authors injected a solution of streptokinase and streptodornase subcutaneously into the flexor side of the forearm. The response was read at 24 hours (hr) and again at 48 hr after injection. Eighty percent of the controls had an induration of 5 mm or more in diameter 24 or 48 hr after they were injected; only 43% of the exposed group responded similarly. All of the poisoned patients had dermal lesions, and the percentage of patients with a positive response decreased with increasing severity of the skin lesions (chloracne). Furthermore, the degree of the dermal lesions appeared to be associated with the whole blood PCB concentrations. Patients with minor skin lesions that were classified as grade 1 appeared to have a normal skin response. The same authors found that PCBs caused a decreased concentration of IgA and IgM, but not of IgG, in serum.

Furthermore, the percentages of total T cells, active T cells, and T mu cells decreased, whereas the percentage of B cells and T gamma cells were not affected (100). These two reports are the first in which the effect on the immune response was actually correlated with body burdens of PCBs and in which only severely poisoned patients showed this effect. This finding is consistent with the findings from animal studies in which relatively high doses of PCBs affected the immune response and also caused some other adverse effects.

In the Japanese and the Taiwanese Yusho and Yucheng poisoning outbreaks, sensory neuropathy was reported in a number of patients for whom nerve conduction velocities were measured (101, 102). The blood levels of the various chemicals (PCBs, PCDFs, PCQs) were negatively correlated with the lowered nerve conduction velocity, suggesting that these types of chemicals affect nerve conduction velocity. (It is not quite clear why most investigators measure nerve conduction velocity to detect sensory neuropathy. Other tests that would measure the detection of vibration, touch, and temperature would be more useful from a clinical perspective.)

Seppalainen et al (103) examined 16 men working in a cardboard plant who were exposed to fumes that resulted from the explosion of 15 capacitors containing Clophen A-30. The first PCB air concentrations, measured 5.5 hr after the explosion, were 8,000 to 16,000 $\mu g/m^3$ air. PCDFs were also formed. The soot samples contained tetrachlorodibenzofuran up to 90 $\mu g/g$, of which 6.5 $\mu g/g$ was 2,3,7,8-tetrachlorodibenzofuran. In addition, monochloropyrenes and dichloropyrenes were found. Most of the men had a transient sensory neuropathy in their lower extremities.

Chang et al (104) reported increased urinary δ-aminolevulinic acid uroporphyrin excretion in 69 Yucheng patients over that of 20 controls. No information on the patients' clinical conditions or on how these findings related to degree of exposure was given. No such observations have been reported from Japan.

POLYBROMINATED BIPHENYLS

Since the toxicity of PBBs both in laboratory animals and livestock was recently reviewed (105), we do not review it here in detail. In laboratory animals, PBBs generally cause effects similar to those that the PCBs cause. They produce morphological changes in the liver, affect reproduction, and promote biochemical changes, such as hepatic porphyria and induction of mixed-function oxidases. Teratogenic effects have also been noted. In addition, atrophy of the thymus has been reported, and hepatocellular carcinomas have been produced in both rats and mice. The overall findings reported in animal studies are similar to those that have been reported for PCBs.

Although the PCB contamination of the environment is a more general problem, the PBB contamination primarily affects certain areas within the state of Michigan. Most persons living within the lower peninsula of Michigan have had slight exposure, since the contamination resulted from dairy products and since normal marketing channels for these products involved the mixing of milk from many producers in relatively few processing facilities. In addition, most cull dairy cattle are used for hamburgers and processed meat products that would also receive wide distribution. Thus, the marketing system diluted the degree of exposure for the individual; however, it increased the number of those exposed. In 1978, the distribution of PBBs was comprehensively studied in a probability sample of 1,738 persons. PBB levels in serum were determined, and 844 adipose tissue samples were also analyzed for PBBs. PBBs were detected in 97.3% of the adipose tissue samples, in 68% of the adult serum samples, and in 72.7% of the serum samples from children. The mean PBB concentration in adipose tissue was 400 ppb (μg/kg); in serum it was 1.3 ppb (μg/kg) for adults and 1.8 ppb (μ/gkg) for children. The highest adipose tissue concentration was 37 ppm (mg/kg) (18). In additional studies, when cohorts of PBB-exposed residents of Michigan were compared with residents of the state of Wisconsin, a higher prevalence of a variety of symptoms and complaints was noted in the Michigan residents (106). Similarly, in comparative neurobehavioral studies, the Michigan population was found to be affected more than that in Wisconsin (107).

Since the findings were not correlated with body burdens of PBB in any of these studies, determining whether other factors may be responsible for these differences is difficult. In 1976, the Michigan Department of Public Health established a cohort of farmers who had been exposed to varying concentrations of PBBs in their products and their environment. A total of 3,877 persons were enrolled. They included farm residents, direct recipients of farm products, chemical workers and their families, and a few persons who had been originally studied in a smaller previous study.

The serum PBB levels in this entire group ranged from no detectable levels to 1,900 ppb (μg/l), with a mean of 21.2 ppb (μg/l) and a median of 3 ppb (μg/l). Because of the wide range of exposure and because results could be analyzed by regression analyses with exposure as a variable, a comparison group for acute health effects was not included. This cohort was found to have various symptoms and conditions; however, these symptoms did not correlate with PBB body burdens. Symptom prevalence rates were slightly higher in persons with no detectable PBBs in serum than in those with measurable quantities. In all groups, including chemical workers and quarantined farm residents, the highest prevalence rates were in persons with the lowest serum PBB levels (22).

Similarly, in this study and in a previous immunologic study (108) no dose-related depression of lymphocyte function in persons exposed to PBBs could be demonstrated. All these findings suggest that there may be no causal relationship between the abnormal lymphocyte functions observed in some persons or the prevalence of other symptoms and exposure to PBBs. This cohort of Michigan residents is still being followed by the Michigan Department of Health in collaboration with the Centers for Disease Control. Several studies of subgroups of this population and surveys for chronic health effects have been conducted since the cohort was first assembled (109, 19). When serum and adipose tissue concentrations were compared, a significant correlation was found. The serum:adipose tissue concentration ratios ranged from 1 to 140 to 1 to 260 for pregnant women and male chemical workers, respectively. Males from farms had a significantly different ratio of 1 to 325 to 329. Potential transplacental passage of PBBs was demonstrated, since they could also be found in the fetus and newborn. Cord blood contained one-tenth of the concentration found in the maternal serum, which indicated partial placental passage. Human milk contained PBBs at 107–119 times the quantity found in maternal serum. PBBs were also detected in bile and feces, which indicates that these materials can be transferred into the intestinal tract. All of these concentrations were measured long after the population had first been exposed to PBBs (19). Concentrations of PBBs observed in bile and feces were about one half to seven-tenths of the serum levels and are probably about 0.5% of the adipose tissue levels. These findings indicate that PBBs are very slowly excreted, which is consistent with the findings of Tuey & Matthews in rats (110). The estimated half-life for PBB is 6.5 years.

More recently, two groups of Michigan residents—those with high PBB serum levels and those with PBB serum levels around 1 ppb—were matched for age, sex, and smoking. For both groups, various clinical laboratory tests were conducted, blood pressure was measured, and height and weight were determined. In this study, 83 participants had PBB serum levels of 50 ppb (μg/l) or more. In the middle group, 83 had PBB levels of 5–49 ppb and 96 had PBB levels of 0–44 ppb (μg/l) in serum. Urinary porphyrins were also measured in all of the participants. Thus far, the final results of this study have not been reported. For most of the parameters studied—which included serum glucose, triglycerides, high-density lipoproteins, various liver functions, creatinine, uric acid, thyroid function, proteins, calcium and phosphorus in serum, and also measurement of various porphyrins—no differences of clinical significance were found among different groups (M. Barone, personal communication). (Note: Even though significantly more women in the high PBB group used birth-control pills than women in the low PBB group, too few were using them to affect urine porphyrin levels.) In none of a variety of other studies conducted on this population as well as other groups in Michigan did any findings indicate that exposure to PBB had impaired the health of the exposed group. All of these studies have been reviewed by Fries (105).

Although this population was exposed during a 9-month period in 1973 and 1974, whether it will have chronic health effects is unknown. This particular cohort needs to be followed for 30 to 40 years before the question of chronic health effects can be intelligently addressed. Two problems with assessing chronic health effects are that the cohort, in spite of its size, is still relatively small and that the amount of exposure it has received varied widely. Although some members of the group exposed to PBBs have relatively high body burdens, these burdens are still appreciably lower than those of rats in which liver cancer developed.

In the study by Kimbrough et al (111), liver cancer developed in the rats that received a dose of 1,000 mg/kg body weight. This dose for humans would roughly translate into a dose of 70 grams per person. These amounts are much greater than the estimated mean total exposure per person. The highest exposure was about 11.7 grams, and the mean was 170 mg per person. In rats given 200 mg/kg, a dose that for humans would be between 12 and 14 grams, only neoplastic nodules developed in their livers; there was no evidence of hepatocellular carcinomas. Of course, whether humans would be more or less susceptible to the toxic effects of PBBs and whether their response would be similar to that of rats is not known.

In conclusion, various toxic effects of PBBs and PCBs have been described in laboratory animals. In humans, acute poisoning outbreaks have only occurred following exposure to a combination of PCBs and PCDFs. When humans were exposed only to PCBs or PBBs, the only observed acute effects have generally been minor. So far, no significant chronic health effects have been causally associated with exposure to PCBs or PBBs.

Use of trade names is for identification only and does not constitute endorsement by the Public Health Service or the US Department of Health and Human Services.

Literature Cited

1. Jensen, S. 1966. Report of a new chemical hazard. *New Sci.* 32:612
2. 1982. Polychlorinated biphenyls (PCBs): manufacturing, processing, distribution in commerce, and use prohibitions: use in electrical equipment. *Fed. Regist.* 47:37342–60
3. 1982. Polychlorinated biphenyls (PCBs): manufacturing, processing, distribution in commerce, and use prohibitions: use in closed and controlled waste manufacturing processes. *Fed. Regist.* 47:46980–96
4. McLeod, K. E. 1981. Polychlorinated biphenyls in indoor air. *Environ. Sci. Technol.* 15:926–28
5. Kutz, F. W., Yang, H. S. C. 1976. A note on polychlorinated biphenyls in air. In *Proc. Natl. Conf. Polychlorinated Biphenyls, Chicago, 1975,* EPA-560/6-75-004, p. 182. Washington, DC: Environ. Prot. Agency
6. Cordle, F., Locke, R., Springer, J. 1982. Determination of human risk in regulating polychlorinated biphenyls (PCBs)—a case study. *CRC Toxicol. Risk Assess.* 2:211–25
7. Cordle, F., Locke, R., Springer, J. 1982. Risk assessment in a federal regulatory agency: an assessment of risk associated with the human consumption of some species of fish contaminated with polychlorinated biphenyls (PCBs). *Environ. Health Perspect.* 45:171–82

8. Sullivan, J. R., Delfino, J. J., Buelow, C. R., Sheffy, T. B. 1983. Polychlorinated biphenyls in the fish and sediment of the Lower Fox River, Wisconsin. *Bull. Environ. Contam. Toxicol.* 30:58–64

9. Schwartz, P. M., Jacobson, S. W., Fein, G. G., Jacobson, J. L., Price, H. A. 1983. Lake Michigan fish consumption as a source of polychlorinated biphenyls in human cord serum, maternal serum, and milk. *Am. J. Public Health* 73:293–96

10. Tatsukawa, R. 1976. PCB pollution of the Japanese environment. In *PCB Poisoning and Pollution*, ed. K. Higuchi, pp. 147–79. Tokyo: Kodansha

11. Morita, M., Nakagawa, J., Rappe, C. 1978. Polychlorinated dibenzofuran (PCDF) formation from PCB mixture by heat and oxygen. *Bull. Environ. Contam. Toxicol.* 19:665–70

12. O'Keefe, P. W., Silkworth, J. B., Gierthy, J. F., Smith, R. M., DeCaprio, A. P., et al. 1985. Chemical and biological investigations of a transformer accident at Binghamton, New York. *Environ. Health Perspect.* 60:201–9

13. Hutzinger, O., Ghulam, G. C., Brock, G. C., Johnston, L. E. 1985. Formation of polychlorinated dibenzofurans and dioxins during combustion, electrical equipment fires and PCB incineration. *Environ. Health Perspect.* 60:3–9

14. Carter, L. 1976. Michigan PBB incident. Chemical mix-up leads to disaster. *Science* 192:240–43

15. Willett, L. B., Liu, T. T. Y., Durst, H. I., Cardwell, B. D., Renkie, E. D. 1985. Quantification and distribution of polychlorinated biphenyls in farm silos. *Bull. Environ. Contam. Toxicol.* 35:51–60

16. Kimbrough, R. D. 1985. Laboratory and human studies on polychlorinated biphenyls (PCBs) and related compounds. *Environ. Health Perspect.* 59:99–106

17. Smith, A. B., Schloemer, J., Lowry, L. K., Smallwood, A. W., Ligo, R. N., et al. 1982. Metabolic and health consequences of occupational exposure to polychlorinated biphenyls (PCBs). *Br. J. Ind. Med.* 39:361–69

18. Wolff, M. S., Anderson, H. A., Selikoff, J. J. 1982. Human tissue burdens of halogenated aromatic chemicals in Michigan. *J. Am. Med. Assoc.* 247:2112–16

19. Eyster, J. T., Humphrey, H. E. B., Kimbrough, R. D. 1983. Partitioning of polybrominated biphenyls (PBB) in serum, adipose tissue, breast milk, placenta, cord blood, biliary fluid and feces. *Arch. Environ. Health* 38:47–53

20. Jensen, A. A. 1983. Chemical contaminants in human milk. *Residue Rev.* 89:1–128

21. Jensen, R. G., Clark, R. M., Ferris, A. M. 1980. Composition of the lipids in human milk, a review. *Lipids* 15:345–55

22. Landrigan, P. J., Wilcox, K. R. Jr., Silva, J. Jr., Humphrey, H. E. B., Kauffman, C., Heath, C. W. Jr. 1979. Cohort study of Michigan residents exposed to polybrominated biphenyls: epidemiologic and immunologic findings. *Ann. N. Y. Acad. Sci.* 320:284–94

23. Kuratsune, M., Yoshimura, T., Matsuzaka, J., Yamaguchi, A. 1972. Epidemiologic study on Yusho, a poisoning caused by ingestion of rice oil contaminated with a commercial brand of polychlorinated biphenyls. *Environ. Health Perspect. Exp.* No. 1:119–28

24. Yoshimura, T., Hayabuchi, H. 1985. Relationship between amount of rice oil ingested by patients with Yusho and their subjective symptoms. *Environ. Health Perspect.* 59:47–51

25. Kimbrough, R. D., Buckley, J., Fishbein, L., Flamm, G., Kasza, L., et al. 1978. Animal toxicology. *Environ. Health Perspect.* 24:173–85

26. Vos, J. G., Faith, R. E., Luster, M. I. 1980. Immune alterations. In *Halogenated Biphenyls, Terphenyls, Naphthalenes, Dibenzodioxins and Related Compounds. Topics in Environmental Health*. ed. R. D. Kimbrough, 4:241–58 Amsterdam: Elsevier Biomedical Bio.

27. Linder, R. E., Gaines, T. B., Kimbrough, R. D. 1974. The effect of polychlorinated biphenyls on rat reproduction. *Food Cosmet. Toxicol.* 12:63–77

28. McNulty, W. P., Becker, G. M., Cory, H. T. 1980. Chronic toxicity of 3,4,3'4'- and 2,5,2',5'-tetrachlorobiphenyls in rhesus macaques. *Toxicol. Appl. Pharmacol.* 56(2):182–90

29. Matthews, H. B., Anderson, M. W. 1975. Effect of chlorination on the distribution and excretion of polychlorinated biphenyls. *Drug. Metab. Dispos.* 3:371–80

30. Matthews, H. B., Kato, S. 1979. The metabolism and disposition of halogenated aromatics. *Ann. N. Y. Acad. Sci.* 320:131–38

31. Parkinson, A., Robertson, L., Uhlig, L., Campbell, M. A., Safe, S. 1982. 2,3,4,4',5-Pentachlorobiphenyl: differ-

ential effects on C57BL/6J and DBA/2J inbred mice. *Biochem. Pharmacol.* 31:2830–33

32. Poland, A., Glover, E. 1977. Chlorinated biphenyl induction of arylhydrocarbon hydroxylase activity: a study of structure activity relationship. *Mol. Pharmacol.* 13:924–38

33. Schaeffer, E., Greim, H., Goessner, W. 1984. Pathology of chronic polychlorinated biphenyl (PCB) feeding in rats. *Toxicol. Appl. Pharmacol.* 75:278–288

34. Norback, D. H., Weltman, R. H. 1985. Polychlorinated biphenyl induction of hepatocellular carcinoma in the Sprague-Dawley rat. *Environ. Health Perspect.* 60:97–105

35. Kimbrough, R. D., Squire, R. A., Linder, R. E., Strandberg, J. D., Montali, R. J., Burse, V. W. 1975. Induction of liver tumors in Sherman strain rats by polychlorinated biphenyl Aroclor 1260. *J. Natl. Cancer Inst.* 55:1453–59

36. National Cancer Institute. 1977. Bioassay of Aroclor (trademark) 1254 for possible carcinogenicity. Springfield, VA: Natl. Tech. Inf. Serv. as PB-279 624/IGA, NCI-CG TR-38. Chem. Abstr. Serv. No. 27323-18-8. DHEW Publ. NIH-78-838

37. Ward, J. M. 1985. Proliferative lesions of the glandular stomach and liver in F 344 rats fed diets containing Aroclor 1254. *Environ. Health Perspect.* 60:89–96

38. Morgan, R. W., Ward, J. M., Hartmann, P. E. 1981. Aroclor 1254 induced intestinal metaplasia and adenocarcinoma in the glandular stomach of F344 rats. *Cancer Res.* 41:5052–59

39. Safe, S., Bandiera, S., Sawyer, T., Robertson, L., Safe, L., et al. 1985. PCB: structure-function relationships and mechanism of action. *Environ. Health Perspect.* 60:47–56

40. McConnell, E. E. 1980. See Ref. 26, pp. 109–90

41. McNulty, W. P. 1985. Toxicity and fetotoxicity of TCDD, TCDF, and PCB isomers in rhesus macaques *(Macaca mulatta). Environ. Health Perspect.* 60:77–88

42. Thunberg, T. 1984. Effect of TCDD on vitamin A and its relation to TCDD toxicity. *Banbury Rep. 18: Biol. Mech. Dioxin Action.* New York: Cold Spring Harbor Lab

43. Brouwer, A., Van den Berg, K. J., Kukler, A. 1985. Time and dose responses of the reduction in retinoid concentrations in C57B1/Rij and DBA/2 mice induced by 3,4,3'4'-tetrachlorobi-

phenyl. *Toxicol. Appl. Pharmacol.* 78: 180–89

44. Kutz, F. W., Strassman, S. C. 1976. Residues of polychlorinated biphenyls in the general population of the United States. See Ref. 5, pp. 139–48

45. Juskiewicz, T., Niewiadowska, A., Radomanski, T. 1977. Polychlorinated biphenyl residues in human adipose tissue. *Pol. Tyg. Lek.* 32:173–175

46. Kreiss, K. 1985. Studies on populations exposed to polychlorinated biphenyls. *Environ. Health Perspect.* 60:193–199

47. Mes, J., Davies, D. J., Turton, D. 1982. Polychlorinated biphenyl and other chlorinated hydrocarbon residues in adipose tissue of Canadians. *Bull. Environ. Contam. Toxicol.* 28:97–104

48. Sahl, J. D., Crocker, T., Gordon, R. J., Faeder, E. J. 1985. Polychlorinated biphenyls in the blood of personnel from an electric utility. *J. Occup. Med.* 27:639–43

49. Unger, M., Olsen, J. 1980. Organochlorine compounds in the adipose tissue of deceased people with and without cancer. *Environ. Res.* 23:257–63

50. Unger, M., Olsen, J., Clausen, J. 1982. Organochlorine compounds in the adipose tissue of deceased persons with and without cancer: a statistical survey of some potential confounders. *Environ. Res.* 29:371–76

51. Unger, M., Kiaer, H., Blichert-Toft, M., Olsen, J., Clausen, J. 1984. Organochlorine compounds in human breast fat from deceased with and without breast cancer and in a biopsy material from newly diagnosed patients undergoing breast surgery. *Environ. Res.* 34:24–28

52. Lawton, R. W., Brown, J. F., Ross, M. R., Feingold, J. 1985. Comparability and precision of serum PCB measurements. *Arch. Environ. Health* 40:29–37

53. Kreiss, K., Zack, M., Kimbrough, R. D., Needham, L. L., Smrek, A. L., Jones, B. T. 1981. Cross-sectional study of a community with exceptional exposure to DDT. *J. Am. Med. Assoc.* 245:1926–30

54. National Center for Health Statistics. 1978. Blood pressure levels of persons 6–74 years, US, 1971–1974. HRS 78-1648, series 11, No. 203. Hyattsville, Md, Natl. Cent. Health Stat., DHEW

55. Kreiss, K., Zack, M., Kimbrough, R. D., Needham, L. L., Smrek, A. L., Jones, B. T. 1981. Association of blood pressure and polychlorinated biphenyl levels. *J. Am. Med. Assoc.* 245:2505–9

56. Kutz, F. W., Yobs, A. R., Strassman, S. C., Viar, J. F. 1977. Effects of reducing DDT usage on total DDT storage in humans. *Pestic. Monit. J.* 11:61–63
57. Davies, J. E., Edmundson, W. F., Raffonelli, A., et al. 1972. The role of social class in human pesticide pollution. *Am. J. Epidemiol.* 96:334–41
58. Lawton, R. W., Ross, M. R., Feingold, J., Brown, J. F. 1985. Effects of PCB exposure on biochemical and hematological findings in capacitor workers. *Environ. Health Perspect.* 60:165–84
59. Chase, K. H., Wong, O., Thomas, D., Stal, B. W., Berney, B. W., Simon, R. K. 1982. Clinical and metabolic abnormalities associated with occupational exposure to polychlorinated biphenyls. *J. Occup. Med.* 24:109–14
60. Akagi, K., Okumura, M. 1985. Association of blood pressure and PCB level in Yusho patients. *Environ. Health Perspect.* 59:37–39
61. Brown, J. F. Jr. 1984. Polychlorinated biphenyl (PCB) partitioning between adipose tissue and serum. *Bull. Environ. Contam. Toxicol.* 33:277–80
62. Emmett, E. A. 1985. Polychlorinated biphenyl exposure and effects in transformer repair workers. *Environ. Health Perspect.* 60:185–92
63. Humphrey, H. E. B., Price, H. A., Budd, M. I. 1976. Evaluation of changes of the level of polychlorinated biphenyls (PCB) in human tissue. *Final Rep. FDA Contract No. 223-73-2209.* Washington, DC: DHEW, FDA
64. Baker, E. L. Jr., Landrigan, P. J., Glueck, C. J., Zack, M. M. Jr., Liddle, J. A., et al. 1980. Metabolic consequences of exposure to polychlorinated biphenyls in sewage sludge. *Am. J. Epidemiol.* 112:553–63
65. Warshaw, R., Fishbein, A., Thornton, J., Miller, A., Selikoff, I. J. 1979. Decrease in vital capacity in PCB exposed workers in a capacitor manufacturing facility. *Ann. N. Y. Acad. Sci.* 320:277–83
66. Sak, M., Ahlers, I. 1977. Serum lipid changes under conditions of occupational exposure to chlorinated biphenyls. *Cesk. Dermatol.* 52:62–65
67. Kimbrough, R. D. 1980. Occupational exposure. See Ref. 26, pp. 373–97
68. Jones, J. W., Alden, H. S. 1936. An acneform dermatergosis. *Arch. Dermatol. Syphilol.* 33:1022–34
69. National Institute for Occupational Safety and Health (NIOSH). 1977. Criteria for a recommended standard. Occupational exposure to polychlorinated biphenyls (PCBs). Washington, DC: Superintendent of Documents, US Govt. Printing Office. USDHEW (NIOSH) Publ. No. 77-225
70. Meigs, J. W., Albom, J. J., Kartin, B. I. 1954. Chloracne from an unusual exposure to Arochlor. *J. Am. Med. Assoc.* 154:1417–18
71. Ouw, H. K., Simpson, G. R., Siyali, D. S. 1976. Use and health effects of Aroclor 1242, a polychlorinated biphenyl in an electrical industry. *Arch. Environ. Health* 31:189–94
72. Alvares, A. P., Fischbein, A., Anderson, K. E., Kappas, A. 1977. Alterations in drug metabolism in workers exposed to polychlorinated biphenyls. *Clin. Pharmacol. Ther.* 22:140–46
73. Taylor, P. R., Lawrence, C. L., Hwang, H. L., Patterson, A. S. 1984. Polychlorinated biphenyls influence on birthweight and gestation. *Am. J. Public Health* 74:1153–54
74. Jacobson, J. L., Jacobson, S. W., Schwartz, P. M., Fein, G. G., Dowler, J. K. 1984. Prenatal exposure to an environmental toxin: a test of the multiple effects model. *Dev. Psychol.* 20:523–32
75. Fein, G. G., Jacobson, J. L., Jacobson, S. W., Schwartz, P. M., Dowler, J. K. 1984. Prenatal exposure to polychlorinated biphenyls: effects on birth size and gestational age. *J. Pediatr.* 102:315–20
76. Jacobson, S. W., Jacobson, J. L., Schwartz, P. M., Fein, G. G. 1983. Intrauterine exposure of human newborns to PCBs: measures of exposure. In *PCBs: Human and Environmental Hazards.* ed. F. M. D'Itri, M. Kamrin, pp. 311–43. Boston: Butterworth
77. Rogan, W., Gladen, B. 1982. Duration of breast-feeding and environmental contaminants in milk. *Am. J. Epidemiol.* 116:565A
78. Rogan, W. J., Gladen, B. C., McKinney, J. D., Carreras, N., Hardy, P., et al. 1986. Polychlorinated biphenyls (PCBs) and dichlorodiphenyl dichloroethene (DDE) in human milk: effects of maternal factors and previous lactation. *Am. J. Public Health* 76:172–77
79. Gellert, R. J., Heinrichs, W. L., Swerdloff, R. S. 1972. DDT homologs. Estrogen-like effects on the vagina, uterus, and puberty of the rat. *Endocrinology* 91:1095–100
80. Bahn, A. K., Rosenwaike, I., Herrmann, N., Grover, P., Stellman, J., O'Leary, K. 1976. Melanoma after exposure to PCB. *N. Engl. J. Med.* 295:450

81. Brown, D. P., Jones, M. 1981. Mortality and industrial hygiene study of workers exposed to polychlorinated biphenyls. *Arch. Environ. Health* 36: 120–29

82. Brown, D. P. 1986. Mortality of workers exposed to polychlorinated biphenyls—an update. *Arch. Environ. Health* In press

83. Bertazzi, P. A., Zocchetti, C., Guercilena, S., Foglia, M. D., Pesatori, A., Ribaldi, L. 1981. Mortality study of male and female workers exposed to PCBs. Presented at *Int. Symp. Prev. Occup. Cancer, Helsinki*

84. Kuratsune, M., Morikawa, Y., Hirohata, T., Nishizumi, M., Kohchi, S., et al. 1969. An epidemiologic study on Yusho or chlorobiphenyls poisoning. *Fukuoka Acta Med.* 60:513–32 (In Japanese)

85. Miyata, H., Kashimoto, T., Kunita N. 1977. Detection and determination of polychlorinated dibenzofurans in normal human tissues and Kanemi rice oil caused Kanemi Yusho. *J. Food Hyg. Soc.* 18:260–65

86. Buser, H. R., Rappe, C., Gara, A. 1978. Polychlorinated dibenzofurans (PCDFs) found in Yusho oil and in used Japanese PCB. *Chemosphere* 5:439–49

87. Miyata, H., Kashimoto, T. 1978. Studies on the compounds related to PCB (IV). Investigation on polychlorodibenzofuran formation. *J. Food Hyg. Soc.* 19:78–84 (In Japanese)

88. Kamps, L. V. R., Trotter, W. J., Young, S. J., Carson, I. J., Roach, J. A. G., et al. 1978. Polychlorinated quaterphenyls identified in rice oil associated with Japanese 'Yusho' poisoning. *Bull. Environ. Contam. Toxicol.* 20:589–91

89. Kuratsune, M. 1980. Yusho. See Ref. 26, pp. 287–302

90. Kikuchi, M. 1984. Autopsy of patients with Yusho. *Am. J. Ind. Med.* 5:19–30

91. Urabe, H., Asahi, M. 1985. Past and current dermatological status of Yusho patients. *Environ. Health Perspect.* 59:11–15

92. Masuda, Y. 1985. Health status of Japanese and Taiwanese after exposure to contaminated rice oil. *Environ. Health Perspect.* 60:321–25

93. Hsu, S. T., Mac, I., Hsu S., K-H., Wu, S-S, Hsu, NH-M, Yeh, C-C, Wu, S-B. 1985. Discovery and epidemiology of PCB poisoning in Taiwan: a four-year follow-up. *Environ. Health Perspect.* 30:5–10

94. Chen, P. H., Wong, C. K., Rappe, C., Nygren, M. 1985. Polychlorinated biphenyls, dibenzofurans and quaterphenyls in toxic rice-bran oil and in the blood and tissues of patients with PCB poisoning (Yu-Cheng) in Taiwan. *Environ. Health Perspect.* 59:59–65

95. Abdel-Hamid, F. M., Moore, J. A., Matthews, H. B. 1981. Comparative study of 3,4,3',4' tetrachlorobiphenyl in male and female rats and female monkeys. *J. Toxicol. Environ. Health* 7:181–91

96. Hara, T. 1985. Health status and PCBs in blood of workers exposed to PCBs and of their children. *Environ. Health Perspect.* 59:85–90

97. Rappe, C., Bergqvist, P. A., Hansson, M., Lars-Owe, K., Lindström, G., et al. 1984. Chemistry and analysis of polychlorinated dioxins and dibenzofurans in biological samples. *Banbury Report 18: Biological mechanisms of dioxin action.* Cold Spring Harbor Laboratory 17–25

98. Schecter, A., Schaffner, F., Tiernan, T., Taylor, M. 1984. Ultrastructural alterations of liver mitochondria in response to dioxins, furans, PCBs, and biphenylenes. See Ref. 42, pp. 177–90

99. Chang, K. J., Hsieh, K. H., Tang, S. Y., Tung, T. C. 1982. Immunologic evaluation of patients with polychlorinated biphenyl poisoning: evaluation of delayed-type skin hypersensitive response and its relation to clinical studies. *J. Toxicol. Environ. Health* 9:217–23

100. Chang, K. J., Hsieh, K. H., Lee, T. P., Tang, S. Y., Tung, T. C. 1981. Immunologic evaluation of patients with polychlorinated biphenyl poisoning: determination of lymphocyte subpopulations. *Toxicol. Appl. Pharmacol.* 61(1):58–63

101. Chen, R. C., Tang, S. Y., Miyata, H., Kashimoto, T., Chang, Y. C., et al. 1985. Polychlorinated biphenyl poisoning: correlation of sensory and motor nerve conduction, neurologic symptoms, and blood levels of polychlorinated biphenyls, quarterphenyls, and dibenzofurans. *Environ. Res.* 37, 340–48

102. Murai, Y., Kuroiwa, Y. 1971. Peripheral neuropathy in chlorobiphenyls poisoning. *Neurology* 21:1173–76

103. Seppalainen, A. M., Vuojolahti, P., Elo, O. 1985. Reversible nerve lesions after accidental polychlorinated biphenyl exposure. *Scand J. Work Environ. Health* 11:91–95

104. Chang, K. J., Lu, F. J., Tung, T. C., Lee, T. P. 1980. Studies on patients with polychlorinated biphenyl poisoning. 2. Determination of urinary coproporphyrin, uroporphyrin, delta-aminolevulinic acid and porphobilinogen.

Res. Commun. Chem. Pathol. Pharmacol. 30(3):547–54
105. Fries, G. 1985. The PBB episode in Michigan: an overall appraisal. *CRC Crit. Rev. Toxicol.* 16:105–56
106. Anderson, H. A., Lillis, R., Selifkoff, J. J., Rosenman, K. D., Valciukas, J. A., et al. 1978. Unanticipated prevalence of symptoms among dairy farmers in Michigan and Wisconsin. *Environ. Health Perspect.* 23:217–26
107. Valciukas, J. A., Lillis, R., Wolff, M. S., Anderson, H. A. 1978. Comparative neurobehavioral study of a polybrominated biphenyl-exposed population in Michigan and a nonexposed group in Wisconsin. *Environ. Health Perspect.* 23:199–210
108. Bekesi, J. G., Holland, J. F., Anderson, H. A., Fischbein, A. S., Rom, W., et al. 1978. Lymphocyte function of Michigan dairy farmers exposed to polybrominated biphenyls. *Science* 199:1207–9
109. Kreiss, K., Roberts, C., Humphrey, H. E. B. 1982. Serial PBB levels, PCB levels, and clinical chemistries in Michigan's PBB cohort. *Arch. Environ. Health* 37(3):141–47
110. Tuey, D. B., Matthews, H. B. 1980. Distribution and excretion of 2,2',4,4',5,5' hexabromobiphenyl in rats and man: pharmacokinetic model predictions. *Toxicol. Appl. Pharmacol.* 53(3):420–31
111. Kimbrough, R. D., Groce, D. F., Korver, M. P., Burse, V. W. 1981. Induction of liver tumors in female Sherman strain rats by polybrominated biphenyls. *J. Natl. Cancer Inst.* 66:535–42

Ann. Rev. Pharmacol. Toxicol. 1987. 27:113–36

DRUGS AFFECTING MOVEMENT DISORDERS

Giuseppe Campanella[1], Madeleine Roy, and André Barbeau

Department of Neurobiology, Clinical Research Institute of Montreal, Montreal, Quebec, Canada H2W 1R7

INTRODUCTION

In 1974 Barbeau (1) reviewed drugs affecting movements disorders in this journal. This review updates the previous one, covering the considerable expansion of pharmacological tools for studying these disorders in the last few years. Unfortunately, Dr. Barbeau was only able to draw the outline for this article before his premature death. We hope that the completed version reflects his extraordinary experience and skill in the treatment of movement disorders.

In the previous review Barbeau (1) defined "movement disorders," a term that could include most, if not all, neurological diseases. Currently, movement disorders are defined as the so-called extrapyramidal diseases in which either the exclusive, the primary, or the essential lesion is located in the basal ganglia. We refer the reader to the 1974 article for more discussion of these introductory remarks. That review centered on the main extrapyramidal symptoms: akinesia, tremor, rigidity, and dyskinesias. In this review we report the considerable number of new drugs according to the main clinical disorders: Parkinson's disease, dystonic syndromes, Huntington's disease, Wilson's disease, and Gilles de la Tourette's disease. In fact, although drugs for movement disorders are mainly symptom specific, some drugs display a disease-specific dose and treatment pattern. This pattern occurs, for example, with anticholinergic drugs in Parkinson's disease and dystonic syndromes. Furthermore, levodopa (L-DOPA), which in the early 1970s was used on a symptom-based rationale (2) to treat several extrapyramidal disorders with

---

[1]On leave from the Department of Neurology, Second School of Medicine, University of Naples, Naples, Italy.

0362-1642/87/0415-0113$02.00

different results, is today used almost exclusively for treating Parkinson's disease. To avoid repetition, general considerations of each drug are reported only the first time it is mentioned.

PARKINSON'S DISEASE

Since L-DOPA was introduced in the treatment of Parkinson's disease (PD) we have gradually reached an understanding of both its mechanism of action and the consequences of its long-term use. More recently other dopamine agonists, particularly ergot derivatives, have considerably increased our therapeutic arsenal. At present, the treatment of PD results from careful evaluations of the following aspects: (a) the type of PD syndrome (akineto rigid, tremor dominant, balanced); (b) the stage of the illness (early, intermediate, advanced); (c) the patient's age (onset may range from the mid-twenties to late old age); and (d) the individual response to the different drugs. Conflicting points of view remain concerning the implications of the stage of the illness and patient's age in PD treatment. We cannot provide a detailed examination of these clinical problems here and refer the reader to a recent paper for a review of this topic (3). However, we emphasize that the increased number of drugs for treating PD has also increased the need for the physician to possess a thorough knowledge of their properties, side effects, and interactions. Achieving good therapeutic results with as few adverse effects as possible is today a fairly complex procedure that requires enduring and skillful care. Patients with PD must be regularly followed as outpatients throughout their illness, at two–six month intervals according to the treatment phase. On one hand, the neurologist must modify the pharmacological regimen when necessary, but on the other hand he must sometimes counteract the attraction of some patients for frequent drug changes and therapeutical novelties.

We now describe the different drugs for PD.

Levodopa

Barbeau reported much about L-DOPA in the previous review (1). After 13 years L-DOPA is still the most useful and effective treatment for PD, although several important side effects of its long-term administration are now recognized. At present L-DOPA is most often given in a combined form, i.e. with a peripheral decarboxylase inhibitor (PDI) that increases its availability in brain tissue. The term "peripheral" indicates that the commonly used dose of PDI is effective on dopa-decarboxylase of peripheral tissues, mainly the small intestine. PDI does not, at that dose, affect brain capillary decarboxylase, i.e. the enzymatic blood-brain barrier (4–6). The two PDIs currently available in commercial preparations are benserazide and carbidopa, the former in a 1:4

ratio, the latter in 1:4 and 1:10 ratios, to L-DOPA. The clinical efficacy of L-DOPA plus benserazide and L-DOPA plus carbidopa does not differ significantly, except in individual cases (7, 8). The combined administration of L-DOPA plus a PDI eliminates or greatly reduces the peripheral side effects of L-DOPA, but does not change the central, i.e. neurological and psychiatric, side effects. The 1:4 ratio of a PDI to L-DOPA reduces peripheral side effects more effectively than 1:10 ratio (8, 9).

We discuss next some important aspects of the treatment with L-DOPA.

FACTORS INFLUENCING BRAIN AVAILABILITY OF L-DOPA   Many factors influence L-DOPA bioavailability in brain tissue. Several studies demonstrate that plasma levels of L-DOPA and modification of parkinsonian symptoms are correlated (10, 11). "Off" fluctuations and episodic unresponsiveness are related to low plasma levels of L-DOPA (10, 12). Therefore, absorption from the gut and plasma levels of L-DOPA appear very important in the clinical fluctuations during L-DOPA therapy of parkinsonian patients. The following factors reduce the gut absorption and/or availability of L-DOPA in the brain: (*a*) several aromatic and branched amino acids from dietary proteins (i.e. protein-rich meals) compete with L-DOPA for the transport carrier system at two subsequent levels, the intestinal mucosa and the brain capillary endothelial cells (13–16); (*b*) some factors reducing gastric emptying time, such as meals, anticholinergic drugs, dopamine agonists, and antidepressants with anticholinergic properties, increase the gastric absorption of L-DOPA (17, 18); (*c*) an increase of gastric acidity also increases absorption of L-DOPA (16); (*d*) physical exercise in patients who are still active reduces mesenteric blood flow and, consequently, the intestinal absorption of the drug (19); and (*e*) 3-O-methyldopa, a metabolite formed from L-DOPA by catechol-O-methyl-transferase, competes with L-DOPA for brain uptake and can also inhibit L-DOPA metabolism in rat brain (20, 21). Parkinsonian "nonresponders" have high plasma levels of 3-*O*-methyldopa (22), which are not modified by addition of a PDI (6).

The following factors increase the absorption and/or availability of L-DOPA: (*a*) a carbohydrate-rich meal reduces the plasma concentration of branched chain amino acids, indirectly favoring the uptake of aromatic amino acids such as L-DOPA by the brain (23); (*b*) metoclopramide, a neuroleptic drug used to improve gastro-intestinal motility, enhances gastric emptying increasing intestinal absorption of L-DOPA (24). However metoclopramide, because of its central action, is also a parkinsongenic drug (25); and (*c*) gastrectomy favors the intestinal absorption of L-DOPA (26, 27).

EFFECT OF LEVODOPA ON THE NATURAL COURSE OF THE DISEASE   In the years after its introduction as a substitution therapy for PD, it was unclear whether L-DOPA could affect the natural course of the disease. Subsequently, some aspects of this question have been well documented. First, disease progression after the initial clinical improvement with the drug is similar to that observed before the initiation of treatment, suggesting that L-DOPA does not interfere with the natural course of the disease (28, 29). Second, overall clinical improvement declines slowly over several years of treatment, with an increasing sensitivity to the drug. Daily dosage must be reduced and/or subdivided and redistributed over 24 hours (28, 30). Similarly, length of clinical effect after a single dose gradually decreases with later onset ("start-up" periods; 31) and earlier ending ("wearing-off" phenomenon; 32). Also, daily fluctuations in clinical improvement can be managed by i.v. infusion of L-DOPA (33). Finally, L-DOPA increases the life span of patients with PD, giving them a greater resistance to intercurrent illnesses (29, 30).

Another point is still widely discussed. After several years of treatment some psychiatric symptoms appear, such as dementia, psychosis, and a psychiatric symptom complex heralded by sleep disruption (34). These symptoms were relatively rare before L-DOPA was used. Whether these symptoms belong to the natural course of the disease (disclosed by the increased life span) or are caused by L-DOPA is unclear. The answer probably lies midway between these two possibilities. The symptoms are probably triggered by a dopaminergic overactivity on a background of advanced neuronal degeneration. This problem is one aspect of the "long-term Levodopa syndrome" we discuss below.

THE LONG-TERM LEVODOPA SYNDROME   After a variable period in which clinical results are evident with or without peripheral side effects, the parkinsonian patient treated with L-DOPA begins to experience "central" side effects, in particular abnormal involuntary movements (AIM's; 35). AIM's are mainly of choreic and dystonic type, but athetotic and ballic dyskinesias can also be observed (30). According to their time of occurrence they can be divided in two main groups, peak-dose dyskinesia and diphasic, or onset and end-of-dose, dyskinesia. The relationship with plasma levels of L-DOPA is evident: peak-dose dyskinesia occurs in close relation with L-DOPA peak in plasma, diphasic dyskinesia occurs at the beginning and at the end of the therapeutic effect when plasma level of L-DOPA is within a critical range either before or after the peak. An increased striatal homovanillic acid/dopamine ratio (HVA/DA) indicates that in PD patients treated with L-DOPA the remaining nigrostriatal neurons are overactive (36). Klawans et al (37) proposed that the development of AIM's is dependent on supersensitivity of the striatal DA receptors. However, in untreated parkinsonian patients the density of D_2 receptors in the striatum is increased, and treatment with L-DOPA reverses this pattern (38, 39). Agid et al (40) pointed out that a decrease of presynaptic autoreceptors might mask a high density of postsynaptic receptors. Therefore, the possibility that AIM's depend on a supersensitivity of striatal DA receptors is not ruled out. Agid et al (40) proposed that diphasic dyskinesias are explained by the activation of one type of supersensitive DA receptor with a high affinity for L-DOPA. In this case AIM's would cease when another type of receptor with a low affinity inhibited the high-affinity receptors. AIM's seem to occur more frequently in young patients; these AIM's include a disabling akineto-rigid variant of PD and a high degree of initial improvement with L-DOPA (33). Another type of AIM, early morning dystonia, which occurs late in the long-term L-DOPA syndrome, is not related to plasma peak of L-DOPA and probably has a different pathogenesis (41).

AIM's are closely correlated with fluctuations or oscillations in performance. At the beginning of treatment with L-DOPA the patient often experiences an even level of improvement during the whole day. Later, parkinsonian symptoms reappear between two consecutive doses (wearing-off phenomenon and start-up delay) with increasingly clear-cut limits. These oscillations in performance are commonly called on-off phenomena, but this term was originally used to indicate a particular type of oscillation[2]. We prefer the term *wearing-off* as a general, comprehensive designation. When wearing-off begins to appear, AIM's may still be absent or if present, they appear briefly in a randomized fashion during "well" periods. In an advanced stage, AIM's start and end in close relation to the reduced length of "well" periods.

Oscillations in performance are considered as a function of the pharmacokinetics of L-DOPA. In fact, i.v. infusion of L-DOPA greatly reduces or abolishes oscillations (33). However, an additional mechanism might play a role. Experimental data in animals show that apomorphine and L-DOPA have a dual effect, i.e. low doses decrease, and high doses increase, motor activity (45). L-DOPA may have a similar effect in patients with PD, thus enhancing "off" periods when its level in plasma is not high enough to improve the patient's condition. To counter their oscillations in performance, some patients become L-DOPA abusers, taking high daily doses of the drug in spite of severe AIM's (46).

MANAGEMENT OF THE LONG-TERM LEVODOPA SYNDROME   We already mentioned that a useful way to manage both AIM's and oscillations in performance is fractionating, redistributing, and eventual reducing L-DOPA

[2]Dr. Barbeau described the on-and-off phenomenon as characterized by a rapid changeover from the free to the rigid condition, or the inverse changeover. He described also another phenomenon called hypotonic freezing or akinesia paradoxica. These changes occur in a continuous flow of fluctuations during chronic L-DOPA treatment. Barbeau summarized those changes in four graphs (1, 30, 32, 42–44). For these and his other contributions to our knowledge of the "long-term Levodopa syndrome," we would like to suggest that Dr. Barbeau's name be attached to it: *Barbeau's syndrome*.

daily dosage. In some patients small doses every two hours, sometimes even during the night, are helpful. However, in our experience the best treatment is prevention: low doses of L-DOPA must generally be administered from the beginning of treatment. These doses should rarely exceed 600 mg of L-DOPA and 150 mg of PDI per day. If the improvement is not sufficient, other drugs can be added (see next sections). A similar preventive stategy may be used to avoid some psychiatric side effects. In general, sleep disrupted by vivid dreams, nightmares, and night terrors precedes the onset of hallucinations. The patient maintains a clear sensorium and remains critical of his hallucinations (hallucinosis). In the following stage it is possible to observe a delusion of paranoid type, in some instances accompanied by a confusional state (47). When such a progression is becoming evident, it is worthwhile to reduce or withdraw drugs in the therapeutic regimen in the following order: (a) anticholinergic drugs; (b) ergot derivatives; (c) amantadine; and (d) L-DOPA. This order reflects an increasing therapeutic index. Sometimes it is necessary to continue the treatment with only L-DOPA at a reduced dose. It has been suggested that, if it is not possible to reduce dopaminergic drugs without a worsening of parkinsonian symptoms, a "drug holiday" of four to seven days is worthwhile (48). This procedure is not free of dangers and must be carried out with hospitalized patients only. (For a review of practical guidelines, benefits, and risks, see 47.)

A few drugs were reported to be helpful in the management of some side effects of the long-term L-DOPA syndrome. It was reported that baclofen reduces foot dystonia (49), naloxone decreases AIM's (50), methysergide counteracts acute psychotic symptoms, and amitriptyline relieves symptoms of sleep disruption and emotional depression (51). However, we think that prevention, and not the addition of another drug, is the best avenue by which to treat Barbeau's syndrome.

LEVODOPA WITHDRAWAL   Acute withdrawal of L-DOPA may be very dangerous. Several reports indicated that an acute withdrawal, caused by lack of drug, negligence, psychiatric problems, or intercurrent illnesses, may induce a syndrome similar to that observed in neuroleptic malignant syndrome (52–55). If absolutely necessary, L-DOPA withdrawal must be carried out gradually over several days under medical supervision.

LEVODOPA AND MELANOMA   At least nine parkinsonian patients treated with L-DOPA were reported to have developed cutaneous or uveal melanoma after a mean treatment length of 46 months (see 3). Another three patients showed a relapse of a skin melanoma diagnosed before L-DOPA treatment. It is not clear whether L-DOPA administration and melanoma are causally related because experimental data point to an antimelanoma effect of L-DOPA

(56). Until this issue is clarified, L-DOPA treatment should be avoided in patients with a previous diagnosis of melanoma.

Anticholinergic and Antihistamine Drugs

Anticholinergic drugs introduced in the 1940s were the first modern drugs for PD. Nevertheless, we still know relatively little about their pharmacokinetics and mechanism of action. They are able to block central muscarinic receptors (57), and some of them inhibit dopamine uptake in striatal synaptosomes (58). Anticholinergic drugs used commonly in the treatment of PD are benztropine mesylate, trihexyphenidyl HCl, procyclidine HCl, cycrimine HCl, biperiden HCl, ethopropazine HCl, bornaprine HCl, and methixene HCl. It is impossible to state, from a clinical point of view, the order of their relative potency. They differ slightly in their target symptom also, although they mainly act on rigidity and tremor. Trihexyphenidyl is more potent than L-DOPA on parkinsonian tremor (59). The overall clinical benefit given by anticholinergics is mild (about 30% improvement) but they can be very useful in the initial stages of PD and in a combined treatment with other drugs. The simultaneous administration of more than one anticholinergic drug is not useful.

The therapeutic index of anticholinergic drugs is sometimes low because of their side effects. The side effects happen mainly in patients over 65 years of age. The most dangerous and insidious of the side effects is mental deterioration with memory loss, which can evolve into a dementialike syndrome. In several patients with PD, choline acetyltransferase levels decrease to 60% of normal central levels in the frontal cortex (60); this cholinergic deficit can be exacerbated by anticholinergic drugs to a symptomatic state (61). Therefore the use of anticholinergics must be avoided in patients who have a previous history of psychiatric symptoms and/or who are over 65 years old. Other relevant contraindications are prostatic hypertrophy, glaucoma, and stenosis of the pylorus, which can be acutely worsened by these drugs.

The combined treatment of anticholinergic drugs plus L-DOPA may have two side effects: (a) by slowing gastric emptying, they reduce intestinal absorption of L-DOPA (18), and (b) by potentiating L-DOPA effect and cholinergic hypofunction, they can increase AIM's (62). An acute withdrawal of anticholinergics may be dangerous, and may bring on a sudden worsening of parkinsonian symptoms, even when their effect appeared to be mild or absent (63, 64). Acetylcholine receptor supersensitivity with increased density of muscarinic receptors in the frontal cortex (60) probably plays a role in this exacerbation of parkinsonian symptoms on anticholinergic withdrawal.

Antihistamines are similar to, but less potent drugs than, anticholinergics. Since their side effects are considerably limited, antihistamines can be used instead of anticholinergics when it is necessary to withdraw the latter drugs. Antihistamines used commonly for PD are diphenhydramine HCl, chlorphenoxamine HCl, and orphenadrine HCl. They belong to the H_1 receptor blocking agents and also have a mild antimuscarinic effect. Their central mechanisms of action and distribution are not well known.

Amantadine

Amantadine HCl was reviewed in the previous article (1), to which we refer the reader. Since its introduction in 1969 amantadine has been a valid pharmacological tool with a well-defined place in the treatment of PD. Its mechanism of action has been investigated in recent years. Amantadine increases dopamine (DA) release and synthesis (65, 66), inhibits DA reuptake (67) and probably has also a direct stimulating effect on DA receptors (68, 69). However, these actions were observed in animals with high doses not comparable with the commonly used dose in humans. Furthermore, amantadine does not modify homovanillic acid (HVA) levels in cerebrospinal fluid of patients with PD (70). Its mechanism of action in man remains controversial, even if several beneficial effects and side effects suggest its inclusion among DA agonists. An argument in favor of the dopaminomimetic effect of amantadine in man is its ability to antagonize partially the neuroleptic-induced extrapyramidal syndrome (71, 72). The increase of DA release seems to be the pharmacological action of amantadine that fits well with its clinical effect in parkinsonian patients. In fact, amantadine tends to lose a part of its efficacy within a few months of treatment (70). It can again elicit some benefit after a withdrawal period (73).

Many clinical results support the statement that the dose of amantadine with a good therapeutic index is between 100 and 200 mg per day. The drug has a long plasma half-life of 10–28.5 hours (hr) (74), and 200 mg can be given in two administrations at 8–12 hr intervals. With doses higher than 200 mg, side effects are frequent. The more long-lasting and dangerous side effects are ankle edema and livedo reticularis (75, 76), and psychiatric symptoms, such as hallucinations and confusion (77). With psychiatric symptoms, amantadine can cause the same side effects induced by anticholinergic drugs (77). This effect must be remembered when a combined treatment is started and the dose of anticholinergics should be reduced or kept low. We observed AIM's analogous to those caused by L-DOPA in one patient treated with 300 mg of amantadine (70).

The percentage of benefit obtained with amantadine in PD is similar to that given by anticholinergics, but amantadine probably works more uniformly on all parkinsonian symptoms, including bradykinesia. There is not a general agreement about the decay of efficacy of the drug (75). However, amantadine can be used alone in the initial stages of PD (stages I–III of Hoehn & Yahr, 78) or can be added to L-DOPA in severely affected patients with whom L-DOPA dosage must be kept at suboptimal levels because of its side-effects.

Ergot Derivatives

A new category of potent antiparkinsonian drugs was developed in the last decade after the first reports of Calne et al on the action of bromocriptine (79). These drugs are ergolines or ergot derivatives with dopaminergic activity (80). They act on postsynaptic DA receptors by a hormonelike action that is independent of the production of axonal impulse (81). This mechanism of action seemed a promising complement to L-DOPA action, particularly in patients with an advanced degeneration of the nigrostriatal pathway. Ergot derivatives have partially met these expectations. In fact, when given in combination with L-DOPA they can reduce oscillations in performance (wearing-off) and AIM's (82). However, they gradually lose efficacy over several years of treatment and cannot counteract disease progression. A striatal receptor down-regulation may also explain this decay of efficacy (83).

Such ergolines as bromocriptine mesylate and lisuride hydrogen maleate are agonists of D_2 dopamine receptors and antagonists of D_1 receptors. Only pergolide mesylate is an agonist of both D_1 and D_2 receptors (81). An oral dose equivalent has been established for the commonly used drugs: 30 mg bromocriptine = 2.5 mg lisuride = 2.5 mg pergolide (81). Other ergot derivatives with a well-defined antiparkinsonian effect are no longer used for human treatment because they have some dangerous side effects. Lergotrile mesylate cannot be used because it shows alterations in liver function tests (84); mesulergine HCl was withdrawn because it induces testicular tumors in one strain of rats (80).

Bromocriptine is the ergoline most thoroughly investigated clinically. Several authors reported that bromocriptine must be given in high doses (i.e. 30–130 mg/day) for maximum efficacy in PD, with a dose–disease stage relationship (85, 86). Unfortunately, severe side effects may impair these beneficial effects, requiring reduction of daily dose or withdrawal of the drug. Side effects of bromocriptine are similar to those of L-DOPA and other dopaminomimetic drugs, but AIM's are rare and psychiatric symptoms are relatively frequent. Nausea and vomiting may be particularly severe, but domperidone, a blocker of peripheral DA receptors, effectively reduces them (87). Also, orthostatic hypotension may be particularly severe. In this case, slow rise from supine position, elastic stockings, and an increase in sodium intake may help the patient. For these problems a slow titration of bromocriptine has been suggested, increasing the dose from 1.25 to 2.5 mg per week (88). Several authors also claimed that low doses of bromocriptine (5–15 mg) are useful (88), but there is no general agreement on this point. A relatively low dose is probably sufficient when bromocriptine is added to L-DOPA. Rinne (82) obtained better results after three years of treatment with the combination of L-DOPA and bromocriptine at a mean daily dose of 16.6 mg than with L-DOPA alone at a higher dose. When bromocriptine is added to L-DOPA in advanced cases, the clinical results are controversial (89, 90). Lander et al (91) reported that a single dose of bromocriptine at bedtime relieves morning akinesia and dystonia.

In recent years lisuride and pergolide joined bromocriptine as effective ergolines in the treatment of PD. Lisuride and bromocriptine have comparable clinical effects, but the effective dose of lisuride is about one-twelfth that of bromocriptine (81, 92). A disadvantage of lisuride is its additional property as a central serotonin agonist, which probably causes enhanced psychiatric side effects in comparison to bromocriptine (92). The most interesting use of lisuride seems to be its continuous subcutaneous administration by means of a portable miniinfusion pump, in addition to oral L-DOPA plus a peripheral decarboxylase inhibitor (PDI) (93). Oscillations in performance and the overall parkinsonian picture were considerably reduced in three patients with an advanced long-term L-DOPA syndrome (93). Pergolide in acute studies has a powerful and long-lasting effect, which lasts more than twice as long as that induced by L-DOPA (94). Its therapeutical dose is equal to, or somewhat smaller than, that of lisuride. There is some controversy about the loss of efficacy of pergolide in chronic treatment of PD. Goetz et al (95) found that pergolide was still effective after five years of treatment; Lieberman et al (96) reported a 35% decrease of efficacy after a mean of 16 months of treatment in a large population of patients. Since such a decrease of efficacy is not dose related and is not restored after a drug holiday, it seems caused by the natural course of the disease more than by receptor down-regulation (97). Side effects of pergolide are similar to those of the other dopamine agonists. A particular drawback seems to be the occurrence of episodes of sudden freezing (97). On the other hand, pergolide lacks cardiac toxicity in parkinsonian patients with cardiac disease (98).

In conclusion, ergot derivatives are a new, important class of antiparkinsonian drugs. Their relatively long-lasting action on postsynaptic DA receptors, essentially of D_2 type, is a useful complement to the pharmacological action of the other antiparkinsonian drugs, in particular L-DOPA. A treatment with one ergoline plus one or more of L-DOPA, amantadine, and an anticholinergic drug is possible and useful in certain circumstances, once the previously mentioned indications, side effects, and interaction of these drugs are considered.

Other Drugs

Several drugs with a potent antiparkinsonian effect were dropped from clinical use in the last few years for different reasons. For instance, apomorphine HCl is not used because of its short duration of action and side effects, whereas MIF [PLG (Pro-Leu-Gly-NH$_2$)], a synthetic tripeptide that potentiates L-DOPA effects, is not used because it is effective only intravenously, not orally (99). Moreover the cost of these drugs is high, and in light of their clinical usefulness, it does not justify their current use.

Other drugs have not yet been submitted to a thorough pharmacological and clinical evaluation. A new, interesting approach to the therapy of PD is based on the introduction of an inhibitor of monoamine oxidase-B (MAO-B), L-deprenyl. L-Deprenyl selectively inhibits DA catabolism (100), and a single oral dose induces a long-lasting (up to three days) dopaminergic potentiation (101). Some clinical studies demonstrated that L-deprenyl, when added to L-DOPA, potentiates L-DOPA's effect. This further improvement is still evident after several years of combined treatment (101, 102). L-Deprenyl is administered orally in a 5–10 mg dose, and the dose of L-DOPA in this combined treatment may be reduced to avoid an increase of AIM's. But some recent experimental data challenge these clinical results. 1-Methyl-4-phenyl-1,2,3,6-tetrahydropyridine (MPTP), a potent neurotoxin, causes a typical parkinsonian syndrome in man and animals (see 103 for a review), and MAO-B is essential to transform MPTP to its active metabolite MPP^+. L-Deprenyl is a good candidate to counteract this transformation. However, Bradbury et al (104) showed that L-deprenyl potentiates DA depletion caused by MPP^+ in mouse striatum. Therefore, these experimental data seem to conflict with clinical experience and require further investigation of the pharmacological properties of this drug.

Another drug, DL-threo-dihydroxyphenylserine (DOPS), a β-hydroxylated form of DOPA that is converted to norepinephrine (NE) by DOPA-decarboxylase, was suggested to improve transient freezing (105), but a subsequent report did not confirm these results (106). The usefulness of a central NE stimulant for some particular symptoms of PD is still uncertain. Recently, Stoessl et al (107) reported that (+)-4-propyl-9-hydroxynaph-thoxazine (PHNO) is an effective antiparkinsonian drug. This observation is interesting and deserves further attention, since PHNO is a new type of DA agonist, not related structurally to morphine and ergolines.

Some drugs introduced many years ago for indications other than PD can help in the management of PD, particularly tremor. Propranolol HCl, a well-known β-adrenergic blocker useful in the treatment of essential tremor, is effective on the postural tremor that sometimes occurs in PD (108). Also nadolol, a β-blocker active only peripherally, has a therapeutic effect on the different types of tremor in PD (109). This finding raises the possibility that parkinsonian tremor can be influenced by a peripherally acting drug. Finally, clonazepam, a benzodiazepine thoroughly used for the treatment of epilepsy, relieves PD tremor when given at a dose of 3 mg per day (110).

In conclusion, the pharmacological means of treating PD have been continuously increasing in the last twenty years. Today, the neurologist has the responsibility of choosing the treatment properly and making the decision of when to give a drug, at which dose, and with what combination of other drugs. Mistakes in the treatment are giving too many drugs at the same time or increasing one drug to the maximum tolerated level to obtain the best result possible. Since PD is a chronic disease, we must be careful in trying to achieve perfect results immediately. A 60–70% improvement should be considered a satisfying and prudent achievement, and the physician should aim to keep the improvement as stable as possible in the following years. Patients with PD sometimes appear to tolerate AIM's very well, but they do indeed become seriously handicapped. Therefore, long-term treatment of PD is essentially a problem of maintaining equilibrium between the present and the future: the easily achievable, immediate benefit and the long-term functional results.

DYSTONIC SYNDROMES

Dystonic syndromes (DS) are fairly common, heterogeneous disorders that may occur idiopathically, as an inherited trait, or secondarily to various brain lesions. They are also encountered within a number of complex degenerative diseases (111). The more frequent idiopathic syndromes are torsion dystonia, cranial dystonia (Meige's syndrome), spasmodic torticollis, and focal dystonia (writer's cramp). The pathological bases and the biochemical abnormalities of DS are unknown. Therefore, the pharmacology of these syndromes is very limited and developed essentially from clinical observations and therapeutic trials. Since some drugs may be beneficial, we report these attempts.

Barbeau (112) suggested that L-DOPA in low doses could improve some DS. He based this suggestion on the well-known dystonic reactions that occur mainly in young people after the administration of neuroleptic drugs and on the consideration that dystonic symptoms are a common feature in postencephalitic parkinsonism. Several clinical trials demonstrated that L-DOPA is not useful in most DS, but in the hereditary Segawa variant with diurnal fluctuations, the drug was reported to cause a sustained improvement of dystonia (113, 114). L-DOPA seems effective in young patients at low doses, not combined with a PDI. A DA agonist, bromocriptine, was reported to have improved three patients with DS when given at high doses (115, 116). Bassi et al (117) obtained a significant improvement in 6 out of 7 patients with DS with another ergot derivative, lisuride (see "Ergot Derivatives"). These results were confirmed by Quinn et al (118), who observed improvement of 8 of 31 patients with idiopathic DS (26%) when they were given lisuride at doses ranging from 0.4 to 5 mg (mean = 3 mg). These authors suggested, however, that lisuride could act on DS because of its serotonergic effect, not because of its dopaminergic properties. Since little is known about the possible involvement of the serotonergic system in DS, this question remains open.

The results with L-DOPA and DA agonists appear to contradict various reports on the beneficial effects of neuroleptics such as haloperidol and tetrabenazine (119–121). Tolosa & Lai (122) based their hypothesis of a striatal DA preponderance in a particular form of dystonia, Meige's syndrome, on this effect. However, neuroleptic drugs may have a highly aspecific, sedative-type effect, which is observed to varying degrees in all the hyperkinetic syndromes.

The most interesting and extensive reports on the treatment of DS concern anticholinergic drugs (AC). Fahn (123) matched the observations on the dystonic reactions caused by neuroleptics (which are reversed by AC) with the therapeutic principle of a slow dose titration to avoid side effects. He also treated 75 patients with DS with trihexiphenidyl (THP) and ethopropazine (EP) (see "Anticholinergic and Antihistamine Drugs") and found significant benefit in 61% of children and 38% of adults. Several reports followed Fahn's contribution, confirming his positive findings in almost the same percentage of patients. We calculated the overall results of 11 reports on patients with idiopathic DS (119, 121, 124–132). Out of 245 patients treated with THP, EP, or benztropine (BT) 105 (43%) showed a clear-cut improvement. The dose of AC varied considerably; for instance, for THP its range was between 2 and 80 mg per day. The main conclusions that can be drawn from these studies are the following: (a) improvement is more frequent in children than in adults because children can tolerate higher doses of AC. (b) THP seems most effective, but it is very difficult to go beyond the dose of 30 mg per day in patients over 40 years old. EP and BT can be used in adults, when THP is not well tolerated. However, the maximum dose tolerated must be very gradually obtained by increases over several months of treatment. (c) The treatment with AC is less effective in patients with symptomatic or secondary DS (such cases are not included in the data given above). (d) Spasmodic torticollis, torsion dystonia, and Meige's syndrome show the best results, while writer's cramp responds less often to AC. (e) The clinical result appears inversely correlated with the length of the disease (132). (f) The value of i.v. AC administration as a predictive test of response to oral administration is controversial. Probably several factors, dose, difference between oral and i.v. administration, patients studied, affect the results. In patients with severe dystonia where THP is not effective, Marsden et al (130) suggested a combined treatment of THP with tetrabenazine and pimozide. In conclusion, although unpredictable and of benefit to a limited percentage of patients only, AC treatment appears the most effective pharmacological tool for DS at the moment. The effect of AC suggests that a cholinergic overactivity occurs in

DS. However, from the available data we cannot infer which neurotransmitter imbalance would be responsible for this "functional" overactivity.

HUNTINGTON'S DISEASE

The main pathological changes in Huntington's disease (HD), i.e. a degeneration of the small cholinergic and GABAergic neurons in the striatum, have been known for several years. We also know that the concentrations of GABA, glutamic acid decarboxylase (GAD), and choline acetylase (ChAc) are lowered in several regions of the HD brain (133, 134). Nevertheless, several therapeutic approaches similar to the "replacement" strategy used in Parkinson's disease, i.e. increasing brain levels of GABA and acetylcholine (ACh), have failed to give substantial results to date. Moreover, the administration of GABA and acetylcholine receptor agonists, which are active in the absence of nerve impulse from degenerated axons, failed to improve choreic hyperkinesias and dementia, the two cardinal symptoms of HD. We briefly review these reports.

Growdon et al (135) gave choline, the ACh precursor, in high doses of 8 to 20 g per day to 10 patients with HD. Although choline levels in cerebrospinal fluid (CSF) were increased, no consistent clinical improvement was observed after 19–125 days (mean = 50 days) of treatment. Arecoline, a potent, short-acting muscarinic agonist, was given to 6 patients in another study and resulted in the exacerbation of choreic movements (136). On the contrary in acute studies physostigmine, an anticholinesterase agent, was reported to improve chorea in 13 out of 23 patients (see 137 for references). Nutt (138) reported that some AC, such as scopolamine and benztropine, paradoxically improve chorea, but he pointed out that the effect of both physostigmine and AC may depend on their aspecific sedative effect, not on their cholinergic or anticholinergic action. In fact, scopolamine and benztropine reduced chorea but worsened incoordination in patients with HD, showing that these effects are dissociated. In therapeutic trials scoring only chorea, not coordination, an important component of the dyskinetic syndrome is certainly missed. In conclusion, the results obtained with drugs active on central cholinergic systems show that this approach cannot presently be used for HD. However, most of these results were obtained in acute, short-term studies in which drug action was observed on abnormal movements, not on psychiatric symptoms.

The GABAergic approach has not been more encouraging than the cholinergic one. Perry and coworkers (139) gave high doses of isoniazide (INH) to 6 patients with HD. They observed a gradual benefit on both dyskinetic and psychiatric symptoms in 3 patients. INH dose was related to the acetylation phenotype of each patient, e.g. a lower dose was given to slow acetylators. The same authors reported a limited improvement, in only 1 out of 9 patients, in a subsequent controlled trial with INH (140). Stober et al (141) confirmed a significant effect of INH in 4 out of 10 patients with classic, hyperkinetic HD. They emphasized the importance of maintaining the trial for at least two-to-three months before evaluating its success. It is unclear why only a limited number of patients responded to the treatment with INH, but the results of these studies (139–141) are probably the most interesting for the practical management of HD. INH increases the brain GABA content by an inhibition of its degradative enzyme GABA-aminotransferase (GABA-T). Other inhibitors of GABA-T, sodium valproate, gamma-acetylenic GABA and gamma-vinyl GABA, which are also inhibitors of GABA-synthetizing enzyme GAD, failed to elicit any clinical improvement (142–145). 4,5,6,7-Tetrahydroisoxazolo-[5,4-6]pyridin-3-ol (THIP), a GABA receptor agonist, was not effective, and interestingly, during the treatment with THIP, CSF content of HVA was increased (146). This finding is in agreement with previous studies of Waddington & Cross (147). These authors predicted the failure of treatment with GABA agonists in HD because these drugs would induce a striatal dopaminergic hyperfunction by acting on the supersensitive GABA receptors in the substantia nigra. In our opinion, further studies with proper dosage and duration of treatment are required to confirm if INH is useful in a subpopulation of patients with HD.

All clinical conditions with AIM's of different types, chorea, dystonia, tics, ballismus, are relieved by neuroleptics. In HD, where there is a preponderance of dopamine, the effect of neuroleptics is particularly pronounced, at least in the first stages of the disease. An important side effect of neuroleptics in HD is mood depression, since these patients are prone to this condition that can lead to suicide. Reserpine, haloperidol, fluphenazine and tetrabenazine are among the first drugs used successfully in HD (1,120). Recently fenfluramine, an inhibitor of serotonin reuptake, has been claimed to be effective in a short-term, open trial on 7 patients with HD (148). Lithium carbonate was also reported to improve dyskinesias in HD (149). A combined treatment of lithium and haloperidol at low doses (1 mg/day) may be useful for both dyskinesias and mood stabilization (150). However, pulse rate must be regularly checked because lithium may cause severe bradycardia in patients with HD (G. Campanella et al, unpublished information). In advanced stages of HD, no drug can help the severely disabled patients.

GILLES DE LA TOURETTE'S SYNDROME

Gilles de la Tourette's syndrome (GTS) begins in childhood and is characterized by multiple tics and inapposite vocalizations. It is often accompanied by complex mannerisms and antics, echophenomena, and coprolalia. The biochemical basis of GTS is unknown, as is its anatomopathology, if any. The pharmacological approach to the treatment of GTS has long been disappointing. In spite of its serious drawbacks, haloperidol, the all-purpose drug, was the most used neuroleptic until recent years, with a fair, but often short-lived, response in 60–90% of patients (151). Specifically, patients treated with haloperidol complain of the "zombie syndrome," i.e. difficulty in thinking adequately and intellectual dulling (152). The effect of haloperidol was supported by the theory of a DA receptor supersitivity in GTS (153). Tetrabenazine and fluphenazine are alternative treatments, with fewer side effects than haloperidol (154, 155). Gillmann & Sandyk (156) recently reported the effectiveness of nitrous oxide (N_2O), an opioid receptor agonist, in controlling tics in one patient with GTS. On the basis of this observation and other experimental data on the link between dopaminergic and opioid systems, they suggested that an opioid underactivity may cause the clinical symptoms of GTS. Further studies are required to validate this therapeutic approach.

Another interesting alternative drug for GTS is clonidine HCl, an antihypertensive agent with an α-adrenergic agonistic effect in the brain. Since 1979 (157) several studies have confirmed the efficacy of clonidine in GTS (see 158 for references). About 46–62% of patients improve with clonidine, and the initial severity of GTS can lead to a positive response (158). Even at the high dosage required in GTS, i.e. 0.125–0.3 mg per day, clonidine has relatively few side effects, mainly sedation and orthostatic hypotension. The mechanism of action of clonidine in GTS is still unknown, but it probably is not simply based on its central adrenergic effect. Treatment with methylphenidate HCl and other central stimulants is contraindicated in GTS (159).

WILSON'S DISEASE

Hepatolenticular degeneration or Wilson's disease (WD) is a rare but important illness. It was the first neurological disease to be successfully managed in the 1950s. The well-known results, treatment scheme, and side effects of therapy with D-penicillamine, (β,β-dimethylcystein) can be found in several comprehensive reviews (160–162). We summarize some points that thirty years of therapeutic experience with this drug have emphasized with increasing clarity. D-Penicillamine is a very active drug that can completely reverse the symptoms of WD and stop its progression. The sooner the diagnosis is made and the treatment started, the better are the results. It is never superfluous to repeat what Sternlieb & Scheinberg (163) and Walshe (160) recommended, that the diagnosis of WD in the presence of signs of chronic hepatitis should always be suspected, particularly in patients under age 40. Recent reports showed that WD is still considerably underdiagnosed or that diagnosis is often dangerously delayed (164, 162). The chelating effect on copper of D-penicillamine must be constant and life-long. In this type of long-term treatment, a patient's compliance is a very delicate problem. Many patients, after experiencing a complete remission of their symptoms for several years, abandon their medication, often with severe and irreversible damage and even a fatal outcome (165). The maintenance dose of D-penicillamine depends on the time of its administration and on the concomitant dietary restriction of copper-rich foods. The drug must be taken about half an hour before meals to avoid saturation of copper sites by copper contained in the food ingested. If a low-copper diet is observed (160–162), 600–750 mg per day are sufficient as a maintenance dose. In Walshe's and our experience, side effects of D-penicillamine are much less frequent in WD than in other diseases such as rheumatoid arthritis.

Although D-penicillamine is the most effective and specific drug for WD, other medications have been introduced in recent years that are valuable alternatives, particularly when D-penicillamine is not well tolerated. The drugs are trientine dihydrochloride (trien) and zinc salts. Trien is as effective as D-penicillamine, and its only side effect is iron deficiency that can be overcome by iron supplements (166). Zinc sulfate or acetate induce a negative copper balance, increasing fecal copper excretion (167, 168). Zinc salts are also useful in addition to D-penicillamine to counteract the hypogeusia caused by the latter drug (164). Finally, if treatment with D-pencillamine is started late and does not alleviate the neurological symptoms, L-DOPA (169) and anticholinergic drugs (164) may help in decreasing akinesia, rigidity, and dystonia.

CONCLUSION

In 1974 Barbeau (1) concluded his review on drugs affecting movement disorders with an important statement that could not have been made several years before: chronic neurological movement disorders *can* be treated. After 13 years we can conclude by emphasizing two outstanding aspects: (*a*) we have much better knowledge of the mechanism of action, indications, and long-term effects of drugs that had already been discovered in 1974, such as L-DOPA, anticholinergics, and penicillamine; (*b*) many new drugs have subsequently been introduced that represent important pharmacologic approaches for treating these disorders. The growing therapeutic arsenal requires a thorough knowledge of the properties of these drugs and thus increases the physician's responsibility.

ACKNOWLEDGMENT

Dr. Campanella's work during his sabbatical year spent in Dr. Barbeau's department was supported by the Fondation Parkinson du Québec.

Literature Cited

1. Barbeau, A. 1974. Drugs affecting movement disorders. *Ann. Rev. Pharmacol.* 14:91–113
2. Barbeau, A. 1972. L'emploi de la Levodopa en dehors de la maladie de Parkinson. *Union Med. Can.* 101:849–52
3. Barbeau, A., Campanella, G., Roy, M. 1987. Treatment of Parkinson's disease. A review. *Clin. Neuropharmacol.* In press
4. Nutt, J. G., Woodward, W. R., Anderson, W. L., Hammerstad, J. P. 1983. What is the function of carbidopa in the treatment of parkinsonism? *Ann. Neurol.* 14:133–34
5. Nutt, J. G., Woodward, W. R., Anderson, J. L. 1985. The effect of carbidopa on the pharmacokinetics of intravenously administered levodopa. The mechanism of action in the treatment of parkinsonism. *Ann. Neurol.* 18:537–43
6. Fahn, S. 1974. "On-off" phenomenon with Levodopa therapy in parkinsonism. *Neurology* 24:431–41
7. Diamond, S. G., Markham, C. H., Treciokas, L. J. 1978. A double-blind comparison of Levodopa, Madopa and Sinemet in Parkinson's disease. *Ann. Neurol.* 3:267–72
8. Rinne, U. K., Mölsä, P. 1979. Levodopa with benserazide or carbidopa in Parkinson's disease. *Neurology* 29:1584–89
9. Tourtelotte, W. W., Syndulko, K., Potvin, A. R., Hirsch, S. B., Potvin, J. H. 1980. Increased ratio of carbidopa to levodopa in treatment of Parkinson's disease. *Arch. Neurol.* 37:723–26
10. Tolosa, E. S., Martin, W. E., Cohen, H. P., Jacobsen, R. L. 1975. Patterns of clinical response and plasma dopa levels in Parkinson's disease. *Neurology* 25:177–83
11. Campanella, G., Algeri, S., Cerletti, C., Dolfini, E., Jori, A., Rinaldi, F. 1977. Correlation of clinical symptoms, HVA and 5-HIAA in CSF and plasma L-DOPA in parkinsonian patients treated with L-DOPA and L-DOPA + Ro 4-4602. *Eur. J. Clin. Pharmacol.* 11:255–61
12. Melamed, E., Bitton, V., Zelig, O. 1986. Episodic unresponsiveness to single doses of L-dopa in parkinsonian fluctuators. *Neurology* 36:100–3
13. Pearce, L. A., Waterbury, L. D. 1974. L-Methionine: A possible L-DOPA antagonist. *Neurology* 24:640–41
14. Weitbrecht, W. U., Nuber, B., Sandritter, W. 1976. Der Einfluss von L-Tryptophan auf die L-DOPA Resorption. *Dtsch. Med. Wochenschr.* 101:20–22
15. Nutt, J. G., Woodward, W. R., Hammerstad, J. P., Carter, J. H., Anderson, J. C. 1984. "On-off" phenomenon in Parkinson's disease: relationship to L-DOPA absorption and transport. *N. Engl. J. Med.* 310:483–88
16. Mena, I., Cotzias, C. G. 1975. Protein intake and treatment of Parkinson's disease with levodopa. *N. Engl. J. Med.* 292:181–84
17. Morgan, J. P., Rivera-Calimlim, L., Messiha, F., Sundaresan, P. R., Trabert, N. 1975. Imipramine-mediated interference with levodopa absorption from the gastrointestinal tract in man. *Neurology* 25:1029–34
18. Algeri, S., Cerletti, C., Curcio, M., Morselli, P. L., Bonollo, L., et al. 1976. Effect of anticholinergic drugs on gastro-intestinal absorption of L-DOPA in rats and in man. *Eur. J. Pharmacol.* 35:293–99
19. Nutt, J. G., Fellman, J. H. 1984. Pharmacokinetics of levodopa. *Clin. Neuropharmacol.* 7:35–49
20. Wade, L. A., Katzman, R. 1975. 3-O-Methyldopa uptake and inhibition of L-DOPA at the blood-brain barrier. *Life Sci.* 17:131–36
21. Reches, A., Fahn, S. 1982. 3-O-Methyldopa blocks DOPA metabolism in rat corpus striatum. *Ann. Neurol.* 12:267–71
22. Rivera-Calimlim, L., Deepak, T., Anderson, R., Joynt, R. 1977. The clinical picture and plasma levodopa metabolite profile of parkinsonian nonresponders. *Arch. Neurol.* 34:228–32
23. Martin-DuPan, R., Mauron, C., Gleaser, B., Wurtman, R. J. 1982. Effect of various oral glucose doses on plasma neutral amino acid levels. *Metabolism* 31:937–43
24. Mearrick, P. T., Wade, D. N., Birkett, D. J., Morris, J. 1974. Metoclopramide, gastric emptying and L-DOPA absorption. *Aust. N. Z. J. Med.* 4:144–48
25. Indo, T., Ando, K. 1982. Metoclopramide-induced parkinsonism—Clinical characteristics of ten cases. *Arch. Neurol.* 39:494–96
26. Rivera-Calimlim, L., Morgan, J. P., Dujovne, C. A., Bianchine, J. R., Lasagna, L. 1970. L-DOPA absorption and metabolism by the human stomach. *J. Clin. Invest.* 49:79a
27. Bianchine, J. R., Rivera-Calimlim, R., Morgan, J. P., Dujovne, C. A., Lasagna, L. 1971. Metabolism and absorption of L-3,4-dihydroxyphenylalanine in patients with Parkinson's

disease. *Ann. N. Y. Acad. Sci.* 179:126–40

28. Barbeau, A. 1976. L-DOPA and Parkinson's disease. In *Brain Metabolism and Cerebral Disorders*, ed. H. C. Himwich, 12:283–361. New York: Spectrum. 2nd ed.

29. Markham, C. H., Diamond, S. G. 1986. Long-term follow-up of early dopa treatment in Parkinson's disease. *Ann. Neurol.* 19:365–72

30. Barbeau, A. 1976. Neurological and psychiatric side-effects of L-DOPA. In *International Encyclopedia of Pharmacology and Therapeutics, Part C, Pharmacology & Therapeutics*, ed. O. Hornykiewicz, 1:475–94. Oxford/New York/ Frankfurt/Paris: Pergamon

31. Melamed, E., Bitton, V. 1984. Delayed onset of responses to individual doses of L-DOPA in parkinsonian fluctuators: An additional side-effect of long-term L-DOPA therapy. *Neurology* 34(2):270 (Abstr.)

32. Barbeau, A. 1976. Pathophysiology of the oscillations in performance after long-term therapy with L-DOPA. In *Advances in Parkinsonism*, ed. W. Birkmayer, O. Hornykiewicz, pp. 424–34. Basel, Switzerland: Roche

33. Quinn, N., Marsden, C. D., Parkes, J. D. 1982. Complicated response fluctuations in Parkinson's disease: Response to intravenous infusion of levodopa. *Lancet* 2:412–15

34. Nausieda, P. A., Weiner, W. J., Kaplan, L. R., Weber, S., Klawans, H. L. 1982. Sleep disruption in the course of chronic levodopa therapy: an early feature of the levodopa psychosis. *Clin. Neuropharmacol.* 5:183–94

35. Barbeau, A. 1970. Importance and pathogenesis of abnormal movements during L-DOPA therapy of Parkinson's disease. *Neurology* 20:377 (Abstr.)

36. Bokobza, B., Ruberg, M., Scatton, B., Javoy-Agid, F., Agid, Y. 1984. [3H]-Spiperone binding, dopamine and HVA concentrations in Parkinson's disease and supranuclear palsy. *Eur. J. Pharmacol.* 99:167–75

37. Klawans, H. L., Goetz, C. G., Nausieda, P. A., Weiner, W. J. 1977. Levodopa-induced dopamine receptor hypersensitivity. *Ann. Neurol.* 2:125–29

38. Rinne, U. K., Koskinen, V., Lonnberg, P. 1980. Neurotransmitter receptors in the parkinsonism brain. In *Parkinson's disease. Current Progress, Problems and Management*, ed. U. K. Rinne, M. Klinger, M. Stamm, pp. 93–107. Amsterdam: Elsevier

39. Guttman, M., Seeman, P. 1985. L-DOPA reverses the elevated density of D_2 dopamine receptors in Parkinson's diseased striatum. *J. Neural Transm.* 64:93–103

40. Agid, Y., Bonnet, A.-M., Rubert, M., Javoy-Agid, F. 1985. Pathophysiology of levodopa induced abnormal involuntary movements. In *Dyskinesia, Research and Treatment*, ed. D. Casey, T. N. Chase, V. Christensen, J. Gerlach, 1:145–59. Berlin: Springer-Verlag

41. Melamed, E. 1979. Early-morning dystonia. A late side-effect of long-term levodopa therapy in Parkinson's disease. *Arch. Neurol.* 36:308–10

42. Barbeau, A. 1971. Long term side-effects of levodopa. *Lancet* 1:395

43. Barbeau, A. 1972. Contributions of Levodopa therapy to the neuropharmacology of akinesia. In *Parkinson's disease: rigidity, akinesia, behavior*, ed. J. Siegfried, 1:151–74. Bern, Switzerland: Huber

44. Barbeau, A. 1974. The clinical physiology of side-effects in long-term levodopa therapy. In *Advances in Neurology*, ed. F. McDowell, A. Barbeau, 5:347–65. New York: Raven

45. Paalzow, G. H. M., Paalzow, L. K. 1986. L-DOPA: How it may exacerbate parkinsonian symptoms. *Trends Pharmacol. Sci.* 7:15–19

46. Nausieda, P. A. 1985. Sinemet "Abusers." *Clin. Neuropharmacol.* 8:318–27

47. Klawans, H. L. 1984. What to do when Sinemet fails: Part One. *Clin. Neuropharmacol.* 7:121–33

48. Direnfeld, L. K., Feldman, R. G., Alexander, M. P., Kelly-Hayes, M. 1980. Is Levodopa drug holiday useful? *Neurology* 30:785–88

49. Nausieda, P. A., Weiner, W. J., Klawans, H. L. 1980. Dystonic foot response of parkinsonism. *Arch. Neurol.* 37:132–36

50. Sandyk, R., Snider, S. R. 1986. Naloxone treatment of L-DOPA-induced dyskinesia in Parkinson's disease. *Am. J. Psychiat.* 143:118 (Lett.)

51. Klawans, H. L. 1982. Behavioral alterations and the therapy of parkinsonism. *Clin. Neuropharmacol.* 5(1):S29–S37

52. Toru, M., Matsuda, O., Makiguchi, K., Sugano, K. 1981. Neuroleptic malignant syndrome-like state following a withdrawal of antiparkinsonian drugs. *J. Nerv. Ment. Dis.* 169:324–27

53. Sechi, G. P., Tanda, F., Mutani, R. 1984. Fatal hyperpyrexia after withdrawal of levodopa. *Neurology* 34:249–51

132   CAMPANELLA, ROY & BARBEAU

54. Figa-Talamanca, L., Gualandi, C., Di Meo, L., Di Battista, G., Neri, G., Lo Russo, F. 1985. Hyperthermia after discontinuance of levodopa and bromocriptine therapy: impaired dopamine receptors a possible cause. *Neurology* 35:258–61
55. Gibb, W. R. G., Griffith, D. N. W. 1986. Levodopa withdrawal syndrome identical to neuroleptic malignant syndrome. *Postgrad. Med. J.* 62:59–60
56. Wick, M. M., Byers, L., Frei, E. 1977. III: Selective toxicity of L-DOPA for melanoma cells. *Science* 197:468–69
57. Duvoisin, R. C. 1967. Cholinergic-anticholinergic antagonism in parkinsonism. *Arch. Neurol.* 17:124–36
58. Coyle, J. T., Snyder, S. H. 1969. Antiparkinsonian drugs: inhibition of dopamine uptake in the corpus striatum as a possible mechanism of action. *Science* 166:899–901
59. Koller, W. C. 1986. Pharmacologic treatment of parkinsonian tremor. *Arch. Neurol.* 43:126–27
60. Ruberg, M., Ploska, A., Javoy-Agid, F., Agid, Y. 1982. Muscarinic binding and choline acetyltransferase activity in parkinsonian subjects with reference to dementia. *Brain Res.* 232:129–39
61. De Smet, Y., Ruberg, M., Serdaru, M., Dubois, B., Lhermitte, F., Agid, Y. 1982. Confusion, dementia and anticholinergics in Parkinson's disease. *J. Neurol. Neurosurg. Psychiat.* 45:1161–64
62. Bullpitt, C. J., Shaw, K., Clifton, P., Stern, G., Davies, J. B., Reid, J. L. 1985. The symptoms of patients treated for Parkinson's disease. *Clin. Neuropharmacol.* 8:175–83
63. Hughes, R. C., Polgar, J. G., Weightman, D., Walton, J. N. 1971. Levodopa in parkinsonism: The effects of withdrawal of anticholinergic drugs. *Brit. Med. J.* 2:487–91
64. Horrocks, P. M., Vicary, D. J., Rees, J. E., Parkes, J. D., Marsden, C. D. 1973. Anticholinergic withdrawal and benzhexol treatment in Parkinson's disease. *J. Neurol. Neurosurg. Psychiat.* 36:936–41
65. Scatton, B., Cheramy, A., Besson, M. J., Glowinski, J. 1970. Increased synthesis and release of dopamine in the striatum of the rat after amantadine treatment. *Eur. J. Pharmacol.* 13:131–33
66. Stromberg, V., Svensson, T. H., Waldeck, B. 1970. On the mode of action of amantadine. *J. Pharm. Pharmacol.* 22:959–62
67. Heikkila, R. E., Cohen, G. 1972. Evaluation of amantadine as a releasing agent or uptake blocker for H³-dopamine in rat brain slices. *Eur. J. Pharmacol.* 20:156–60
68. Pycock, C., Milson, J. A., Tarsy, D., Marsden, C. D. 1976. The effects of blocking catecholamine uptake on amphetamine-induced circling behavior in mice with unilateral destruction of striatal dopaminergic nerve terminals. *J. Pharm. Pharmacol.* 28:530–32
69. Randrup, A., Mogilnicka, E. 1976. Spectrum of pharmacological actions on brain dopamine. Indications for development of new psychoactive drugs. Discussion of amantadines as examples of new drugs with special actions on dopamine systems. *Pol. J. Pharmacol. Pharm.* 28:551–56
70. Buscaino, G. A., Campanella, G., Zallone, E. 1971. Sei mesi di trattamento con amantadina e con L-DOPA. Confronto in due gruppi di parkinsoniani. *Minerva Med.* 62:3974–78
71. Kelly, J. T., Zimmerman, R. L., Abuzzahab, F. S., Schiele, B. C. 1974. A double-blind study of amantadine hydrochloride versus benztropine mesylate in drug-induced parkinsonism. *Pharmacology* 12:65–73
72. Borison, R. L. 1983. Amantadine in the management of extrapyramidal side-effects. *Clin. Neuropharmacol.* 6(1):S57–S63
73. Fahn, S., Isgreen, W. P. 1975. Long-term evaluation of amantadine and Levodopa combination in parkinsonism by double-blind crossover analyses. *Neurology* 25:695–700
74. Pacifici, G. M., Nardini, M., Ferrari, P., Latini, R., Fieschi, C., Morselli, P. L. 1976. Effect of amantadine on drug-induced parkinsonism: relationship between plasma levels and effect. *Br. J. Clin. Pharmacol.* 3:883–89
75. Butzer, J. F., Silver, D. E., Sahs, A. L. 1975. Amantadine in Parkinson's disease. *Neurology* 25:603–6
76. Timberlake, W. H., Vance, M. A. 1978. Four-year treatment of patients with parkinsonism using amantadine alone or with levodopa. *Ann. Neurol.* 3:119–28
77. Postma, J. V., Tilburg, W. V. 1975. Visual hallucinations and delirium during treatment with amantadine (Symmetrel). *J. Am. Geriatr. Soc.* 23:212–15
78. Hoehn, M. M., Yahr, M. D. 1967. Parkinsonism: onset, progression, and mortality. *Neurology* 17:427–42
79. Calne, D. B., Teychenne, P. F., Claveria, L. E., Eastman, R., Greenacre, J. K., Petrie, A. 1974. Bro-

mocriptine in parkinsonism. *Br. Med. J.* 4:442–44

80. Pfeiffer, R. F. 1985. The pharmacology of mesulergine. *Clin. Neuropharmacol.* 8:64–72

81. Calne, D. B., Burton, K., Beckman, J., Martin, W. R. W. 1984. Dopamine agonists in Parkinson's disease. *Can. J. Neurol. Sci.* 11:221–24

82. Rinne, U. K. 1986. Early combination of bromocriptine and levodopa in the treatment of Parkinson's disease. In *Recent Developments in Parkinson's Disease*, ed. S. Fahn, C. D. Marsden, P. Jenner, P. Teychenne, pp. 267–71. New York: Raven. 375 pp.

83. Reches, A., Fahn, S. 1982. 3-*O*-Methyldopa blocks DOPA metabolism in rat corpus striatum. *Ann. Neurol.* 12:267–71

84. Klawans, H. L., Goetz, C. G., Volkman, P., Nausieda, P. A., Weiner, W. J. 1978. Lergotrile in the treatment of parkinsonism. *Neurology* 28:699–702

85. Barbeau, A., Roy, M., Gonce, M., Labrecque, R. 1979. Newer therapeutic approaches in parkinson's disease. In *Advances in Neurology*, ed. L. J. Poirier, T. L. Sourkes, P. J. Bédard, 24:433–50. New York: Raven

86. Lees, A. J., Stern, G. M. 1981. Sustained bromocriptine therapy in previously untreated patients with Parkinson's disease. *J. Neurol. Neurosci. Psychiatry* 44:1020–23

87. Agid, Y., Bonnet, A.-M., Pollak, P., Signoret, J. L., Lhermitte, F. 1979. Bromocriptine associated with a peripheral dopamine blocking agent in treatment of Parkinson's disease. *Lancet* 1:570–72

88. Teychenne, P. F., Bergsrud, D., Racy, A., Elton, R. L., Vern, B. 1982. Bromocriptine: low dose therapy in Parkinson's disease. *Neurology* 32:577–83

89. Caraceni, T. A., Celano, I., Parati, E., Girotti, F. 1977. Bromocriptine alone or associated with L-DOPA plus benserazide in Parkinson's disease. *J. Neurol. Neurosurg. Psychiatry* 40:1142–46

90. Lees, A. J., Haddad, S., Shaw, K. M., Kohout, L. J., Stern, G. M. 1978. Bromocriptine in parkinsonism. A long-term study. *Arch. Neurol.* 35:503–5

91. Lander, C. M., Lees, A., Stern, G. 1979. Oscillations in performance in levodopa-treated parkinsonians: treatment with bromocriptine and L-deprenyl. *Clin. Exp. Neurol.* 16:197–203

92. LeWitt, P. A., Gopinathan, G., Ward, C. D., Sanes, J. N., Dambrosia, J. M.

1982. Lisuride versus bromocriptine treatment in Parkinson's disease: a double-blind study. *Neurology* 32:69–72

93. Obeso, J. A., Luquin, M. R., Martinez-Lage, J. M. 1986. Lisuride infusion pump: a device for the treatment of motor fluctuations in Parkinson's disease. *Lancet* 1:467–70

94. Mear, J.-Y., Barroche, G., de Smet, Y., Weber, M., Lhermitte, F., Agid, Y. 1984. Pergolide in treatment of Parkinson's disease. *Neurology* 34:983–86

95. Goetz, C. G., Tanner, C. M., Glantz, R. H., Klawans, H. L. 1985. Chronic agonist therapy for Parkinson's disease: A 5-year study of bromocriptine and pergolide. *Neurology* 35:749–81

96. Lieberman, A., Gopinathan, G., Neophytides, A., Nelson, J., Hiesiger, E., et al. 1986. Pergolide in Parkinson's disease. See Ref. 82, pp. 323–30

97. Jankovic, J. 1985. Long-term use of dopamine agonists in Parkinson's disease. *Clin. Neuropharmacol.* 8(2):131–40

98. Tanner, C. M., Chhablani, R., Goetz, C. G., Klawans, H. L. 1985. Pergolide mesylate: Lack of cardiac toxicity in patients with cardiac disease. *Neurology* 35:918–21

99. Barbeau, A., Roy, M., Kastin, A. J. 1976. Double-blind evaluation of oral L-propyl-L-leucyl-glycine amide in Parkinson's disease. *Can. Med. Assoc. J.* 114:120–22

100. Knoll, J., Magyar, K. 1972. Some puzzling pharmacological effects of monoamine oxidase inhibitors. *Adv. Biochem. Psychopharmacol.* 5:393–408

101. Birkmayer, W., Riederer, P., Youdim, M. B. H. 1982. (–)Deprenyl in the treatment of Parkinson's disease. *Clin. Neuropharmacol.* 5:195–230

102. Lees, A. J., Shaw, K. M., Kohout, L. J., Stern, G. M., Elsworth, J. D., et al. 1977. Deprenyl in Parkinson's disease. *Lancet* 1:791–95

103. Barbeau, A. 1987. Parkinson's disease: Clinical features, and etio-pathology. In *Handbook of Clinical Neurology, Extrapyramidal Disorders*, ed. G. W. Bruyn, H. L. Klawans. Amsterdam: Elsevier. In press

104. Bradbury, A. J., Costall, B., Jenner, P. G., Kelly, M. E., Marsden, C. D., Naylor, R. J. 1985. The neurotoxic actions of 1-methyl-4-phenyl-pyridine (MPP$^+$) are not prevented by deprenyl treatment. *Neurosci. Lett.* 58:177–81

105. Narabayashi, H., Kondo, T., Nagatsu, T., Hayashi, A., Suzuki, T. 1984. L-Threo-3,4-dihydroxyphenylserine for freezing symptom in parkinsonism. In

Advances in Neurology, ed. R. G. Hassler, J. F. Christ, 40:487–502. New York: Raven

106. Quinn, N. P., Perlmutter, J. S., Marsden, C. D. 1984. Acute administration of DL-threo-DOPS does not affect the freezing phenomenon in parkinsonian patients. *Neurology* 34:149A

107. Stoessl, A. J., Mak, E., Calne, D. B. 1985. (+)-4-Propyl-9-hydroxynaphthoxazine (PHNO), a new dopaminomimetic, in treatment of parkinsonism. *Lancet* 2:1330–31

108. Kissel, P., Tridon, P., André, J. M. 1974. Levodopa-propanolol therapy in parkinsonian tremor. *Lancet* 1:403–4 (Lett.)

109. Foster, N. L., Newman, R. P., LeWitt, P. A., Gillespie, M. M., Larsen, T. A., Chase, T. N. 1984. Peripheral beta-adrenergic blockade treatment of parkinsonian tremor. *Ann. Neurol.* 16:505–8

110. Loeb, C., Priano, A. 1977. Preliminary evaluation of the effects of clonazepam on parkinsonian tremor. *Eur. Neurol.* 15:143–45

111. Fahn, S., Eldridge, R. 1976. Definition of dystonia and classification of the dystonic states. In *Advances in Neurology,* ed. R. Eldridge, S. Fahn, 14:1–5. New York: Raven

112. Barbeau, A. 1970. Rationale for the use of L-DOPA in the torsion dystonias. *Neurology* 20 (11; part 2):96–102

113. Segawa, M., Hosaka, A., Miyagawa, F., Nomura, Y., Imai, H. 1976. Hereditary progressive dystonia with marked diurnal fluctuation. See Ref. 111, pp. 215–33

114. Richards, C. L., Bedard, P. J., Fortin, G., Malouin, F. 1983. Quantitative evaluation of the effects of L-DOPA in torsion dystonia: a case report. *Neurology* 33:1083–87

115. Sabouraud, P., Allain, H., Pinel, J. F., Menault, F. 1978. Dystonie familiale transformée par la bromocriptine. *Nouv. Presse Med.* 7:3370

116. Gautier, J. C., Awada, A. 1983. Dystonia musculorum deformans. Effet favorable de la bromocriptine. *Rev. Neurol.* 139:6–7

117. Bassi, S., Ferraresi, C., Frattola, L., Sbacchi, M., Trabucchi, M. 1982. Lisuride in generalized dystonia and spasmodic torticollis. *Lancet* 1:514–15 (Lett.)

118. Quinn, N. P., Lang, A. E., Sheehy, M. P., Marsden, C. D. 1985. Lisuride in dystonia. *Neurology* 35:766–69

119. Gollomp, S. M., Fahn, S., Burke, R. E., Reches, A., Ilson, J. 1983.

Therapeutic trials in Meige syndrome. In *Advances in Neurology,* ed. S. Fahn, D. B. Calne, I. Shoulson, 37:207–13. New York: Raven. 319 pp.

120. Jankovic, J. 1983. Tetrabenazine in the treatment of hyperkinetic movement disorders. See Ref. 119, pp. 277–89

121. Marsden, C. D., Lang, A. E., Sheehy, M. P. 1983. Pharmacology of cranial dystonia. *Neurology* 33:1100–1 (Lett.)

122. Tolosa, E. S., Lai, C. 1979. Meige disease: striatal dopaminergic preponderance. *Neurology* 29:1126–30

123. Fahn, S. 1979. Treatment of dystonia with high-dosage anticholinergic medication. *Neurology* 29:605 (Abstr.)

124. Sheehy, M. P., Marsden, C. D. 1982. Writer's cramp—A focal dystonia. *Brain* 105:461–80

125. Tanner, C. M., Glantz, R. H., Klawans, H. L. 1982. Meige disease: Acute and chronic cholinergic effects. *Neurology* 32:783–85

126. Duvoisin, R. C. 1983. Meige syndrome. Relief on high-dose anticholinergic therapy. *Clin. Neuropharmacol.* 6:63–66

127. Fahn, S. 1983. High dosage anticholinergic therapy in dystonia. *Neurology* 33:1255–61

128. Fisher, C. M. 1983. Pharmacology of cranial dystonia. *Neurology* 33:1101 (Lett.)

129. Ortiz, A. 1983. Neuropharmacological profile of Meige's disease: Overview and a case report. *Clin. Neuropharmacol.* 6:297–304

130. Marsden, C. D., Marion, M.-H., Quinn, N. 1984. The treatment of severe dystonia in children and adults. *J. Neurol. Neurosurg. Psychiatry* 47:1166–73

131. Nutt, J. G., Hammerstad, J. P., de Garmo, P., Carter, J. 1984. Cranial dystonia: double-blind crossover study of anticholinergics. *Neurology* 34:215–17

132. Lang, A. E. 1986. High dose anticholinergic therapy in adult dystonia. *Can. J. Neurol. Sci.* 13:42–46

133. Perry, T. L., Hansen, S., Kloster, M. 1973. Huntington's chorea: Deficiency of γ-aminobutyric acid in brain. *N. Engl. J. Med.* 288:337–42

134. McGeer, P. L., McGeer, E. G., Fibiger, H. C. 1973. Choline acetylase and glutamic acid decarboxylase in Huntington's chorea. *Neurology* 23:912–17

135. Growdon, J. H., Cohen, E. L., Wurtman, R. J. 1977. Huntington's disease: Clinical and chemical effects of choline administration. *Ann. Neurol.* 1:418–22

136. Nutt, J. G., Rosin, A., Chase, T. N. 1978. Treatment of Huntington's disease

with a cholinergic agonist. *Neurology* 28:1061–64

137. Nutt, J. G., Morgan, N. T. 1983. Acute effects of scopolamine in Huntington's disease. See Ref. 119, pp. 291–97

138. Nutt, J. G. 1983. Effect of cholinergic agents in Huntington's disease: A reappraisal. *Neurology* 33:932–35

139. Perry, T. L., Wright, J. M., Hansen, S., Macleod, P. M. 1979. Isoniazid therapy of Huntington's disease. *Neurology* 29:370–75

140. Perry, T. L., Wright, J. M., Hansen, S., Baker, T. S. M., Allan, B. M., et al. 1982. A double-blind clinical trial of isoniazid in Huntington's disease. *Neurology* 32:354–58

141. Stober, T., Schimrigk, K., Holzer, G., Ziegler, B. 1983. Quantitative evaluation of functional capacity during ioniazid therapy in Huntington's disease. *J. Neurol.* 229:237–45

142. Shoulson, I., Kartzinel, R., Chase, T. N. 1976. Huntington's disease: Treatment with dipropylacetic acid and gamma-amino-butyric acid. *Neurology* 26:61–63

143. Pearce, I., Heathfield, K. W. G., Pearce, J. M. S. 1977. Valproate sodium in Huntington's chorea. *Arch. Neurol.* 34:308–9

144. Tell, G., Böhlen, P., Schechter, P. J., Koch-Weser, J., Agid, Y., et al. 1981. Treatment of Huntington's disease with gamma-acetylenic GABA, an irreversible inhibitor of GABA-transaminase: increased CSF GABA and homocarnosine without clinical amelioration. *Neurology* 31:207–11

145. Scigliano, G., Giovannini, P., Girotti, F., Grassi, M. P., Caraceni, T., Schechter, P. J. 1984. Gamma-vinyl GABA treatment of Huntington's disease. *Neurology* 34:94–96

146. Foster, N. L., Chase, T. N., Denaro, A., Hare, T. A., Tamminga, C. A. 1983. THIP treatment of Huntington's disease. *Neurology* 33:637–39

147. Waddington, J. L., Cross, A. J. 1980. Pathophysiology and therapeutic strategies in Huntington's chorea. *Lancet* 2:206–7 (Lett.)

148. Roccatagliata, G., Pizio, N., Farinini, D., Firpo, M. P., Bartolini, A., et al. 1983. Effect de la fenfluramine dans la chorée de Huntington. *Rev. Neurol.* 139:589–92

149. Dalén, P. 1973. Lithium therapy in Huntington's chorea and tardive dyskinesia. *Lancet* 1:107 (Lett.)

150. Candalino, G., Fragassi, N. A., Campanella, G. 1977. Utilità del litio carbo-

nato nel trattamento della corea di Huntington. *Acta Neurol.* 32:862–71

151. Shapiro, A. K., Shapiro, E., Eisenkraft, G. J. 1983. Treatment of Gilles de la Tourette syndrome with clonidine and neuroleptics. *Arch. Gen. Psychiatry* 40:1235–40

152. Barbeau, A. 1980. Therapeutic controversies in movement disorders. *Ther. Controversies Movement Disord. Trans. Am. Neurol. Assoc.* 104:31–51

153. Butler, I. J., Koslow, S. H., Seifert, W. E., Caprioli, R. M., Singer, M. S. 1979. Biogenic amine metabolism in Tourette syndrome. *Ann. Neurol.* 6:37–39

154. Jankovic, J., Glaze, D. G., Frost, J. D. 1984. Effect of tetrabenazine on tics and sleep of Gilles de la Tourette's syndrome. *Neurology* 34:688–92

155. Goetz, C. G., Tanner, C. M., Klawans, H. L. 1984. Fluphenazine and multifocal tic disorders. *Arch. Neurol.* 41:271–72

156. Gillman, M. A., Sandyk, R. 1984. Tourette syndrome: Effect of analgesic concentrations of nitrous oxide and naloxone. *Br. Med. J.* 288:114(Lett.)

157. Cohen, D. J., Young, J. G., Nathanson, J. A., Shaywitz, B. A. 1979. Clonidine in Tourette's syndrome. *Lancet* 2:551–53

158. Leckman, J. F., Detlor, J., Harcherik, D. F., Ort, S., Shaywitz, B. A., Cohen, D. J. 1985. Short- and long-term treatment of Tourette's syndrome with clonidine: A clinical perspective. *Neurology* 35:343–51

159. Price, R. A., Leckman, J. F., Pauls, D. L., Cohen, D. J., Kidd, K. K. 1986. Gilles de la Tourette's syndrome: Tics and central nervous system stimulants in twins and nontwins. *Neurology* 36:232–37

160. Walshe, J. M. 1976. Wilson's disease (hepatolenticular degeneration). In *Handbook of Clinical Neurology*, ed. P. J. Vinken, G. W. Bruyn, 27:379–402. Amsterdam: North-Holland

161. Barbeau, A. 1981. Treatment of Wilson's disease. In *Disorders of Movement*, ed. A. Barbeau, 8:209–20. Lancaster, England: MTP Press

162. Campanella, G., Buscaino, G. A. 1985. Morbo di Wilson. In *Terapia Medica delle Malattie del Sistema Nervoso*, ed. V. Bonavita, A. Quattrone, pp. 557–77. Padova: Piccin

163. Sternlieb, I., Scheinberg, I. H. 1968. Prevention of Wilson's disease in asymptomatic patients. *New Engl. J. Med.* 278:352–59

164. Shoulson, I., Goldblatt, D., Plassche, W., Wilson, G. 1983. Some therapeutic observations in Wilson's disease. See Ref. 119, pp. 239–46

165. Walshe, J. M., Dixon, A. K. 1986. Dangers of non-compliance in Wilson's disease. *Lancet* 1:845–47

166. Walshe, J. M. 1982. Treatment of Wilson's disease with trientine (triethylene tetramine) dihydrochloride. *Lancet* 1: 643–47

167. Hoogenraad, T. V., Loevoet, R., De Ruyter Korver, E. G. W. M. 1979. Oral zinc sulphate as long-term treatment in Wilson's disease (hepatolenticular degeneration). *Eur. Neurol.* 18:205–11

168. Brewer, G. J., Hill, G. M., Prasad, A. S., Cossack, Z. T., Rabbani, P. 1983. Oral zinc therapy for Wilson's disease. *Ann. Int. Med.* 93:314–20

169. Barbeau, A., Friesen, H. 1970. Treatment of Wilson's disease with L-DOPA after failure with penicillamine. *Lancet* 1:1180–81 (Lett.)

Ann. Rev. Pharmacol. Toxicol. 1987. 27:137–56

ACETYLCHOLINE AND THE REGULATION OF REM SLEEP: BASIC MECHANISMS AND CLINICAL IMPLICATIONS FOR AFFECTIVE ILLNESS AND NARCOLEPSY[1]

Priyattam J. Shiromani and J. Christian Gillin

Department of Psychiatry (V-116A), VA Medical Center and University of California, San Diego, California 92161

Steven J. Henriksen

The Research Institute of Scripps Clinic, La Jolla, California 92037

INTRODUCTION

Despite over half a century of scientific inquiry into the basic brain processes underlying the alternation of mammalian states of arousal and sleep, we have little understanding of the mechanisms subserving this basic behavior. More recent experimental and theoretical reviews have proposed multicenter, interdigitated anatomical systems, with multiple neurochemical signatures, involved in the elaboration of the sleep state (1–3). However, no construct has yet successfully described the natural processes underlying sleep initiation, sleep maintenance, sleep stage alternation, or the subsequent relationship of sleep stage alternation to the processes underlying wakefulness and its maintenance or sleep-wake pathologies. Recent evidence suggests that particular subsets of brain stem cholinoceptive neurons are involved in the elaboration

[1]The US Government has the right to retain a nonexclusive, royalty-free license in and to any copyright covering this paper.

137

of major behavior and are physiological constituents of rapid-eye-movement (REM) sleep (1, 2). To date these collective studies provide the most complete description of the potential anatomical and neurochemical substrate for the initiation and maintenance of mammalian states of arousal and sleep.

In this review we focus on and summarize the evidence for the role of cholinergic mechanisms in REM sleep. Interest in this neurochemical system has increased during the past ten years, and important advances have been made in histochemically identifying the cholinergic neuron. New anatomical techniques have been useful in elucidating the role of the cholinergic system in REM sleep generation. We review the evidence that a diffuse network of cholinoceptive neurons in the medial pontine reticular formation (PRF) primes, initiates, and maintains the consolidated state of REM sleep. Neither the origin of the cholinergic input to cholinoreceptive neurons nor the chemical identity of these neurons is fully established at this time.

The realization that cholinergic mechanisms play an important role in the initiation and maintenance of REM sleep coincides with increased interest in states or conditions in which REM sleep occurs earlier, or more, than usual (4). These conditions include clinical disorders such as major depressive disorder, narcolepsy, and, perhaps, other disorders such as obsessive-compulsive disorder and some schizophrenias in which short REM latency (elapsed time from onset of sleep to onset of the first REM period) occurs. These observations raise the possibility that abnormal activation of central cholinergic mechanisms may be part of the pathophysiology of these clinical conditions.

THE NEUROANATOMICAL ORGANIZATION OF THE CHOLINERGIC SYSTEM

Acetylcholine is a neurotransmitter in the central nervous system, as was experimentally determined over a decade ago (5). However, lack of accurate mapping procedures comparable to those used to localize serotonin and the catecholamines has hindered progress in determining the organization of acetylcholine. New procedures, such as autoradiography to locate cholinergic receptors (6), immunohistochemical labeling of the acetylcholine-synthesizing enzyme, choline-acetyltransferase (ChAT) (7), and identification of acetylcholine in neurons (8), are only now providing information on the organization of the acetylcholine system and its potential role in sleep and other behaviors such as information processing (9).

Earlier methods for identifying cholinergic neurons involved detection of acetylcholinesterase (AchE), the enzyme that metabolizes acetylcholine. This procedure, developed by Koelle & Friedenwald (10), was used by Lewis & Shute (11) to provide early maps of the cholinergic system. Conclusions from this procedure have been questioned, as this approach provides a limited, indirect method of localizing cholinergic pathways. Moreover, AchE is found in places devoid of acetylcholine, such as the zona incerta, hypothalamic arcuate and dorsomedial nuclei, lateral posterior hypothalamus, and substantia nigra (12, 13). This procedure, therefore, falsely indicates many positive sites.

A more direct histochemical marker of cholinergic pathways has been developed. Recently, immunohistochemical procedures have been used to label ChAT. Using this immunohistochemical technique, Mesulam and coworkers (14) have identified six major cholinergic groups. Cholinergic groups 1 and 2 (Ch 1 and 2) lie within the medial septal nucleus and the vertical limb nucleus of the diagonal band, respectively. Neurons from these two groups innervate the hippocampus. Group Ch 3 is partly contained in the horizontal limb nucleus of the diagonal band and innervates the olfactory bulb. The largest collection of cholinergic cells is located within the nucleus basalis of Meynert and in the nucleus of the ansa lenticularis, in the nucleus of the ansa peduncularis, and in the medullary laminae of the globus pallidus and substantia innominata. Collectively, these cholinergic neurons are referred to as the Ch 4 group, and they are the principal cause of the cholinergic innervation of the amygdala and neocortex. Loss of these cholinergic neurons has been hypothesized to cause the cognitive deterioration observed in Alzheimer's disease (15).

In the brain stem the largest collection of cholinergic cells occurs in the pedunculo-pontine nucleus (Ch 5), which borders the brachium conjunctivum, and the lateral dorsal tegmental nucleus (Ch 6), which is medial to the locus coeruleus. These two groups, which form the ascending cholinergic pathway of Lewis & Shute (11, see also 16), innervate the thalamus, hippocampus, hypothalamus, and cingulate cortex (14, 16–18). In the brain stem, cholinergic neurons are also found in the cranial motor nerve nuclei and the solitary nucleus.

ACETYLCHOLINE AND THE TONIC AND PHASIC COMPONENTS OF REM SLEEP

REM sleep was first discovered with the observation of a wakelike EEG associated with bursts of rapid eye movements during behavioral sleep in man (19, 20). When subjects were awakened from this state, they frequently reported dreaming (20). Since then sleep and REM sleep have been identified in virtually all mammals, some birds, and, perhaps, in reptiles (21).

REM sleep is composed of both tonic (occurring throughout the REM sleep episode) and phasic (occurring only sporadically during REM sleep) events. The major tonic events include cortical desynchronization, loss of muscle tone in antigravity musculature, and theta activity in the dorsal hippocampus. The phasic events include monophasic waves in pons, lateral geniculate nucleus, and occipital cortex (these waves are called ponto-geniculo-occipital waves, i.e. PGO waves), and rapid eye movements. As we review below, data from lesion, transection, pharmacological, and single-unit studies indicate that the various tonic and phasic components of REM sleep are controlled by discrete reticular formation (RF) nuclei. Moreover, a collection of neurons in the medial pontine reticular formation (PRF) may trigger the discrete reticular nuclei individually responsible for the various tonic and phasic components of REM sleep.

Acetylcholine and Cortical Desynchronization

Cortical EEG desynchronization is an important, distinguishing tonic feature of REM sleep. During both REM sleep and waking the cortical EEG typically shows low-voltage, fast activity, whereas orthodox (NREM) sleep is characterized by the presence of slow (1–3 Hz), high-amplitude waves, sleep spindles (12–14 Hz), and K-complexes.

Moruzzi & Magoun (22) showed that the mesencephalic reticular formation was important for desynchronizing the cortex. Over the years various RF nuclei, particularly the norepinephrine-containing locus coeruleus (LC), have been implicated in cortical EEG desynchronization (23). Data from lesion and single unit studies, however, show that the LC is not necessary for cortical desynchronization during waking and REM sleep (3, 24–26).

Cholinergic mechanisms, on the other hand, do appear to play an important role in cortical desynchronization. Systemically administered atropine, a cholinergic antagonist, readily produces slow, high-amplitude waves, even during behavioral waking (27). Local infusion of cholinergic agonists, such as carbachol, bethanechol, or oxotremorine, into the RF increases cortical desynchronization (28–32). Intense behavioral and EEG arousal is noted with carbachol injections into the mesencephalic RF (28, 33, 34).

Acetylcholine and Rapid Eye Movements

Evidence from lesion studies (35) indicates that the vestibular nuclei may be involved in rapid eye movements during REM sleep. Evidence supporting this hypothesis comes from studies that show that phasic changes in firing rates of vestibular neurons occur during REM sleep in intact cats (36), in the decerebrate preparation (37, 38), and in acute decerebrate animals treated with acetylcholine-potentiating agents such as physostigmine (37, 38). Furthermore, Mergner & Pompeiano (39) showed that increased discharge rates of medial vestibular neurons and abducens motoneurons, which innervate the lateral rectus muscles of the eye, occur 11–15 msec prior to activity in the lateral rectus muscle. Vestibular lesions, however, abolish bursts of rapid eye movements but do not interfere with isolated, slow eye movements or with REM sleep per se.

The excitation in vestibular and abducens motoneurons may be generated by nuclei located within the paramedian RF (40, 41). Indeed, reticular units do show bursts preceding saccadic eye movements (40–44). Moreover, cells in the giganto-cellular tegmental field show cyclic changes in discharge rates before rapid eye movements, not only in intact animals (45) but also in decerebrate animals treated with acetylcholine-potentiating agents (46, 47).

Acetylcholine and PGO Waves

Ponto-geniculo-occipital (PGO) waves are slow, monophasic potentials that occur either singly or in clusters of three to four just prior to and during REM sleep. These waves are recorded in cats, from the pons, lateral geniculate nucleus (LGN), and occipital cortex, areas directly related to the visual system.

The neurons responsible for PGO waves are hypothesized (for review see 48) to be located in and around the brachium conjunctivum (which Sakai (48) calls the "X" area), the rostral part of the lateral parabrachial nucleus, which is just caudal to the "X" area, and the rostral part of the locus coeruleus. Some neurons in these areas fire in phasic bursts (3–5 spikes) as much as 5–25 msec before the onset of a PGO wave (48, 49). During wakefulness some of these units also fire in conjunction with eye movements. Electrical stimulation of this area induces PGO waves, whereas electrical ablation abolishes the PGO waves (48).

The neurons responsible for PGO potentials appear to be cholinergic or at least cholinoceptive in nature. Atropine significantly reduces PGO bursts (50), whereas physostigmine triggers PGO bursts in collicular or pontine-transected cats (51). Significantly, microinfusions of carbachol in the dorso-lateral pontine tegmentum induce PGO activity selectively (28, 31). A vestibular component also appears to be involved because carbachol microinfusion into the vestibular region can evoke PGO waves tightly coupled to stereotyped eye movements (P. J. Shiromani, personal observations).

The elaboration and discharge of PGO waves are not exclusively under cholinergic control; noradrenergic and serotonergic inputs from the locus coeruleus and dorsal raphe nucleus (DRN) are hypothesized to inhibit the cholinergic PGO executive neurons (48). Evidence in support of the inhibitory influence is provided by studies showing that electrical stimulation of DRN inhibits PGO waves (52), whereas lesions or cooling of DRN immediately releases PGO activity (53). Treatments that decrease serotonin or norepinephrine also release PGO activity immediately (53). Moreover, DRN and LC neurons stop activity just prior to, and in temporal contiguity with, PGO activity (54–57).

The anatomical profile of the PGO neuronal network confirms the electrophysiological and pharmacological evidence. Using retrograde tracer and immunohistochemical studies, Sakai (for review see 53) demonstrated that neurons in the "X" area project directly to the LGN (where PGO waves are most easily recorded) and stain positively for ChAT, a specific marker of cholinergic neurons. In turn, the neurons in the "X" area receive norepinephrine and serotonin afferents from the DRN and LC.

Acetylcholine and Atonia

Much evidence supports the hypothesis that the cataplectic episodes of narcoleptic humans and dogs are related to the muscle atonia of normal REM sleep. The inhibition of antigravity musculature is hypothesized (48) to result from activation of a discrete group of nonmonoaminergic cells located ventrally in the LC complex. These peri-LC neurons (48) may exert an excitatory influence on magnocellular neurons located in the medullary RF. The magnocellular neurons correspond to the medullary inhibitory center previously described by Magoun & Rhines (58) and are postulated to induce a nonreciprocal inhibition of spinal motoneurons by exciting spinal inhibitory interneurons (47, 59–62).

Electrical stimulation of the medullary RF, especially the magnocellular, elicits generalized inhibition of spinal motoneurons (48), whereas bilateral electrical ablation of the peri-LC and medial LC abolishes the atonia during REM sleep (63). Moreover, neuronal activity within the peri-LC and the magnocellular is high during periods of atonia in REM sleep (48, 64). The dorso-lateral pontine tegmentum, which contains the peri-LC, exhibits intense metabolic activity, as determined by the 2-deoxyglucose (2-DG) method, during concussion-induced behavioral suppression (65). Investigators suggested (65, 66) that a common mechanism underlies the atonia of REM sleep and the behavioral suppression that follows concussion. Horseradish peroxidase technique (HRP) studies (67, 68) show connections between the peri-LC, the magnocellular, nucleus, and the spinal cord.

The cholinergic mechanism is also implicated in the phenomena of atonia. Infusion of carbachol into the pontine tegmentum readily induces cataplexy in cats (28, 29, 31, 34, 66, 69–71). In acute decerebrate cats, systemic infusion of physostigmine induces cataplexy; such a loss of decerebrate rigidity occurs at regular intervals only with a chronic preparation (72). In narcoleptic dogs, systemically administered cholinomimetics precipitate cataplectic episodes, whereas muscarinic receptor blockers delay these episodes, and nicotinic agents have no effect (73, 74). Moreover, in narcoleptic dogs, increased muscarinic receptor binding is found in several pontine sites (73). In addition, ChAT is found in these areas (7, 75, 76).

ACETYLCHOLINE AND REM SLEEP GENERATION

Although discrete RF nuclei may be responsible for generating the major tonic and phasic components of REM sleep, we suggest that a PRF cholinoceptive mechanism primes the various RF nuclei. Historically, the cholinergic system was the first neurotransmitter system implicated in REM sleep generation. Indeed, Jouvet (77) initially hypothesized that cholinergic mechanisms served an executive function in REM sleep generation. However, he subsequently formulated the "mono-aminergic theory of sleep" (23) when the development of the Falck–Hillarp histofluorescence technique (78) revealed that monoamine pathways originating from the brainstem regions were implicated in arousal, sleep, and REM sleep. The finding that the monoamine system innervated almost the entire brain and spinal cord suggested that this system was involved in orchestrating widespread electrophysiological changes associated with the sleep-wake cycle. Considerable research shows that dopamine, norepinephrine, and serotonin play important roles in sleep and arousal (23, 79). These neurotransmitters are also implicated in the regulation of the REM sleep process but may not be directly involved in REM sleep generation. Instead, these neurotransmitters are currently hypothesized to exert an inhibitory control on a diffusely represented neuronal system responsible for the initiation and maintenance of REM sleep (1). Considerable work has been done on establishing the inhibitory role of the catecholamines (principally norepinephrine) and serotonin in REM sleep, however very little is known about the diffuse REM sleep generating system.

Pharmacological studies show that cholinergic mechanisms in the medial PRF play an important role in the generation of REM sleep. For example, in cats and rats administration of cholinergic agonists, e.g. carbachol, directly into the PRF evokes elements of REM sleep (atonia, PGO waves, rapid eye movements) or complete REM sleep, which may be unusually long (28–32, 34, 69, 70, 80–82). Infusions into midbrain or medullary sites fail to induce REM sleep (28, 34, 70), whereas local infusion of scopolamine blocks the cholinomimetic-induced and physiologic REM sleep (31, 82). Recently, Shiromani & McGinty (70) found that some medial PRF neurons increase discharge in conjunction with the carbachol-induced REM sleep. The medial PRF appears to be unique because blood pressure changes during the carbachol-induced REM sleep (when the cabachol infusions are made in the medial PRF) are similar to those during physiological REM sleep (34). During REM sleep increased release of acetylcholine occurs in cortex (83, 84) and striatum (85) of normal cats and in ventricular perfusates of conscious dogs (86). In human subjects, intravenous infusions of physostigmine or arecoline during non-REM sleep decrease the latency to REM sleep, although infusions during or immediately after REM sleep produce arousal (87–91). In addition, an orally active muscarinic agonist (RS-86) shortens REM latency in normal volunteers (92).

The cholinomimetic-induced and normal REM sleep may be mediated by muscarinic receptor activation because scopolamine and atropine block normal and cholinomimetic-induced REM sleep (28, 31, 82, 91). In narcoleptic dogs, as mentioned, muscarinic receptor agonists readily trigger cataplexy, whereas nicotinic agonists have no effect (74). In narcoleptic dogs, increased muscarinic receptors are located in the medial PRF regions implicated in REM sleep generation (73, 93, 94). In normal human subjects, a three-consecutive-morning treatment with scopolamine decreases the latency to REM sleep at night (95). In rats, REM sleep augmentation occurs in conjunction with muscarinic receptor up-regulation during withdrawal from a seven-day chronic scopolamine treatment (96). In this study increased muscarinic density was found in the caudate and hippocampus but unchanged density was observed in the cortex, brainstem, and cerebellum. Finally, increased REM sleep is found in a strain of rats genetically inbred for increased numbers of central cholinergic receptors (P. J. Shiromani, D. Overstreet & J. C. Gillin, unpublished observations).

Numerous pharmacological studies implicate cholinergic mechanisms in REM sleep generation, however, they only indicate that neurons sensitive to acetylcholine can generate REM sleep. Indeed, we find no cholinergic cell bodies in the medial PRF, an area traditionally implicated in REM sleep generation (97). Also, we show that some neurons in the medial PRF show a progressive increase in discharge from waking to REM sleep (97). Previously, Sakai (48) had identified some "REM-on" neurons and suggested that they are important for REM sleep generation, since they show a unique firing increase related to REM sleep.

Few, if any, cholinergic cell bodies are located in the medial PRF. Therefore, the control system in the medial PRF responsible for REM sleep generation is apparently not mediated by intrinsic PRF cholinergic neurons. As an alternate hypothesis, we suggest that an extrinsic cholinergic input "primes" the cholinoceptive REM sleep neurons in the medial PRF. Thus, the medial PRF may actually represent a final common path in a sequence of events originating elsewhere. Now, we must determine the source of the cholinergic input to the medial PRF.

Two cholinergic groups are the possible source of cholinergic afferents to the medial PRF. The first choice of a group is the cholinergic cells in the pedunculo-pontine (PPG) and lateral dorsal tegmental (LDT) groups. These cells form the largest collection of cholinergic cells in the PRF (7, 14, 75, 98), and considering that REM sleep originates from the PRF, this collection of cells is a logical choice of a possible source. These two groups form the ascending cholinergic pathway of Shute and Lewis (11, 16), which innervates the thalamus, hippocampus, hypothalamus, and cingulate cortex (14–18). The PPG and LDT may also be a component of the ascending reticular-activating system described by Moruzzi & Magoun (22).

Much evidence indicates that cholinergic cells in the PPG and LDT play a very important role in some tonic and phasic components of REM sleep. For example, Steriade et al (99) suggest that EEG activation during waking and REM sleep may be result from a tonic activation of an ascending cholinergic system in the rostral reticular core. Steriade et al (99) suggest that midbrain-subthalamic-thalamic-cortical loops underlie the ascending activating reticular influences. The PPG and LDT innervate the thalamus (for review see 16), and microinfusion of carbachol into the rostral portions of the PPG induces a sustained behavioral arousal characterized by EEG desynchronization (28, 34). Indeed, acetylcholine is released from the cerebral cortex during REM sleep (84). PGO activity is another component of REM sleep hypothesized to be under the control of cholinergic cells in the PPG and LDT (48, 53). PGO waves are a phasic component of REM sleep, and they occur just before and during REM sleep. The PPG and LDT project to the LGN (where PGO waves are recorded easily) (48, 53, 100–102). Some neurons in the PPG and LDT fire before and with PGO, leading some investigators to suggest that these are PGO executive neurons (48, 53, 103). Finally, the muscle atonia that accompanies REM sleep may be a result of descending cholinergic neurons in the more medial-caudal portions of the PPG located in the nucleus sub-coeuruleus and locus coeruleus-alpha (48, 53, 68).

The other possible source of cholinergic afferents to the medial PRF is the cholinergic cells in the basal forebrain. Since rostral transection does not eliminate REM-like states in the isolated pons, we postulate that cholinergic inputs from the basal forebrain or other rostral sites might exert modulation control over REM sleep rather than be the sole regulation of REM sleep. This region along with the raphe is considered to be one of the somnogenic sites (104). Electrolytic (104, 105) and kainic acid (106) lesions of the basal forebrain produce long-lasting insomnia, and electric stimulation produces sleep (107). Diathermic warming in this region also produces sleep (108). More importantly, Szymusiak & McGinty (109) found that some basal fore-brain neurons discharge only during sleep. The chemical identity of this type of basal forebrain neuron is unknown, but since these cells are localized in areas found to contain cholinergic cells (7), the cells causing sleep may be cholinergic.

Most studies have examined the ascending projections of the cholinergic neurons. The descending projections of the basal forebrain are not thoroughly examined. Recently, retrograde studies demonstrated that there is a descending projection from the basal forebrain to the PRF in rats (110). However, these studies did not determine whether cholinergic neurons innervated the PRF. This determination is vitally important considering that the basal forebrain represents a somnogenic center whereas the PRF is important for arousal and REM sleep. The interplay between cholinergic basal forebrain cells and cholinoceptive medial PRF cells may be responsible for the regular transition from waking to sleep to REM sleep. For example, we noted earlier that some basal forebrain neurons discharge selectively during non-REM sleep. If these neurons are cholinergic, then increased discharge during non-REM sleep could release acetylcholine in the medial PRF and prime the medial PRF cholinoceptive neurons responsible for REM sleep. Subsequent interplay between acetylcholine, catecholamine, and indoleamine neuronal systems, and other chemically unidentified neurons in the pons, may then be responsible for the initiation and maintenance of REM sleep (1, 111).

Even though we suggest that a cholinergic input primes the cholinoceptive medial PRF, the medial PRF neurons may have an intrinsic property to exhibit a tonic or bursting firing pattern similar to that seen in thalamic neurons (112–114). Indeed, Greene & McCarley (115) have begun to examine, in pontine slices, the firing pattern of medial PRF neurons, and they find similarities with thalamic neurons.

SUMMARY OF BASIC MECHANISMS

Considerable evidence indicates that discrete brain stem nuclei are responsible for the various tonic and phasic components of REM sleep. The preponderance of evidence suggests that these discrete nuclei are activated and REM sleep ensues when a group of medial PRF neurons begin to fire. The evidence derived from pharmacological and anatomical studies indicates that the medial PRF neurons instrumental to REM sleep generation are cholinoceptive and are dependent on a cholinergic input for activation. Although we focus on the cholinergic system in this review, we stress that the catecholamine and serotonin systems also play very important roles and that the interplay between these transmitter systems may be responsible for the orderly transition between waking, sleep, and REM sleep. In addition, the chemical identity of the apparent cholinoreceptive cells in medial PRF remains unknown; they are not cholinergic, serotonergic, or catecholaminergic.

CHOLINERGIC REGULATION OF REM SLEEP: CLINICAL IMPLICATIONS

The evidence for cholinergic involvement in REM sleep, reviewed above, has implications for conditions in which short REM latency occurs. The two best-documented clinical disorders with short REM latency are depression and narcolepsy, which we briefly review.

Short REM latency has been reported in some patients with severe obsessive-compulsive disorder, schizophrenia, alcoholism, anorexia nervosa, and attention-deficit disorder. Controversy exists regarding some of these later conditions, and the significance of the reports is not yet clear. Further research is needed to determine the clinical specificity of short REM latency and other sleep disorders in depression.

In addition, short REM latency may occur in normal subjects under certain conditions, such as withdrawal from drugs that suppress REM sleep, following deprivation of REM sleep, and under altered sleep-wake patterns, such as naps, free-running conditions in which the subject lives in an environment free of time cues, and on experimental "short days" (i.e. 30 minutes sleep and 60 minutes wake). A circadian rhythm of REM latency and REM sleep exists, which is roughly in phase with the core body-temperature rhythm. REM latency tends to be longest and REM percentage lowest when body temperature is highest, for example, in the early evening. In contrast, REM latency is shortest and REM percentage highest when temperature is lowest, for example, at the end of the normal rest period. REM latency also varies with age; it is highest in early adolescence and tends to decline moderately after midlife.

Many studies from around the world demonstrate that short REM latency is a state-dependent characteristic of patients with moderate-to-severe depression, particularly those with endogenous, melancholic, or primary subtypes (for reviews see 116, 117). In addition, some, but not all, studies report increased duration of the first REM period and increased ocular activity during REM periods (increased REM density). Loss of total sleep time, poor sleep efficiency (percentage time asleep in bed), and low amounts of delta (Stages 3 & 4) sleep are also commonly reported. The sleep alterations in depression tend to be worse in older than in younger patients compared with age-matched controls.

Short REM latency in depression appears to be associated with hypercortisolemia in depression, as manifested either by an elevated concentration of plasma cortisol (118) or with "escape" on the dexamethasone-suppression test (DST) (119–122).

Many biochemical theories of affective disorder have been proposed. Included is the cholinergic-aminergic imbalance hypothesis, originally proposed by Janowsky et al (123). Based on inferences from pharmacological studies, they suggest that depression results from an increased ratio of central cholinergic to aminergic activity, while mania results from the opposite. For example, physostigmine and other cholinomimetics drugs have antimanic effects in manic patients and depressogenic effects in normal controls and depressed patients, especially in depressives.

The cholinergic-aminergic balance hypothesis of affective disorders provides an explanatory mechanism for both short REM latency and hypercortisolemia in depression. As reviewed already, considerable evidence suggests that cholinergic mechanisms help regulate REM latency and REM density in normal sleep. In addition, cholinergic mechanisms facilitate release of plasma ACTH and cortisol. Physostigmine has been reported to elevate plasma ACTH levels to a greater extent in depressives than in normals (124) and to reverse dexamethasone suppression of cortisol in normal subjects (125).

It has not been possible to test the cholinergic-aminergic hypothesis directly. Nevertheless, depressive sleep patterns, short REM latency, elevated REM density, and poor sleep efficiency, can be induced in normal volunteers by the administration of scopolamine for three consecutive mornings (126). In addition, following this treatment, sleep records of normal volunteers were chosen as "depressed" by a discriminant function analysis that had previously separated depressed, insomniac, and normal sleep records successfully (127). As stated, administration of scopolamine in this fashion may induce muscarinic receptor supersensitivity (95). These observations suggest that a central, functional muscarinic supersensitivity is present in patients with affective disorders.

To test this hypothesis, we developed the Cholinergic REM Induction Test (CRIT), which was originally used to demonstrate muscarinic supersensitivity in normal volunteers following administration of scopolamine (91, 128). In the CRIT, arecoline (0.5 or 1.0 mg) is administered during the second NREM period of the night, and the latency to the second REM period is measured. Our original studies indicated that patients with bipolar depression (both in a state of clinical remission and ill) responded more rapidly than normal controls (91, 129, 130). Further studies in identical twins suggested that the response on the CRIT might be partially under genetic control (131). Since the original study, Sitaram and his colleagues have confirmed the general cholinergic muscarinic supersensitivity in patients with endogenous depression using the CRIT (132–134). Our own recent preliminary results confirm a faster REM induction in patients with major depressive disorder and bipolar depression with an arecoline dose of 1.0 mg than with a 0.5-mg dose.

Using another sleep measure to assess cholinergic supersensitivity in depression, Berger et al (135) found that depressed patients were more likely than normal controls to awaken following an infusion of physostigmine (0.5 mg), administered shortly after sleep onset. Since we had previously shown time- and dose-dependent arousal to intravenously administered physostigmine in sleep, this result may be consistent with increased responsiveness to cholinomimetics in depressives compared to controls.

More recently, Berger et al (136) reported that the experimental muscarinic agonist, RS-86, shortens REM latency to a greater extent in depressives than in normal controls. All of these sleep studies, employing a variety of cholinergic agonists (arecoline, physostigmine, and RS-86), support the hypothesis that REM sleep can be induced more rapidly with cholinomimetics in patients with depression than in normal volunteers. Although no studies provide direct evidence of increased muscarinic receptor density in patients with depression, these data from sleep studies suggest that functional muscarinic supersensitivity may be a feature of depression.

The other disorder characterized by short REM latency is narcolepsy, a chronic disease in man, characterized by excessive daytime sleepiness and attacks of cataplexy, often precipitated by emotional arousal (137–139). The clinical symptoms of narcolepsy probably represent dissociated features of normal REM sleep. For example, cataplexy may be the normal muscle atonia accompanying REM sleep. Genetics play an important role in narcolepsy and virtually all patients with narcolepsy have the HLA antigen DR2 (140). Narcolepsy also occurs in certain animals. Recent evidence suggests that muscarinic receptor density is increased in brainstem of narcoleptic dogs (73, 93, 94). Furthermore, dopamine turnover appears to be reduced in narcoleptic dogs (141).

As mentioned above, short REM latency also occurs when normal subjects sleep near the low point of their circadian temperature rhythm. Studies of autopsied brain tissue in man (142) and rat (143) suggest that various neurotransmitter receptors, including muscarinic receptor density, have a circadian rhythm. Thus, the circadian rhythm of muscarinic receptor density in selected brain regions may underlie the circadian rhythm of REM latency and REM sleep.

Finally, in the context of circadian rhythms, cholinergic nicotinic mechanisms may be involved in mediating the phase position of the suprachiasmatic nucleus (SCN), the best-established circadian clock in mammalian brain. Nicotinic agonists, like light, can advance or delay the phases of circadian rhythms, depending upon the time of administration of the stimulus (creating the classical phase-response curve) (144).

CONCLUSION

A role for cholinergic neurons in the control of REM sleep and its physiological components seems firmly established. The anatomical basis for this cholinergic involvement needs further investigation. The role of other neurotransmitter systems in the general control of sleep and circadian rhythms also needs investigation. In terms of clinical implications, the involvement of cholinergic mechanism in normal sleep may provide clues to pathophysiological mechanisms in certain disorders.

ACKNOWLEDGMENTS

The research was supported by grants from the American Narcolepsy Association to P. J. Shiromani, and VAMC Research and NIMH-38738 grants to J. C. Gillin.

Literature Cited

1. Hobson, J. A., Lydic, R., Baghdoyan, H. 1986. Evolving concepts of sleep cycle generation: From brain centers to neuronal populations. *Behav. Brain Sci.* In press
2. McGinty, D. J., Drucker-Colin, R. R. 1982. Sleep mechanisms: Biology and control of REM sleep. *Int. Rev. Neurobiol.* 23:391–436
3. Vertes, R. P. 1984. Brainstem control of the events of REM sleep. *Prog. Neurobiol.* 22:241–88
4. McCarley, R. W. 1982. REM sleep and depression: common neurobiological control mechanisms. *Am. J. Psychiatry* 139:569–70
5. Krnjevic, K. 1974. Chemical nature of synaptic transmission in vertebrates. *Physiol. Rev.* 54:418–540
6. Wamsley, J. K., Lewis, M. S., Young, W. S., Kuhar, M. J. 1981. Autoradiographic localization of muscarinic cholinergic receptors in rat brainstems. *J. Neurosci.* 1:176–91
7. Kimura, H., McGeer, P. L., Peng, J. H., McGeer, E. G. 1981. The central cholinergic system studied by choline acetyltransferase immuno-histochemistry in the cat. *J. Comp. Neurol.* 200: 151–201
8. Geffard, M., McRae-Degueurce, A., Souan, M. L. 1985. Immunocytochemical detection of acetylcholine in the rat central nervous system. *Science* 229:77–79
9. Bartus, R. T., Dean R. L., Beer, B., Lippa, A. S. 1982. The cholinergic hypothesis of geriatric memory dysfunction. *Science* 217:408–17
10. Koelle, G. B., Friedenwald, J. S. 1949. A histochemical method for localizing cholinesterase activity. *Proc. Soc. Exp. Biol. Med.* 70:617–22
11. Lewis, P. R., Shute, C. C. D. 1967. The cholinergic limbic system: Projections to hippocampal formation, medial cortex, nuclei of the ascending cholinergic reticular system, and subfornical organ and supra-optic crest. *Brain* 110:521–40
12. Butcher, L. L., Talbot, K., Bilezikjian, L. 1975. Acetylcholinesterase neurons in dopamine-containing regions of the brain. *J. Neural Transm.* 37:127–53
13. Eckenstein, F., Sofroniew, M. V. 1983. Identification of central cholinergic neurons containing both choline acetyltransferase and acetylcholinesterase and of central neurons containing only acetylcholinesterase. *J. Neurosci.* 3:2286–91
14. Mesulam, M. M., Mufson, E. J., Wainer, B. H., Levey, A. I. 1983. Central cholinergic pathways in the rat: An overview based on an alternative nomenclature. *Neuroscience* 10:1185–201
15. Coyle, J. T., Price, D. L., DeLong, M. R. 1983. Alzheimer's disease: A disorder of cortical cholonergic innervation. *Science* 219:1184–90
16. Wilson, P. M. 1985. A photographic perspective on the origins, form, course and relations of the acetylcholinesterase containing fibres of the dorsal tegmental pathway in the rat brain. *Brain Res. Rev.* 10:85–118
17. Saper, C. B., Loewy, A. D. 1982. Projections of the pedunculopontine tegmental nucleus in the rat: Evidence for additional extrapyramidal circuitry. *Brain Res.* 252:367–72
18. Sofroniew, M. V., Priestley, J. V., Consolazione, A., Eckenstein, F., Cuello, A. C. 1985. Cholinergic projections from the midbrain and pons to the thalamus in the rat, identified by combined retrograde tracing and choline acetyltransferase immunohistochemistry. *Brain Res.* 329:213–23
19. Aserinsky, E., Kleitman, N. 1953. Regularly occurring periods of eye motility and concomitant phenomena during sleep. *Science* 28:273–74
20. Dement, W., Kleitman, N. 1957. Cyclic variations in EEG during sleep and their relations to eye movement, body motility, and dreaming. *Electroencephalogr. Clin. Neurophysiol.* 9:673–90
21. Campbell, S. C., Tobler, I. 1984. Animal sleep: A review of sleep duration across phylogeny. *Neurosci. Biobehav. Rev.* 8:269–300
22. Moruzzi, G., Magoun, H. W. 1949. Brain stem reticular formation and

activation of the EEG. *Electroencephalogr. Clin. Neurophysiol.* 1:455–73
23. Jouvet, M. 1972. The role of monoamines and acetylcholine-containing neurons in the regulation of the sleep-waking cycle. *Ergeb. Physiol.* 64:166–308
24. Jones, B. E., Harper, S. T., Halaris, A. 1977. Effects of locus coereuleus lesions upon cerebral monoamine content, sleep-wakefulness states and the response to amphetamine in the cat. *Brain Res.* 124:473–96
25. Robinson, T. E., Vanderwolf, C. H., Pappas, B. A. 1977. Are the dorsal noradrenergic bundle projections from the locus coeruleus important for neocortical or hippocampal activation? *Brain Res.* 138:75–98
26. Ramm, P. 1979. The locus coeruleus, catecholamines, and REM sleep: A critical review. *Behav. Neurol. Biol.* 25:415–48
27. Longo, V. G. 1966. Behavioral and electroencephalographic effects of atropine and related compounds. *Pharmacol. Rev.* 18:965–96
28. Baghdoyan, H. A., Rodrigo-Angula, M. L., McCarley, R. W., Hobson, J. A. 1984. Site-specific enhancement and suppression of desynchronized sleep signs following cholinergic stimulation of three brainstem sites. *Brain Res.* 306:39–52
29. Baghdoyan, H. A., Monaco, A. P., Rodrigo-Angula, M. L., Assens, F., McCarley, R. W., Hobson, J. A. 1984. Microinjection of neostigmine into the pontine reticular formation of cats enhances desynchronized sleep signs. *J. Pharmacol. Exp. Ther.* 312:173–80
30. George, R., Haslett, W. L., Jenden, D. J. 1964. A cholinergic mechanism in the brainstem reticular formation: Induction of paradoxical sleep. *Int. J. Neuropharmacol.* 3:541–52
31. Shiromani, P., McGinty, D. J. 1983. Pontine sites for cholinergic PGO waves and atonia: Localization and blockade with scopolamine. *Soc. Neurosci.* 9(2):1203 (Abstr.)
32. Silberman, E., Vivaldi, E., Garfield, J., McCarley, R. W., Hobson, J. A. 1980. Carbachol triggering of desynchronized sleep phenomena: Enhancement via small volume infusions. *Brain Res.* 191:215–24
33. Baxter, B. L. 1969. Induction of both emotional behavior and a novel form of REM sleep by chemical stimulation ap-
plied to cat mesencephalon. *Exp. Neurol.* 23:220–30
34. Shiromani, P. J., Siegel, J., Tomaszewski, K., McGinty, D. J. 1986. Alterations in blood pressure and REM sleep after pontine carbachol microinfusion. *Exp. Neurol.* 91:285–92
35. Morrison, A. R., Pompeiano, O. 1966. Vestibular influences during sleep. IV. Functional relations between vestibular nuclei and lateral geniculate nucleus during desynchronized sleep. *Arch. Ital. Biol.* 104:425–58
36. Bizzi, E., Pompeiano, O., Somogyi, I. 1964. Spontaneous activity of single vestibular neurons of unrestrained cats during sleep and wakefulness. *Arch. Ital. Biol.* 102:308–20
37. Thoden, U., Magherini, P. C., Pompeiano, O. 1972. Cholinergic mechanisms related to REM sleep. II. Effects of an anticholinesterase on the discharge of central vestibular neurons in the decerebrate cat. *Arch. Ital. Biol.* 110:260–83
38. Thoden, U., Magherini, P. C., Pompeiano, O. 1972. Cholinergic activation of vestibular neurons leading to rapid eye movements in the mesencephalic cat. *Biol. Opthalmol.* 82:99–108
39. Mergner, T., Pompeiano, O. 1977. Neurons in the vestibular nuclei related to saccadic eye movements in the decerebrate cat. In *Control of Gaze by Brainstem Neurons,* ed. R. Baker, A. Bertholz, pp. 243–52. Amsterdam: Elsevier/North-Holland
40. Cohen, B., Henn, V. 1972. Unit activity in the pontine reticular formation associated with eye movements. *Brain Res.* 46:403–10
41. Henn, V., Cohen, B. 1975. Activity in eye muscle motoneurons and brainstem units during eye movements. In *Basic Mechanisms of Ocular Motility and Their Clinical Implications,* ed. C. Lennestrand, P. Bach-y-Rita, pp. 305–45. Oxford: Pergamon
42. Keller, E. L. 1974. Participation of medial pontine reticular formation in eye movement generation of monkeys. *J. Neurophysiol.* 37:316–32
43. Luschei, E. S., Fuchs, A. F. 1972. Activity of brain stem neurons during eye movements of alert monkeys. *J. Neurophysiol.* 35:445–61
44. Sparks, D. L., Travis, R. P. 1971. Firing patterns of reticular formation neurons during horizontal eye movements. *Brain Res.* 33:477–81
45. Pivik, R. T., McCarley, R. W., Hob-

son, J. A. 1977. Eye movement associated discharge in brainstem neurons during desynchronized sleep. *Brain Res.* 121:59–76
46. Hoshino, K. Pompeiano, O., Magherini, P. C., Mergner, T. 1976. Oscillatory activity of pontine neurons related to the regular occurrence of REM bursts in the decerebrate cat. *Brain Res.* 116:125–30
47. Pompeiano, O. 1980. Cholinergic activation of reticular and vestibular mechanisms controlling posture and eye movements. In *The Reticular Formation Revisited,* ed. J. Allan Hobson, Mary Brazier, pp. 473–512. New York: Raven
48. Sakai, K. 1980. Some anatomical and physiological properties of ponto-mesencephalie-tegmental neurons with special reference to the PGO waves and postural atonia during paradoxical sleep in the cat. See Ref. 47, pp. 427–47
49. McCarley, R. W., Nelson, J. P., Hobson, J. A. 1978. Ponto-geniculo-occipital (PGO) burst neurons: correlative evidence for neuronal generators of PGO waves. *Science* 201:269–72
50. Henriksen, S. J., Jacobs, B. L., Dement, W. C. 1972. Dependence of REM sleep PGO waves on cholinergic mechanisms. *Brain Res.* 48:412–16
51. Magherini, P. C., Pompeiano, O., Thoden, U. 1971. The neurochemical basis of REM sleep: A cholinergic mechanism responsible for rhythmic activation of the vestibulo-oculomotor system. *Brain Res.* 35:565–69
52. Jacobs, B. L., Asher, R., Dement, W. C. 1973. Electrophysiological and behavioral effects of electrical stimulation of the raphe nuclei in cats. *Physiol. Behav.* 11:489–96
53. Sakai, K. Anatomical and physiological basis of paradoxical sleep. 1985. In *Brain Mechanisms of Sleep,* ed. D. McGinty, A. Morrison, R. R. Drucker-Colin, P. L. Parmeggiani, pp. 111–38. New York: Spectrum
54. Chu, N. S., Bloom, F. E. 1973. Norepinephrine containing neurons: changes in spontaneous discharge patterns during sleeping and waking. *Science* 179:908–10
55. Chu, N. S., Bloom, F. E. 1974. Activity patterns of catecholamine pontine neurons in the dorso-lateral tegmentum of unrestrained cat. *J. Neurobiol.* 5:527–44
56. McGinty, D. J., Harper, R. M. 1976. Dorsal raphe neurons: Depression of firing during sleep in cats. *Brain Res.* 101:569–75

57. Sheu, Y. S., Nelson, J. P., Bloom F. E. 1974. Discharge patterns of cat raphe neurons during sleep and waking. *Brain Res.* 73:263–76
58. Magoun, H. W., Rhines, R. 1946. An inhibitory mechanism in the bulbar reticular formation. *J. Neurophysiol.* 9:165–71
59. Fung, S., Boxer, P. A., Morales, F., Chase, M. 1982. Hyperpolarizing membrane responses induced in lumbar motoneurons by stimulation of the nucleus reticularis pontis oralis during active sleep. *Brain Res.* 248:267–73
60. Glenn, L. L., Foutz, A. S., Dement, W. C. 1978. Membrane potential of spinal motoneurons during natural sleep in cats. *Sleep* 1:199–204
61. Morales, F. R., Chase, M. K. 1978. Intracellular recording of lumbar motoneuron membrane potential during sleep and wakefulness. *Exp. Neurol.* 62:821–27
62. Pompeiano, O. 1976. Mechanisms responsible for spinal inhibition during desynchronized sleep: experimental study. In *Narcolepsy,* ed. C. Guilleminault, W. C. Dement, P. Passouant. pp. 411–49. New York: Spectrum
63. Henley, K., Morrison, A. D. 1974. A re-evaluation of the effects of lesions of the pontine tegmentum and locus coeruleus on phenomena of paradoxical sleep in the cat. *Acta Neurobiol. Exp.* 34:215–32
64. Kanamori, N., Sakai, K., Jouvet, M. 1980. Neuronal activity specific to paradoxical sleep in the ventromedial medullary reticular formation of restrained cats. *Brain Res.* 189:251–55
65. Hayes, R. L., Pechura, C. M., Katayama, Y., Povlishock, J. T., Giebel, M. L., Becker, D. P. 1984. Activation of pontine cholinergic sites implicated in unconsciousness following cerebral concussion in the cat. *Science* 223: 301–3
66. Katayama, Y., DeWitt, D. S., Becker, D. P., Hayes, R. L. 1984. Behavioral evidence for a cholinoceptive pontine inhibitory area: Descending control of spinal motor output and sensory input. *Brain Res.* 296:241–62
67. Sakai, K., Touret, M., Salvert, D., Jouvet, M. 1978. Afferents to the cat locus coeruleus as visualized by the horseradish peroxidase technique. In *Interactions Between Putative Neurotransmitters in the Brain,* ed. S. Garattini, J. P. Pujol, R. Samanin, pp. 319–42. New York: Raven
68. Sakai, K., Sastre, J. P., Salvert, D.,

CHOLINERGIC REGULATION OF REM SLEEP   153

Torret, M., Tohyama, M., Jouvet, M. 1979. Tegmento—reticular projections with special reference to the muscular atonia during paradoxical sleep: An HRP study. *Brain Res.* 176:233–54

69. Mitler, M., Dement, W. C. 1974. Cataplectic-like behavior in cats after microinjection of carbachol in pontine reticular formation. *Brain Res.* 68:335–43

70. Shiromani, P., McGinty, D. J. 1986. Pontine neuronal responses to local cholinergic infusion: Relation to REM sleep. *Brain Res.* In press

71. Van Dongen, P. A., Broekamp, L. E., Coola, A. R. 1978. Atonia after carbachol microinjections near the locus coeruleus in cats. *Pharmacol. Biochem. Behav.* 8:527–32

72. Hoshino, K., Pompeiano, O. 1976. Selective discharge of pontine neurons during the postural atonia produced by an anti-cholinesterase in the decerebrate cat. *Arch. Ital. Biol.* 114:244–77

73. Baker, T. L., Dement, W. C. 1985. Canine narcolepsy-cataplexy syndrome: Evidence for an inherited monoaminergic-cholinergic imbalance. See Ref. 53, pp. 199–234

74. Delashaw, J. B., Foutz, A. S., Guilleminault, C., Dement, W. C. 1979. Cholinergic mechanisms and cataplexy in dogs. *Exp. Neurol.* 66:745–57

75. Armstrong, D. M., Saper, C. B., Levey, A. I., Wainer, B. I., Terry, R. D. 1983. Distribution of cholinergic neurons in the rat brain: Demonstrated by the immunocytochemical localization of choline acetyltransferase. *J. Comp. Neurol.* 216:53–68

76. Kimura, H., Maeda, T. 1982. Aminergic and cholinergic systems in the dorsolateral pontine tegmentum. *Brain Res. Bull.* 9:403–99

77. Jouvet, M. 1962. Recherches sur les structures nerveuses et les méchanismes responsales des differéntes du sommeil physiologique. *Arch. Ital. Biol.* 100:125–206

78. Dahlstrom, A., Fuxe, K. 1964. Evidence for the existence of monoamine neurons in the central nervous system. I. Demostration of monoamines in the cell bodies of brain stem neurons. *Acta Physiol. Scand.* 62:1–55

79. Jacobs, B. L., Jones, B. E. 1978. The role of central monoamine and acetylcholine systems in sleep-wakefulness states: mediation or modulation. In *Cholinergic-Monoaminergic Interactions in the Brain*, ed. L. L. Butcher, pp. 271–90. New York: Academic

80. Amatruda, T. T., Black, D. A., McKenna, T. M., McCarley, R. W., Hobson, J. A. 1975. Sleep cycle control and cholinergic mechanisms: Differential effects of carbachol at pontine brainstem sites. *Brain Res.* 98:501–15

81. Hobson, J. A., Goldberg, M., Vivaldi, E., Riew, D. 1983. Enhancement of desynchronized sleep signs after pontine microinjections of the muscarinic agonist bethanechol. *Brain Res.* 275:127–36

82. Shiromani, P., Fishbein, W. 1986. Long-term pontine cholinergic microinfusions via mini-pump induces sustained alterations in rapid eye movement sleep. *Pharmacol. Biochem. Behav.* In press

83. Celesia, G. G., Jasper, H. H. 1966. Acetylcholine released from cerebral cortex in relation to state of activation. *Neurology* 16:1053–64

84. Jasper, H. H., Tessier, J. 1971. Acetylcholine liberation from cerebral cortex during paradoxical (REM) sleep. *Science* 172:601–2

85. Gadea-Ciria, M., Stadler, H., Lloyd, K. G., Bartholini, G. 1973. Acetylcholine release within the cat striatum during the sleep-wakefulness cycle. *Nature* 243:518–19

86. Haranath, P. S., Venkatakrishna-Bhatt, H. 1973. Release of acetylcholine from perfused cerebral ventricles in unanesthetized dogs during waking and sleep. *Jpn. J. Physiol.* 23:241–50

87. Sitaram, N., Wyatt, R. J., Dawson, S., Gillin, J. C. 1976. REM sleep induction by physostigmine infusion during sleep in normal volunteers. *Science* 191:1281–83

88. Sitaram, N., Mendelson, W. B., Wyatt, R. J., Gillin, J. C. 1977. The time-dependent induction of REM sleep and arousal by physostigmine infusion during normal human sleep. *Brain Res.* 122:562–67

89. Sitaram, N., Moore, A. M., Gillin, J. C. 1978. Experimental acceleration and slowing of REM ultradian rhythm by cholinergic agonist and antagonist. *Nature* 274:490–92

90. Sitaram, N., Moore, A. M., Gillin, J. C. 1978. Induction and resetting of REM sleep rhythm in normal man by arecoline: Blockade by scopolamine. *Sleep* 1:83–90

91. Sitaram, N., Gillin, J. C. 1980. Development and use of pharmacological probes of the CNS in man: Evidence for cholinergic abnormality in primary affective illness. *Biol. Psychiatry* 15:925–55

92. Spiegel, R. 1984. Effects of RS-86, an orally active cholinergic agonist, on sleep in man. *Psychiatr. Res.* 11:1–13

93. Boehme, R. E., Baker, T. L., Mefford, I. N., Barchas, J. D., Dement, W. C., Ciaranello, R. D. 1984. Narcolepsy: Cholinergic receptor changes in an animal model. *Life Sci.* 34:1825–28

94. Kilduff, T. S., Bowersox, S., Kaitin, K., Baker, T. L., Ciaranello, R. D., Dement, W. C. 1986. Muscarinic cholinergic receptors and the canine model of narcolepsy. *Sleep* 9:102–6

95. Sitaram, N., Moore, A. M., Gillin, J. C. 1979. Scopolamine-induced muscarinic supersensitivity in normal man: changes in sleep. *Psychiatr. Res.* 1:9–16

96. Sutin, E. L., Shiromani, P., Kelsoe, J., Storch, F., Gillin, J. C. 1985. REM sleep and muscarinic receptor binding in rats are augmented during withdrawal following chronic scopolamine treatment. *Sleep Res.* 14:61

97. Shiromani, P., Armstrong, D. M., Groves, P. M., Gillin, J. C. 1986. Combined neurophysiological and immunohistochemical mapping of the medial-lateral pontine reticular formation: Relation of REM-on cells with cells containing choline acetyltransferase. *Sleep Res.* 15:12

98. Satoh, K., Armstrong, D. M., Fibiger, H. C. 1983. A comparison of the distribution of central cholinergic neurons as demonstrated by acetylcholinesterase pharmacohistochemistry and choline acetyltransferase immunohistochemistry. *Brain Res. Bull.* 11:693–720

99. Steriade, M., Ropert, N., Kitsikis, A., Oakson, G. 1980. Ascending activating neuronal networks in midbrain reticular core and related rostral systems. See Ref. 47, pp. 125–67

100. Kayama, Y. 1985. Ascending, descending and local control of neuronal activity in the rat lateral geniculate nucleus. *Vision Res.* 25:339–47

101. Kayama, Y., Negi, T., Sugitani, M., Iwama, K. 1982. Effects of locus coeruleus stimulation on neuronal activities of dorsal lateral geniculate nucleus and perigeniculate reticular nucleus of the rat. *Neuroscience* 7:655–66

102. Tohyama, M., Satoh, K., Sakumoto, T., Kimoto, Y., Takahashi, Y., et al. 1977. Organization and projections of the neurons in the dorsal tegmental area of the rat. *J. Hirnforschung* 19:165–76

103. Nelson, J. P., McCarley, R. W., Hobson, J. A. 1983. REM sleep burst neurons, PGO waves, and eye movement information. *J. Neurophysiol.* 50:784–97

104. McGinty, D. J., Sterman, M. B. 1968. Sleep suppression after basal forebrain lesions in the cat. *Science* 160:1253–55

105. Szymusiak, R., Satinoff, E. 1984. Ambient temperature-dependence of sleep disturbances produced by basal forebrain damage in rats. *Brain Res. Bull.* 12:295–305

106. Szymusiak, R., McGinty D. J. 1985. Sleep-suppression after kainic acid–induced lesions of the basal forebrain in cats. *Sleep Res.* 14:2

107. Sterman, M. B., Clemente, C. 1962. Forebrain inhibitory mechanisms: Sleep patterns induced by basal forebrain stimulation in the behaving cat. *Exp. Neurol.* 6:103–17

108. Roberts, W., Robinson, T. C. 1969. Relaxation and sleep induced by warming of preoptic region and anterior hypothalamus in cats. *Exp. Neurol.* 25:282–94

109. Szymusiak, R., McGinty, D. J. 1986. Sleep-related neuronal discharge in the basal forebrain of cats. *Brain Res.* 370:82–92

110. Shammah-lagnado, S. J., Negrao, N., Silva, B. A., Silva, J. A., Ricardo, J. A. 1985. Afferent connections of the magnocellular reticular formation: A horseradish peroxidase study in the rat. *Neurosci. Abstr.* 11:1026

111. McCarley, R. W., Hobson, J. A. 1975. Neuronal excitability modulation over the sleep cycle: A structural and mathematical model. *Science* 189:58–60

112. Llinas, R., Jahnsen, H. 1982. Electrophysiology of mammalian thalamic neurones in vitro. *Nature* 297:406–8

113. Jahnsen, H., Llinas, R. 1984. Electrophysiological properties of guinea-pig thalamic neurones: An in vitro study. *J. Physiol.* 349:205–26

114. Jahnsen, H., Llinas, R. 1984. Ionic bases for the electroresponsiveness and oscillatory properties of guinea-pig thalamic neurones in vitro. *J. Physiol.* 349:227–47

115. Greene, R. W., McCarley, R. W. 1986. Initial membrane potential determines two firing patterns of mPRF neurons recorded in vitro. *Sleep Res.* 15:4

116. Gillin, J. C., Sitaram, N., Wehr, T. 1984. Sleep and affective illness. In

Neurobiology of Mood Disorders, ed. R. M. Post, J. C. Ballenger, pp. 157–89. Baltimore: Williams & Wilkins

117. Thase, M. E., Kupfer, D. J., Spiker, D. G. 1984. Electroencephalographic sleep in secondary depression: A revisit. *Biol. Psychiatr.* 19:805–14

118. Asnis, G. M., Halbreich, U., Sachar, E., Nathan, R. S., Ostrow, L. C., et al. 1983. Plasma cortisol secretion and REM period latency in adult endogenous depression. *Am. J. Psychiatr.* 140:(6): 750–53

119. Ansseau, M., Scheyvaerts, M., Donmont, A., Poirrier, R., Legros, J. J., Franck, G. 1984. Concurrent use of REM latency and dexamethasone suppression as markers of endogenous depression: a pilot study. *Psychiatr. Res.* 12:261–72

120. Feinberg, M., Carroll, B. J. 1984. Biological "markers" for endogenous depression. *Arch. Gen. Psychiatr.* 41: 1080–85

121. Mendlewicz, J., Kerkhofs, M., Hoffman, G., Linkowski, P. 1984. Dexamethasone suppression test and REM sleep in patients with major depressive disorder. *Br. J. Psychiatr.* 145:383–88

122. Rush, J., Giles, G. E., Roffwarg, H. P., Parker, C. R. 1982. Sleep EEG and dexamethasone suppression test findings in outpatients with unipolar major depressive disorder. *Biol. Psychiatr.* 17: 327–41

123. Janowsky, D. C., El-Yousef, M. K., Dans, J. M. 1972. A cholinergic-adrenergic hypothesis of mania and depression. *Lancet* 2:632–25

124. Risch, S. C., Cohen, R. M., Janowsky, D. S., Kalin, N. H., Murphy, D. L. 1980. Plasma beta-endorphin and cortisol elevations accompany the mood and behavioral effects of physostigmine in man. *Science* 209:1545–46

125. Carroll, B., Greden, J. F., Haskett, R. 1980. Neurotransmitter studies of neuroendocrine pathology in depression. *Acta Psychiatr. Scand. Suppl.* 280:183–99

126. Gillin, J. C., Sitaram, N., Duncan, W. 1979. Muscarinic supersensitivity: A possible model for the sleep disturbance of primary depression. *Psychiatr. Res.* 1:17–22

127. Gillin, J. C., Duncan, W. C., Pettigrew, K., Frankel, B. L., Synder, F. 1979. Successful separation of depressed, normal, and insomniac subjects by EEG sleep data. *Arch. Gen. Psychiatr.* 36: 85–90

128. Gillin, J. C., Sitaram, N., Nurnberger, J. I., Gershon, E. S., Cohen, R., et al. 1983. The cholinergic REM induction test (CRIT). *Psychopharmacol. Bull.* 19:668–70

129. Sitaram, N., Kaye, W. H., Nurnberger, J. I., Ebert, M., Gershon, E. S., Gillin, J. C. 1982. Cholinergic REM sleep induction test: A trait marker of affective illness? In *Biological Markers in Psychiatry and Neurology*, ed. E. Usdin, I. Hanin, pp. 397–404. New York: Pergamon

130. Sitaram, N., Nurnberger, J. I., Gershon, E. S., Gillin, J. C. 1982. Cholinergic regulation of mood and REM sleep: A potential model and marker for vulnerability to affective disorder. *Am. J. Psychiatry* 139:571–76

131. Nurnburger, J. Jr., Sitaram, N., Gerson, E. S., Gillin, J. C. 1983. A twin study of cholinergic REM induction. *Biol. Psychiatr.* 18:1161–65

132. Dube, S., Kumar, N., Etledgui, E., Pohl, R., Jones, D., Sitaram, N. 1985. Cholinergic REM induction response: separation of anxiety and depression. *Biol. Psychiatr.* 20:208–18

133. Jones, D., Kelwala, S., Bell, J., Dube, S., Jackson, E., Sitaram, N. 1985. Cholinergic REM sleep induction response correlation with endogenous depressive subtype. *Psychiatr. Res.* 14:99–110

134. Sitaram, N., Dube, S., Jones, D., Pohl, R., Gershon, S. 1984. Acetylcholine and alpha-1 adrenergic sensitivity in the separation of depression and anxiety. *Psychopathol. Suppl. 3* 17:24–39

135. Berger, M., Lund, R., Bronisch, T., von Zerssen, D. 1983. REM latency in neurotic and endogenous depression and the cholinergic REM induction test. *Psychiatr. Res.* 10:113–23

136. Berger, M., Hochli, D., Zulley, J., Lauer, C., von Zerssen, D. 1985. Cholinomimetic drug RS-86, REM sleep and depression. *Lancet* 1:1385–86

137. Guilleminault, C. 1976. Cataplexy. See Ref. 62, pp. 125–43

138. Hishikawa, Y., Kaneku, Z. 1965. Electroencephalographic study on narcolepsy. *Electroencephalogr. Clin. Neurophysiol.* 18:249–59

139. Rechtschaffen, A., Wolpert, W., Dement, W. C., Mitchell, S., Fisher, C. 1963. Nocturnal sleep of narcoleptics. *Electroencephalogr. Clin. Neurophysiol.* 15:599–609

140. Langdon, N., Walsh, K. F., van Dam, M., Vaughan, R., Parkes, D. 1984. Ge-

netic markers in narcolepsy. *Lancet* 2:1178–80
141. Mefford, I., Baker, T., Boehme, R., Foutz, A., Ciaranello, R., et al. 1983. Narcolepsy: Biogenic amine deficits in an animal model. *Science* 220:629–32
142. Perry, E. K., Perry, R. H., Tomlinson, B. E. 1977. Circadian variations in cholinergic enzymes and muscarinic receptor binding in human cerebral cortex. *Neuroscience* 4:185–89

143. Kafka, M. S., Wirz-Justice, A., Wehr, T. A. 1981. Circadian acetylcholine receptor rhythm in rat brain and its modification by imipramine. *Neuropharmacology* 20:421–25
144. Zatz, M., Brownstein, M. J. 1979. Intraventricular carbachol mimics the effects of light on the circadian rhythm in the rat pineal gland. *Science* 203:358–61

Ann. Rev. Pharmacol. Toxicol. 1987. 27:157–67

SAFETY EVALUATION OF POLYMER MATERIALS

Thomas D. Darby

Department of Pharmacology, School of Medicine, University of South Carolina, Columbia, South Carolina 29208

INTRODUCTION

Polymer materials have made important contributions to human well-being during the last fifty years. The different chemical formulas and syntheses of polymers supply an enormous number of materials of widely differing composition. Continuous research and development in the health industry have led to an increased life span and improved quality of life for many patients by providing improved materials for medical devices. Both elastomers and plastics have been devised to furnish materials with every conceivable type of physical response. Yet, ideas for new and better materials to replace existing materials are proposed each day.

As with other products, safety evaluation of polymer materials and the devices made from them begins with concerns for toxic or adverse reaction associated with the raw materials for the product and ends with the safe disposal of the end materials from product use. One has only to review the problems associated with the production of vinyl chloride monomer to be concerned about manufacture of products with polyvinyl chloride (1, 2). If the monomer had been removed from production, many polyvinyl chloride products would no longer be in the market place. In addition, traces of contaminants from the manufacture of raw materials often contribute to the potential toxicity of a product (3). Naturally, most concern in safety assessment is directed toward the manufacture and use of products. However, shipping and storage can also contribute to toxic effects at time of use. Also, disposal of end materials of product use causes environmental concerns. Polyvinyl chloride is also a good example in this case because the release of hydrochloric acid during pyrolysis causes adverse reactions ranging from eye irritation to pulmonary problems including asthma (4, 5).

157

0362-1642/87/0415-0157$02.00

This review analyzes the test systems used to evaluate the toxic risk potential for polymer materials and discusses the general concepts used in these evaluations. The test systems are generally intended to assure safety as well as to investigate the range of toxicity for plasticizers and other substances contained in the polymer material.

In vitro test systems and in vivo animal studies are often considered indicative of the risks to man. Therefore, these investigations require well-designed standard operating procedures. Also important are protocol studies that consider all relevant parameters prior to actual test, so that the resulting data can be analyzed and applied to human safety concerns.

Tests used in safety assessment of plastic materials need to be sensitive and inexpensive, and must provide comparative data for competing materials. The time in which the data are collected should be minimal. Therefore, investigators have devised a series of sensitive screening tests that attempt to eliminate false-negative safety data while allowing a fairly substantial number of false-positive results. These simple screening tests that include both chemical and biological measurements are not intended to eliminate valuable new materials but to indicate, when positive, that additional protocol tests must be designed. The object of these additional tests is to determine whether the plastic material will be safe to manufacture and use and whether its end products can be disposed of safely (6).

SCREENING TEST

The tests listed in the *United States Pharmacopeia* (USP/NF Volume I, 1980) are frequently used to screen materials for safety. The description of the sample preparation and the test protocol is not detailed enough to allow the user to determine many important parameters of the test. Therefore, review of the data generated by these standard USP tests depends on the standard operation procedures (SOP) of the laboratory where the test is conducted.

Table 1 illustrates the test procedures used for medical-grade plastic materials. The tests are listed in order of procedure. The sample preparation is important to the SOP of the test procedures. Plastic materials are usually a mixture of ingredients. Substances involved in the manufacture of the plastic may appear as contaminants (7). Tests are most useful when the test specimen is as close as possible in composition to the final material that will be used in device manufacture. In any case, raw materials for devices should be screened at periods that allow statistical assurance of safety for the material or materials used in current manufacture of devices.

Physico-Chemical Test

USP tests are designed to determine physical and chemical properties of plastics and their extracts. When testing extracts, the designated amount of

Table 1   Screening test sequence

Chemical Screening Tests
  USP analysis
    Nonvolatile residue
    Residue on ignition
    Heavy metal analysis
    Buffering capacity
  Other analyses
    IR spectrum analysis
    Ammonia test for nitrogen
  Decision to stop or continue testing
Biological Tests
  USP procedures
    Systemic injection test
    Intracutaneous test
    Implantation test
  Other procedures
    Ames test
    Cell culture and Ames test with enzyme additives, e.g. S-9 liver cell fraction
  Decision to stop or continue testing
Protocol Tests
  Safety studies
    With the device
    With chemical compounds knows to be potentially toxic
  Toxicity Studies
    With extracts from the device
    With chemical compounds known to be potentially toxic
  Safety and risk assessment associated with decision to market device

---

the plastic must be used and the specified surface area must be available for extraction at the designated temperature (8, 9). The ingredients of a plastic material migrate to the surface in a complicated process controlled by several factors. Rate of removal from the surface is one such factor (7).

In these tests the extract is usually tested. Naturally, a certain amount of the plastic may often be tested directly. These tests are designed to estimate potential toxic effects, based on the known potential toxic characteristics of extracts. Nonvolatile residue and ash provide an estimate of the amount of extractable material contained in the specimen. The quantity of extractable substances is related to the dose upon patient exposure. Since dose is important to toxicity, especially in the case of functional toxicity, these tests are extremely important. Heavy metals are toxic, especially lead and tin. Certain organotin compounds cause extensive toxic reactions (10, 11).

Changes in buffering capacity of the extraction medium indicate that acids or bases have been extracted from the specimens. These potentially reactive compounds could cause adverse reactions. Likewise, a simple test for ammonia can indicate the presence of nitrogen-containing compounds that are leached from the specimen. Infrared spectra indicate activity sites such as double bonds. As more chemically reactive substances are extracted from the plastic sample or contained in the plastic matrix, potentials for toxic reactions in the biosphere are greater.

These data, along with a list of chemical substances in the formulation, are most helpful when selecting from a list of potential materials. During manufacture of a medical device, however, other chemicals may be incorporated into the plastic. Substances such as solvents, detergents, lubricants, sterilizing agents, etc are often found in the finished product (8, 9, 11).

As Table 1 indicates, a choice between competing materials can often be made at this early point in the testing procedure. Since a major goal of each product is to provide the maximum benefit at a minimum risk, the material with the lowest amount of extractable material and the least potential for chemical reaction is the most favorable.

Biological Tests

These USP tests examine a plastic's suitability for incorporation into a product. These tests of the plastic or its extracts provide information that is often useful in assessing worker safety and evaluating concerns for environmental pollution effects following disposal.

USP tests are preliminary in nature and are screening tests only. Protocol tests are necessary to determine safety. These tests are based on the interpretation of data in making toxicity and safety judgments about plastics in a particular device. Many factors must be analyzed, including plastic composition, processing, and cleaning procedures, contacting media, inks, adhesives, absorption, preservatives, conditions of storage, stability of the plastic, and specific conditions of use (8, 9).

The tests procedures (except for the implantation test) are based on the use of extracts. Temperature determines the class designation for the plastic material. USP Class I plastics are extracted at 50°C. The class of the plastic and the temperature of extraction are usually included in the test results; for example, Class IV has a temperature extraction of 121°C. Systemic injection and intracutaneous tests are carried out with predetermined volumes of the extraction medium containing plastic extracts. Extraction medium is used as a negative control (8, 9).

SYSTEMIC INJECTION TEST   The USP systemic injection test is insensitive and therefore fails to meet the criteria for a screening test. It was designed to detect toxic substances that might be leached from a container used for products intended for large volume parental administrations. The use of this test for other purposes is doubtful.

In the systemic injection test five mice comprise the test group and five control mice are used for comparison. The dose administered is usually 50 ml of the extract per kilogram of body weight of the mouse. The rate of injection is important and is adjusted to approximately 0.1 ml per second.

Extracts from plastics obtained under the conditions established above are injected either intravenously or intraperitoneally. The extraction medium can be physiological saline, ethanol in saline, or an oil such as vegetable oil or cotton seed oil. The extracts provide both hydrophilic and lipophilic extraction of chemicals from the plastic matrix. The total time of the extraction can be varied depending on the use of the medical device. However, in the general screening test it is desirable to use a standard procedure and build a data base on a particular raw material. Thus, the data base becomes generic and can be used to compare materials for many different intended uses.

The mice are observed during the first hour (hr) following the test and then for short periods at 24, 48, and 72 hr. This three-day observation is time-consuming and only overt signs of toxicity can be observed. Certainly if the mice die the material tested is very suspect. Because of the small number of animals used in the test, euthanasia and examination of the tissues are of little value.

INTRACUTANEOUS TEST   The USP intracutaneous test is essentially an in vivo cell culture toxicity test. Extracts from the plastic are injected and the site of injection is observed for tissue changes such as edema and erythema. One major problem with both this test and the implantation test is that the reaction to the plastic extract is judged against a negative control called the "blank." The blank is a sample of the extraction medium. Both false negatives and false positives result from this procedure. Edema and erythema can be randomly caused by the injection so that positive tissue reactions can occur at blank injection-sites. Since these screening tests emphasize positive reactions to the specimen, a large number of samples would be needed to reduce the likelihood of false-negative results confounding the data.

The intracutaneous test uses New Zealand White rabbits. At least two rabbits of either sex are used for each type of extraction media. The test area on the back of the rabbit is prepared by closely clipping the hair and carefully cleaning the area with dilute alcohol. Ten injection sites on each side of the spinal processes are used. The volume of the extraction fluid injected is 0.2 ml. Control sites and test sites may be divided into areas. The injected sites are examined at 24, 48, and 72 hr. The sites are graded on a numerical scale from zero, for no reaction, to four for lesion formation. If longer periods of observation are needed care must be taken in removing hair from the site of the injection before observation. The multiple injections allow averaging of the test scores for the test medium and the control medium. When undetermined differences in the test and control medium give positive results, retest is necessary. The retest should contain data from at least three rabbits.

IMPLANTATION TEST   The implantation test is an excellent tissue toxicity test in that the tissue fluids extract substances from the plastic. The test is similar to the tissue culture or cell culture tests in which the culture overlays the plastic material.

The negative control material implanted with the specimen material is used for a comparison of the tissue effects of implantation. The use of the negative control plastic material can lead to false-negative results when the time of reading is three days or less from the time of the implant. Seven-day readings appear to give better results.

Table II illustrates this point. Usually trauma of implantation clears up quickly. However, longer leaching times correlate with increased toxicity from the implant.

Naturally, surface extraction of toxic substances may be higher at the time of the implant. The time required for migration of toxic substances to the surface can affect the degree of toxic effects. If the delivery time is sufficiently long the reaction resembles the slow release of active ingredients from time-released dose forms. Cell culture toxicity tests where larger concentrations of extracted substances can be obtained have the advantage of fewer false-negative responses.

The intramuscular injection sites are similar in location to the sites chosen for the intracutaneous test. The methods used for reading the test results are also similar. Here again the SOP for the laboratory is needed to make judgments regarding the test. Procedural differences are possible, and round robin test results demonstrate both false-positive and false-negative results.

The injection site is best evaluated by removal of the tissue at the site of the implant and microscopic examination of the tissue. Staining preparations may be used to aid in determining the degree of tissue injury.

Table 2   False positive and false negative responses[a]

	Scores		
	3-day Reading	5-day Reading	7-day Reading
Material A	+2	+4	+4
Control A	+3	+1	0
Material B	+4	0	0
Control B	+1	+1	0
Material C	0	0	+3
Control C	+2	+1	0

[a]Three examples of types of readings of implant and intracutaneous scores. Material A could be considered nontoxic at day 3, but at days 5 and 7 the readings are positive. Material B is toxic at day 3, but would be judged nontoxic at days 5 and 7. Material C failed to show toxicity until day 7. If Control B were used to judge Control A or Control C, these two control nontoxic materials could be judged toxic.

Cell Culture and Tissue Culture Tests

Cell culture and tissue culture tests best meet the criteria of the screening test procedures. These tests are very sensitive to cell toxicity, and they screen for potential toxic effects rather than measure directly the toxicity occurring under conditions of use. When a specimen material passes the screening test under standard operating conditions, it is very unlikely that it will cause adverse effects under use conditions because the concentration of the extractants and the sensitivity of the test should be sufficient to provide this assurance (10, 12).

However, when a specimen material fails a screening test, protocol safety evaluations are necessary to assure that the screening test result was a false-positive result and that the material is not toxic in the intended application. The positive screening test results also alert the investigators to the possibility of toxic responses at points other than the end use of the product.

The in vitro test sensitivity can be improved by choice of cell lines and choice of cell culture response evaluated. Biochemical methods can measure such cell functions as DNA synthesis, protein synthesis, and ATP activity. Cell function tests such as adhesion and phagocytosis are highly sensitive but have low toxicity-ranking agreement and reproducibility. Measuring ATP activity with CCL76 or mouse-embryo cell cultures, DNA synthesis with CCL76 or CCL 1 cultures, and protein synthesis with CCL 1 or mouse-embryo cultures might be appropriate for biomaterial toxicity screening. Each of these assays demonstrates high relative sensitivity in discernment of test materials with known toxicity. Reproducibility and predictability of cellular response were good with these tests (10). Less complicated and more subjective means of measuring cellular response are also functionally acceptable as a screening system (12).

For example, the Ames test allows evaluation of specimen materials for genotoxic responses (13). When the S-9 liver enzyme fraction is added to the culture medium, the metabolic alteration of the parent compounds can be tested (14). The metabolic system can also be used with other enzyme testing methods. The choice of the SOP is based on the chemical structure of the ingredients of the material and on their metabolism. While false-negative responses can also occur here, the concentration of the extractable materials can be increased to levels that overrule low dose considerations. A positive Ames test warrants further tests for potential chemical carcinogenesis as well as for potential effects on reproduction.

PROTOCOL TESTS

The USP tests and the cell culture and tissue culture tests will likely fail to detect function toxicity, especially that related to metabolites of the leached compound. Since patient exposure dose can be estimated from the chemical tests and these doses are generally very low, concerns for functional toxicity related to phase I biotransformations or to failure of the phase II detoxication processes are not important (15). However, both toxicological testing and safety testing frequently require test procedures other than those in the screening test for benefit-risk assessments. These test protocols can be used to discover functional toxicity as well as tissue toxicity. As for devices with blood-material interactions, special protocol tests may be needed to evaluate effects on blood functions, clotting, calcification of the materials, and other hematological responses (16). Toxicity due to large-dose exposures (such as those occurring with feeding) in which doses of two to four percent of the diet weight is common, where the toxicity is related to biotransformations or failure of the phase II reactions (15). Often toxicity occurs when the capacity of detoxication mechanisms is exceeded. For example, large oral doses of di(2-ethylhexyl)phthalate (DEHP) cause an increase in hepatic peroxisome proliferation in rat feeding studies (17). Hypolipidemic responses associated with hepatic peroxisome proliferators are reported to form a novel class of chemical carcinogens (18, 19). The response following DEHP administration is actually a response to MEHP, a metabolite of DEHP (20, 21). In cases where DEHP is used to plasticize materials contained in medical devices the exposure dose is low even for hemodialysis patients, and MEHP, which is water soluble, is rapidly cleared by the body. However, human patients differ in their hepatic and other reaction to DEHP exposure according to the lipid level of their plasma.

Laboratory test systems provide us with excellent products, but noticeable failures have occurred after long-term human exposure in the ability of these test systems to predict adverse effects.

Immunological responses and allergic reactions are the most difficult to detect with animal systems. Yet, with long-term hemodialysis, anaphylactic-type reactions have occurred (22). These reactions are thought to be related to residual ethylene oxide from sterilization procedures. Although these patients have elevated levels of immunoglobulins, animal test systems fail to demonstrate a cause-effect relationship for any known chemical found in devices used for human dialysis.

These and other laboratory protocol test systems used to assess the risk of human exposure to chemical substances need to be validated. The method used and the means of data analysis should consistently detect a response directly related to a human response. Whole-life carcinogenesis tests, with their multiple organ examinations at regular intervals during the test period, are often biologically confounded (23). Unlike pharmacological or toxicological response detection, where drug receptor response can be determined to occur in each animal at some dose, the animal carcinogenesis test is like an epidemiology test. Prediction of carcinogenesis in other species has been less than exciting.

With each standard operation procedure or test protocol, dose form, route of exposure, whole body distribution, species metabolism, and elimination differences are important. Studies conducted with DEHP have certainly proven this importance (24). The use of whole body autoradiography to indicate in which organs or tissues chemical-receptor responses are possible can certainly aid in protocol study design (25).

Improved biochemical procedures for study of chemical-receptor binding have greatly improved our understanding of receptor occupation responses (26). Application of these techniques to toxicity mechanism studies can improve dose-response assessments of human risk. Stephenson (27) supplies the following postulates:

1. A maximum effect can be produced by an agonist when it occupies only a small proportion of the receptors.

2. The response is not linearly proportional to the number of receptors occupied.

3. Different drugs may have varying capacities to initiate a response and may consequently occupy different proportions of the receptors when producing equal responses. This property was referred to as the efficacy of the drug. In this setting, a pure antagonist would have zero efficacy.

These postulates help to clarify some of the problems associated with toxicity assessment. In cases of toxicity both efficacy or intrinsic activity and affinity are important (28). Binding and metabolism are also useful detoxification mechanisms. In carcinogenesis studies the genetic specific target (GST) is recognized as the receptor, and certainly "a maximum effect can be produced by an agonist when occupying only a small proportion of the receptors" (1). Naturally the higher the number of people exposed to a given concentration of a toxic substance the greater the probability of an agonist receptor reaction.

The most important aspect of protocol design for safety and toxicity assessment is the analytical chemical determinations. The formulation of the material must be known. Also, analytical procedures can provide qualitative and quantitative data about substances that become incorporated in the polymer matrix during manufacturing processes. These investigations of risk assessment are greatly improved over previous procedures.

CONCLUSIONS

A group of screening tests has been suggested that allows comparisons of materials proposed for use in medical devices. Whereas certain organizations have proposed the division of medical devices into classes and the selection of the screening procedure based on the intended use of the device, the generic use of these tests must be considered. When these screening tests are considered as a battery, the sensitivity of the system is sufficient to prevent false-negative results. Because of the ubiquity of medical devices, the diversity of biological states of the patients, and the range of benefit to risk ratios, protocol studies are needed that provide convincing evidence for the safety and efficacy of medical devices. The risk reported in animal toxicity studies involving monomers, polymers, plasticizers, and other substances contained in a material must be evaluated in light of the multiple factors that affect human response during the beneficial use of the device.

ACKNOWLEDGMENTS

The author thanks R. Van Essche, DVM, and R. F. Wallin for their assistance in the preparation of this review.

Literature Cited

1. Infante, P. F., Wagoner, J. K., Wax-weiler, R. J. 1976. Carcinogenic, mutagenic and teratogenic risks associated with vinyl chloride. *Mutat. Res.* 41:131–32

2. Selikoff, I. J., Hammond, E. C., eds. 1975. *Ann. N.Y. Acad. Sci.* Vol. 246

3. Darby, T. D., Johnson, H. J., Northup, S. J. 1978. An evaluation of a polyurethane for use as a medical grade plastic. *Toxicol. Appl. Pharmacol.* 46:449–53

4. Clark, C. A. 1972. Gases from burning PVC. *Soc. Plastics Eng. Tech.* 18:623–26

5. Sokol, W. N., Aelony, Y., Beal, G. N. 1973. Meat Wrappers Asthma. *J. Am. Med. Assoc.*, 226:639–41

6. Darby, T. D. 1978. Pharmacological considerations in the design of toxicology experiments. *Clin. Toxicol.* 12:229–38

7. Henne, W., Dietrich, W., Pelger, M., von Sengbusch, G. 1984. Residual ethylene oxide in hollow-fiber dialyzers. *Artif. Organs* 8:306–9

8. Henry, T. J., ed. 1985. Guidelines for the preclinical safety evaluation of materials used in medical devices. *HIMA Rep.* 85-1, Washington, DC: Health Ind. Manufactures Assoc.

9. Committee on Standards. 1982. Standard practice for selecting generic biological test methods for materials and devices. *Ann. Book ASTM Standards,* Vol. 13.01. F-748-82

10. Johnson, H. J., Northup, S. J., Seagraves, P. A., Garvin, P. J., Wallin, R. F. 1983. Biocompatibility test procedures for materials evaluation, in vitro. I. Comparative test system sensitivity. *J. Biomed. Mater. Res.* 17:571–86

11. Autian, J. 1980. Plastics. In *Toxicology, The Basic Science of Poisons,* ed. J. Doull, C. D. Klaassen, M. O. Amdur, p. 531. New York: Macmillan

12. Johnson, H. J., Northup, S. J., Seagraves, P. A., Atallah, M., Garvin P. J., Darby, T. D. 1985. Biocompatibility test procedures for materials evaluation, in vitro. II. Objective methods of toxicity assessment. *J. Biomed. Mater. Res.* 19:489–508

13. McCann, J., Choi, E., Yamasaki, E., Ames, B. N. 1975. Detection of carcinogens as mutagens in the Salmonella/microsome test: assay of 30 chemicals. *Proc. Natl. Acad. Sci. USA* 72:5135–39

14. Maron, D. M., Ames, B. N. 1983. Revised methods for the Salmonella mutagenicity test. *Mutat. Res.* 113:173–215

15. Neal, R. A. 1980. Metabolism of toxic Substances. See Ref. 11, p. 56

16. McIntire, L. V., ed. 1985. Guidelines for blood-material interactions. *US Dep. Health Human Serv. NIH Publ.* No. 85-2185

17. Reddy, J. K., Moody, D. E., Azarnoff, D. L. 1976. Di-(2-ethyl) phthalate: An industrial plasticizer induces hypolipidemia and enhances hepatic catalase

and carnitine acetyltransferase activities in rats and mice. *Life Sci.* 18:941–45

18. Reddy, J. K., Azarnoff, D. L., 1980. Hypolipidemic hepatic proliferatiors form a novel class of chemical carcinogens. *Nature* 283:397–98

19. Reddy, J. K., Warren, J. R. 1981. Toxicological implications of hepatic peroxisome proliferation in rodents: Possible role of oxygen radical toxicity in hypolipidemic drug-induced carcinogenesis. *Toxicologist* 1:131

20. Albro, P. W., Thomas, R., Fishbein, L. 1973. Metabolism of diethylhexyl phthlate by rats. Isolation and characterization of the urinary metabolites. *J. Chromatogr.* 76:321–30

21. Albro, P. W., Corbett, J. T., Schroeder, J. 1981. The fate di-(2-ethylhexyl) phthalate in rats. *Toxicologist* 1:55

22. Grammer, L. C., Roberts, M., Nicholls, A. J., Platts, M. M., Patterson, R. 1984. IgE against ethylene oxide-altered human serum albumin in patients who have had acute dialysis reactions. *J. Allergy Clin. Immunol.* 74:544–46

23. Hart, R. W., Turturro, A., Weisburger, E. 1985. Chemical carcinogens; A review of the science and its associated principles. *Fed. Reg.* March 14, p. 49–52

24. Thomas, J. A., Darby, T. D., Wallin, R. F., Garvin, P. J., Martis, L. 1978. A review of the biological effects of di-2(ethyl hexyl) phthalate. *Toxicol. Appl. Pharmacol.* 45:1–27

25. Waddell, W. J., Marlowe, C., Miripol, J. E., Garvin, P. J. 1977. The distribution in mice of intravenously administered 14C-di-2-(ethyl hexyl) phthalate (14C DEHP) determined by whole-body autoradiography. *Toxicol. Appl. Pharmacol.* 39:339–53

26. Limbird, L. E. 1986. *Cell Surface Receptors: A Short Course on Theory and Methods.* Boston: Nijhoff 196 pp.

27. Stephenson, R. P. 1956. A modification of receptor theory. *Br. J. Pharmacol.* 11:379–93

28. van Rossum, J. M., Ariens, E. J. 1962. Receptor reserve and threshold phenomena. II. Theories on drug-action and a quantitative approach to spare receptors and threshold values. *Arch. Int. Pharmacodyn.* 136:385–13

Ann. Rev. Pharmacol. Toxicol. 1987. 27:169–91

EXTRACORPOREAL REMOVAL OF DRUGS AND POISONS BY HEMODIALYSIS AND HEMOPERFUSION

Ralph E. Cutler,[1,2] *Steven C. Forland,*[1] *Paul G. St. John Hammond,*[1,2] *J. Robert Evans*[1,2]

Department of Medicine,[1] Nephrology Section,[2] Loma Linda Veterans Administration Hospital, Loma Linda, California 92357

INTRODUCTION

Accidental or intentional overdose and poisoning cause much sickness and death. Agents involved in overdoses include illicit drugs such as opiates and cocaine, prescribed drugs such as antiepileptics and cardiovascular agents (digoxin, antiarrhythmics), and poisons (metals, herbicides). Overdose and poisoning also occur by deliberate ingestion of carbon monoxide, barbiturates, alcohol, psychotherapeutics, analgesics (acetaminophen, salicylates), and autonomic agents.

Treatment of overdoses or poisoning includes prevention of further drug absorption, antidotal therapy if available, support of vital organ function, and enhancement of drug elimination. This article reviews drug elimination, with an emphasis on extracorporeal methods.

Although approximately 40% of patients recognizably poisoned require hospitalization, few die. These impressive statistics are of recent origin and are based on the body's potential for detoxification and elimination of a wide spectrum of chemical agents. Clemmensen & Nilsson documented that intensive supportive care, without massive gastric lavage or analeptic agents, produced a mortality rate of 1.5% (1). Only about 10% of these patients need intensive medical assistance to maintain vital function; the rest recover with adequate nursing care. Methods to increase poison elimination are either feasible or appropriate in fewer than 5% of cases (2). Forced urinary diuresis

169

0362-1642/87/0415-0169$02.00

Table 1 Poisons responsive to hemodialysis or hemoperfusion

Hemodialysis	Hemoperfusion
Salicylates	Salicylates
Phenobarbitol	Phenobarbitol
Methanol/ethanol	Other barbiturates
Ethylene glycol	Ethchlorvynol
Lithium	Glutethimide
Isopropanol	Meprobamate
Theophylline	Methaqualone
	Trichloroethanol derivatives
	Disopyramide
	Theophylline

and/or extracorporeal removal (Table 1) are directed toward this small group of patients. The safety and efficacy of these techniques in poisonings remain unproven, since most studies reported neither control nor randomized selection of therapy. Extracorporeal devices may be applied under the following conditions (2). (*a*) The drug or toxic substance should either diffuse easily through the dialysis membrane or be readily taken up by an absorbent. (*b*) A significant proportion of the poison should be present in plasma water or capable of rapid equilibration with it. (*c*) The pharmacological effect of the toxin should be directly related to the blood concentration. (*d*) Dialysis or hemoperfusion should add significantly to other body mechanisms of elimination.

PHARMACOKINETIC CONCEPTS

Pharmacokinetic principles indicate why dialysis or hemoperfusion is infrequently useful in treating drug overdose (3–5). The rate of removal of any substance from a single body compartment parallels its plasma clearance (Cl_p), which is the product of the apparent volume of distribution (V_d) of the agent and the elimination rate constant (K_{el}):

$$Cl_p = V_d \cdot K_{el}. \qquad\qquad 1.$$

Volume of Distribution

The V_d is the volume of water in which a specific amount of an agent would yield the concentration found in plasma. A large V_d implies that most of the agent is tissue bound and not readily accessible for removal from the blood by dialysis or hemoperfusion. The V_d corresponds to a physiological compartment only for substances like lithium and methanol that distribute in body water without significant tissue binding. Agents with high lipid solubility usually have a large V_d, diffuse rapidly into the brain and fat depots, and are slowly removed from these sources because of poor partitioning into plasma water and relatively low blood flow.

Certain diseases may alter the V_d of some agents, e.g. renal failure increases the V_d for phenytoin but decreases it for digoxin. Impairment of major organs of chemical excretion, such as the liver and kidneys, causes significant reduction in the overall elimination rate of many agents. Digoxin, a drug commonly associated with toxicity, illustrates these concepts. In individuals with normal renal function, digoxin has a V_d of 7.1 liter (l)/kg body weight, a Cl_p of 165 ml/min with more than 90% of a loading dose excreted unchanged in the urine. In those with end-stage renal disease (ESRD), the V_d is decreased to 4.2 l/kg, and the Cl_p falls to 35 ml/min (6). This marked reduction of Cl_p of digoxin in ESRD is caused by both the decreased V_d and the reduced renal elimination.

Protein Binding

Only unbound substances participate in diffusion and are dialyzable. In contrast to hemodialysis, plasma protein binding and water solubility have little influence on the efficiency of hemoperfusion (3). Protein binding occurs in plasma, mostly to albumin, and in tissues to intracellular proteins. The affinity of most chemicals for proteins is low and readily reversible, but some interactions may be covalent and relatively irreversible. As noted by Gibaldi (7), the fraction of unbound agent in blood and tissues influences the V_d:

$$V_d = V_B + V_T (F_B/F_T), \qquad\qquad 2.$$

where V_B and V_T are the actual volumes of water in blood and tissues and F_B and F_T are the fractions of free drug in blood and tissues, respectively. Consequently, an increase in the free fraction of an agent in blood without a corresponding increase in the free fraction in tissue would produce an increase in V_d. This situation may occur in renal failure with drugs like phenytoin and clofibrate, but the opposite occurs with methotrexate and digoxin, where V_d falls by 30% to 50%, respectively.

Distributive Kinetics

Most substances introduced into the body are not confined to the vascular compartment but are distributed at varying rates to extravascular tissues. After the initial distribution phase (indicated by a rapid decline in plasma concentration following intravenous injection), the fall of concentration over time is usually linear when plotted semilogarithmically. This linearity indicates that a pseudoequilibrium exists between movement from extravascular tissues into the blood and elimination from the vascular space. Rapid removal of an agent from the blood by an extracorporeal device may disrupt this pseudoequilibrium. If the rate of distribution of the agent from extravascular tissues is slower than the overall elimination rate, the agent will be removed from the blood more rapidly than it can be replaced from tissue stores. This occurrence results in a rebound in blood concentration of the agent on cessation of extracorporeal removal. Such rebounds are common when the V_d of an agent is large (>1 l/kg). Unfortunately, most reported studies have not considered these principles. Thus, reported declines of blood concentrations following the use of extracorporeal devices are useless for evaluating a significant reduction in total body stores of an agent unless the amount of drug removed in the effluent is measured.

Extracorporeal Elimination

The contribution of dialysis or hemoperfusion to the overall clearance of a drug $(Cl_p + Cl_d)$ must be determined by first considering the intrinsic plasma clearance of the drug without extracorporeal removal. Amitriptyline, a tricyclic antidepressant, illustrates this requirement. The V_d of this agent is 20 l/kg; thus 1 gram of amitriptyline in a 70-kg subject yields a plasma concentration of 0.7 mg/l. Assuming complete extraction of amitriptyline by an extracorporeal device, with a 200 ml/min blood flow through the device, clearance would theoretically be 200 ml/min. However, the actual amount of drug removed would be a negligible 0.14 mg/min or 33.6 mg in 4 hours (hr) of treatment. Although extracorporeal removal is highly efficient in this example, the clinical results are ineffective.

Measurement of the total amount of drug removed in the dialysate effluent or absorbed to the hemoperfusion column is the best method of determining the efficiency of treatment. However, the tables in this review are a compromise; they contain the calculated fractional removal of the body stores of certain therapeutic agents and poisons during 4 hr of hemodialysis or hemoperfusion treatment based upon reported data obtained largely from changes in plasma concentrations. Fractional removal without and with hemodialysis or hemoperfusion is calculated to show the contribution of extracorporeal removal.

Concentration-Dependent Kinetics

With an overdose it is possible that first-order kinetics of an agent may become concentration dependent and approach zero-order kinetics (4). Saturation kinetics may be a consequence of decreased metabolic clearance at high plasma concentrations as occurs, for example, with capacity-limited hepatic metabolism of ethchlorvynol, or changes in protein binding similar to alterations in V_d seen with phenytoin. Since many drugs may be subject to concentration-dependent kinetics, and only limited pharmacokinetic data are available for toxic doses of many drugs, it is perhaps incorrect to extrapolate kinetics during overdose from data derived during therapeutic dosage studies. Therefore, whenever possible, determination of the elimination half-life or Cl_p of a drug should be made in intoxicated patients to indicate the benefit derived from dialytic or hemoperfusion therapy.

EXTRACORPOREAL DEVICES

Dialysis

The dialyzability of a drug depends upon physicochemical properties of the agent and the dialysis system. The specific properties of a chemical that predict the efficacy of dialysis are molecular weight or size, lipid or water solubility, and protein binding.

Removal by dialysis of an agent from either peritoneal fluid or blood decreases as the molecular weight of the agent increases: a small solute such as lithium (74 daltons) is dialyzable, but a larger drug such a vancomycin (1800 daltons) is not, despite its low protein binding (10%). Further, solutes insoluble in water do not diffuse from the blood into aqueous dialysates. For example, despite a low molecular weight of 252 daltons, phenytoin is insoluble in water at a pH of 7.4, highly protein bound, and not dialyzed.

In conventional dialysis, unbound solute removal is principally accomplished by diffusion down a concentration gradient between plasma water and dialysate. Therefore, as the protein binding of a solute increases, the dialysis clearance decreases. With this ratio the possible benefit of dialysis can be predicted. However, customary protein binding of a drug may be altered in a patient with intoxication. If saturation of binding sites occurs, then an increased unbound fraction is available for diffusion. This situation happens with salicylic acid and disopyramide, where plasma protein-binding capacity may be exceeded even when the concentration of either drugs is within the therapeutic range (5). The presence of renal disease is also commonly associated with reduction of drug protein binding, which increases the amount of unbound drug available for diffusion (8).

Specific properties of the dialysis system that affect solute or drug removal are the permeability and surface area of the membrane and the flow rates of both blood and dialysate. Small molecules (<500 daltons) exhibit high membrane permeability with a rapid decline in blood to dialysate gradient; the limiting determinants of clearance are blood and dialysate flow rates. In contrast, large molecules exhibit low membrane permeability, maintain a gradient across the membrane, and their clearance is dependent on membrane surface area rather than the rate of blood or dialysate flow. Therefore, a low cardiac output in the intoxicated patient may preclude the effectiveness of either peritoneal or hemodialysis by reducing blood flow rates and compromising the effective membrane surface area.

Whereas estimation of plasma clearance is fairly simple, the measurement of Cl_d is complicated. Over thirty years ago, Wolf et al (9) suggested using the Fick principle:

$$Cl_d = Q(A-V)/A \qquad\qquad 3.$$

where Q is the dialyzer blood flow, A and V the concentration of any substance entering and leaving the dialyzer, respectively. Several derivatives from this general equation are possible, including

$$Cl_d = Q_p(A_p-V_p)/A_p, \qquad\qquad 4.$$

$$Cl_d = Q_b(A_b-V_b)/A_b, \text{ and} \qquad\qquad 5.$$

$$Cl_d = Q_b(A_p-V_p)/A_p, \qquad\qquad 6.$$

where p is plasma, b is blood, Q_p is plasma flow $[(1-hct)Q_b]$, and hct is the hematocrit.

Because concentrations of drugs and other agents are usually measured in plasma, Equation 4 can be used to estimate Cl_d. However, this relationship only holds if the agent is confined to plasma alone and is neither within, on, nor removed from, blood cells. A possible solution to this complication would be to use whole-blood assays and Equation 5. However, since Cl_p is usually calculated from plasma concentration data, Equation 5 will not relate to Cl_p unless corrections are made for the fraction of red cells to plasma and the free fraction of the agent in plasma.

Unfortunately, both past studies and many recent reports use, inappropriately Equation 6. In this calculation whole blood-flow rate is combined with the plasma-extraction ratio. An overestimate of Cl_d occurs if the agent is only removed from plasma; an underestimate occurs if the agent is carried on or in blood cells, and is removed from them as well as from the plasma. Other important assumptions that are made when Equation 6 is used are often invalid under certain circumstances and are discussed elsewhere (10–12).

Equations 4–6 assume accurate measurement of dialyzer blood flow, a major potential weakness. Errors in this measurement can be as much as 30–40% if based on bubble transit time or if using pumps that are not calibrated before and after any study of dialyzer clearance. In addition, the ultrafiltration of plasma water during dialysis may proceed at a rate greater than that of the agent of interest, producing a relative increase of concentration in the dialyzer outlet port. This change can be estimated:

$$V_{p'} = V_p[1-(V_{hct}-A_{hct})/V_{hct}], \qquad\qquad 7.$$

where p' is the corrected venous plasma concentration and p is the observed plasma concentration. Changes in plasma protein concentration could also be used in place of changes in hematocrit.

Although somewhat more difficult, the benchmark for measurement of dialyzer clearance is

$$Cl_d = R/AUC_d, \qquad\qquad 8.$$

where R is the total recovery of unchanged agent in the expended dialysate and AUC_d is the area under the curve of the plasma concentration vs time plot during hemodialysis. Plasma measurements are done on blood entering the dialyzer. This equation is independent of changes in dialyzer blood flow, alterations in plasma concentration produced by ultrafiltration, and the effects of any blood cell uptake of the agent. Not surprisingly, Cl_d measured by this technique can exceed actual blood or plasma flow rate if the agent is present in, and removed from, blood cells.

Peritoneal Dialysis

Peritoneal dialysis clearances are considerably less than those of hemodialysis and rarely exceed 10 ml/min. This technique is, therefore, rarely useful for treating poisonings unless conducted over prolonged intervals.

Hemoperfusion

Hemoperfusion removes substances from the blood by direct contact with an adsorbent material. Any material that has greater affinity than blood for a given substance removes both native and foreign substances. The concept, first applied by Muirhead & Reid in 1948 with mixed ion exchange resins, was used to remove "uremic toxins" from animals (13). Early column use was plagued with complications including febrile reactions, destruction of blood cells, embolization of charcoal particles, electrolyte disturbances, and thrombosis (14). The development in the early 1970s of coated charcoal, fixed-bed charcoal, and the discovery of newer polymer resins overcame these technical problems (15).

Properties intrinsic to the adsorbent and the substance being removed, as well as certain technical factors, influence the efficacy of hemoperfusion (Table 2). Of the two basic types, charcoal and polymer resin, only charcoal devices are commercially available in the United States. Charcoal

Table 2 Factors Influencing Substance Removal by Hemoperfusion

Factor	Adsorbent	Pharmacokinetics	Technical
Surface properties	Surface properties	Distributive kinetics	Blood flow
Affinity for sorbent	Pore size:	Distribution volune	pH
Configuration	macro 50 nm		Temperature
Lipophilicity	micro 2 nm		Viscosity
Plasma protein binding	Pore configuration		
Size/molecular weight	Saturation		
Water solubility	Surface area		
	Adsorbent capacity		
	Affinity for substance		
	Coating (membrane)		

hemoperfusers use either fixed, uncoated, or coated particulate columns. The coating, although decreasing embolization, forms a membrane barrier (.05–5 μm), the effect of which is negligible except with high-molecular-weight substances (16). Activated charcoal, a nonspecific adsorbent, removes both water and lipid soluble substances from 113 to 40,000 daltons in size (14).

The adsorptive capacity of most charcoal columns is large, but the nonspecificity allows many bloodborne substances to adhere to the charcoal, which quickly reduces its capacity to adsorb desired toxins. Consequently, removal rate declines progressively with prolonged use, necessitating column replacement.

Assessing Total Body Removal

Although the efficiency of extracorporeal agent removal is commonly measured in terms of dialysis or hemoperfusion clearance, such measurements do not directly correlate with the amount of agent removed from body stores. Gwilt recently reported an equation that allows calculation of changes in body stores produced by extracorporeal removal (17). If the mass balance of a substance is considered, then

$$X_s = X_d + X_{el} + X_f, \qquad\qquad 9.$$

where X_s and X_f are the amounts of drug in the body at the beginning and the end of extracorporeal removal, respectively, and X_d and X_{el} are the amounts of an agent eliminated by extracorporeal removal and by the body during usual elimination routes during extracorporeal procedures. Equation 9 may be expressed as:

$$X_s = (Cl_d \cdot AUC_1) + (Cl_p \cdot AUC_1) + (Cl_p \cdot AUC_2), \qquad\qquad 10.$$

where AUC_1 is the area under the plasma concentration versus time curve during extracorporeal removal and AUC_2 is the area under the plasma concentration versus time curve from the termination of extracorporeal removal to infinity. The fraction of drug in the body at the start of extracorporeal removal that is removed by the device is given by:

$$f = X_d/X_s \qquad\qquad 11.$$

which, from Equation 9 may be expressed as:

$$f = (Cl_d \cdot AUC_1)/[(Cl_p + Cl_d)AUC_1 + (Cl_p \cdot AUC_2)]. \qquad 12.$$

SPECIFIC DRUG OR AGENT REMOVAL

Central Nervous System Agents

ALCOHOLS   Ethanol, methanol, isopropanol, and ethylene glycol are readily dialyzable because of their diffusibility, water solubility, nonprotein binding, and small V_d. Consequently, hemodialysis is the treatment of choice in intoxication states rather than hemoperfusion. As noted in Table 3, the fractional removal of all these agents by dialysis is substantial and clinically useful.

Ethanol Levels in excess of 350 mg/dl are potentially dangerous, but concentrations greater than 500 mg/dl may be fatal. Ethanol is eliminated primarily by hepatic metabolism and demonstrates concentration-dependent kinetics. Its metabolism increases by 25% following intravenous administration of fructose (18). Body clearance increases 50% with hemodialysis to 300–400 ml/min; removal rate of ethanol is increased to 280 mg/min (19).

Isopropanol Since the acute effects of simple alcohols on the central nervous system increase in correlation to their molecular weight, isopropanol may be twice as potent as ethanol. About 80% of an absorbed dose is metabolized, predominantly to acetone. Acetone is excreted along with the unchanged form by the kidneys and lungs. Whereas the ingestion of 20 ml may cause mild symptoms, 150–240 ml can be lethal. Hemodialysis is indicated in cases with hypotension and hypothermia (coma) or serum alcohol concentration exceeding 400–500 mg/dl (20).

Methanol Intoxication with methanol is characterized by central nervous system depression or coma and formate production, which mediates retinal

Table 3 Pharmacokinetic properties of selected drugs and poisons

Drug name	Apparent volume of distribution (l/kg)	Plasma clearance (ml/min)	Plasma protein binding (%)	Hemodialyzer clearance (ml/min)	Hemoperfusion clearance (ml/min)	Fractional removal in 4 hr (%) Normal patient	With hemodialysis	With hemoperfusion
Central nervous system agents								
Alcohols								
Ethanol	0.6	170–320	0	120–160	—	76	87	—
Isopropanol	0.6		0	—	—	—	79	—
Methanol	0.6	44	0	98–176	—	22	56	—
Ethylene glycol	0.8	64	—	—	—	—	—	—
Sedative hypnotics								
Chloral hydrate	6	600	35–41	120	157–238	29	34	37
Ethchlorvynol	2.8	90	30–50	64	125–300	10	17	23
Glutethimide	2.7	180	45	50	60–250	20	25	32
Meprobamate	0.75	60	0–20	60	85–150	24	42	56
Methyprylon	—		20–80	5–171	25–171	50	—	—
Methaqualone	6	140	80	23	216	8	9	18
Pentobarbital	1	36	66	22	50–300	12	18	27
Phenobarbital	0.75	9	25–60	80	80–290	4	33	39
Secobarbital	1.42	5	70	NS[a]	20–119	1	1	16
Analgesics								
Acetaminophen	1	400	10–21[b]	120	125	75	83	83
Aspirin	0.21	45	73–94	20	90	52	65	89

Anticonvulsant drugs								
Carbamazepine	1	59	70–80	NS	80–129	17	17	36
Ethosuximide	0.7	10	0	140	—	5	52	—
Phenytoin	0.57[c]	25	87–93	NS	76–189	14	14	61
Primidone	0.6	40	0	98	98	20	55	55
Sodium Valproate	0.15–0.4	10	90–95	23	—	12	33	—
Psychotherapeutic drugs								
Amitriptyline	20	—	96	NS	14–210	—	—	—
Chlordiazepoxide	0.3	25	86–93	NS	—	—	—	—
Chlorpromazine	—	—	90	NS	—	—	—	—
Desipramine	0.74[d]	35	69–76	NS	—	15	15	—
Diazepam	23	1330	90	NS	—	—	—	—
Haloperidol	11	1000	90	NS	—	—	—	—
Imipramine	—	—	86–96	18	—	27	27	—
Lithium carbonate	0.79	20	0	150	—	8	52	12
Nortriptyline	21	740	94	NS	14–210	11	11	—
Cardiovascular agents								
Antiarrhythmic drugs								
Bretylium	7	725	1–6	NS	—	—	—	—
Disopyramide	0.83	93	5–65[e]	123	—	32	40	—
Flecainide	8.7	567	40	NS	—	—	—	86
Lidocaine	1.2	606	66	NS	75–90	82	82	—
Mexiletine	7–10	846	70	NS	—	29	29	—
Procainamide	2	810	15	65	—	75	78	—
NAPA[f]	1.5	200	10	41–97	125	37	49	40
Quinidine	2	270	80–85	11–18	24	37	39	—
Tocainide	3.2	182	10–15	25	—	18	20	—
Antihypertensive drugs								
Acebutolol	1.4	665	11–19	43	—	80	82	—
Atenolol	1.2	176	<5	29–39	—	40	45	—
Diazoxide	0.12	7	94	25	—	18	60	—
Nadolol	2	135	20–30	46–102	—	21	30	—

Table 3 (*continued*)

Drug name	Apparent volume of distribution (l/kg)	Plasma clearance (ml/min)	Plasma protein binding (%)	Hemodialyzer clearance (ml/min)	Hemoperfusion clearance (ml/min)	Fractional removal in 4 hr (%)		
						Normal patient	With hemodialysis	With hemoperfusion
Cardiotonic agents								
Digitoxin	0.5	3	90	NS	19	2	2	14
Digoxin	7.1	160	20–30	20	80	7	8	11
Spasmolytic agents								
Theophylline	0.45	46	60	70	100–225	30	59	74
Antineoplastic agent								
Methotrexate	0.64[g]	52	50–70	—	54–137	24	—	64
Metals and minerals								
Fluoride	0.5	100	—	100–188	—	—	—	—
Mercury	—	—	99	NS	—	—	—	—
Methylmercury	—	—	99	50–150[h]	—	—	—	—
Herbicides and insecticides								
Paraquat	2.8	28	—	NS	57–156	—	—	—
Demeton-s-methyl-sulfoxide	—	—	—	53	84	—	—	—

[a]NS = not significant.
[b]Data are for the metabolite trichlorethanol.
[c]Concentration dependent.
[d]V_d in uremia is 1.4 l/kg body weight.
[e]V_d in uremia is 2.2 l/kg body weight.
[f]Binding is concentration dependent.
[g]N-acetylprocainamide.
[h]Volume of distribution reduced to 0.42 l/kg in ESRD.
[i]With concurrent L-cysteine infusion.

cell injury and severe metabolic acidosis. Formate concentrations, rather than methanol, correlate clinically with, and are a more direct indicator of, toxicity and the need for intervention therapy (21). Ethanol and folate provide the preliminary therapy and may be fully effective in mild intoxication. Folate enhances formate oxidation, and ethanol competitively inhibits alcohol dehydrogenase and reduces the formation of formate from methanol. Early hemodialysis treatment is indicated particularly as the clearances of both methanol and formate are enhanced tenfold by this method. Hemodialysis clearance of methanol is 98–176 ml/min (22). During ethanol therapy hemodialysis achieves about 90% of total body clearance (23). Sorbent systems for dialysate regeneration are not effective, as is presumably also true of hemoperfusion devices (24). Postethanol rebound in serum formate concentrations has been recorded. The ethanol dose should be increased during dialysis to 7 g/hr above the predialysis infusion rate to maintain adequate blood ethanol concentrations.

Ethylene glycol   Alcohol dehydrogenase is involved in the metabolism of ethylene glycol to aldehyde, oxalate, and organic acids. Oxalate formation produces renal and cerebral dysfunction with hypocalcemia secondary to calcium oxalate deposition, whereas citric acid–cycle inhibition results in lactic acidosis. Initial therapy consists of an ethanol infusion of 10–20 g/hr, increasing by 7 g/hr during dialysis to maintain a blood concentration of 100–200 mg/dl, which competitively inhibits ethylene glycol metabolism. Hemodialysis shortens the plasma half-life from 9 to 2.5 hours (25, 26). Hemodialysis is critical in removing the toxic alcohol, aldehyde metabolites, and organic acids (27). Postdialysis rebound in plasma ethylene glycol concentration is attributed to either a continuation of gastrointestinal absorption or redistribution from the peripheral to central compartment.

SEDATIVES AND HYPNOTICS

Barbiturates   Most barbiturates are rapidly absorbed from the gastrointestinal tract, and therefore induction of emesis, gastric lavage, or administration of activated charcoal should be done immediately. Indications for extracorporeal intervention are high drug concentrations, prolonged coma, or cardiorespiratory complications that are unresponsive to intensive care.

Barbiturates can be divided into short- and long-acting varieties by their differing physiochemical properties that also correspond to contrary detoxification procedures. Long-acting compounds like phenobarbital have a low pK_a value, increased water solubility, decreased protein binding, and effective removal by hemodialysis. The short-acting barbiturates are lipid soluble, highly protein bound, and more effectively removed by charcoal and resin hemoperfusion (28). Resin hemoperfusion is more efficient, since the clearance is limited by blood flow rather than adsorbent capacity of the column or the affinity of the drug to the adsorbent (29). However, rebound distribution from the peripheral compartment to the blood and to highly perfused organs such as the brain results in deterioration after discontinuing perfusion. Therefore, dialytic or perfusion treatments should be prolonged or repeated.

Ethchlorvynol   The lethal dose of ethchlorvynol is from 10–25 g but may be as little as 2.5 g if alcohol is also ingested. Because of a large V_d, hemodialysis removes a small amount despite clearances of 20–82 ml/min (30). Of the two, resin is more effective than charcoal hemoperfusion, with 100% extraction of the drug by a single pass using Amberlite XAD-4 resin perfusion (29, 31, 32). Hemoperfusion clearance is about 3-fold that of the plasma clearance. Despite this removal rate, reduction of body stores is slow, and prolonged extracorporeal treatment is needed to achieve any benefit.

Chloral hydrate   The lethal dose of chloral hydrate ranges between 4 and 30 g. It is rapidly absorbed and metabolized by alcohol dehydrogenase to trichloroacetic acid and trichloroethanol, the latter of which is the pharmacologically active metabolite. In therapeutic doses the half-life of trichloroethanol is 8 (4–12) hr, but in toxic levels the half-life increases to 35 hr, possibly due to saturation kinetics. Hemodialysis removes trichloroethanol effectively with an average clearance of 162 ml/min, removing 34% of body stores over 4 hr (33). Charcoal hemoperfusion is also effective with comparable clearances (34).

Glutethimide   This substance, structurally similar to, but more lipid soluble than, phenobarbital, is almost entirely metabolized. Its erratic gastric absorption, enterohepatic circulation, and large V_d make the use of extracorporeal devices controversial (35). Hemoperfusion is preferred since hemodialysis is limited by protein binding and lipid solubility (29, 36). Patient deterioration may result from rebound in drug concentration after extracorporeal removal secondary to drug redistribution or enterohepatic recirculation.

Methyprylon   Although therapeutic and toxic plasma concentrations have not been definitely established for methyprylon, plasma concentrations of 10 mg/l reportedly produce therapeutic effect; concentrations of 30 mg/l or greater may produce coma; and those in excess of 100 mg/l are potentially lethal. Overdose prolongs the usual half-life of 4 hr to 7–50 hours, probably because of saturation kinetics. Hemodialysis, and especially hemoperfusion, is effective in removing the drugs from the blood (37, 38), but body elimination is low because of the presumed large V_d.

Meprobamate Deep coma occurs at a serum concentration of 12 mg/dl of meprobamate, and death occurs at about 24 mg/dl. Protein binding is low, and clearances using hemodialysis average 60 ml/min (39). With charcoal hemoperfusion, clearances average 153 ml/min (40). Extraction of the drug is almost complete (82–100%), with resin (XAD-4) hemoperfusion and clearance ranges between 162–222 ml/min (41). Despite high rates of removal by hemoperfusion, only about 50% of body stores are removed by 4–6 hr treatments.

Methaqualone This drug, related to both glutethimide and methyprylon, is rapidly absorbed, highly protein bound, and metabolized by the liver. Hemodialysis clearance is 23 ml/min, and charcoal hemoperfusion clearances averaged 137 ml/min (42, 43). Hemoperfusion is suggested when the plasma concentration exceeds 40 mg/l (2), but its effectiveness is unproven.

ANALGESICS Although useful for salicylates, extracorporeal removal of acetaminophen, propoxyphene, or any of the nonsteroidal antiinflammatory drugs is ineffective.

Salicylates Unlike barbiturates, most deaths from salicylates occur after hospital admission and are, therefore, potentially avoidable with appropriate treatment.

The V_d of salicylates is small (0.21 l/kg), and removal of substantial quantities by extracorporeal devices or renal excretion is excellent. Animal toxicity studies with salicylates show a marked reduction in mortality when hemoperfusion is used (44, 45). Thus, hemoperfusion or hemodialysis (which also may correct any underlying acid-base defects), are appropriate when forced diuresis is contraindicated or inadequate.

Acetaminophen Increasing acute poisoning with high mortality rate is associated with this salicylate substitute. Although hemodialysis and hemoperfusion plasma clearance rates are high (100–125 ml/min), the large V_d, and frequent associated circulatory insufficiency, severely limits drug removal. The maximum amount removed has never exceeded 13% of the known quantity of acetaminophen ingested (46, 47). However, anecdotal experience suggests that drug removal may be of value in some cases (48).

Early intervention with the antioxidant *N*-acetylcysteine is effective. Although unproven, combined treatment of *N*-acetylcysteine with hemoperfusion or hemodialysis may be more beneficial than antioxidant treatment alone.

Currently, extracorporeal removal should be considered only adjunctive treatment.

ANTICONVULSANTS   Because plasma protein binding exceeds 70% for carbamazepine, phenytoin, and valproic acid, hemodialytic removal is negligible. However, the fractional 4-hr removal is about 50% for ethosuximide and 55% for primidone during hemodialysis. These percentages represent an increase of 10-fold and 2.5-fold, respectively, above nondialysis removal rates (49, 50). With hemoperfusion clearances about 100 ml/min, the 4-hr fraction removal is increased 2-fold for carbamazepine and 4-fold for phenytoin (51, 52). Such enhancements may be of clinical benefit for overdose.

PSYCHOTHERAPEUTIC AGENTS

Antidepressants   Tricyclic agents such as amitriptyline, imipramine, and nortriptyline are extremely lipid soluble, are highly tissue and protein bound, and have very large V_d. As anticipated, active elimination techniques including hemodialysis and hemoperfusion are ineffective even if instituted within hours of drug ingestion.

Benzodiazepines   These drugs, including diazepam, flurazepam, lorazepam, and chlordiazepoxide are generally benign when taken in excess. However, their depressor effect may persist despite insignificant concentrations of the parent drug because much of the drug is converted in the liver to several active metabolites. Both the parent drug and its metabolites are widely distributed into body tissues and are highly bound to plasma proteins. A 57% decrement in plasma benzodiazepine concentration occurs with in vitro hemoperfusion (53). Clinical reports regarding the value of hemoperfusion, however, are lacking.

Lithium   Hemodialysis is a very effective means of lithium removal but is limited by the large V_d and slow equilibration between central and peripheral compartments, necessitating prolonged treatment (54, 55). Extended hemodialysis (8–12 hr) is indicated in the treatment of patients with severe clinical symptoms or serum lithium levels greater than 4 mEq/l.

Cardiovascular Agents

CARDIAC GLYCOSIDES   In a recent study of iatrogenic hospitalizations, digitalis products were surpassed only by aspirin as a cause. The large V_d of digoxin and the extensive plasma protein binding of digitoxin preclude extensive removal of these agents by hemodialysis. The current treatment of choice for digoxin toxicity is administration of a specific antibody to bind and inactivate the drug (56). Data suggest that significant amounts of digitoxin can be removed by hemoperfusion. Although clearance of digitoxin by a charcoal (about 30 ml/min) or resin (about 20 ml/min) column is low, its small V_d makes removal of significant quantities of drug possible. Hemoperfusion increases total body clearance 8–20 times, producing a significant fall in total body store of the drug (57).

ANTIARRHYTHMIC DRUGS   The large V_d, extensive plasma protein binding, and/or rapid biotransformation of amiodarone, bretylium, flecainide, lidocaine, mexiletine, procainamide, propranolol, and tocainide confirm the inadequacy of extracorporeal removal for toxicity. The low plasma clearance, particularly in renal failure, and small V_d of disopyramide, N-acetylprocainamide, and possibly quinidine suggest that extracorporeal removal may be feasible.

Disopyramide   Plasma protein binding falls as the concentration of disopyramide rises. Hemodialysis removal during overdose is effective, with a rate about 30 ml/min (58). Hemoperfusion removal rates may be three times greater and produce a substantial reduction in plasma concentrations and body stores (59).

Procainamide and N-acetylprocainamide (NAPA)   The hemodialysis clearance of procainamide (65 ml/min) and its active metabolite NAPA (45 ml/min) is substantial (60). However, as the metabolic clearance of procainamide is much greater, hemodialysis or hemoperfusion does not contribute significantly to total body removal. However, hemodialysis and particularly hemoperfusion substantially increase the removal of NAPA, especially in renal sufficiency, since NAPA is normally excreted at a rate comparable to the glomerular filtration rate (GFR) (61).

ANTIHYPERTENSIVES: ATENOLOL AND NADOLOL   Overdoses with atenolol and nadolol have yet to be reported. As with other beta-blockers, adverse hemodynamic effects are best treated with glucagon. Although protein binding is not high, V_d is >1 l/kg, making fractional removal by extracorporeal devices not very effective. However, with diminished renal function, the major route of elimination of these drugs is impaired, and extracorporeal removal could be a significant form of overdose treatment. Hemodialysis clearance is 29–39 ml/min for atenolol and 46–102 ml/min for nadolol (6). No hemoperfusion data are available.

Antimicrobial Agents

Extracorporeal removal has little effect on the plasma clearance of most antibiotics when hepatic and renal function are normal because 80–90% of the dose is eliminated by these normal routes. However, charcoal hemoperfusion improves removal of chloramphenicol when intoxication occurs in newborns (62). This problem is unlikely to occur in adults because of greater intrinsic metabolism of chloramphenicol.

Spasmolytic Drugs: Theophylline

Although hemodialysis removes theophylline, hemoperfusion is more efficient. With charcoal, the extraction was 75–100%, depending on blood flow. A single 3-hr hemoperfusion removes approximately 60% of the total body load of theophylline without serum concentration rebound (39, 63, 64).

Antineoplastic Agents: Methotrexate

About 80% of a dose of methotrexate appears unchanged in the urine; therefore, toxicity may occur when renal function is compromised unless appropriate adjustments are made. Hemoperfusion is more efficient than hemodialysis in drug removal because of 50–70% plasma protein binding. Extracorporeal removal may enhance the rate of elimination 2- or 3-fold when renal function is normal, with fractional elimination of about 60% of body stores over 4 hr (65).

Metals and Minerals

GENERAL   No pertinent data concerning extracorporeal removal in humans are available for antimony, barium, cadmium, chromium, magnesium, manganese, selenium, or zinc. Where applicable, urinary and/or intestinal elimination of most metals is enhanced by the use of chelation. Only with iron and aluminum overload in ESRD has extracorporeal removal been found useful in addition to chelation.

ALUMINUM   Kinetics of aluminum have not been extensively studied. At plasma concentrations found in healthy subjects, aluminum is primarily excreted through bile. Urine elimination increases when plasma concentrations become elevated (66). Toxic aluminum loads are associated with ESRD when the dialysate is contaminated, or when patients are given chronic, high doses of aluminum salts for the chelation of oral phosphates. Intravenous deferoxamine can chelate aluminum, increase plasma concentrations, and allow increased elimination by either hemodialysis or hemoperfusion, although hemoperfusion is more effective (66).

ARSENIC   Poisoning is treated with supportive measures and chelation therapy using dimercaprol or penicillamine. Acute intoxication may be associated with renal failure. Hemodialysis has been used to remove arsenic; clearances of 76–87 ml/min have been recorded (67). Although kinetic data are not available, substantial tissue binding would probably prevent significant fractional removal of this toxin. The use of chelation in addition to dialysis or hemoperfusion has not been described.

COPPER   Chelation and excretion by customary elimination routes are the main treatment for copper poisoning. Addition of albumin to the dialysate enhances peritoneal dialysis removal (68). Because of extensive plasma protein binding, hemodialysis is ineffective; no data are available for hemoperfusion or the combination of chelation plus extracorporeal devices.

FLUORIDE   The V_d of flouride is 0.5 l/kg, plasma protein binding is negligible, and the molecular weight is low. Thus, hemodialysis is effective in removing over 80% of body stores of this agent within 4 hr (29, 69). No data are currently available for the effectiveness of hemoperfusion, but it is expected to be less effective than hemodialysis.

IRON   Acute or chronic iron overload is best treated by phlebotomy or chelation using deferoxamine (70). Chelation therapy increases iron elimination through the kidney and gut. Deferoxamine and extracorporeal devices replace phlebotomy, which cannot be used in renal failure. Elimination kinetics of iron following deferoxamine chelation and maintenance hemodialysis in ESRD have not been reported but must be low, as it takes months, in our experience, to substantially reduce serum ferritin concentrations with an iron overload.

LEAD   Hemodialysis without concurrent chelation is of no value in removal of body stores of lead (71). When hemodialysis is used with EDTA chelation the plasma half-life decreased from 96 to 9 hr, as compared to elimination with EDTA alone in one study (72).

MERCURY   Poisoning with elemental and inorganic mercury is treated with dimercaprol chelation for symptomatic patients and penicillamine for less severe exposures (73). Concurrent chelation with hemodialysis does enhance removal when compared with coincident excretion through the urine and gut (74). However, the extensive distribution of the agent suggests that fractional removal of body stores will be small.

METHYLMERCURY   Hemodialysis has been combined with regional (infusion into the dialyzer inflow port) chelation therapy using L-cystine and

N-acetylcysteine for treating methylmercury poisoning (75, 76). Both chelators enhance removal by dialysis, but clearances are low and fractional removal of body stores is trivial. Hemoperfusion using polymercaptal microspheres shows promise (77).

Herbicides and Insecticides

PARAQUAT AND DIQUAT   Paraquat poisoning is associated with a mortality rate of approximately 70%. Although extracorporeal removal has often been attempted along with gastric lavage and forced diuresis, the extensive tissue distribution of these agents and evidence of rebound in plasma concentrations after stopping hemoperfusion suggests that fractional removal of these toxins is clinically insignificant (78, 79).

ORGANOPHOSPHATES   Organophosphates have cholinesterase-inhibiting activity. Parathione is a nondialyzable, lipophilic drug. It is metabolized to paraxon, which is probably the actual toxic agent in parathione poisoning. Unlike parathione, paraxon is removable by hemodialysis, and both agents are removable by charcoal hemoperfusion (80, 81). Two other organophosphates, demeton-S-methyl sulfoxide and dimethoate, have been reported to be removed by hemodialysis, charcoal, and resin hemoperfusion in laboratory studies (81, 82). In a clinical case report, 70% of the total body load of the poison was removed during 5 hr of hemoperfusion (82).

Mushroom Poisoning

The death cap *(Amanita phalloides)* and the destroying angel *(Amanita verna)* are appropriately named, for death follows in about 30% of those who ingest these toxins. The toxins are dialyzable and have a high affinity for charcoal (83, 84). Case reports provide strong circumstantial evidence that charcoal hemoperfusion is effective in removing toxins from the blood even 24 hr after ingestion (84). Seven patients who had ingested more than 3 death caps each received hemoperfusion within 16–24 hr following ingestion; all recovered.

Literature Cited

1. Clemmensen, C., Nilsson, E. 1961. Therapeutic trends in the treatment of barbiturate poisoning: The Scandinavian Method. *Clin. Pharmacol. Ther.* 2:220–29
2. Vale, A., Meredith, T., Buckley, B. 1984. ABC of poisoning: Eliminating poisons. *Brit. Med. J.* 289:366–69
3. Blye, E., Lorch, J., Cortell, S. 1984. Extracorporeal therapy in the treatment of intoxication. *Am. J. Kidney Dis.* 3:321–38

4. Takki, S., Gambertoglio, J. G., Honda, D. H., Tozer, T. N. 1978. Pharmacokinetic evaluation in acute drug overdose. *J. Pharmacokinet. Biopharm.* 6:427–42
5. Lunde, K. K. M., Skuterud, B. 1977. Pharmacological principles in the diagnosis and treatment of acute intoxications. *Acta Pharmacol. Toxicol. Suppl.* 41:26–37
6. Cutler, R. E., Forland, S. C., Davis, G. M., Misson, R. T. 1984. Pharmacology

of drugs in renal failure. In *Current Nephrology*, ed. H. C. Gonick, 7:131–71. New York: Wiley

7. Gibaldi, M. 1977. Drug distribution in renal failure. *Am. J. Med.* 62:471–474

8. Cutler, R. E., Kirchman, K. H., Blair, A. D. 1979. Pharmacology of drugs in renal failure. In *Current Nephrology*, ed. H. C. Gonick, 3:397–435. Boston: Houghton Mifflin

9. Wolf, A. V., Kemp, D. G., Kiley, J. E. 1951. Artificial kidney function. Kinetics of hemodialysis. *J. Clin. Invest.* 30:1062–70

10. Nichols, C. Jr., Nichols, N. 1953. Electrolyte equilibria in erythrocytes during acidosis. *J. Clin. Invest.* 32:113–20

11. Nolph, K. D., Bass, O. E., Maher, J. F. 1974. Acute effects of hemodialysis on removal of intracellular solutes. *Trans. Am. Soc. Artif. Intern. Organs* 20:622–27

12. Murdaugh, H. V. Jr., Doyle, E. M. 1964. Effect of hemoglobin on erythrocyte urea concentration. *J. Lab. Clin. Med.* 57:759–69

13. Muirhead, E. E., Reid, A. F. 1948. Resin artificial kidney. *J. Lab. Clin. Med.* 33:841–44

14. Winchester, J. F., Gelfand, M. C., Tilstone, W. F. 1978. Hemoperfusion in drug intoxication: clinical and laboratory aspects. *Drug Metab. Rev.* 8:69–104

15. Gelfand, W. C., Winchester, J. F. 1980. Hemoperfusion in drug overdosage: a technique when conservative management is not sufficient. *Clin. Toxicol.* 17:583–602

16. Andrade, J. D., Van Wagenen, R. A., Chen, C., Ghavamian, M., Volder, J., Kirkham, R. 1972. Coated adsorbents for direct blood perfusion, II. *Trans. Am. Soc. Artif. Intern. Organs* 18:473–83

17. Gwilt, P. R. 1981. General equation for assessing drug removal by extracorporeal devices. *J. Pharm. Sci.* 70:345–46

18. Levy, R., Eco, T., Hanenson, I. B. 1977. Intravenous fructose treatment of acute alcohol intoxication. *Arch. Intern. Med.* 137:1175–77

19. Elliott, R. W., Hunter, P. R. 1974. Acute ethanol poisoning treated by hemodialysis. *Postgrad. Med. J.* 50:515–17

20. Lacouture, P. G., Wason, S., Abrams, A., Lovejoy, F. H. Jr., 1983. Acute isopropyl alcohol intoxication. *Am. J. Med.* 75:680–86

21. Osterloh, J. D., Pond, S. M., Grady, S., Becker, C. E. 1986. Serum formate con-

centrations in methanol intoxication as a criterion for hemodialysis. *Ann. Intern. Med.* 104:200–3

22. Gonda, A., Gault, H., Churchill, D., Hollomby, D. 1978. Hemodialysis for methanol intoxication. *Am. J. Med.* 64:749–58

23. Jacobsen, D., Janse, H., Wiik-Larsen, E., Bredesen, J. E., Halvorse, S. 1982. Studies on methanol poisoning. *Acta Med. Scand.* 212:5–10

24. Whalen, J. E., Richards, C. J., Ambre, J. 1979. Inadequate removal of methanol and formate using the sorbent based regeneration hemodialysis delivery system. *Clin. Nephrol.* 11:318–21

25. Hagstam, K. E., Ingvar, D. H., Patela, M., et al. 1965. Ethylene glycol poisoning treated by hemodialysis. *Acta Med. Scand.* 178:599–606

26. Stokes, J. B., Aueron, F. 1980. Prevention of organ damage in massive ethylene glycol ingestion. *J. Am. Med. Assoc.* 243:2065–66

27. Bobbitt, W. H., Williams, R. M., Freed, C. R. 1986. Severe ethylene glycol intoxication with multisystem failure. *West. J. Med.* 144:225–28

28. Vale, J. A., Rees, A. J., Widdop, B., Goulding, R. 1975. Use of charcoal haemoperfusion in the management of severely poisoned patients. *Br. Med. J.* 1:5–9

29. Burgess, E. D., Blair, A. D., Cutler, R. E. 1982. Dialysis and hemoperfusion of drugs and poisons. In *Current Nephrology*, ed. H. C. Gonick, 5:309–32. New York: Wiley

30. Tozer, T. N., Witt, L. D., Gee, L., Tong, T. G. 1974. Evaluation of hemodialysis for ethchlorvynol (Placidyl) overdose. *Am. J. Hosp. Pharm.* 31:986–89

31. Benowitz, N., Abolin, C., Tozer, T., Rosenberg, J., Rogers, W., et al. 1980. Resin hemoperfusion in ethchlorvynol overdose. *Clin. Pharmacol. Ther.* 27:236–42

32. Kathpalia, S. C., Haslitt, J. H., Lim, V. S. 1982. Charcoal hemoperfusion for treatment of ethchlorvynol overdose. *Artif. Organs* 7:246–56

33. Stalker, N. E., Gambertoglio, J. G., Fukumitsu, C. J., Naughton, J. L., Benet, L. Z. 1978. Acute massive chloral hydrate intoxication treated with hemodialysis: A clinical pharmacokinetic analysis. *J. Clin. Pharmacol.* 18:136–42

34. Gerretsen, M., deGroot, G., van Heijst, A. N. P., Maes, R. A. 1979. Chloral hydrate poisoning: Its mechanism and

therapy. *Vet. Hum. Toxicol.* 21:53–56 (Suppl.)
35. Chazan, J. A., Garella, S. 1971. Glutethimide intoxication (A prospective study of 70 patients treated conservatively without hemodialysis). *Arch. Intern. Med.* 128:215–19
36. Maher, J. F., Schreiner, G. E. 1961. Acute glutethimide poisoning. II. The use of hemodialysis. *Trans. Am. Soc. Artif. Intern. Organs* 7:100–9
37. Mandelbaum, J. M., Simon, N. M. 1971. Severe methyprylon intoxication treated by hemodialysis. *J. Am. Med. Assoc.* 216:139–40
38. Koffler, A., Bernstein, M., LaSette, A., Massry, S. G. 1978. Fixed-bed charcoal hemoperfusion—treatment of drug overdose. *Arch. Intern. Med.* 138:1691–94
39. Lobo, P. L., Spyker, D., Surrat, P., Westervelt, F. B. 1977. Use of hemodialysis in meprobamate overdose. *Clin. Nephrol.* 7:73–75
40. Crome, P., Higgenbottom, T., Elliott, J. A. 1977. Severe meprobamate poisoning: successful treatment with haemoperfusion. *Postgrad. Med. J.* 53:698–99
41. Hoy, W. E., Rivero, A., Marin, M., Rieders, F. 1980. Resin hemoperfusion for treatment of a massive meprobamate overdose. *Ann. Intern. Med.* 93:455–56
42. Proudfoot, A. T., Noble, J., Nimmo, J., Brown, S. S., Cameron, J. C. 1967. Peritoneal dialysis and hemodialysis in methaqualone poisoning. *Scot. Med. J.* 13:232–36
43. Gelfand, M. C. 1977. Symposium on sorbents in uremia: Part 3. Charcoal hemoperfusion in treatment of drug overdosage. *Dialysis Transplant.* 6(8):8–15
44. Schreiner, G. E., Maher, J. F., Marc-Aurele, J. 1959. The dialysance of exogenous poisons and some common metabolites in the twin-coil artificial kidney. *J. Clin. Invest.* 38:1040–45
45. de Torrente, A., Rumack, B. H., Blair, D. T., Anderson, R. J. 1979. Fixed-bed uncoated charcoal hemoperfusion in the treatment of intoxications: animal and patient studies. *Nephron* 24:71–77
46. Winchester, J. F., Tilstone, W. J., Edwards, R. O., Gilchrist, T., Kennedy, A. C. 1974. Hemoperfusion for enhanced drug elimination—a kinetic analysis in paracetamol poisoning. *Trans. Am. Soc. Artif. Organs* 20:358–63
47. Gazzard, B. G., Willson, R. A., Weston, M. J., Thompson, R. P., Williams, R. 1974. Charcoal haemoperfusion for

paracetamol overdose. *Br. J. Clin. Pharmacol.* 1:271–75
48. Helliwell, M. 1980. Severe barbiturate and paracetamol overdose: the simultaneous removal of both poisons by haemoperfusion. *Postgrad. Med. J.* 56:363–65
49. Marbury, T. C., Lee, C. C., Perchalski, R. J., Wilder, B. J. 1981. Hemodialysis clearance of ethosuximide in patients with chronic renal disease. *Am. J. Hosp. Pharm.* 38:1757–60
50. van Heijst, A. N. P., de Jong, W., Selderijk, R., van Dijk, A. 1983. Coma and crystalluria: a massive primidone intoxication treated with haemoperfusion. *J. Toxicol. Clin. Toxicol.* 20:307–18
51. de Groot, G., van Heijst, A. N. P., Maes, R. A. A. 1984. Charcoal hemoperfusion in the treatment of two cases of acute carbamazepine poisoning. *Clin. Toxicol.* 22:349–62
52. de Groot, G., Maes, R. A. A., van Heijst, A. N. P. 1977. The use of hemoperfusion in the elimination of absorbed drug mixtures in acute intoxications. *Neth. J. Med.* 20:142–48
53. Winchester, J. F., Gelfand, M. C., Knepshield, J. H., Schreiner, G. E. 1977. Dialysis and hemoperfusion of poisons and drugs—update. *Trans. Am. Soc. Artif. Intern. Organs* 23:762–842
54. Hansen, H. E., Amdisen, A. 1978. Lithium intoxication—report of 23 cases and review of 100 cases from the literature. *Q. J. Med.* 186:123–44
55. Jaeger, A., Sauder, Ph., Kopferschmitt, J., Jaegle, M. L. 1986. Toxicokinetics of lithium intoxication treated by hemodialysis. *Clin. Toxicol.* 23:501–17
56. Smith, T. W., Haber, E., Yeatman, L., Butler, V. P. 1976. Reversal of advanced digoxin intoxication with Fab fragments of digoxin-specific antibodies. *N. Engl. J. Med.* 294:797–800
57. Shah, G., Nelson, H. A., Atkinson, A. J., Okita, G. T., Ivanovich, P., et al. 1979. Effect of hemoperfusion on the pharmacokinetics of digitoxin in dogs. *J. Lab. Clin. Med.* 93:370–80
58. Burgess, E. D., Blair, A. D., Cutler, R. E. 1981. Disopyramide pharmacokinetics in normal and end-stage renal failure subjects. *Clin. Res.* 29:81A
59. Hayler, A. M., Medd, R. K., Holt, D. W., O'Keeffe, B. D. 1979. Experimental disopyramide poisoning: treatment by cardiovascular support and with charcoal hemoperfusion. *J. Pharmacol. Exp. Ther.* 21:491–95
60. Atkinson, A. J., Krumlovsky, F. A., Huang, C. M., del Greco, F. 1976.

Hemodialysis for severe procainamide toxicity: clinical and pharmacokinetic observations. *Clin. Pharmacol. Ther.* 20:585–92

61. Braden, G. L., Fitzgibbons, J. P., Germain, M. J., Ledewitz, H. M. 1986. Hemoperfusion for treatment of N-acetylprocainamide intoxication. *Ann. Intern. Med.* 105:64–65

62. Mauer, S. M., Chavers, B. M., Kjellstrand, C. M. 1980. Treatment of an infant with severe chloramphenicol intoxication using charcoal-column hemoperfusion. *J. Pediatr.* 96:136–39

63. Ehlers, S. M., Zaske, D. E., Sawchuck, R. J. 1978. Massive theophylline overdose—rapid elimination by charcoal hemoperfusion. *J. Am. Med. Assoc.* 240:474–75

64. Muir, K. T., Pond, S. M. 1979. Removal of theophylline from the body by haemoperfusion. *Clin. Pharmacokinet.* 4:320–21

65. Djerassi, I., Ciesielka, W., Kim, J. S. 1977. Removal of methotrexate by filtration absorption using charcoal filters or by hemodialysis. *Cancer Treat. Rep.* 61:751–52

66. Lione, A. 1985. Aluminum toxicology and the aluminum-containing medications. *Pharmacol. Ther.* 29:255–85

67. Vaziri, N. D., Upham, T., Barton, C. H. 1980. Hemodialysis clearance of arsenic. *Clin. Toxicol.* 17:451–56

68. Agarwal, B. N., Bray, S. H., Bercz, P., Plotker, R., Labovitz, E. 1975. Ineffectiveness of hemodialysis in copper sulphate poisoning. *Nephron* 15:74–77

69. Berman, L., Taves, D., Mitra, S., Newmark, K. 1973. Inorganic fluoride poisoning: treatment by hemodialysis. *N. Engl. J. Med.* 289:922 (Lett.)

70. Lovejoy, F. J. Jr. 1983. Chelation therapy in iron poisoning. *J. Toxicol. Clin. Toxicol.* 19:871–74

71. Smith, H. D., King, L. R., Marzolin, E. G. 1965. Treatment of lead encephalopathy. *Am. J. Dis. Child.* 109:322–24

72. Pedersen, R. S. 1978. Lead poisoning treated with haemodialysis. *Scand. J. Urol. Nephrol.* 12:189–90

73. Klaassen, C. D. 1985. Heavy metals and heavy-metal antagonists. In *The Pharmacological Basis of Therapeutics*, ed. A. G. Gilman, L. S. Goodman, T. W. Rall, F. Murad, pp. 1605–27. New York: Macmillan

74. Leuman, E. P., Brandenberger, H. 1977. Hemodialysis in a patient with acute mercuric cyanide intoxication. Concentrations of mercury in blood, dialysate, urine, vomitus and feces. *Clin. Toxicol.* 11:301–8

75. Bakir, F., Rustam, H., Tikriti, S., Al-Damluji, S. F., Shihristani, H. 1980. Clinical and epidemiological aspects of methylmercury poisoning. *Postgrad. Med. J.* 56:1–10

76. Lund, M. E., Banner, W., Clarkson, T. W., Berlin, M. 1984. Treatment of acute methylmercury ingestion by hemodialysis with N-acetylcysteine (Mucomyst) infusion and 2,3-dimercaptopropane sulfonate. *Clin. Toxicol.* 22:31–49

77. Margel, S. 1981. A novel approach for heavy metal poisoning treatment, a model. Mercury poisoning by means of chelating microspheres: hemoperfusion and oral administration. *J. Med. Chem.* 24:1263–66

78. Powell, D., Pond, S. M., Allen, T. B., Portale, A. A. 1983. Hemoperfusion in a child who ingested disquat and died from pontine infarction and hemorrhage. *Exp. Toxicol. Clin. Toxicol.* 20:405–20

79. Fairshter, R. D., Dabir-Vaziri, N., Smith, W. R., Glauser, F. L., Wilson, A. F. 1979. Paraquat poisoning: an analytical toxicologic study of three cases. *Toxicology* 12:259–66

80. Okonek, S. 1977. Hemoperfusion with coated activated charcoal in the treatment of organophosphate poisoning. *Acta Pharmacol. Toxicol. Suppl.* 41:85–89

81. Okonek, S., Boelcke, G., Hollmann, H. 1976. Therapeutic properties of haemodialysis and blood exchange transfusion in organophosphate poisoning. *Eur. J. Intensive Care Med.* 2:13–18

82. Okonek, S., Tonnis, H. J., Baldamus, C. A., Hofmann, A. 1979. Hemoperfusion versus hemodialysis in the management of patients severely poisoned by organophosphorus insecticides and bipyridyl herbicides. *Artif. Organs* 3: 341–49

83. Editorial. 1980. Mushroom poisoning. *Lancet* 2:351–53

84. Wauters, J. P., Rossel, C., Farquet, E. T. C. 1978. *Amanita phalloides* poisoning treated by early charcoal hemoperfusion. *Br. Med. J.* 2:1465

Ann. Rev. Pharmacol. Toxicol. 1987. 27:193–213

COMPUTER-AIDED DRUG DESIGN

Garland R. Marshall

Department of Pharmacology, Washington University School of Medicine, St. Louis, Missouri 63110

INTRODUCTION

Molecular modeling and computational chemistry are assuming an increasingly important role in understanding the basis of drug–receptor interactions and assisting the medicinal chemist in the design of new therapeutic agents. Computer graphics has emerged as a cost-effective tool, and adequate computational power is now available, which removes limitations that have crippled computational chemistry. These advances have stimulated the development of software tools for probing the three-dimensional aspects of specificity. Several recent reviews by Cohen (1, 2), Hopfinger (3), and Marshall & Motoc (4) offer more detailed coverage of this area.

To gain insight into the application of these approaches, we focus on recent studies and emphasize the range of techniques. Which technique is chosen is dictated by the knowledge of the molecular therapeutic target, whether enzyme or receptor. We emphasize the inherent limitations of each technique so that the reader may temper his enthusiasm in the face of the masterful and, sometimes artistic, applications of these approaches.

KNOWN ACTIVE SITES

Detailed information on the three-dimensional structure of macromolecules is available for an increasing number of enzymes and nucleic acids (the latest edition of the Brookhaven database contains over 290 structures). With the rapid developments in genetic engineering, it is possible to isolate and clone enough target macromolecules for experimental investigation. The increased speed of new detectors in X-ray crystallography [along with advances in nuclear magnetic resonance (NMR) spectroscopy that allow the determination of three-dimensional structure on noncrystalline materials] places an increas-

193

0362-1642/87/0415-0193$02.00

ing emphasis on the determination of the three-dimensional structure of the target as the prelude to rational drug design. The three-dimensional solution structure of a 75-residue protein, tendamistat, determined by NMR, resembles closely its crystal structure, which was determined independently (6). The determination of this structure in solution marks the beginning of a new era.

The Wellcome group [see reviews by Beddell (7) and Goodford (8)] pioneered the designing of compounds to effect the oxygen dissociation of hemoglobin based on the known allosteric effector, 2,3-diphosphoglycerate (DPG). The three-dimensional structure of the complex has inspired a number of other such efforts. The work of the Abraham group on sickle cell anemia (9) resulted in the design of novel chemical structures with good affinity that were subsequently shown to bind as predicted by determination of the crystal structure of the drug–hemoglobin complex. In both of these studies, however, the predictions were qualitative and based on placing groups on an appropriate three-dimensional framework for potential interaction with complementary groups in the receptor. Analogs with enhanced affinity for dihydrofolate reductase (DHFR) have also been designed by Kuyper et al (10) using a similar rationale.

In cases such as these, computer modeling has simply replaced the physical model of the enzyme that formed the basis of the original work. Binding affinity is estimated by counting the enhanced interactions (e.g. hydrogen bonds) and multiplying this number by some average energy of interaction, which should approximate the enhanced affinity. Compounds have also been designed to affect the solubility of insulin by influencing the crystal structure (11). Andrews et al (12) analyzed the binding affinities of a large set of drugs to partition these affinities into groups based on average interactions for each functional group. These average values provide a scheme to evaluate how well a drug binds to its receptor. If the observed affinity is greater than that predicted from a summation of average fragment contributions, then the drug–receptor complex must have greater than average complementarity. Such analyses may also provide some insight into entropy loss on binding (13). Goodford (14) developed a method of identifying optimal sites for interaction by probing the surface of known structures with different chemical fragments. This method correctly identifies known sites for bound water and other ligands. Kuntz et al (15) developed an efficient procedure to determine complementarity between rigid ligands and potential binding clefts on known crystal structures. This procedure generates a set of spheres that fill the pockets and the grooves on the surface of a receptor molecule. These spheres are then subdivided into sites. A similar representation is used for the ligand. Correspondence that does not require explicit rotation and translation of one structure into the other is sought between the distance matrixes for the sets of spheres representing the ligand and the presumptive site.

Hansch and coworkers have compared the parameters derived from quantitative structure-activity relationship (QSAR) analyses of ligands that bind to enzymes. The structures of dihydrofolate reductase (16), papain (17), actinidin (18), chymotrypsin (19), trypsin (20), carboxypeptidase (unpublished work cited in 17), alcohol dehydrogenase (22), and carbonic anhydrase (23) have been determined. Generally the terms derived in the QSAR equations do bear a relationship to the three-dimensional structure. In spite of the flexibility in conformation available to enzymes, the data obtained in solution and summarized by the correlation equation agree quite well with the static view of the active site. In QSAR, steric effects are often modeled by continuous variables that show that contact between the ligand and the enzyme does not preclude activity, but rather reduces it in proportion to the size of the substituent. The coefficient of the hydrophobic term, log P or pi, in the QSAR equation can be roughly related to the extent of desolvation of the ligand. A coefficient of 1 would suggest binding in a pocket, while a coefficient of 0.5 might suggest binding of the substituent to a flat surface requiring only partial desolvation. QSAR can offer insight, therefore, into the nature of the receptor site adjacent to the substituent under study.

A word of caution comes from the studies by Perutz et al (24) of the crystal structure of hemoglobin complexed with four compounds, each of which affects the polymerization of deoxyhemoglobin S. These compounds bound at different sites between the alpha chains far from the DPG site, implying that the same molecular event, a change in the allosteric equilibrium of the receptor, can occur by different molecular mechanisms. The binding sites were generally characterized as niches in the protein with available van der Waals space and complementary electrostatic interactions. The binding site of p-bromobenzyloxyacetic acid, however, was located in a position closely packed with sidechains in the uncomplexed structure. This observation emphasizes the dynamic nature of protein structure and the ability of drug-receptor interactions to induce complementarity.

Qualitative Applications

Vedani & Meyer (25) qualitatively analyzed the interactions of 28 sulfonamide inhibitors of human carbonic anhydrase, and suggested two binding modes for the heterocyclic ring in the active site. A hydrophobic pocket more than 10 Å from the active site zinc contributes important binding interactions. Smith et al (26) examined the mechanism of action and inhibition of thermolysin as a prelude to inhibitor design and more quantitative studies. DNA has been intensively targeted as a binding site. Many antibiotics such as actinomycin D and daunomycin bind by intercalation; the helix expands so that the flat polycyclic drug can occupy a site between two adjacent base pairs. Hendry and coworkers (27) postulated a similar mechanism to explain the hormonal activity of steroids. Other antitumor drugs bind within the minor groove of the DNA double helix (28). Kopka et al (29) determined the crystal structure of a netropsin-B DNA double-helix complex. Based on the mode of binding observed, Goodsell & Dickerson (30) analyzed the geometrical requirements for complementarity with the minor groove for 14 candidate monomer units to determine the optimal length for the oligomeric drug.

Thermodynamics of Binding

A second level of sophistication develops when one attempts to calculate the affinity of the ligand for the presumed site. Molecular mechanics is used to calculate the energy of the complex; from this number the energy of the free ligand and the free receptor are subtracted. The difference is the approximate enthalpy of binding. To understand the problems associated with these calculations, a short digression is in order. The first problem arises from the fact that calculations often approximate the enthalpy (ΔH) of binding in vacuo, when the quantity that should correlate with experimental observation is the free energy (ΔG) of binding in solution. The omission of solvation and entropy effects in theoretical approach of most studies is clearly an error, and reflects inadequate methodology for their estimation. A recent paper by Lybrand et al (31) using molecular dynamics with the explicit inclusion of the solvent and calculation of the entropic effect shows agreement within experimental error for the selectivity of the chloride complex of a macrotricyclic compound SC24 compared with the bromide complex. Considering the computational complexity of this approach, one cannot yet judge its practicality for large molecules in the near future. A preliminary report on trypsin by Wong & McCammon (32) is encouraging, but longer simulation is necessary to evaluate the agreement with experimental data. The assumption that entropy and solvation effects are similar for analogs is often used to justify comparison of the differences in binding activity between analogs, or the $\Delta\Delta$G. Another effect that makes correlations between calculated ΔH and binding affinities likely is the entropy–enthalpy compensation seen in aqueous solvents (33). Because of this relationship between the two components of free energy, one of the components should correlate with the other, with appropriate scaling.

These problems exist regardless of the quality of the force field used in the energy evaluation. Unfortunately, several reservations about current application of molecular mechanics must be mentioned. Parameters for novel structures are not readily available and require extensive theoretical or experimental study. In addition, the effects of electrostatics at the molecular level are unclear unless one can apply quantum mechanics in a fairly rigorous manner. The dielectric constant that screens the strength of interaction is, in fact, a variable that depends on the intervening atoms and their polarizability (34, 35). Currently the popular approach is to use a distance-dependent dielectric, 1/R, which simplifies the computation by eliminating a square root calculation. These practical limitations cause uncertainty in the interpretation of calculated binding affinities. Reliable accuracies of the order of a Kcal/mole would still lead to inaccuracies in predicted potency of a factor of ten, since at room temperature, 1.4 Kcal/mole reflects a tenfold concentration difference in binding affinity.

Applications

The binding of the thyroid hormones, T3 and T4, to prealbumin has been studied extensively as a model system, as the crystal structures of the complexes have been determined. Oatley et al (36) used the AMBER force field to refine the energy of the complexes. The calculated relative energy of binding (T4 to T3) was −2.9 Kcal/mole after a simple empirical correction for the solvation differences of the two hormones, whereas the observed differences are −1.4 Kcal/mole. Considering the reservations expressed above regarding the omission of entropy and force field uncertainties, this result is encouraging. Application to a large series of analogs would offer a firmer basis for evaluation. Zakrzewska et al (37) analyzed the binding energy of six antibiotics that bind in the minor groove of B-DNA. Introduction of a correction for solvent effect was essential to reproduce correctly the relative affinity and to scale the calculated energy to an appropriate level. Crystal structure analysis of the netropsin-DNA complex confirms (29) the prediction of the location of the charged nitrogen groups. Caldwell & Kollman (38) modeled this complex using NMR data as a guide. The major discrepancy with the crystal structure was the position of the charged headgroups of netropsin that were closely associated with the phosphate backbone in the calculated structure. This discrepancy reflects the omission of solvent and counterions in this study. Rao et al (39) explored several alternate DNA-binding modes for mitomycins and favor major groove binding for this drug. Lybrand & Kollman (40) compared a united atom force field with consideration of each atom of the intercalation drug, ethidium, with DNA fragments. Excellent agreement with experimental data was found with the all-atom representation. Besides a minimum energy complex corresponding to a model derived from crystal structures, a second minimum with a strong hydrogen bond between a phosphate oxygen and an amino hydrogen of ethidium was observed. This finding may reflect the absence of solvent in the calculations, which compounds the problem with electrostatics.

One major difficulty is the assumption of a common binding mode for compounds with similar structures. Even if one assumes rigid geometry for both the drug and the receptor, one must still explore six parameters (three translation and three orientation variables) to ensure that the global minimum for the complex has been determined. Adding internal flexibility to both the drug and the site to accommodate induced fit increases the computational complexity to the point that technological limitations preclude systematic search for optimal binding modes. Naruto et al (41) combined systematic search for productive binding modes with energy minimization for a series of mechanism-based inhibitors of chymotrypsin. The calculated enthalpies of binding predicted the order of affinity as well as a lack of stereoselectivity which was subsequently confirmed by resolution and enzymatic assay. The alternate binding modes found for the stereoisomers with equivalent affinity would not have been discovered by minimization from equivalent starting geometries. The success of this study probably reflects both the similar contributions to electrostatics, solvation, and entropy in a congeneric series as well as the enthalpy–entropy correlation referred to above.

RECEPTOR SITE BY HOMOLOGY

In a number of cases of therapeutic interest, the amino acid sequence of the target protein is known and homologous proteins exist whose three-dimensional structure has been determined. Computer modeling has been used to transform the known structure into the target by a combination of sidechain replacement and energy minimization. Obviously, when the structure of the target protein is close to the known structure, one has a greater chance of success. Aspartyl proteases are probably most widely studied. With these structures, renin inhibitors are the target (42). Several investigators have attempted to evaluate the likelihood of success of such studies. The Alberta group (43) made the most critical evaluation. They determined the crystal structure of an enzyme that had previously been modeled by homology. Drug design usually focuses on the active site; specificity for the particular enzyme is a design goal. Unfortunately, it is the residues that differ between the two proteins that cause the specificity. The successful design of renin inhibitors that resulted from this approach may be due to the same medicinal chemical logic that inspired so many angiotensin-converting enzyme (ACE) inhibitors in the absence of three-dimensional information. In that case, mechanistic arguments generated a framework on which to base designs, as the sequence of ACE was not available—even though the structures of carboxypeptidase A and thermolysin might have served as a rough template (44).

RECEPTOR SITE BY INDUCTION

With the advent of DNA sequencing, determining the sequence of proteins by inference has become routine, and a project to sequence the entire human genome is under consideration. Unfortunately, knowing the sequence of the therapeutic target does not aid the medicinal chemist. Progress in understanding the process of protein folding continues at an enhanced rate, with genetic engineering techniques offering a powerful experimental adjunct to theoretical studies. What hope do we have of predicting the three-dimensional structure based on sequence information alone? Whereas it is clear the tertiary information resides in the sequence, the translation rules have defied definition. Predictive methodology based strictly on statistical approaches is only approximately 60% accurate in secondary structure prediction (45). Even if one could correctly predict secondary structure, the correct folding is a combinatorial problem whose complexity should not be underestimated. A heuristic approach by Cohen et al (46) claims a high success rate (approximately 90%) in turn prediction. Sheridan et al (47, 48) have correlated amino acid composition and hydrophobicity patterns with the structure of protein domains. Their results may allow the prediction of the structural class with some degree of certainty and offer increased hope that such methodology may allow systematic exploration of possible folded structures by energy minimization. The same caveats expressed with regard to force fields, entropy, solvation, and local minima apply, of course, and become even more dominant due to the size of the structures considered.

Finer-Moore & Stroud (49) and Guy (50) proposed models for the acetylcholine receptor alpha subunit that contains the acetylcholine binding site. Mishina et al (51) described 26 analogs of this over-400-residue subunit prepared by site-directed mutagenesis that support the overall features of the models. Several models (52) of the sodium channel have also been proposed based on secondary structure predictions. McCormick et al (53) proposed a model for p21, the product of the *ras* oncogene, which Pincus & Scheraga (54) also studied. Blanar et al (55) used the techniques developed by Cohen et al (46) to model the RecA protein of *Escherichia coli*. A model of the apolipoprotein B-E receptor was developed by De Loof et al (56), who used hydrophobicity profiles to determine protein domains. In each of these cases, many more experimental data are required to refine, and, perhaps, redefine these models.

RECEPTOR SITE BY DEDUCTION

The problem most familiar to the medicinal chemist is the one in which the therapeutic target (the receptor) can by inferred only by binding studies or pharmacological studies. Systematic variation of the chemical structure leads quickly to the conclusion that some parts of the molecule are critical for activity, whereas others can be changed, causing only minor variations in affinity. These qualitative differences in results led to the concept of the pharmacophore at the turn of the century.

The inherent conformational freedom associated with most drugs hampered efforts to interpret structure-activity information in a three-dimensional framework. The work of Hansch and others in developing the QSAR paradigm showed that a common frame of reference based on a congeneric series offered a basis for rational interpretation. Comparison of binding modes at known active sites with the correlation equations developed with QSAR show clearly that the coefficients of the parameters can be interpreted with some degree of assurance in terms of the binding site (22, 23). While this approach is essentially topological, a topographical, or three-dimensional, equivalent must exist. This realization led Marshall and his coworkers (57–59) to develop the Active Analog Approach in which the pharmacophore provides the frame of reference analogous to the congeneric framework as a basis for comparison of molecules.

The pharmacophoric pattern must be defined before congeneric series can be compared. With rigid molecules and sufficient modification, inference of the pharmacophore should be straightforward. Unfortunately, most systems of therapeutic interest do not limit themselves to rigid structures, and the conformational problem must be confronted. Many approaches to this problem have been suggested. Most center around convenience and available methodology. Many have focused on energy minima as the key to biological activity. Certainly, most methodologies such as molecular mechanics, crystallography, or spectroscopy are aimed at determining the minimum under the experimental conditions of the investigation. The absence of the receptor in these studies clearly compromises their relevance on theoretical grounds. Several systems have been studied in sufficient detail to confirm this inadequacy (4). Nevertheless, papers continue to be published in which biological relevance is claimed, when no correlation of any observed phenomena with biological activity has been demonstrated. Hopefully, the availability of receptors by isolation and cloning will allow both experimental determination of the receptor-bound conformation, as well as measurement of difference between the solution ensemble of conformers and those limited sets capable of binding with high affinity.

The determination of the pharmacophore in the Active Analog Approach requires the initial examination of each three-dimensional pattern of candidate functional groups resulting from an energetically accessible conformation. If the premise of a pharmacophore, or common electronic message, is tenable, then each active analog must be capable of presenting that pattern that must appear in the set of possible patterns determined for each compound. Several approaches to pharmacophore identification have been suggested. Naruto et al (60) have applied the concept of constrained minimization of active compounds (in which the pharmacophoric groups are forced to assume a similar geometric arrangement) to histamine antagonists. Sheridan et al (61) cleverly apply distance geometry and use the simultaneous constraints presented by an ensemble of active molecules to find common geometric patterns, as demonstrated with the nicotinic pharmacophore. Both of these paradigms have the inherent limitation of minimization procedures that find a solution without regard to uniqueness, and that depends on the formulation of the problem. Multiple applications with different starting points can indicate the validity of the solution. Systematic exploration of the conformations available to an active compound determines the set of possible three-dimensional patterns that the pharmacophoric groups can present. Finding this set of patterns requires determining the logical intersection of the patterns available to each of the active compounds.

One must make an arbitrary decision regarding the energetics of conformations rejected from consideration. In some cases, the conformation presenting the pharmacophore may be near a local minimum energetically, but no a priori assumptions exclude perturbation of the energy surface of the isolated drug by the binding interaction. For example, 28 different chemical classes of ACE inhibitors were determined (D. Mayer, I. Motoc, C. B. Naylor & G. R. Marshall, unpublished information) to be capable of binding to a unique active site with a maximum energy distortion of 4 Kcal/mole upon binding. In other words, if the energy cutoff for consideration had been set at less than 3 Kcal/mole, then no active site would be capable of optimally binding these inhibitors. Conformers less stable than 2 Kcal/mole have little chance of being detected by most experimental techniques, as their abundance is less than 1% at room temperature.

Once a pharmacophoric hypothesis is proven valid by the experimental data, it can be further tested for consistency by examining compounds that have the prerequisite functional groups, but show little or no activity. Each compound can be checked to see if it can assume an energetically reasonable conformation in which the pharmacophoric groups are correctly aligned for activity. For those in which such alignment is possible, alternative explanations for inactivity must be sought. These explanations could include differences in distribution or metabolism, as well as negative steric interaction with the receptor. The technique of receptor mapping has been developed (59) to determine the volume adjacent to the pharmacophore that must exist for drug binding. Addition of the volume essential for each active drug when bound appropriately determines the minimal available space. One plausible explanation for inactivity arises when an inactive compound, capable of presenting the pharmacophore, requires a novel volume. Part of this novel volume may be occupied by the receptor and may preclude binding of the compound in question.

This approach suffers from several limitations. First, analysis of crystal structures of enzyme–ligand complexes shows clearly that alternate binding modes often exist, and that the hypothesized overlap of functional groups of the ligand is an oversimplification. If the data are sufficiently diverse, assumptions can be made with regard to the types of functionality in the receptor responsible for binding. Then, supermolecules can be constructed with such groups attached to those complementary groups of the ligand by idealized geometry. The investigator can search systematically for all geometrical arrangements of the hypothetical receptor site capable of interacting with the set of ligands. In the case of ACE, whose three-dimensional structure has yet to be determined, D. Mayer, I. Motoc, C. B. Naylor & G. R. Marshall (unpublished information) determined a unique active-site geometry for the postulated zinc, hydrogen bond donor, and positively charged groups based on 28 different chemical classes of inhibitors. For each chemical class, the energy difference between the bound conformer and the nearest local minimum was determined by energy minimization, with 4 Kcal/mole being the maximum decrease. In the pharmacophoric model of Wender et al (63) for the activation of protein kinase C, the conformation of 1,2-diacylglycerol corresponding to the C-4, C-9, and C-20 hydroxyl of phorbol is approximately 4 Kcal/mole above the global minimum. Previous efforts to determine the relative geometry of the active site of ACE were limited to a few chemical classes, and focused extensively on energetic minima to limit the computational complexity of the problem (64–66).

Knowledge of the chemistry at an enzyme active site often places severe stereochemical constraints on the relative orientation of groups. These restraints simplified greatly the consideration of possible binding modes in the analysis of mechanism-based inhibitors of chymotrypsin (41). Lim & Spirin (67) analyzed the stereochemistry of transpeptidation on the ribosome. They determined that a unique conformation of the tetrahedral intermediate is consistent with the formation of each of the 400 pairs of amino acids possible, which implies a particular geometry for the active site.

Another limitation concerns the lack of quantitation and the loss of information sustained by ignoring the relative affinities of the different compounds. A method for three-dimensional quantitative structure-activity studies remains to be completed. Several approaches being developed merit attention. A logical extension of the receptor-mapping approach by Hopfinger (68) begins with a congeneric series and relates overlap in molecular volume for the assumed receptor-bound conformation to other QSAR parameters to establish a correlation equation. Extensions (69–70) of this approach have focused on overlaps in the potential fields generated by probing the volume adjacent to the receptor with various probes, such as proton, water, and methyl. The loss of geometrical information by integration of the field is an inherent limitation in this procedure that defies the experience in specific directional interactions obtained by analysis of receptor-drug complexes. Wise et al (71) developed an approach that overcomes this objection. In this approach the potential field is sampled on a lattice adjacent to the drug. The lattice is oriented according to a set of rules, i.e. a pharmacophore hypothesis. A correlation is then sought by statistical evaluation of combinations of grid point values. While the number of parameters involved probably assures that such a correlation will be found, newer statistical methods developed by Wold et al (72) allow one to analyze this problem with some security. The only published application involves inhibitors of GABA uptake (73).

Motoc & Marshall (74) have also extended the volume mapping approach in a quantitative manner by subdividing the volume occupied by a drug and classifying each segment according to its contribution to affinity. This approach combines a recognition of the positive contribution to affinity by occupancy of the receptor site, as well as of negative contributions by competition with the receptor for volume and of a neutral portion that does not change its solvation state on binding. Only fragmentary aspects of this approach have been published (75), and an application of the completed procedure is not yet available.

In a quite distinctive approach, Ghose & Crippen (76) used the methodology of distance geometry and the concepts of QSAR to generate a hypothetical site with properties whose calculated affinity for sets of analogs reproduced the experimental affinities. This approach, however, does not appear to be deterministic and requires interaction and guidance from the user to devise a model active site. Nevertheless, such a site model offers help in the selection of compounds for screening and synthesis as well as an opportunity for continued refinement as new data are obtained. It appears a more refined approach than that constructing a hypothetical receptor site analogous to that advocated by Kier (77) or those built from amino acid fragments by Holtje & Tintelnot (78) and whose affinity for drugs correlated strongly with experimental data. Linschoten et al (79) developed a nine-point geometric representation of the turkey erythrocyte beta receptor with six energy parameters whose affinity for 58 diverse structures correlated well with observed affinity. With this representation these authors predicted different binding sites for the phenyl rings of phenethanolamines and phenoxypropanolamines.

The concept of pharmacophore, or three-dimensional mimicry, has guided the interpretation of activity of diverse chemical compounds as well as the development of several new classes for therapeutic development (1–4). Lloyd & Andrews (80) published a provocative study in which a common pharmacophoric mode was found for 14 classes of CNS-active drugs. A common precursor biogenic amine receptor could be responsible for this common binding mode, and different receptors could distinguish between molecules based on differences in accessory binding sites. Jeffrey & Liskamp (81) explained the tumor-promoting activity of phorbol esters, teleocidin B, and aplysiatoxin by the pharmacophoric concept. Wender et al (63) have analyzed similar compounds, including the natural activator of protein kinase C, 1,2-diacylglycerol. Based on the pharmacophoric model deduced, two novel structures with the predicted activity were prepared. Griffith et al (82) developed a novel atypical antidepressant based on a three-dimensional model of classical tricyclic antidepressants and mianserin. Martin & Kim (83) described the application of molecular modeling and QSAR reasoning that aided the development of a new class of diuretics (84). Loew and coworkers attempted to define receptor-site requirements that would explain activity at the benzodiazepine receptor (85, 86). The recent development of a nonpeptide antagonist of cholecystokinin by Evans et al (87) led to the suggestion that the benzodiazepine ring may exploit some feature common to peptide receptors. Two attempts (88, 89) to rationalize dopamine structure-activity relations based on receptor-site models have appeared.

On the other hand, emphasis on minimum energy structures continues in the literature. Robson & Finn (90) describe an approach that includes solvation effects, but still dwells on minimum energy conformers as exemplified in work on thyrotropin-releasing hormone (TRH) (91). Momany & Chuman (92) reviewed their work on morphiceptin and enkephalin analogs. These small peptides received attention from Loew et al (93), Hall & Pavitt (94), Maigret et al (95), and Paine & Scheraga (96). Using the Active Analog Approach, Nelson & Marshall (97) and Nelson et al (98) have clearly defined the receptor-bound conformation of morphiceptin by the use of analogs containing amino acids with defined conformational constraints. Font (99) also defined three alternatives for the receptor-bound conformation of TRH. Wong et al (100) presented their conformational analysis on a set of anticonvulsant drugs without consideration of a previous similar study by Klunk et al (101) of a different set of anticonvulsant compounds.

DETERMINATION OF SOLUTION CONFORMATION

The recent advances in NMR spectroscopy added to algorithmic advances in combining constraints from experiments with conformational calculations will clearly have a dramatic impact on drug design. Experimental measurements of spin-spin coupling constants, nuclear Overhauser effects (NOE), and hydrogen bonding determine sets of distances within a molecule that must be satisfied in any model. In the case of the small protein, tendamistat, 401 distant constraints from NOE measurements, 50 torsion angle constraints, and 168 distance constraints from hydrogen bonds and disulfide bridges were used (5). Rigid geometry was assumed to determine the three-dimensional structure according to the method of Braun & Go (102). Havel & Wuthrich (103) developed a similar methodology around the distance geometry paradigm.

Clore et al (104) explored the use of molecular dynamics with experimental constraints in determining the solution conformation of DNA binding F helix of cAMP receptor protein of *Escherichia coli*. In this case, 87 approximate distances from NOE measurements were used to define the alpha helical structure of this 17-residue fragment.

The three-dimensional structure of a novel antibiotic, aridicin A of the vancomycin-ristocetin family, was determined by a combination of two-dimensional NMR, systematic search, and energy minimization (105). In this case, the stereochemistry was also assigned in an unambiguous manner. The structure was determined as the only one consistent with the experimental data by systematic examination of conformational possibilities. Mildvan and coworkers (106, 107) pioneered the substitution of paramagnetic ions in metallo-enzymes as a probe to determine the enzyme-bound conformation of substrates and cofactors as well as the active-site residues adjacent to the metal. Two recent examples are the ATP-binding site of adenylate kinase (106) and the conformation of glutathione analogs bound to glyoxalase I (107).

METHODOLOGY

The application of various approaches is intimately related to the current stage of methodology development. Any comments are only relevant to the current state, as reflected by the experience of the author. Newer developments which may impact the applicability will be stressed.

Molecular Mechanics

The lack of parameters for many molecular fragments limits molecular mechanics. Development of parameters can be tedious, depending on the predictive accuracy required, but improvements in force fields continue (108–109). The increasing use of quantum mechanics (110) combined with analysis of experimental data (111) offers a strategy that should be generally used. Application to transition states has been attempted in the past (112, 113), but recent results by Houk (114) in which traditional methods are used to calculate the force field parameters for molecular mechanics offer considerable agreement with experimental observations. Weiner et al (115) studied trypsin hydrolysis by a hybrid approach.

Quantum Mechanics

The increasing computational power available makes the use of quantum mechanics more possible. Conjugated systems and transition states require consideration at this level. An increasing role as the basis for parameter determination for force fields is an obvious prediction. Clementi (116) and

Gresh & Pullman (117) developed parameters for larger molecular fragments such as amino acid residues by quantum methods and fit empirical functions to reproduce the energy surfaces. These energy functions are used to evaluate ion binding and hydration of nucleic acid oligomers (118) and other complex systems by Monte Carlo techniques. Questions concerning reactivity and mechanisms often require application of these techniques (119–121).

Molecular Dynamics

Molecular dynamics, a simulation technique, offers considerable insight into the vibrational modes accompanying transitions between conformational states. The computational requirements to simulate molecular behavior given the derivative of the potential energy field, the force, requires summation and mass weighting to determine the acceleration, which is added iteratively. The time steps necessary to simulate molecular motions are extremely small, femtoseconds, and the computational requirements to simulate phenomena of chemical and biological interest are enormous because of the large number of steps required. Another problem is the random walk of the procedure that occurs unless one is attempting to determine the energetics along a known transition path. Explicit inclusion of solvent offers an exciting approach to understanding solvation. The major caveat is the difficulty of ascertaining the extent of conformational space explored, the extreme computational demands, and the inherent limitations in current force field representations of electrostatics. Applications to numerous areas of chemistry are being reported (122–124) and are helping to establish confidence in this approach.

Monte Carlo Sampling

In the Monte Carlo sampling method, random conformations are generated and their energy is evaluated. By sufficient sampling, an overview of the energy surface is obtained and confidence limits may be placed on the relevance of the minimum energy conformation found to the global minimum. The Metropolis algorithm is normally used to reject conformers from the statistical sample whose energies are greater than would be predicted by the Boltzmann distribution (125–126). Paine & Scheraga (96) suggested a new approach. The application to the backbone conformation of the pentapeptide enkephalin produced results agreeing with those from energy minimization procedures.

Systematic Search

A systematic search is a uniform grid search of torsional space in which each conformation corresponding to a grid point is generated and its energy evaluated. The major advantage of this method is that all minima are located within the space examined and to the accuracy of the grid space. As this procedure is combinatorial, its computational demands restrict its use to problems with limited torsional degrees of freedom (ten rotatable bonds) or in which constraints can be used to limit the search. The determination of the three-dimensional structure of the antibiotic aridicin A by Jeffs et al (105) combined constraints such as coupling constants and NOE measurements from NMR with systematic search to arrive at a unique structure. This method is basic to pharmacophore identification with the Active Analog Approach.

Distance Geometry

The distance geometry method is a mathematical transformation in which the geometrical constructs are expressed in terms of relative distances. One obvious advantage is direct comparison of objects without concern about rotational and translational transformations. This procedure has become an integral part of the Ghose & Crippen approach (76) to receptor site modeling, as well as to the determination of three-dimensional solution structure by NMR as exemplified by the procedure of Havel & Wuthrich (103). A novel and important application has been to pharmacophore identification by Sheridan et al (61). The major disadvantage is that the procedure as implemented relies on minimization, which identifies only the nearest solution and provides no information regarding the uniqueness of the solution. Crippen (127) and Purisima & Scheraga (128) suggested approaches to alleviating the local minima problem.

SUMMARY

Progress in genetic engineering has increased the need for, while advances in computational hardware have removed barriers impeding, the development of appropriate computational tools to assist in the understanding of molecular interactions. Advancements both in techniques and in broadening application have been clearly demonstrated. Further development requires progress in the fundamental aspects of theoretical chemistry as well as an increased base of experience in choosing the appropriate set of assumptions for a particular problem. Computer-aided drug design is a current reality, but one that, at its best, supplements an incomplete methodology with the traditional insight and wisdom of an experienced medicinal chemist. In the next few years progress in developing a sound theoretical foundation will make molecular design a realistic aid to the medicinal chemist and protein engineer.

ACKNOWLEDGMENTS

For providing a stimulating environment that has focused many of the relevant issues, the students, fellows, and colleagues associated with the Computer-Aided Drug Design group over the past twenty years of molecular modeling all deserve credit for their many contributions. Melissa Taylor and Melissa Marshall assisted admirably with the logistics of compiling this review, as did the National Institutes of Health by their support of this research area (GM 24483). To those colleagues whose work has not been adequately considered, my sincere apologies for both my prejudices and oversight. I believe this article is an honest attempt at an impossible task.

Literature Cited

1. Cohen, N. C. 1985. Rational drug design and molecular modeling. *Drugs Future* 10(4):311–28
2. Cohen, N. C. 1985. Drug design in three dimensions. In *Advances in Drug Research*, ed. B. Testa, 14:41–145. London: Academic
3. Hopfinger, A. J. 1985. Computer-assisted drug design. *J. Med. Chem.* 28(9):1133–39
4. Marshall, G. R., Motoc, I. 1986. Approaches to the conformation of the drug bound to the receptor. In *Molecular Graphics and Drug Design*, ed. A. S. V. Burgen, G. C. K. Roberts, M. S. Tute, pp. 115–56. Amsterdam: Elsevier
5. Kline, A. D., Braun, W., Wuthrich, K. 1986. Studies by ¹H nuclear magnetic resonance and distance geometry of the solution conformation of the α-amylase inhibitor tendamistat. *J. Mol. Biol.* 189:377–82
6. Pflugrath, J. W., Wiegand, G., Huber, R., Vertesy, L. 1986. Crystal structure determination, refinement and the molecular-model of the alpha-amylase inhibitor Hoe-467A. *J. Mol. Biol.* 189(2):383–86
7. Beddell, C. R. 1984. Designing drugs to fit a macromolecular receptor. *Chem. Soc. Rev.* 13:279–319
8. Goodford, P. J. 1984. Drug design by the method of receptor fit. *J. Med. Chem.* 27(5):557–64
9. Abraham, D. J., Gazze, D. M., Kennedy, P. E., Mokotoff, M. 1984. Design, synthesis, and testing of potential antisickling agents. 5. Disubstituted benzoic acids designed for the donor site and proline salicylates designed for the acceptor site. *J. Med. Chem.* 27(12):1549–59
10. Kuyper, L. F., Roth, B., Baccanari, D. P., Ferone, R., Beddell, C. R., et al. 1985. Receptor-based design of dihydrofolate reductase inhibitors: Comparison of crystallographically determined enzyme binding with enzyme affinity in a series of carboxy-substituted

trimethoprim analogues. *J. Med. Chem.* 28(3):303–11
11. Manallack, D. T., Andrews, P. R., Woods, E. F. 1985. Design, synthesis, and testing of insulin hexamer-stabilizing agents. *J. Med. Chem.* 28(10):1522–26
12. Andrews, P. R., Craik, D. J., Martin, J. L. 1984. Functional group contributions to drug-receptor interactions. *J. Med. Chem.* 27(12):1648–57
13. Andrews, P. 1986. Functional groups, drug-receptor interactions and drug design. *Trends Pharmacol. Sci.* 7(4):148–51
14. Goodford, P. J. 1985. A computational procedure for determining energetically favorable binding sites on biologically important macromolecules. *J. Med. Chem.* 28(7):849–56
15. Kuntz, I. D., Blaney, J. M., Oatley, S. J., Langridge, R., Ferrin, T. E. 1982. A geometric approach to macromolecule-ligand interactions. *J. Mol. Biol.* 161:269–88
16. Hansch, C., Li, R., Blaney, J. M., Langridge, R. 1982. Comparison of the inhibition of *Escherichia coli* and *Lactobacillus casei* dihydrofolate reductase by 2,4 - diamino - 5 - (substituted - benzyl)pyrimidines: Quantitative structure-activity relationships, X-ray crystallography, and computer graphics in structure-activity analysis. *J. Med. Chem.* 25(7):777–84
17. Carotti, A., Casini, G., Hansch, C. 1984. Structure-activity relationship of the ficin hydrolysis of phenyl hippurates. Comparison with papain, actinidin, and bromelain. *J. Med. Chem.* 27(11):1427–31
18. Carotti, A., Hansch, C., Mueller, M. M., Blaney, J. M. 1984. Actinidin hydrolysis of substituted-phenyl hippurates: A quantitative structure-activity relationship and graphics comparison with hydrolysis by papain. *J. Med. Chem.* 27(11):1401–5
19. Hansch, C., Blaney, J. M. 1984. The new look to QSAR. In *Drug Design:*

Fact or Fantasy?, ed. G. Jolles, K. R. H. Wooldridge, pp. 185–208. London: Academic

20. Recanatini, M., Klein, T., Yang, C., McClarin, J., Langridge, R., et al. 1986. Quantitative structure-activity relationships and molecular graphics in ligand receptor interactions: Amidine inhibition of trypsin. *Mol. Pharmacol.* 29:436–46

21. Deleted in proof

22. Hansch, C., Klein, T., McClarin, J., Langridge, R., Cornell, N. W. 1986. A quantitative structure-activity relationship and molecular graphics analysis of hydrophobic effects in the interactions of inhibitors with alcohol dehydrogenase. *J. Med. Chem.* 29(5):615–20

23. Hansch, C., McClarin, J., Klein, T., Langridge, R. 1985. A quantitative structure-activity relationship and molecular graphics study of carbonic anhydrase inhibitors. *Mol. Pharmacol.* 27:493–98

24. Perutz, M. F., Fermi, G., Abraham, D. J., Poyart, C., Bursaux, E. 1986. Hemoglobin as a receptor of drugs and peptides: X-ray studies of the stereochemistry of binding. *J. Am. Chem. Soc.* 108(5):1064–78

25. Vedani, A., Meyer, E. F. Jr. 1984. Structure-activity relationships of sulfonamide drugs and human carbonic anhydrase C: Modeling of inhibitor molecules into the receptor site of the enzyme with an interactive computer graphics display. *J. Pharm. Sci.* 73:352–58

26. Smith, G. H., Hangauer, D. G., Andose, J. D., Bush, B. L., Fluder, E. M., et al. 1984. Intermolecular modeling methods in drug design/Modeling the mechanism of peptide cleavage by thermolysin. *Drug Inf. J.* 18:167–78

27. Hendry, L. B., Bransome, E. D. Jr., Lehner, A. F., Muldoon, T. G., Hutson, M. S., et al. 1986. The stereochemical complementarity of DNA and reproductive steroid hormones correlates with biological activity. *J. Steroid Biochem.* 24(4):843–52

28. Dervan, P. B. 1986. Design of sequence-specific DNA-binding molecules. *Science* 232:464–71

29. Kopka, M. L., Yoon, C., Goodsell, D., Pjura, P., Dickerson, R. E. 1985. Binding of an antitumor drug to DNA netropsin and C-G-C-G-A-A-T-T-^{Br}C-G-C-G. *J. Mol. Biol.* 183:553–63

30. Goodsell, D., Dickerson, R. E. 1986. Isohelical analysis of DNA groove-binding drugs. *J. Med. Chem.* 29(5):727–33

31. Lybrand, T. P., McCammon, J. A., Wipff, G. 1986. Theoretical calculation of relative binding affinity in host-guest systems. *Proc. Natl. Acad. Sci. USA* 83:833–35

32. Wong, C. F., McCammon, J. A. 1986. Dynamics and design of enzymes and inhibitors. *J. Am. Chem. Soc.* 108(13):3830–32

33. Lumry, R., Rajender, S. 1970. Enthalpy-entropy compensation phenomena in water solutions of proteins and small molecules: A ubiquitous property of water. *Biopolymers* 9:1125–227

34. Hingerty, B. E., Ritchie, R. H., Ferrell, T. L., Turner, J. E. 1985. Dielectric effects in biopolymers: The theory of ionic saturation revisited. *Biopolymers* 24:427–39

35. Matthew, J. B. 1985. Electrostatic effects in proteins. *Ann. Rev. Biophys. Biophys. Chem.* 14:387–417

36. Oatley, S. J., Blaney, J. M., Langridge, R., Kollman, P. A. 1984. Molecular-mechanical studies of hormone-protein interactions: The interaction of T_4 and T_3 with prealbumin. *Biopolymers* 23:2931–41

37. Zakrzewska, K., Lavery, R., Pullman, B. 1984. The solvation contribution to the binding energy of DNA with non-intercalating antibiotics. *Nucleic Acids Res.* 12(16):6559–74

38. Caldwell, J., Kollman, P. 1986. A molecular mechanical study of netropsin-DNA interactions. *Biopolymers* 25:249–66

39. Rao, S. N., Singh, U. C., Kollman, P. A. 1986. Conformations of the noncovalent and covalent complexes between mitomycins A and C and d(GCGCGCGCGC)$_2$. *J. Am. Chem. Soc.* 108(8):2058–68

40. Lybrand, T., Kollman, P. 1985. Molecular mechanical calculations on the interaction of ethidium cation with double-helical DNA. *Biopolymers* 24:1863–79

41. Naruto, S., Motoc, I., Marshall, G. R., Daniels, S. B., Sofia, M. J., et al. 1985. Analysis of the interaction of haloenol lactone suicide substrates with α-chymotrypsin using computer graphics and molecular mechanics. *J. Am. Chem. Soc.* 107(18):5262–70

42. Sibanda, B. L., Blundell, T., Hobart, P. M., Fogliano, M., Bindra, J. S., et al. 1984. Computer graphics modelling of human renin. *FEBS Lett.* 174:102–11

43. Read, R. J., Brayer, G. D., Jurasek, L., James, M. N. G. 1984. Critical evaluation of comparative model building of

Streptomyces griseus trypsin. *Biochemistry* 23:6570–75

44. Wyvratt, M. J., Patchett, A. A. 1985. Recent developments in the design of angiotensin-converting enzyme inhibitors. *Med. Res. Rev.* 5:483–531

45. Palau, J., Argos, P., Puigdomenech, P. 1982. Protein secondary structure: Studies on the limits of prediction accuracy. *Int. J. Pept. Protein Res.* 19:394–401

46. Cohen, F. E., Abarbanel, R. M., Kuntz, I. D., Fletterick, R. J. 1986. Turn prediction in proteins using a pattern-matching approach. *Biochemistry* 25:266–75

47. Sheridan, R. P., Dixon, J. S., Venkataraghavan, R., Kuntz, I. D., Scott, K. P. 1985. Amino acid composition and hydrophobicity patterns of protein domains correlate with their structures. *Biopolymers* 24:1995–2023

48. Sheridan, R. P., Dixon, J. S., Venkataraghavan, R. 1985. Generating plausible protein folds by secondary structure similarity. *Int. J. Pept. Protein Res.* 25:132–43

49. Finer-Moore, J., Stroud, R. M. 1984. Amphipathic analysis and possible formation of the ion channel in an acetylcholine receptor. *Proc. Natl. Acad. Sci. USA* 81:155–59

50. Guy, H. R. 1984. A structural model of the acetylcholine receptor channel based on partition energy and helix packing calculations. *Biophys. J.* 45(1):249–61

51. Mishina, M., Tobimatsu, T., Imoto, K., Tanaka, K., Fujita, Y., et al. 1985. Location of functional regions of acetylcholine receptor α-subunit by site-directed mutagenesis. *Nature* 313:364–69

52. Greenblatt, R. E., Blatt, Y., Montal, M. 1985. The structure of the voltage-sensitive sodium channel: Inferences derived from computer-aided analysis of the *Electrophorus electricus* channel primary structure. *FEBS Lett.* 193(2):125–34

53. McCormick, F., Clark, B. F. C., La Cour, T. F. M., Kjeldgaard, M., Norskov-Lauritsen, L., et al. 1985. A model for the tertiary structure of p21, the product of the *ras* oncogene. *Science* 230:78–82

54. Pincus, M. R., Scheraga, H. A. 1985. Conformational analysis of biologically active polypeptides, with application to oncogenesis. *Acc. Chem. Res.* 18:372–79

55. Blanar, M. A., Kneller, D., Clark, A. J., Karu, A. E., Cohen, F. E., et al. 1984. A model for the core structure of the *Escherichia coli* recA protein. *Cold Spring Harbor Symp. Quant. Biol.* 49:507–11

56. De Loof, H., Rosseneu, M., Brasseur, R., Ruysschaert, J. M. 1986. Use of hydrophobicity profiles to predict receptor binding domains on apolipoprotein E and the low density lipoprotein apolipoprotein B-E receptor. *Proc. Natl. Acad. Sci. USA* 83:2295–99

57. Marshall, G. R., Barry, C. D., Bosshard, H. E., Dammkoehler, R. A., Dunn, D. A. 1979. The conformational parameter in drug design: The active analog approach. In *Computer-Assisted Drug Design, ACS Symp. 112,* ed. E. C. Olson, R. E. Christoffersen, pp. 205–26. Washington, D.C.: Am. Chem. Soc.

58. Marshall, G. R. 1985. Structure-activity studies: A three-dimensional probe of receptor specificity. *Ann. N. Y. Acad. Sci.* 439:162–69

59. Motoc, I., Dammkoehler, R. A., Marshall, G. R. 1986. Three-dimensional structure-activity relationships and biological receptor mapping. In *Mathematics and Computational Concepts in Chemistry,* ed. N. Trinajstic, pp. 221–51. Chichester, England: Horwood

60. Naruto, S., Motoc, I., Marshall, G. R. 1985. Computer-assisted analysis of bioactivity. I. Active conformation of histamine HI receptor antagonists. *Eur. J. Med. Chem.* 20(6):529–32

61. Sheridan, R. P., Nilakantan, R., Dixon, J. S., Venkataraghavan, R. 1986. The ensemble approach to distance geometry: Application to the nicotinic pharmacophore. *J. Med. Chem.* 29(6):899–906

62. Deleted in proof

63. Wender, P. A., Koehler, K. F., Sharkey, N. A., Dell'Aquila, M. L., Blumberg, P. M. 1986. Analysis of the phorbol ester pharmacophore on protein kinase C as a guide to the rational design of new classes of analogs. *Proc. Natl. Acad. Sci. USA* 83:4214–18

64. Hassall, C. H., Krohn, A., Moody, C. J., Thomas, W. A. 1984. The design and synthesis of new triazolo, pyrazolo-, and pyridazo-pyridazine derivatives as inhibitors of angiotensin converting enzyme. *J. Chem. Soc. Perkin Trans. 1,* pp. 155–64

65. Andrews, P. A., Carson, J. M., Caselli, A., Spark, M. J., Woods, R. 1985. Conformational analysis and active site modelling of angiotensin-converting enzyme inhibitors. *J. Med. Chem.* 28:393–99

66. Thorsett, E. D., Harris, E. E., Aster, S. D., Peterson, E. R., Snyder, J. P., et al. 1986. Conformationally restricted inhibitors of angiotensin converting enzyme: Synthesis and computations. *J. Med. Chem.* 29(2):251–60

67. Lim, V. I., Spirin, A. S. 1986. Stereochemical analysis of ribosomal transpeptidation: Conformation of nascent peptide. *J. Mol. Biol.* 188:565–77

68. Hopfinger, A. J. 1980. A QSAR investigation of dihydrofolate reductase inhibition by Baker triazines based upon molecular shape analysis. *J. Am. Chem. Soc.* 102(24):7196–206

69. Hopfinger, A. J. 1983. Theory and application of molecular potential energy fields in molecular shape analysis: A quantitative structure-activity relationship study of 2,4-diamino-5-benzylpyrimidines as dihydrofolate reductase inhibitors. *J. Med. Chem.* 26(7):990–96

70. Mabilia, M., Pearlstein, R. A., Hopfinger, A. J. 1985. Molecular shape analysis and energetics-based intermolecular modelling of benzylpyrimidine dihydrofolate reductase inhibitors. *Eur. J. Med. Chem.* 20(2):163–74

71. Wise, M., Cramer, R. D., Smith, D., Exman, I. 1983. Progress in three-dimensional drug design: the use of real time colour graphics and computer postulation of bioactive molecules in DYLOMMS. In *Quantitative Approaches to Drug Design,* ed. J. C. Dearden, pp. 145–46. Amsterdam: Elsevier

72. Wold, S., Albano, C., Dunn, W. J. III, Esbensen, K., Hellberg, S., et al. 1984. Modelling data tables by principal components and PLS: Class patterns and quantitative predictive relations. *Analusis* 12(10):477–85

73. Wise, M. 1985. Evolution of QSAR methodology and the role of newer computational techniques. In *QSAR and Strategies in the Design of Bioactive Compounds,* ed. J. K. Seydel, pp. 19–29. Weinheim, Fed. Rep. Germany: VCH Verlag

74. Motoc, I., Marshall, G. R. 1985. Molecular shape descriptors. 2. Quantitative structure-activity relationships based upon three-dimensional molecular shape descriptor. *Z. Naturforsch.* 40a:1114–20

75. Motoc, I., Marshall, G. R., Labanowski, J. 1985. Molecular shape descriptors. 3. Steric mapping of biological receptor. *Z. Naturforsch.* 40a:1121–27

76. Ghose, A. K., Crippen, G. M. 1984. General distance geometry three-dimensional receptor model for diverse dihydrofolate reductase inhibitors. *J. Med. Chem.* 27(7):901–14

77. Kier, L. B. 1968. Receptor mapping using molecular orbital theory. In *Fundamental Concepts in Drug-Receptor Interactions,* ed. J. F. Danielli, J. F. Moran, D. J. Triggle, pp. 15–45. New York: Academic

78. Holtje, H.-D., Tintelnot, M. 1984. Theoretical investigations on interactions between pharmacon molecules and receptor models. V: Construction of a model for the ribosomal binding site of chloramphenicol. *Quant. Struct. Act. Relat. Pharmacol. Chem. Biol.* 3(1):6–9

79. Linschoten, M. R., Bultsma, T., Ijzerman, A. P., Timmerman, H. 1986. Mapping the turkey erythrocyte β receptor: A distance geometry approach. *J. Med. Chem.* 29(2):278–86

80. Lloyd, E. J., Andrews, P. R. 1986. A common structural model for central nervous system drugs and their receptors. *J. Med. Chem.* 29(4):453–62

81. Jeffrey, A. M., Liskamp, R. M. J. 1986. Computer-assisted molecular modeling of tumor promoters: Rationale for the activity of phorbol esters, teleocidin B, and aplysiatoxin. *Proc. Natl. Acad. Sci. USA* 83:241–45

82. Griffith, R. C., Gentile, R. J., Robichaud, R. C., Frankenheim, J. 1984. Cis-1,3,4,6,7,11b-hexahydro-2-methyl-7-phenyl-2H-pyrazino(2,1-a)-isoquinoline: A new atypical antidepressant. *J. Med. Chem.* 27(8):995–1003

83. Martin, Y. C., Kim, K. H. 1984. Application of theoretical drug design methodology to a series of diuretics. *Drug Inf. J.* 18:95–113

84. Plattner, J. J., Martin, Y. C., Smital, J. R., Lee, C., Fung, A. K. L., et al. 1985. [(Aminomethyl)aryloxy]-acetic acid esters. A new class of high-ceiling diuretics. 3. Variation in the bridge between the aromatic rings to complete mapping of the receptor. *J. Med. Chem.* 28(1):79–93

85. Loew, G. H., Nienow, J. R., Poulsen, M. 1984. Theoretical structure-activity studies of benzodiazepine analogues: Requirements for receptor affinity and activity. *Mol. Pharmacol.* 26:19–34

86. Loew, G. H., Nienow, J., Lawson, J. A., Toll, L., Uyeno, E. T. 1985. Theoretical structure-activity studies of β-carboline analogs: Requirements for

benzodiazepine receptor affinity and antagonist activity. *Mol. Pharmacol.* 28:17–31

87. Evans, B. E., Bock, M. G., Rittle, K. E., DiPardo, R. M., Whitter, W. L., et al. 1986. Design of potent, orally effective, nonpeptidal antagonists of the peptide hormone cholecystokinin. *Proc. Natl. Acad. Sci. USA* 83:4918–22

88. Wikstrom, H., Andersson, B., Sanchez, D., Lindberg, P., Arvidsson, L., et al. 1985. Resolved monophenolic 2-aminotetralins and 1,2,3,4,4a,5,6,10b-octahydrobenzo(f)quinolines: Structural and stereochemical considerations for centrally acting pre- and postsynaptic dopamine-receptor agonists. *J. Med. Chem.* 28(2):215–25

89. Seeman, P., Watanabe, M., Grigoriadis, D., Tedesco, J. L., George, S. R., et al. 1985. Dopamine D_2 receptor binding sites for agonists. *Mol. Pharmacol.* 28:391–99

90. Robson, B., Finn, P. W. 1983. Rational design of conformationally flexible drugs. *Alt. Lab. Animals* 11(2):67–78

91. Ward, D. J., Griffiths, E. C., Robson, B. 1986. Conformational study of thyrotropin-releasing hormone. 1. Aspects of importance in the design of novel TRH analogues. *Int. J. Pept. Protein Res.* 27:461–71

92. Momany, F. A., Chuman, H. 1986. Computationally directed biorational drug design of peptides. In *Methods in Enzymology,* ed. P. M. Conn, 124:3–18. London: Academic

93. Loew, G., Keys, C., Luke, B., Polgar, W., Toll, L. 1986. Structure-activity studies of morphiceptin analogs: Receptor binding and molecular determinants of μ-affinity and selectivity. *Mol. Pharmacol.* 29:546–53

94. Hall, D., Pavitt, N. 1985. Conformation of cyclic analogs of enkephalin. III. Effect of varying ring size. *Biopolymers* 24:935–45

95. Maigret, B., Fournie-Zaluski, M., Roques, B., Premilat, S. 1986. Proposals for the μ-active conformation of the enkephalin analog tyr-cyclol(-N^γ-D-A_2-bu-gly-phe-leu-). *Mol. Pharmacol.* 29:314–20

96. Paine, G. H., Scheraga, H. A. 1985. Prediction of the native conformation of a polypeptide by a statistical-mechanical procedure. I. Backbone structure of enkephalin. *Biopolymers* 24:1391–1436

97. Nelson, R. D., Marshall, G. R. 1986. Receptor-bound conformation of peptides: Morphiceptin. In *Peptide Chemis-* *try 1985,* ed. Y. Kiso, pp. 239–44. Osaka, Japan: Protein Res. Found.

98. Nelson, R. D., Gottlieb, D. I., Balasubramanian, T. M., Marshall, G. R. 1986. Opioid peptides: Analysis of specificity and multiple binding modes through computer-aided drug design and structure-activity studies. In *Opioid Peptides: Medicinal Chemistry, NIDA Res. Monogr. Ser. 69,* ed. R. S. Rapaka, G. Barnett, R. L. Hawks, pp. 204–30. Rockville, Md: Natl. Inst. Drug Abuse

99. Font, J. L. 1986. Computer-assisted drug design and the receptor-bound conformation of thyrotropin-releasing hormone. PhD thesis, Washington Univ. St. Louis, Mo.

100. Wong, M. G., Defina, J. A., Andrews, P. R. 1986. Conformational analysis of clinically active anticonvulsant drugs. *J. Med. Chem.* 29(4):562–72

101. Klunk, W. E., Kalman, B. L., Ferrendelli, J. A., Covey, D. F. 1983. Computer-assisted modeling of the picrotoxinin and γ-butryolactone receptor site. *Mol. Pharmacol.* 23:511–18

102. Braun, W., Go, N. 1985. Calculation of protein conformations by proton-proton distance constraints: A new efficient algorithm. *J. Mol. Biol.* 186:611–26

103. Havel, T., Wuthrich, K. 1984. A distance geometry program for determining the structures of small proteins and other macromolecules from nuclear magnetic resonance measurements of intramolecular ^1H-^1H proximities in solution. *Bull. Math. Biol.* 46(4):673–98

104. Clore, G. M., Gronenborn, A. M., Brunger, A. T., Karplus, M. 1985. Solution conformation of a heptadecapeptide comprising the DNA binding helix F of the cyclic AMP receptor protein of *Escherichia coli:* Combined use of ^1H nuclear magnetic resonance and restrained molecular dynamics. *J. Mol. Biol.* 186:435–55

105. Jeffs, P. W., Mueller, L., DeBrosse, C., Heald, S. L., Fisher, R. 1986. Structure of aridicin A. An integrated approach employing 2D NMR, energy minimization, and distance constraints. *J. Am. Chem. Soc.* 108(11):3063–75

106. Fry, D. C., Kuby, S. A., Mildvan, A. S. 1986. ATP-binding site of adenylate kinase: Mechanistic implications of its homology with ras-encoded p21, F_1-ATPase, and other nucleotide-binding proteins. *Proc. Natl. Acad. Sci. USA* 83:907–11

107. Rosevear, P. R., Sellin, S., Mannervik, B., Kuntz, I. D., Mildvan, A. S. 1984.

NMR and computer modeling studies of the conformations of glutathione derivatives at the active site of glyoxalase I. *J. Biol. Chem.* 259(18):11436–47

108. Weiner, S. J., Kollman, P. A., Nguyen, D. T., Case, D. A. 1986. An all atom force field for simulations of proteins and nucleic acids. *J. Comp. Chem.* 7(2):230–52

109. Robson, B., Platt, E. 1986. Refined models for computer calculations in protein engineering: Calibration and testing of atomic potential functions compatible with more efficient calculations. *J. Mol. Biol.* 188:259–81

110. Hopfinger, A. J., Pearlstein, R. A. 1984. Molecular mechanics force-field parameterization procedures. *J. Comp. Chem.* 5(5):486–99

111. Burkert, U., Allinger, N. L. 1982. *Molecular Mechanics, ACS Monograph 177,* Washington, D.C.: Am. Chem. Soc.

112. DeTar, D. F. 1981. Computation of enzyme-substrate specificity. *Biochemistry* 20:1730–43

113. Pincus, M. R., Scheraga, H. A. 1981. Theoretical calculations on enzyme-substrate complexes: The basis of molecular recognition and catalysis. *Acc. Chem. Res.* 14:299–306

114. Houk, K. N. 1986. Modeling stereoselective organic reactions. *Abstr. Am. Chem. Soc.* 191:137

115. Weiner, S. J., Seibel, G. L., Kollman, P. A. 1986. The nature of enzyme catalysis in trypsin. *Proc. Natl. Acad. Sci. USA* 83:649–53

116. Clementi, E. 1980. *Lecture Notes in Chemistry: Computational Aspects for Large Chemical Systems,* Vol. 19. Berlin, Fed. Rep. Germany: Springer-Verlag

117. Gresh, N., Pullman, B. 1986. A theoretical study of the binding of phenothiazine derivatives to residues 82–93 of calmodulin. *Mol. Pharmacol.* 29:355–62

118. Kim, K. S., Clementi, E. 1985. Hydration analysis of the intercalated complex of deoxydinucleoside phosphate and

proflavin: Computer simulations. *J. Phys. Chem.* 89(17):3655–63

119. Maynard, A. T., Pedersen, L. G., Posner, H. S., McKinney, J. D. 1986. An *ab initio* study of the relationship between nitroarene mutagenicity and electron affinity. *Mol. Pharmacol.* 29:629–36

120. Barnett, G. 1986. Alteration of cytosine-guanine interactions due to N7 metal cation binding: A structure-activity relationship for cisplatin analogues. *Mol. Pharmacol.* 29:378–82

121. Weinstein, H., Mazurek, A. P., Osman, R., Topiol, S. 1986. Theoretical studies on the activation mechanism of the histamine H_2-receptor: The proton transfer between histamine and a receptor model. *Mol. Pharmacol.* 29:28–33

122. Karim, O. A., McCammon, J. A. 1986. Dynamics of a sodium chloride ion pair in water. *J. Am. Chem. Soc.* 108(8):1762–66

123. Struthers, R. S., Rivier, J., Hagler, A. T. 1985. Molecular dynamics and minimum energy conformations of GnRH and analogs. A methodology for computer-aided drug design. *Ann. N. Y. Acad. Sci.* 439:81–96

124. Hagler, A. T., Osguthorpe, D. J., Dauber-Osguthorpe, P., Hempel, J. C. 1985. Dynamics and conformational energetics of a peptide hormone: Vasopressin. *Science* 227:1309–15

125. Jorgensen, W. L., Gao, J., Ravimohan, C. 1985. Monte Carlo simulations of alkanes in water: Hydration numbers and the hydrophobic effect. *J. Phys. Chem.* 89(16):3470–73

126. Ranghino, G., Romano, S., Lehn, J. M., Wipff, G. 1985. Monte Carlo study of the conformation-dependent hydration of the 18-crown-6 macrocycle. *J. Am. Chem. Soc.* 107(26):7873–77

127. Crippen, G. M. 1982. Conformational analysis by energy embedding. *J. Comp. Chem.* 3(4):471–76

128. Purisima, E. O., Scheraga, H. A. 1986. An approach to the multiple-minima problem by relaxing dimensionality. *Proc. Natl. Acad. Sci.* 83:2782–86

Ann. Rev. Pharmacol. Toxicol. 1987. 27:215–35

METABOLISM OF ALPHA- AND BETA-ADRENERGIC RECEPTORS IN VITRO AND IN VIVO

Lawrence C. Mahan

Laboratory of Cell Biology, National Institute of Mental Health, Bethesda, Maryland 20892

Ruth M. McKernan and Paul A. Insel

Division of Pharmacology, Department of Medicine, University of California at San Diego, La Jolla, California 92093

INTRODUCTION

In the past decade the development of radioligand-binding techniques for membrane receptors has been a major advance in molecular pharmacology. With these techniques investigators have been able to study drug and neurotransmitter receptors as discrete molecular entities and have described changes in receptor number and affinity in different settings. A variety of drugs, diseases, and physiologic states are associated with increased (up-regulation) or decreased (down-regulation) numbers of receptors for catecholamines (alpha- and beta-adrenergic receptors) in target cells. In spite of the voluminous literature that describes these changes, our understanding of the cellular and molecular mechanisms that mediate alterations in receptor expression is limited. These alterations in the steady-state expression of receptors on target cells must represent perturbations in one or more steps of the metabolism or turnover of receptors. (The schematic model shown in Figure 1 incorporates some general features of this turnover.) Although many parts of the scheme have not been well characterized for adrenergic receptors, this model forms a basis for examining how receptor number changes in target cells. Alterations in receptor number must result from changes in the rate of receptor appearance and/or disappearance from the plasma membrane. Recep-

215

0362-1642/87/0415-0215$02.00

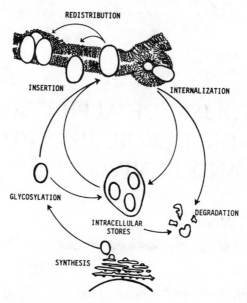

Figure 1   General features of receptor metabolism in cells.

tors appearance includes receptor synthesis, intracellular processing and transport, and membrane insertion or reutilization (recycling) of receptors from intracellular pools. Receptor disappearance includes removal from the cell surface, loss of binding function, and degradation of primary structure.

Adrenergic receptors, which recognize the endogenous catecholamines, epinephrine and norepinephrine, can be divided into four subtypes—$alpha_1$, $alpha_2$, $beta_1$, and $beta_2$—based on agonist and antagonist potencies for a variety of physiological responses (1–3). Although their precise structures are not yet known, each subtype of adrenergic receptor appears to be a distinct integral membrane glycoprotein with subunit molecular weight in mammalian cells between 60,000 and 80,000 (4, 5). Whereas $beta_1$- and $beta_2$-adrenergic receptors both activate adenylate cyclase and stimulate generation of the second messenger cAMP, signal transduction by $alpha_1$- and $alpha_2$-adrenergic receptors may occur through a variety of effector systems. These include inhibition of adenylate cyclase ($alpha_2$), Ca^{2+} mobilization ($alpha_1$ and $alpha_2$), phosphatidylinositol hydrolysis ($alpha_1$), enhancement of Na^+ or K^+ flux ($alpha_1$ and $alpha_2$), and arachidonic acid release ($alpha_1$ and $alpha_2$) (6, 7). Despite such functional heterogeneity, all adrenergic receptors are thought to act via interaction with one or more transduction proteins (the guanine nucleotide–binding (G or N) proteins), which couple the receptors to their respective effector mechanisms.

The extent to which the similarities and differences between adrenergic receptors are reflected in aspects of their cellular metabolism has yet to be elucidated. Thus, whereas much is known about adrenergic receptors and their coupling mechanisms, comparatively little is known of their turnover. In contrast, with other hormone receptors (e.g. insulin and epidermal growth factor receptors), considerably more is known about the receptor turnover than about coupling mechanisms. As discussed below, the limited understanding of the turnover of adrenergic receptors results partly from the use of indirect techniques to assess adrenergic receptor metabolism.

METHODS FOR THE STUDY OF RECEPTOR METABOLISM

A number of methodological approaches exist for the study of receptor metabolism in cells in vitro. Few of these methods can be successfully applied to the study of receptor turnover in vivo. Ideally, when measuring receptor metabolism, the tools used to make the measurements should not interfere with the metabolism of the receptors themselves.

Direct Approaches

Antibodies to receptors can often be used to identify the receptor protein. This method does not require structural integrity of the agonist- or antagonist-binding site. Use of antibodies is a preferred method because immature or partially degraded forms of the receptor can be identified (8). Two approaches to localizing and quantitating receptors are the use of radiolabeled antireceptor antibodies or the labeling of cells with radioactive amino acids and identification of receptors by immunoprecipitation or immunoblotting methods with unlabeled antibodies. Unfortunately, few antibodies for adrenergic receptors exist that can be used for these types of studies.

Isotopically heavy (^{15}N, ^{13}C, ^{2}H) amino acids have been used to study rates of receptor synthesis and degradation in cultured cells. In these studies the proportions of solubilized receptors were determined in "heavy" and "light" fractions on density gradients prepared from labeled cells (9–11). Aside from the considerable expense of heavy amino acids and potential problems of developing appropriate labeling, solubilization, and density gradient methods, these amino acids can have cytotoxic effects on some cells (11).

For classes of receptors other than adrenergic receptors, investigators have combined morphological approaches with biochemical methods to examine receptor metabolism (12). Receptors have been detected in intracellular organelles involved in receptor processing using fluorescently labeled agonists or antibodies tagged with fluorescent or electron-dense markers, or using irreversible binding of radiolabeled agonist or antagonist probes containing covalently reactive groups (chemically or photochemically activatable). This approach has been hindered by the relatively small number of adrenergic receptors expressed on most cells (typically $< 2 \times 10^4$/cell) and the lack of high affinity agonists or other probes that would allow receptors to be studied during the entire turnover process. Decreases in binding affinity for agonists commonly occur after beta- and alpha-adrenergic receptors encounter agonists. These changes make it difficult to use agonists to follow receptors through pathways of intracellular processing. In addition, it has not been shown that agonists are internalized along with adrenergic receptors and thus labeling of receptors with agonists may not be an appropriate approach for tracking receptors.

Indirect Approaches

Measuring receptor metabolism indirectly requires radiolabeled agonists or antagonists of high specific activity and specificity for the receptor studied. To estimate the rate(s) of receptor disappearance, cells or tissues are treated with inhibitors of protein synthesis, and the subsequent loss of receptors is measured by radioligand-binding methods. This technique has several shortcomings: (a) protein synthesis inhibitors may themselves alter receptor metabolism; (b) it cannot easily distinguish reutilization of receptors from intracellular pools; (c) use of agonists and antagonists to identify receptors may contribute to changes in receptor appearance and disappearance, since they can down-regulate or up-regulate receptors, respectively; (d) receptors cannot be measured before the binding site is formed (or in the correct conformation) or after the binding site is lost (or conformationally modified); and (e) some radiolabeled antagonists cross the cell membrane and thus receptors identified in studies with intact cells may include plasma membrane receptors (presumably functional) as well as receptors in intracellular pools.

Another indirect approach well suited for studies of metabolism of certain classes of receptors is the analysis of the reappearance of receptors (by radioligand-binding assays) after treatment of cells or tissues with antagonists capable of irreversible binding to receptors. There are a number of such alpha- and beta-adrenergic antagonists, and this approach has been the one most widely used to study metabolism of adrenergic receptors. Antagonists of high pharmacological specificity are preferred so that low concentrations can be used to achieve substantial blockade of receptors on target cells while facilitating removal of unreacted reagent after treatment. One critical assumption with the use of irreversible blocking agents is that covalently modified receptors do not themselves alter the normal expression of reappearing receptors. As described below, analysis of the kinetics of reappearance of receptors after blockade can provide insights into the potential cellular mechanisms that regulate expression of adrenergic receptors.

Kinetic Analysis of Receptor Metabolism

Kinetic analyses of receptor turnover have been performed for a number of receptors including alpha- and beta-adrenergic receptors (13–18). These studies allow one to define rates and rate constants that characterize general features of receptor metabolism. Generally, two criteria must be met before an adequate analysis can be made: (*a*) receptor production should be constant during the period of study and (*b*) the degradation of receptors, at any time, should be proportional to the concentration of these receptors in the cell. These criteria have been validated for a number of receptor systems, including those for insulin (9), epidermal growth factor (10), and acetylcholine (13). Thus, the kinetics of receptor synthesis and degradation (appearance and disappearance in binding studies) can be described by

$$R(t) = \frac{k_a}{k_d} (1 - \exp^{-k_d t}) + R_0 \exp^{-k_d t}, \qquad 1.$$

where $R(t)$ represents receptor number at time t, k_a, and k_d are the rate of receptor appearance and the rate constant of receptor disappearance, respectively, and R_0 is the initial number of receptors at the start of an experiment (9).

One experimental approach is to measure directly either k_a or k_d and then to derive the other value from the steady-state relationship when receptor levels, R_{ss}, are constant and $R_{ss} = k_a/k_d$. Thus, for example, k_d can be ascertained from the rate of loss of receptor binding sites when cells are treated with a protein synthesis inhibitor. Receptor half-life is then defined as $0.693/k_d$.

An alternative approach is to measure the rate of receptor reappearance after receptors have been blocked with an irreversible antagonist. Analysis of such data by nonlinear regression methods can yield unique values for k_a or k_d and a value for R_{ss} that should be equivalent to the steady-state number of receptors in untreated controls. This approach is probably best applied to studies with cells in vitro. When these analyses are performed on confluent cells that are not dividing, the values obtained apply to a single cell. In continuously growing cultures, cells in different phases of the cell cycle contain different levels of receptors, since as a first approximation, receptor synthesis must lead to a doubling in receptor number during one generation time prior to mitosis. Therefore one must take into account cell growth during the course of such studies, described by

$$C(t) = C_0 \exp^{k_c t}, \qquad 2.$$

where k_c is the rate of cell growth and C_0 is the initial cell density. When equations for receptor turnover and cell growth are combined (17), total receptor production is expressed as

$$R_T(t) = [(k_a C_0)/(k_c + k_d)]\exp^{k_c t} + [R_0 - (k_a C_0)/(k_c + k_d)]\exp^{-k_d t}, \qquad 3.$$

and values for k_a and k_d can then be obtained by nonlinear regression analysis. Use of this equation to obtain unique solutions of k_a and k_d is difficult when both variables are unknown. Total receptor production is a function of two independent exponential processes with disparate rate constants and is later heavily contributed to by cell growth. Thus a reasonable fit of data can be obtained by a series of different values for the two parameters, each combination of which yields an equivalent value for R_{ss}. Precise determination of k_a and k_d requires extensive data in the initial phase of receptor reappearance, where the signal-to-noise ratio is lowest. A more manageable rearrangment of this equation to receptors/cell (i.e. dividing by the cell growth equation) gives an equation similiar to that for confluent cultures except it reflects the influence of the cell growth rate constant:

$$R(t) = [k_a/(k_c + k_d)]\exp^{-(k_c + k_d)t} + (R_0/C_0)\exp^{-(k_c + k_d)t}. \qquad 4.$$

Accurate measurement of k_c in treated cells is necessary for deriving values for receptor appearance and disappearance. In addition, no alterations should occur in cell growth or distribution in cell cycle phases, since such alterations could influence the calculation of receptor number per average cell. Because this analysis describes the average cell in a continuously growing culture, measurements of receptor expression during the cell cycle in a synchronized population of cells can provide a more detailed description of changes that occur in a single cell.

Receptor metabolism studied in the absence of agonists is often termed "basal" metabolism. Experiments in vitro therefore require the use of serum-free media or serum screened for negligible levels of catecholamines. Studies of basal metabolism of receptors in vivo entail assessment of receptor metabolism in the presence of endogenous levels of tissue and plasma catecholamines in animals. Prolonged agonist or antagonist interaction with adrenergic receptors alters receptor expression on a number of target cells. These alterations are perhaps best understood with a knowledge of the basal metabolism of receptors. To date few kinetic analyses have been used to derive rates and rate constants for adrenergic receptor appearance and disappearance, respectively. The fairly straightforward nature of the approach should facilitate its application both in vitro and in vivo.

IN VITRO STUDIES OF ADRENERGIC RECEPTOR METABOLISM

Alpha-Adrenergic Receptors

Most studies on the metabolism of alpha-adrenergic receptors have involved the use of irreversible blockade of receptors, most commonly by administration of the antagonist phenoxybenzamine (POB), although N-ethoxycarbonyl-2-ethoxy-1,2-dihydroquinoline (EEDQ) has also been used (19, 20). Subsequent reappearance of receptors has been assessed using radiolabeled antagonists such as [^{3}H]prazosin for alpha$_1$-receptors or [^{3}H]yohimbine, [^{3}H]rauwolscine, and [^{3}H]clonidine for alpha$_2$-receptors.

Both POB and EEDQ are somewhat nonspecific. POB alkylates proteins through an unstable ethyleniminium ion that may irreversibly couple to negatively charged groups on the receptor protein (19). EEDQ efficiently couples to carboxylic acids either at the C-terminus or through an acidic amino acid, and is used as a coupling agent in peptide synthesis (21). Hence, both compounds rely on the accessibility of suitable chemical groups at, or near the site at which, the ligands bind to a given receptor. POB is reportedly more selective for alpha$_1$- than for alpha$_2$-adrenergic receptors (22, 23), whereas EEDQ appears more selective for alpha$_2$-adrenergic receptors (24). Unfortunately, both these drugs can bind to several classes of receptors in addition to alpha-adrenergic receptors. POB blocks dopaminergic (25, 26), cholinergic (27), gamma–aminobutyric acid (28), and opiate (29) receptors. EEDQ is similarly promiscuous and blocks binding to dopaminergic (30, 31), serotonergic (24), and cholinergic receptors and to various enzymes (32). The radioligand used to quantitate receptors provides some specificity in measuring receptor metabolism. However, different receptor systems may interact, and thus events measured in a given system could include both direct effects as well as indirect changes produced by interacting receptor systems. Also, if an extensive number of proteins are inactivated by POB or EEDQ, the altered protein synthesis in the cell may influence the metabolic turnover of a given receptor.

There are only a few reports on in vitro metabolism of alpha-adrenergic receptors (Table 1). One limiting factor has been that few established cell lines express sufficiently high numbers of alpha$_1$- or alpha$_2$-receptors. Assessment of reappearance of alpha$_1$-receptors after POB treatment has been reported for the BC$_3$H1 muscle cell line (18, 33). Other cell lines expressing high numbers of alpha$_1$-adrenergic receptors, DDT$_1$ cells derived from smooth muscle (34), and MDCK cells derived from renal tubular epithelium (35) are now available as useful models.

Table 1 Turnover of alpha- and beta-adrenergic receptors: in vitro studies

Cell type	$T_{1/2}$ (hr)[a]	Comment	Ref.
Alpha-receptors: Basal			
BC$_3$H1 muscle	24	Confluent	18, 23
Hepatocytes	18	Loss in primary culture	36
Down-regulation			
BC$_3$H1 muscle	3	Recovery CHX[d] sensitive	18
MDCK renal	8		37
Beta-receptors: Basal			
BC$_3$H1 muscle	n.d.[b]	Preconfluent	18
	170–200	Confluent	
C6 glioma	>150	Confluent	48
1321N1 astrocytoma	>100	Preconfluent	51
VA lung	25–30	Confluent	49
S49 lymphoma	30	Continuous growth	17
Down-regulation			
BC$_3$H1 muscle	1	Recovery CHX sensitive	18
S49 lymphoma	3	Recovery CHX sensitive	55, 58
C6 glioma	2	Down-regulation CHX sensitive	48, 57
		Recovery CHX insensitive	
1321N1 astrocytoma	n.m[c]	Recovery CHX/TUN insensitive in preconfluent cells	45, 51
	n.m (<12)	Recovery CHX sensitive, TUN insensitive in postconfluent cells	

[a]receptor half-life, calculated (k_d) or estimated for basal data; estimated half-life for down-regulation data.
[b]n.d. = not detectable
[c]n.m. = measured.
[d]CHX = cycloheximide; TUN = tunicamycin.

Alpha$_1$-adrenergic receptor number increases in BC$_3$H1 cells as a function of cell growth. At confluence, cells maintain a steady-state level of 200–250 fmol receptor/mg membrane protein. Measurements of receptor number in confluent cells after treatment with cycloheximide or POB yielded an identical estimate for receptor half-life of ~24 hr (18, 33). This estimate of receptor turnover is similar to that reported for alpha$_1$-receptor disappearance ($t_{1/2} =$ 18 hr) in hepatocytes that lose receptors in primary culture (36). Reappearance of receptors in BC$_3$H1 cells after POB treatment was inhibited by treatment of cells with cycloheximide, indicating that reappearance was dependent upon protein synthesis (presumably receptor protein) (33).

Incubation of target cells with catecholamine agonists promotes a down-regulation of alpha$_1$-adrenergic receptor number (18, 37). In BC$_3$H1 cells, this decrease in receptor number occurred at a rate substantially faster ($t_{1/2} =$ 3 hr) than that obtained for basal turnover of receptors. This enhanced loss of receptors was unaffected by cycloheximide, implying that an increase in receptor disappearance, and not a decrease in receptor appearance, accounted for down-regulation of receptor number (18). Following removal of agonists, alpha$_1$-receptors in BC$_3$H1 cells returned to control levels within 10 hr, a rate considerably faster than that obtained after POB treatment of cells (18, 33). This result suggests either that receptors down-regulated by agonists are endocytosed but not degraded and are then recycled from an intracellular site, or that agonist treatment increased a rate-limiting step in new receptor synthesis, processing, or insertion. Recovery of down-regulated receptors was inhibited by cycloheximide, indicating that protein synthesis is required. Recovery of functional response (phosphatidyl-inositol turnover) closely paralleled the recovery of alpha$_1$-receptors in these cells after POB or agonist treatment (18). Thus, those receptors measured during the period of reappearance were probably located on the plasma membrane.

Although several cell lines have been reported to express alpha$_2$-adrenergic receptors [including NG108-15, rodent neuroblastoma–glioma hybrid cells (38); HT29, human adenocarcinoma cells (39); HEL, human erythroleukemia cells (40); and RINm5F, rat insulin-secreting cells (41)], studies examining metabolism of these receptors have not been reported.

Beta-Adrenergic Receptors

Most data on the cellular metabolism of beta-adrenergic receptors result from studies using inhibition of protein synthesis or irreversible blockade of receptors in cultured cell lines. Receptors have been identified using radiolabeled antagonists such as [^{3}H]dihydroalprenolol (DHA), [^{125}I]iodocyanopindolol (IYCP), [^{125}I]iodopindolol (IPIN), or [^{125}I]iodohydroxypindolol (IHYP). The pindolol antagonists, IPIN and ICYP, bind with high affinity (pM) and low nonspecific binding ($<20\%$) to both beta$_1$- and beta$_2$-receptors in membrane preparations or in intact cells (42–45). As detailed below, the irreversible antagonists are derivatives of propranolol, alprenolol, or pindolol that undergo alkylation reactions with neighboring thiol, amino, thioether, or imidazole groups on the receptor (46).

Basal rates of beta-receptor turnover have been measured in many cell lines that reach confluence in culture. In BC$_3$H1 muscle cells, turnover of beta$_2$-receptors virtually ceased in confluent cells (18). In preconfluent cultures, receptor appearance paralleled cell growth and receptor turnover was negligible. Estimated half-lives of receptors in confluent cells were 170–200 hr. These half-lives were calculated from rate constants of disappearance in experiments using either inhibition of protein synthesis or irreversible inactivation of receptors with the antagonist N-[2-hydroxy-3-(1-naphthoxy)-propyl]-N'-bromoacetylethylenediamine (NHNP-NBE). This slow rate of receptor disappearance was associated with a very slow receptor appearance rate: <15% of control levels of receptors accumulated over 72 hr. These properties of beta-receptor turnover differ markedly from those for alpha$_1$-receptors on the same cell (Table 1).

In C$_6$ glioma cells, which contain predominantly beta$_1$-receptors, similar results were obtained. In preconfluent cells synchronized by double thymidine block, receptor number increased continuously as cells moved from the G$_1$ through the S phase of the cell cycle (47). By contrast, beta-receptor turnover was negligible in confluent cells (t$_{1/2}$>150 hr); few receptors reappeared after treatment of cells with the irreversible antagonist bromoacetylaminomethyl-pindolol (Br-AAM-pindolol) (48). This reappearance was caused by a transient stimulation of cell growth and was completely blocked by cycloheximide.

In human embryonic lung (VA) cells, turnover of beta$_2$-receptors was more rapid (49). The half-life of reappearance of receptors after blockade with NHNP-NBE was 25–30 hr. However, in this study the steady-state level of receptors attained after blockade was only 60% of that of control cells, which makes this estimate of receptor turnover difficult to interpret. The protein synthesis inhibitor, puromycin, blocked the reappearance of receptors, but more interestingly, receptors reappeared at a faster rate in cells treated with glucocorticoids.

Beta-receptor expression in another cell line that reaches confluence in culture, 1321N1 human astrocytoma cells, is biphasic, i.e. receptor number increases prior to, but then decreases after, confluency is reached (45, 50). The initial receptor expression (80–100 sites/cell/hr) was consistent with cell growth and dependent on receptor glycosylation. Preconfluent cultures treated with cycloheximide lost receptors very slowly (t$_{1/2}$>100 hr) (51). At confluence, receptor number reached a peak of ~4000 sites/cell and then decreased over 48 hr to 800–1000 sites/cell. This slower receptor expression in confluent cultures (~20 sites/cell/hr) was insensitive to inhibition of glycosylation, thus indicating differences in beta-receptor metabolism in pre- and postconfluent cultures.

In a continuously growing cell line, the S49 T-lymphoma, that grows in suspension culture, turnover of beta$_2$-receptors was measured after receptor blockade with the irreversible antagonist, bromoacetylalprenololmenthane (BAAM) and compared to receptor expression during the cell division cycle (17). Receptors appeared at a continuous rate of 75 sites/cell/hr in synchronized cells that maintained an average of 1200–1400 sites/cell when grown in asynchronous culture. This average number of receptors reflects the distribution of cells within the cell cycle phases (G$_1$, S, G$_2$/M). Receptors reappeared on cells treated with BAAM to steady-state levels. When analyzed according to Equation 1, a receptor half-life of ~30 hr was obtained. This estimate of turnover (0.023 hr^{-1}) is less than the value predicted by Equation

4, or $k_c + k_d$. The minimum half-life of receptors would equal the rate constant for S49 cell doubling, $k_c = 0.041$ hr^{-1} if receptor turnover was negligible ($k_d = 0$). (This point was not noted in the report of these data.) Although BAAM produced no apparent alteration in cell growth or cell cycle phase distribution, it may have slowed receptor appearance, possibly through interactions with intracellular receptor pools.

Incubation of cells in culture with beta-adrenergic agonists markedly reduces receptor number as measured by radioligand-binding assays. This agonist-induced down-regulation is distinct from and preceded by a rapid onset of cellular refractoriness, or desensitization, in which total receptor number is unchanged (52–54). During this early phase of refractoriness, receptors have become uncoupled from adenylate cyclase and may be localized in cellular compartments distinct from the plasma membrane. In several cell types studied thus far, agonist-promoted down-regulation of beta-receptors occurs more quickly than basal turnover (Table 1). The estimated half-life of receptor down-regulation in these studies is typically 1–4 hr.

Down-regulation of receptors could result from a marked decrease in receptor appearance or an increase in receptor disappearance. In BC$_3$H1 cells inclusion of cycloheximide had no effect on the rate of agonist-induced down-regulation, suggesting that accelerated clearance (or degradation) of receptors, not decreased synthesis, was the underlying mechanism. Similarly, in S49 cells a decrease in receptor appearance alone could not account for the kinetics of down-regulation (17, 55). In contrast, down-regulation of receptor number by agonists in C6 and C6-2B glioma cells was inhibited by cycloheximide, although in these cells down-regulation is induced by elevation of intracellular cAMP (56, 57). This type of down-regulation is distinct from that observed in studies using clonal variants of wild-type S49 cells that have lesions in the coupling of receptors to adenylate cyclase and the activation of cAMP-dependent protein kinase. Both the rate and extent of down-regulation of receptors by agonists were dependent upon receptor interaction with the alpha subunit of G_s but not upon activation of adenylate cyclase, generation of cAMP, or phosphorylation by cAMP-dependent protein kinase (55). Studies of agonist-induced down-regulation of beta-receptors have not produced direct evidence for the degradation of the primary structure of receptors.

In two cell lines, BC$_3$H1 and S49, recovery of beta-receptors following down-regulation by agonists occurred more rapidly than could be accounted for by basal receptor appearance or cell growth. Following a 16-hr exposure to epinephrine, receptor levels on BC$_3$H1 cells returned to control cell levels after 10 hr, following an initial 2-hr lag (18). In S49 cells, in which ~80% of the receptors were lost by an overnight exposure to isoproterenol, receptors recovered fully by 10–12 hr (55, 58). Recovery in both cell types was inhibited by cycloheximide (18, 58). Interestingly, recovery of receptors from down-regulation occurred at a similiar rate in wild-type S49 cells and in several clonal variants, suggesting that in contrast to down-regulation, recovery was independent of G_s, cAMP, or of cAMP-dependent protein phosphorylation.

Recovery of beta-receptors differed in pre- and postconfluent cultures of 1321N1 cells subjected to agonist-induced down-regulation. In preconfluent cultures, receptors recovered at a rate similar to the rate of receptor expression in untreated cells. Also in preconfluent cultures, recovery was not inhibited by cycloheximide or the glycosylation inhibitor, tunicamycin, suggesting that recycling of receptors may occur (45, 51). In contrast, the rate of recovery of receptors in postconfluent cultures was rapid and occurred during a period when receptor levels in untreated cells fell more than 50%. Inclusion of cycloheximide, but not tunicamycin, inhibited recovery, suggesting that recovery in postconfluent cultures requires protein synthesis but not receptor glycosylation. Subsequent studies using the heavy amino acid/ density-shift method (11), demonstrated clearly that receptors were newly synthesized during recovery from down-regulation in postconfluent cells. Thus both basal metabolism and agonist-altered metabolism of beta-receptors appear to be regulated differently in pre- and postconfluent 1321N1 cells.

In studies on postconfluent C6 glioma cells, the rate of recovery of receptors following down-regulation was faster than that of basal expression of receptors (48). When cells were incubated with Br-AAM-pindolol prior to down-regulation, and receptor reappearance was assessed, however, the resulting increased rate of recovery was not due to an increase in the rate of receptor appearance. In addition, this recovery process was insensitive to cycloheximide. Thus agonists may promote a recycling of beta-adrenergic receptors in this system. The cellular compartment in which down-regulated receptors reside and from which they recycle has not yet been identified in either C6 cells or 1321N1 cells.

IN VIVO STUDIES OF ADRENERGIC RECEPTOR METABOLISM

Alpha-Adrenergic Receptors

More data are available on the metabolism of alpha-adrenergic receptors in vivo than in vitro. To date, most studies have involved administration of POB or EEDQ to rats or rabbits. Reappearance of either $alpha_1$- or $alpha_2$-adrenergic receptors and function has subsequently been measured in peripheral and CNS tissues (Table 2).

In rats treated with POB, reappearance of $alpha_1$-receptors in liver occurred with a half-life of 42 hr (59). Recovery paralleled the return of $alpha_1$-

Table 2   Turnover of alpha- and beta-adrenergic receptors: in vivo studies

Tissue	$T_{1/2}$	Comment	Ref.
Alpha$_1$-receptors: Basal			
Rat			
salivary gland	33 hr	Reappearance cycloheximide sensitive	23
liver	42 hr	Recovery of function parallels receptor reappearance	59
cerebral cortex	5–6 day		22
	8 day	Young rats	
	15 day	Aged rats	62
Rabbit			
spleen	86 hr	Functional recovery (vascular) precedes receptor reappearance	60
cerebral cortex	11 day		61
brainstem	13 day		61
Alpha$_2$-receptors: Basal			
Rat			
cerebral cortex	4–5 day	Differential recovery of functional response	20, 62
	10–14 hr	30% blockade of receptors; no inhibition of function	22, 64
Rabbit			
spleen	38 hr	Vascular response parallels receptor reappearance	60
cerebral cortex	6 day	CNS-mediated function	61
brain stem	4–5 day	precedes receptor reappearance	
Beta-receptors			
Rat			
heart (beta$_1$)	100 hr	Young rats; basal	73
	350 hr	Old rats; basal	74
lung (beta$_2$)	320 hr	Young rats; basal	73
	550 hr	Old rats; basal	74
renal cortex	45 hr	Beta$_1$ recovery from down-regulation	76
	18 hr	Beta$_2$ recovery from down-regulation	
	12 hr	Down-regulation: beta$_1$ and beta$_2$	

adrenergic function, as measured by phenylephrine-stimulated glucose release ($t_{1/2}$ = 49 hr) and $^{45}Ca^{2+}$ efflux ($t_{1/2}$ = 38 hr) in tissue slices. In rat submaxillary glands (23), kinetic analysis of receptor reappearance yielded a similiar value for the half-life of alpha$_1$-receptors ($t_{1/2}$ = 33 hr). In contrast, alpha$_1$-receptors in rabbit spleen reappeared more slowly ($t_{1/2}$ = 86 hr) after POB administration (60). In these studies, however, alpha$_1$-mediated pressor response to phenylephrine and contraction of renal arteries by norepinephrine recovered more quickly ($t_{1/2}$ = 22 hr and 10 hr, respectively). Aside from the potential for tissue-specific differences in the metabolism of alpha$_1$-adrenergic receptors, these results demonstrate the potential difficulty in predicting alterations in function from changes in receptor number in vivo.

Studies thus far in CNS tissues suggest that alpha$_1$-receptors in the brain are more metabolically stable than those in peripheral tissues. After treatment of rabbits with POB, reappearance of alpha$_1$-receptors was slow; observed half-lives for reappearance were 10–11 days in cortex and 13 days in brain stem (61). In rats treated with POB, cortical alpha$_1$-receptors reappeared with a half-life of 5–6 days (22). Results from similar treatments of young (3-months-old) and aged (24-months-old) rats, and measurements of reappearance of [^{3}H]prazosin-binding sites in cerebral cortex and hypothalamus, extend these findings (62). Reappearance of 50% of the number of receptors in controls took approximately 8 days in young rats, but 15 days in old rats. The high lipid content of the brain could serve as a depot for POB, a lipophilic compound, and could potentially affect receptor reappearance. However analysis of the concentration and rate of disappearance of labeled POB in brains from young and old rats were identical and did not account for the differences in rates of reappearance observed in these studies. Thus a decreased turnover of alpha$_1$-receptors in the brain, especially in aged animals, may reflect the generally slower rate of protein synthesis and turnover in brain than in peripheral tissues (63).

Similiar studies have examined the metabolism of alpha$_2$-adrenergic receptors in vivo. In rabbits treated with POB, reappearance of [^{3}H]-clonidine binding sites in the spleen occurred with a $t_{1/2}$ of 38 hr; this rate is in good agreement with the recovery of maximum pressor response to administration of guanabenz, an alpha$_2$-selective agonist (60). The turnover of alpha$_2$-receptors in the CNS is slower and similar to results observed for alpha$_1$-receptors. Analysis of the kinetics of reappearance of alpha$_2$-receptors in cortex and brain stem from rabbits yielded estimates for receptor half-life of 6.1 and 4.6 days, respectively (61). Recovery of central alpha$_2$-mediated depressor response to intracisternally administered clonidine, however, occurred with a half-life of 2.4 days. Comparable estimates of 4–5 days were obtained for the half-life of reappearance of alpha$_2$-receptors in rat cortex (20, 62). Agonist (UK-14,304)-mediated inhibition of release of preloaded [^{3}H]norepinephrine in rat cortical slices (20) recovered more quickly ($t_{1/2}$ = 2.4 days), although alpha$_2$-mediated inhibition of [^{3}H]serotonin release paralleled the reappearance of receptors ($t_{1/2}$ = 4.6 days). These results cannot distinguish, however, whether inhibitory alpha$_2$-receptors exhibit different rates of turnover on noradrenergic and serotonergic neurons or that these inhibitory responses have different receptor occupancy requirements.

An exception to the slow turnover of alpha$_2$-receptors in the CNS has been reported for cortical tissue from rats administered POB (22, 64). In this study, the half-life of reappearance was 10–12 hrs; however, only 25–30% blockade was achieved and no change was observed in clonidine-mediated inhibition of release of preloaded [^{3}H]norepinephrine from synaptosome preparations. Theoretically the extent of blockade does not alter estimates of receptor turnover in a homogeneous population of receptors. This study suggests that cortex may contain subpopulations of alpha$_2$-receptors with different rates of turnover and/or accessibility to POB, however dose-dependent effects on the rate of reappearance of adrenergic receptors after irreversible blockade have been reported in vivo (23), whereas these effects are not observed in vitro (15, 17). Of note, reappearance of alpha-adrenergic receptors in vivo has been blocked in animals treated with inhibitors of protein synthesis such as 5-fluorouracil (61) and cycloheximide (23).

An alternative approach to the study of the metabolism of adrenergic receptors *in vivo* is to examine the recovery of receptor binding sites and function after down-regulation of receptor number. Receptor down-regulation has been indirectly elicited by administration of drugs that elevate plasma levels of catecholamines, such as antidepressants (65–67) and steroids (68), or by denervation (69). In many cases it has been difficult to determine whether elvated catecholamines or other compensatory responses are responsible for changes in receptor number. Administration of agonists in vivo has been successfully used to elicit down-regulation of alpha$_1$-adrenergic receptors. Plasma concentrations of catecholamines have been elevated either by intraveneous administration or by implantation of catecholamine-secreting pheochromocytomas (69–71). Studies of the influence of agonists on receptor turnover, however, have not been performed. This approach has not proved useful for the study of alpha$_2$-receptors in vivo. Agonist-induced down-regulation of these receptors has rarely been observed in tissues thus far examined (72). It is conceivable that after exposure to agoinsts, alpha$_2$-receptors become uncoupled from functional response, and receptors are translocated or sequestered in the membrane, but the binding site remains intact. Thus, as discussed earlier, such changes might not be detected in subsequent radioligand-binding studies.

Beta-Adrenergic Receptors

A limited number of studies have examined the in vivo metabolism of beta-adrenergic receptors. These studies have investigated the reappearance of receptors following either irreversible blockade or treatment with agonists.

Reappearance of [^{3}H]DHA binding to beta-receptors in heart (>beta$_1$) and lung (>beta$_2$) was measured in young rats (1 month old) after treatment with BAAM, which caused an ~90% reduction in receptor number (73). Receptors reached control levels after 8 days ($t_{1/2}$~100 hr) in heart and 27 days

($t_{1/2}\sim 320$ hr) in lung. In a similar series of experiments, reappearance of beta-receptors in the heart and lung was compared in young (1 month old) and senescent (27 month old) rats (74). Reappearance was markedly slower in both tissues from senescent rats ($t_{1/2}$ of ~ 350 hr and ~ 550 hr for heart and lung, respectively). Although BAAM is lipid soluble and could potentially partition in fat tissues or cross the blood-brain barrier, no evidence of residual BAAM in membrane preparations was detected in radioligand binding studies. In studies of blockade of beta-receptors by BAAM in guinea-pig lung, reappearance of antagonist binding sites preceded that of high affinity agonist binding sites and airway responsiveness to beta-agonists (75).

Subtype-selective alterations in the number of beta-adrenergic receptors occur in various tissues from rats implanted with norepinephrine-secreting pheochromocytomas or catecholamine-infusing osmotic minipumps (70, 71). In these studies plasma catecholamines were markedly elevated ($>$50-fold). Using continuous infusion and removal of the agonist isoproterenol, rates of $beta_1$- and $beta_2$-receptor appearance and disappearance were determined in rat renal cortical membranes, which contain 70% $beta_1$- and 30% $beta_2$-subtype (76). Infusion rates of 50–110 μg/kg/hr for 72 hr reduced total beta-receptor number by 50%. A similar reduction in both $beta_1$- and $beta_2$-subtypes (40% and 50%, respectively) was observed. Agonist-induced rate constants of receptor disappearance for both subtypes were identical, yielding an estimate for receptor half-life of 12 hr. $Beta_1$-receptors recovered more slowly ($t_{1/2} = 45$ hr) from down-regulation, however, than did $beta_2$-receptors ($t_{1/2} = 18$ hr). These data were analyzed according to Equation 1 to estimate k_a and k_d. The faster recovery observed for $beta_2$-receptors was associated with a more than a twofold elevation in both the rate of receptor appearance and rate constant of receptor disappearance compared to values observed for $beta_1$-receptors. Although limited in number, these in vivo studies suggest that basal turnover of beta-adrenergic receptors is slow and exhibits age dependency similiar to that observed for alpha-adrenergic receptors. By analogy with in vitro studies, exposure of tissues to elevated concentrations of agonists may accelerate the cellular metabolism of beta-adrenergic receptors.

SUMMARY AND CONCLUSIONS

Despite considerable evidence that changes in number of adrenergic receptors can occur under various conditions, knowledge of the mechanisms mediating these changes is still rudimentary. As discussed, indirect approaches emphasizing the kinetics of receptor turnover have been the principal means of investigation. These indirect methods, which depend on the ability of a radioligand to detect the receptors, are limited by several factors. Even so, the data obtained using indirect approaches, in particular on various model systems in cell culture, lead to several conclusions:

1. Both alpha$_1$- and beta-adrenergic receptors are metabolized rather slowly in vitro under basal conditions, in the absence of exposure to agonists. Typical half-lives are >20 hr, a turnover that is slower than that of several other classes of neurotransmitter and hormone receptors (9, 10, 12, 16). Moreover, alpha$_1$-adrenergic receptors and beta-adrenergic receptors can have substantially different half-lives, even when expressed on the same cell.
2. In view of the relatively slow rate of disappearance of adrenergic receptors under basal conditions, settings in which receptor number increases are almost certainly to result from increases in one or more of the factors that contribute to the rate of receptor appearance on the plasma membrane.
3. Treatment of cells with agonists markedly shortens the half-life of alpha$_1$- and beta-adrenergic receptors. This shortened half-life results primarily from an enhanced loss of receptors from the plasma membrane, and not from agonist-induced attenuation of receptor appearance. In fact, data acquired from studies of receptor recovery after agonist-induced down-regulation suggest that rates of receptor reappearance are markedly enhanced through either receptor recycling or an increase in receptor synthesis.
4. Limited studies conducted in vivo yield qualitatively similar results to those observed in in vitro studies of the metabolism of adrenergic receptors. In general, adrenergic receptors in the CNS turn over more slowly than those in peripheral tissues.

These conclusions help to highlight the many aspects of metabolism of adrenergic receptors that are as yet unknown, including identification and characterization of the cellular machinery responsible for receptor metabolism, elucidation of the molecular events that control metabolism, and assessment of how drugs and other factors influence these events. Future studies are likely to be based on the development of new methodology with antireceptor antibodies, receptor cDNA's, and improved morphological methods (autoradiography, immunohistochemistry, etc). Application of these techniques should help provide the biochemical and morphologic answers to the numerous unresolved aspects of adrenergic receptor metabolism.

ACKNOWLEDGMENTS

Work in the authors' laboratory has been supported by grants from the National Institutes of Health, the National Science Foundation, and the Elsa U. Pardee Foundation.

Literature Cited

1. Ahlquist, R. P. 1948. A study of the adrenotropic receptors. *Am. J. Physiol.* 153:586–600
2. Lands, A. M., Arnold, A., McAuliff, J. P., Luduena, F. P., Brown, T. C. 1967. Differentiation of receptor systems activated by sympathomimetic amines. *Nature* 214:597–98
3. Starke, K. 1981. Alpha-adrenoceptor subclassification. *Rev. Physiol. Biochem. Pharmacol.* 88:199–236
4. Lefkowitz, R. J., Caron, M. G. 1985. Adrenergic receptors: molecular mechanisms of clinically relevant regulation. *Circ. Res.* 35:395–406
5. Homcy, C. J., Graham, R. M. 1985. Molecular characterization of adrenergic receptors. *Circ. Res.* 56:635–50
6. Exton, J. H. 1985. Mechanisms involved in alpha-adrenergic phenomena. *Am. J. Physiol. Endocrinol. Metab.* 248(6):E633–47
7. Limbird, L. E., Sweatt, J. D. 1985. Alpha$_2$-adrenergic receptors: apparent interaction with multiple effector systems. In *The Receptors*, ed. P. M Conn, 2:281–305. Orlando/New York: Academic
8. Anderson, D. J. 1983. Acetylcholine receptor biosynthesis: from kinetics to molecular mechanism. *Trends Neurosci.* 6:169–171
9. Reed, B. C., Lane, D. M. 1980. Insulin receptor synthesis and turnover in differentiating 3T3-L1 preapidocytes. *Proc. Natl. Acad. Sci. USA* 77:285–89
10. Krupp, M. N., Connolly, D. T., Lane, D. M. 1982. Synthesis, turnover, and down-regulation of epidermal growth factor receptors in human A431 epidermoid carcinoma cells and skin fibroblasts. *J. Biol. Chem.* 257:11489–96
11. Waldo, G. L., Doss, R. C., Perkins, J. P., Harden, T. K. 1984. Use of a density shift method to assess beta-adrenergic receptor synthesis during recovery from catecholamine-induced down-regulation in human astrocytoma cells. *Mol. Pharmacol.* 26:424–29
12. Pastan, I. H., Willingham, M. C. 1981. Receptor-mediated endocytosis of hormones in cultured cells. *Ann. Rev. Physiol.* 43:239–50
13. Devreotes, P. N., Fambrough, D. M. 1975. Acetylcholine receptor turnover in membranes of developing muscle fibers. *J. Cell Biol.* 65:335–58
14. Ciechanover, A., Schwartz, A. L., Dautry-Varsat, A., Lodish, H. F. 1983. Kinetics of internalization and recycling of transferrin and the transferrin receptor in a human hepatoma cell line. *J. Biol. Chem.* 258:9681–89
15. Sladeczek, F., Homburger, V., Mauger, J. P., Gozlan, H., Lucas, M., et. al. 1984. Turnover of adrenergic receptors under normal and desensitized conditions. *J. Receptor Res.* 4:69–89
16. Wiley, H. S. 1985. Receptors as models for the mechanisms of membrane protein turnover and dynamics. In *Current Topics in Membranes and Transport*, ed. P. A. Knauf, J. S. Cook, 24:369–412. Orlando/New York: Academic
17. Mahan, L. C., Insel, P. A. 1986. Expression of beta-adrenergic receptors in synchronous and asynchronous S49 lymphoma cells. I. Receptor metabolism after irreversible blockade of receptors and in cells traversing the cell division cycle. *Mol. Pharmacol.* 29:7–15
18. Hughes, R. J., Insel, P. A. 1986. Agonist-mediated regulation of alpha$_1$- and beta$_2$-adrenergic receptor metabolism in a muscle cell line, BC3H-1. *Mol. Pharmacol.* 29:521–30
19. Nickerson, M., Gump, W. S. 1949. The chemical basis for adrenergic blocking activity in compounds related to dibenamine. *J. Pharmacol. Exp. Ther.* 97:25–47
20. Adler, C. H., Meller, E., Goldstein, M. 1985. Recovery of alpha$_2$-adrenoceptor binding and function after irreversible inactivation by N-ethoxycarbonyl-2-ethoxy-1,2-dihydroqunioline (EEDQ). *Eur. J. Pharmacol.* 116:175–78
21. Bodansky, M., Klausner, Y. S., Ondetti, M. A. 1976. Coupling reactions in peptide synthesis. In *Peptide Synthesis,* ed. G. A. Olah, pp. 114–23. New York: Wiley. 2nd ed.
22. McKernan, R. M., Campbell, I. C. 1982. Measurement of alpha-adrenoceptor "turnover" using phenoxybenzamine. *Eur. J. Pharmacol.* 80:279–80
23. Sladeczek, F., Bockaert, J. 1983. Turnover *in vivo* of alpha$_1$-adrenergic receptors in rat submaxillary glands. *Mol. Pharmacol.* 23:282–88
24. Meller, E., Bohmaker, K., Goldstein, M., Friedhoff, A. J. 1985. Inactivation of D$_1$ and D$_2$ dopamine receptors by N-ethoxycarbonyl-2-ethoxy-1,2-dihydroquinoline *in vivo:* selective protection by neuroleptics. *J. Pharmacol. Exp. Ther.* 233:656–62
25. Lehmann, J., Langer, S. Z. 1981. Phenoxybenzamine blocks dopamine auto-

receptors irreversibly: Implications for multiple dopamine receptor hypotheses. *Eur. J. Pharmacol.* 75:247–54

26. Hall, M. D., Jenner, P., Marsden, C. D. 1983. Turnover of specific [³H]spiperone and [³H]*N*,n-propylnorapomorphine binding sites in rat striatum following phenoxybenzamine administration. *Biochem. Pharmacol.* 32:2973–77

27. Blazso, G., Minker, E. 1980. Alkylation of ganglionic cholinergic receptors with haloalkyl amines. *Acta Pharm. Hung.* 50:137–44

28. Smockum, R. W. J. 1983. Inactivation of GABA receptors by phenoxybenzamine: effects on GABA-stimulated benzodiazepine binding in the central nervous system. *Eur. J. Pharmacol.* 86:259–64

29. Robson, L. E., Kosterlitz, H. W. 1979. Specific protection of the binding sites of D-Ala²-D-Leu⁴-enkephalin (delta receptors) and dihydromorphine (mu receptors). *Proc. R. Soc. London Ser. B* 205:425–32

30. Hamblin, M. W., Creese, I. 1983. Behavioral and radioligand binding evidence for irreversible dopamine receptor blockade by *N*-ethoxycarbonyl-2-ethoxy-1,2-dihydroquinoline. *Life Sci.* 32:2247–55

31. Leff, S. E., Gariano, R., Creese, I. 1984. Dopamine receptor turnover rates in rat striatum are age-dependent. *Proc. Natl. Acad. Sci. USA* 81:3910–14

32. Chang, K. J., Moran, J. F., Triggle, D. J. 1970. Mechanisms of cholinergic antagonism by *N*-ethoxycarbonyl-2-ethoxy-1,2-dihydroquinoline (EEDQ). *Pharmacol. Res. Commun.* 2:63–66

33. Mauger, J.-P., Sladeczek, F., Bockaert, J. 1982. Characteristics and metabolism of alpha₁-adrenergic receptors in a nonfusing muscle cell line. *J. Biol. Chem.* 257:875–79

34. Cornett, L. E., Norris, J. S. 1982. Characterization of the alpha₁-adrenergic receptor subtype in a smooth muscle cell line. *J. Biol. Chem.* 257:694–97

35. Meier, K. E., Snavely, M. D., Brown, S. L., Brown, J. H., Insel, P. A. 1983. Alpha₁- and beta₂-adrenergic receptor expression in the MDCK renal epithelial cell line. *J. Cell Biol.* 97:405–25

36. Schwartz, K. R., Lanier, S. M., Carter, E. A., Homcy, C. J., Graham, R. M. 1985. Rapid reciprocal changes in adrenergic receptors in intact isolated hepatocytes during primary cell culture. *Mol. Pharmacol.* 27:200–9

37. Meier, K. E., Sperling, D. N., Insel, P. A. 1985. Agonist-mediated reulation of alpha₁- and beta₂-adrenergic receptors in cloned MDCK cells. *Am. J. Physiol.* 249:C69–77

38. Kahn, O. J., Mitrius, J. C., U'Prichard, D. C. 1982. Alpha₂-adrenergic receptors in neuroblastoma glioma hybrid cells. *Mol. Pharmacol.* 21:17–26

39. Turner, J. T., Ray-Prenger, C., Bylund, D. B. 1985. Alpha₂-adrenergic receptors in the human cell line HT29. Characterization with the full agonist radioligand [³H]UK-14,304 and inhibition of adenylate cyclase. *Mol. Pharmacol.* 28:422–30

40. McKernan, R. M., Motulsky, H. J., Rozansky, D., Insel, P. A. 1986. Alpha₂-adrenergic receptors on a platelet precursor cell line, HEL. *Fed. Proc.* 45(3):562 (Abstr.)

41. Ullrich, S., Wollheim, C. B. 1985. Expression of both alpha₁- and alpha₂-adrenoceptors in an insulin secreting cell line. *Mol. Pharmacol.* 28:100–6

42. Barovsky, K., Brooker, G. 1980. (–)-[¹²⁵I]-Iodopindolol, a new highly selective radioiodinated beta-receptor antagonist: measurement of beta-receptors on intact rat astrocytoma cells. *J. Cyclic Nucleotide Res.* 6:297–307

43. Engel, G., Hoyer, D., Berthold, R., Wagner, H. 1981. (+)-[¹²⁵Iodo]-cyanopindolol, a new ligand for beta-adrenoceptors: identification of subclasses of beta-adrenoceptors in guinea pig. *Naunyn-Schmiedebergs Arch. Pharmakol.* 317:277–285

44. Insel, P. A., Mahan, L. C., Motulsky, H. J., Stoolman, L. M., Koachman, A. M. 1983. Time-dependent decreases in binding affinity of agonists for beta-adrenergic receptors of intact S49 lymphoma cells. *J. Biol. Chem.* 258:13597–605

45. Doss, R. C., Kramarcy, N. R., Harden, T. K., Perkins, J. P. 1985. Effects of tunicamycin on the expression of beta-adrenergic receptors in human astrocytoma cells during growth and recovery from agonist-induced down-regulation. *Mol. Pharmacol.* 27:507–16

46. Means, G. E., Feeney, R. E. 1971. Alkylating and similar reagents. In *Chemical Modification of Proteins*, 6:105–38. San Francisco: Holden-Day

47. Charlton, R. R., Venter, J. C. 1980. Cell cycle–specific changes in beta-adrenergic receptor concentrations in C6 glioma cells. *Biochem. Biophys. Res. Commun.* 94:1221–26

48. Homburger, V., Pantaloni, C., Lucas,

M., Gozlan, H., Bockaert, J. 1984. Beta-adrenergic receptor repopulation of C6 glioma cells after irreversible blockade and down-regulation. *J. Cell. Physiol.* 121:589–97

49. Fraser, C. M., Venter, J. C. 1980. The synthesis of beta-adrenergic receptors in cultured human lung cells: induction by glucocorticoids. *Biochem. Biophys. Res. Commun.* 94:390–97

50. Harden, T. K., Foster, S. J., Perkins, J. P. 1979. Differential expression of components of the adenylate cyclase system during growth of astrocytoma cells in culture. *J. Biol. Chem.* 254:4416–22

51. Doss, R. C., Perkins, J. P., Harden, T. K. 1981. Recovery of beta-adrenergic receptors following long term exposure of astrocytoma cells to catecholamine. *J. Biol. Chem.* 256:12281–86

52. Harden, T. K. 1983. Agonist-induced desensitization of the beta-adrenergic receptor-linked adenylate cyclase. *Pharmacol. Rev.* 35:5–32

53. Hertel, C., Perkins, J. P. 1984. Receptor-specific mechanisms of desensitization of beta-adrenergic receptor function. *Mol. Cell. Endocrinol.* 37:245–56

54. Sibley, D. R., Lefkowitz, R. J. 1985. Molecular mechanisms of receptor desensitization using the beta-adrenergic receptor-coupled adenylate cyclase system as a model. *Nature* 317:124–29

55. Mahan, L. C., Koachman, A. M., Insel, P. A. 1985. Genetic analysis of beta-adrenergic receptor internalization and down-regulation. *Proc. Natl. Acad. Sci. USA* 82:129–33

56. Moylan, R. D., Barovsky, K., Brooker, G. 1982. N^6, O^2-dibutyryl cyclic AMP and cholera toxin-induced beta-adrenergic receptor loss in cultured cells. *J. Biol. Chem.* 257:4947–50

57. Zaremba, T. G., Fishman, P. H. 1984. Desensitization of catecholamine-stimulated adenylate cyclase and down-regulation of beta-adrenergic receptors in rat glioma C6 cells. *Mol. Pharmacol.* 26:206–13

58. Rich, K. A., Iyengar, R. 1984. Down-regulation of the beta-adrenergic receptor of the S49 lymphoma cell. *J. Cell. Biochem. Suppl.* 8A:246 (Abstr.)

59. Lynch, C. R., Deth, R. C., Steer, M. L. 1983. Simultaneous loss and reappearance of alpha₁-adrenergic responses and [³H]-prazosin binding sites in rat liver after irreversible blockade by phenoxybenzamine. *Biochim. Biophys. Acta* 757:156–63

60. Hamilton, C. A., Dalrymple, H. W.,

Reid, J. L., Sumner, D. J. 1984. The recovery of alpha-adrenoceptor function and binding sites after phenoxybenzamine: an index of receptor turnover. *Naunyn-Schmiedebergs Arch. Pharmakol.* 325:34–41

61. Hamilton, C. A., Reid, J. C. 1985. The effects of phenoxybenzamine on specific binding and function of central alpha-adrenoceptors in the rabbit. *Brain Res.* 344:89–95

62. Greenberg, L. H. 1985. Regulation of brain adrenergic receptors during aging. *Fed. Proc.* 45:55–59

63. Dunlop, D. S. 1983. Protein turnover in brain: synthesis and degradation. In *Handbook of Neurochemistry*, ed. A. Lajtha, 5:25–63. New York: Plenum

64. McKernan, R. M., Campbell, I. C. 1986. Phenoxybenzamine partially inhibits alpha₂-adrenoceptors without affecting their presynaptic function. *Neuropharmacology* 25:47–52

65. Campbell, I. C., McKernan, R. M. 1982. Central and peripheral changes in adrenergic receptors in response to chronic antidepressant drug administration. In *New Vistas in Depression. Advances in the Biosciences, Vol. 40*, ed. M. Briley, pp. 153–60. Oxford/New York: Pergammon

66. Cohen, R. M., Aulakh, C. S., Campbell, I. C., Murphy, D. L. 1982. Functional subsensitivity accompanies reductions in yohimbine binding. *Eur. J. Pharmacol.* 81:145–48

67. Wong, D. T., Bymaster, F. P., Reid, L. R., Threlkeld, P. G. 1983. Fluoxetine and two other serotonin uptake inhibitors without affinity for neuronal receptors. *Biochem. Pharmacol.* 32:1287–93

68. Elliot, J. M., Peters, J. R., Grahame-Smith, D. G. 1980. Oestrogen and progesterone change the binding characteristics of alpha-adrenergic and serotonergic receptors on rabbit platelets. *Eur. J. Pharmacol.* 66:21–30

69. Colucci, W. S., Gimbrone, M. A., Alexander, R. W. 1981. Regulation of the post-synaptic alpha-adrenergic receptor in rat mesenteric artery: effects of chemical sympathectomy and epinephrine treatment. *Circ. Res.* 48:104–11

70. Snavely, M. D., Mahan, L. C., O'Conner, D. T., Insel, P. A. 1983. Selective down-regulation of adrenergic receptor subtypes in tissues from rats with pheochromocytoma. *Endocrinology* 113:354–61

71. Snavely, M. D., Ziegler, M. G., Insel, P. A. 1985. Subtype-selective down-

regulation of rat renal cortical alpha- and beta-adrenergic receptors by catecholamines. *Endocrinology* 117:2182–89

72. Insel, P. A., Motulsky, H. J. 1987. Regulation of alpha$_2$-adrenergic receptors. In *The Alpha$_2$-Adrenergic Receptor,* ed. L. E. Limbird. Clifton, NJ: Humana. In press

73. Baker, S. P., Pitha, J. 1982. Irreversible blockade of beta-adrenoreceptors and their recovery in the rat heart and lung *in vivo. J. Pharmacol. Exp. Ther.* 220:247–51

74. Pitha, J., Hughes, B. A., Kusiak, J. W., Dax, E. M., Baker, S. P. 1982. Regeneration of beta-adrenergic receptors in senescent rats: a study using an irreversible binding antagonist. *Proc. Natl. Acad. Sci. USA* 79:4424–27

75. Nelson, C. A., Muther, T. F., Pitha, J., Baker, S. P. 1986. Differential recovery of beta-adrenoreceptor antagonist and high affinity binding sites in the guinea-pig lung after irreversible blockade. *J. Pharmacol. Exp. Ther.* 237:830–36

76. Snavely, M. D., Ziegler, M. G., Insel, P. A. 1985. A new approach to determine rates of receptor appearance and disappearance in vivo. *Mol. Pharmacol.* 27:19–26

Ann. Rev. Pharmacol. Toxicol. 1987. 27:237–55

PLATELET-ACTIVATING FACTOR ANTAGONISTS

Robert N. Saunders and Dean A. Handley

Platelet Department, Sandoz Research Institute, East Hanover, New Jersey 07936

INTRODUCTION

History

In 1966 Barbaro & Zvaifler (1) noted the release of histamine from rabbit platelets in the presence of antigen and leukocytes. This activity was confirmed and described as complement independent (2, 3). Henson (4, 5) demonstrated that this labile factor was released from leukocytes by a calcium- and temperature-dependent process. The parameters surrounding the release of this factor and its potential role in immune complex deposition were described by Benveniste (6, 7) who first coined the term *platelet-activating factor* (PAF). Henson & Pinckard gave PAF a potential role in pathology when they described it as the mediator of IgE anaphylaxis in the rabbit (8, 9). After this early characterization, research interest with PAF focused on the structural determination of the molecule (10–12). In 1979 two laboratories (13, 14) chemically described PAF as acetyl glycerol ether phosphorylcholine (1-O-hexadecyl/octadecyl-2-acetyl-*sn*-glycerol-3-phosphorylcholine; Figure 1). A third laboratory determined that PAF was identical to a renal medullary hypotensive phospholipid (APRL) that was being investigated independently (15). Biosynthetic PAF was determined to be one of a family of active phospholipids of varying potency with structural modifications primarily in the length of the alkyl chain at position one (16). These observations, plus the determination that PAF activates many cells other than platelets, caused investigators to question the appropriateness of the term *platelet-activating factor*. Alternate terms used were *acetyl glycerol ether phosphorylcholine* (AGEPC) or *PAF-acether*. Investigators in the field and the authors of a recent review (17) agree that the term *PAF* should remain in use.

237

0362-1642/87/0415-0237$02.00

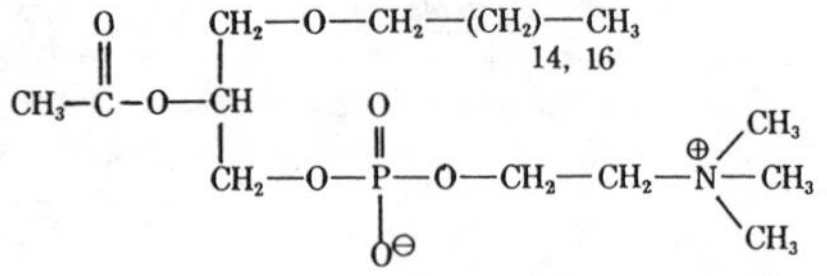

Figure 1   PAF structure.

The structural determination and synthetic preparation of PAF enhanced the interest in, and number of investigators using, this autocoid substance. The short biological half-life (18) and the concurrent release of other mediators in pathological models (19) have impeded the determination of PAF's importance in disease. The possession of specific PAF antagonists would aid the examination of the pathophysiological role of PAF. This review describes the evolution of such antagonists and, where possible, discusses the information on the potential role of PAF provided by their use. We also refer the reader to several recent reviews on this subject (17, 19–21).

Pharmacology of PAF

The association of PAF in serum sickness was postulated (6–8, 22) and substantiated (12), suggesting that this agent was indeed an autocoid mediator of inflammation. The most prominent and species-universal effect of PAF is increased vascular permeability (23–25). Plasma molecules as large as very low density lipoproteins extravasate from the vascular system when PAF is infused (25). This enhanced permeability is suggested to occur at postcapillary venules (24, 26). At low doses the effect of PAF is direct and does not require the participation of leukocytes (26, 27) or platelets (27). The concentration of PAF required to induce extravasation in the guinea pig is severalfold less than that needed for the extravasation of leukotrienes or histamine (28, 29).

Early quantitation of PAF was based on platelet-aggregation and -release reactions (5). The activation of platelets occurs by specific, saturable binding of PAF to a membrane receptor (30, 31). Platelet sensitivity to PAF varies greatly among the species evaluated; the rabbit and guinea pig (13, 32) are the most sensitive. The human, baboon, and canine platelets demonstrate intermediate sensitivity (32), and the rhesus and cebus apella primate platelets have minimal PAF sensitivity (33, 34). Rat (35, 36) and mouse (36) platelets are considered unresponsive to PAF and lack PAF receptors (37). The infusion of PAF into the sensitive species, guinea pig (38), rabbit (39), baboon (40), and man (J. Benveniste, personal communication), results in rapid and pronounced thrombocytopenia, which reverses within one hour. The relationship of this platelet aggregate formation with vascular thrombolic states has not been clearly defined. The topical superinfusion of PAF on the guinea pig mesentery over an injured arterial segment produces a platelet thrombus (41). This observation suggests that local vascular PAF production could lead or contribute to occlusive thrombotic events.

The platelet's sensitivity to PAF also appears related to the potential of this mediator to induce bronchoconstriction (38). Those species with reactive platelets, such as the guinea pig (38), rabbit (39), baboon (40), and man (42–45), also demonstrate bronchoconstriction with PAF infusion. Conversely, those species with minimal or reduced platelet sensitivity, such as the rat (35), rhesus primate, and cebus apella primate (33, 34), also demonstrate reduced or absent bronchoconstrictive responses (46). Platelet accumulation within the guinea pig lung after a one-hour infusion of low PAF concentrations has been suggested to induce airways hyperreactivity (47, 48). The presence of polymorphonuclear neutrophil leukocytes and eosinophils in the lungs (49, 50) after PAF infusion suggests that all of these cells contribute to the pulmonary response induced by PAF. The human eosinophil (51) and neutrophil (31, 52) demonstrate specific saturatable membrane binding of PAF. Pulmonary tissue has a direct contractile response (31, 53–55) to PAF. PAF binds specifically to the smooth muscle membrane (31), and PAF-induced intracellular calcium mobilization in smooth muscle cells can be blocked by a PAF receptor antagonist (56). This contractile effect of PAF on bronchial smooth muscle may be more apparent after aerosol administration (57) than after intravenous infusion (33).

PAF induces hypotension, as was noted early in its investigations (58). This activity is similar to the vascular permeability effect of PAF in that it occurs in all species tested (33, 40, 59) and is a non-platelet-mediated occurrence (60). Permeability and hypotension are independent events, since hypotension occurs at lower doses, and is immediate and reversible (61), whereas the extravasation response requires 4–10 min to peak and several hours to reverse (21, 29, 40). The vascular endothelium has been suggested to be required for the hypotensive activity of PAF in the rat (62, 63), but preliminary experiments in the rabbit do not support this hypothesis (64). The hypotensive response may be the result of arteriolar dilation, especially in the splanchnic vascular bed (65). Low doses of PAF administered by intracoronary injections produce coronary vasodilation in the dog (66), but systemic administration can produce coronary constriction in the same species (67). Investigations of the hypotensive mechanism have ruled out renin inhibition, central mechanism, and α-adrenergic antagonism as possible mechanisms (68). PAF release from isolated rat kidneys (69), and the presence of PAF in urine (70) and blood (71) of control, but not anephric, individuals (71), suggests that PAF may play a role in blood-pressure regulation, as hypothesized by early investigators (58).

TECHNIQUES FOR THE DISCOVERY OF PAF ANTAGONISTS

In Vitro Assays

The interaction of PAF with cells in vitro is accompanied by a variety of responses, which, depending upon the cell type, can include chemotaxis, aggregation, granule release, enzyme secretion, increased phagocytosis, and generation of toxic oxygen radicals. The simplicity of measuring platelet aggregation and the discovery of PAF receptors on platelets (30, 31, 72, 73) have led to the use of the aggregation assay in primary screening of anti-PAF compounds (32). PAF is thought to be the most potent low-molecular-weight platelet-activating agent reported to date (74, 75). Thus, the platelet aggregation assay is a sensitive, easy-to-use receptor-mediated response (32, 74, 76) that evaluates PAF antagonists. However, several antiplatelet agents (mepacrine, PGI_2, aspirin, indomethacin) partially inhibit PAF-induced aggregation and secretion (77).

In Vivo Models

The most prominent biological effects of PAF are observed following intravenous injection. In various species, PAF injections produce thrombocytopenia, neutropenia, hemoconcentration, bronchoconstriction, hypotension, cardiac dysfunction, pulmonary hypertension, and pulmonary edema. Many of the circulatory and pulmonary alterations are identical to those occurring during IgE-mediated anaphylaxis (78). However, not all of these PAF responses are sufficiently sensitive, reproducible, or governed by dose-response relationships to be useful parameters in animal pharmacology models. To date the physiological responses to PAF that are most reproducible and often cited are hypotension, hemoconcentration, and bronchoconstriction. Although the hypotensive response from PAF can be induced in mice (79), rats (58, 59, 61, 80), guinea pigs (59), rabbits (59, 81), and dogs (59, 82), the rat is most commonly used. The first reported PAF antagonist, CV-3988, was described as an inhibitor of PAF-induced hypotension in the rat (83, 84). Other PAF receptor antagonists, including SRI 63-072 (61), ONO-6240 (85), kadsurenone (86), and BN 52021 (87), as well as nonspecific agents such as glucocorticoids (88) and thyrotropin-releasing hormone (89), effectively inhibit PAF-induced anaphylactic lethality and hypotension. Models of endogenous PAF production are gram-negative sepsis (90), endotoxin challenge (84), infusion of immune aggregates (79), and renal artery ligation with contralateral nephrectomy (91). The endotoxin and immune challenges are dose dependent in terms of their hypotensive properties (61) and are effectively inhibited by several PAF antagonists (61, 84–87). The hypotensive response of PAF may be assumed to be receptor mediated in the rat, since specific PAF receptor antagonists immediately raise the depressed blood pressure to pre-PAF values (61, 84, 87).

Hemoconcentration results from a complete loss of selective endothelial permeability (25), leading to extravasation of plasma and elevation of hematocrit levels. Active at the picomolar range, PAF is one of the most potent inducers of increased vascular permeability identified to date (92). PAF can increase systemic (25, 93), microvascular (26, 94), and pulmonary (95–97) permeabilities. The species most sensitive to PAF-induced hemoconcentration are the guinea pig (93, 98, 99) and rabbit (23, 39), although the rat (24, 27), dog (80, 95), and primate (40, 46) exhibit this response at somewhat higher PAF challenges. The hyperpermeability effects of PAF are reproducible when PAF is given by intradermal (12, 27, 100, 101) or intravenous (39, 40, 46, 80, 93) routes. PAF antagonists SRI 63-072 (21, 46, 102), CV-3988 (29, 98, 103), BN 52021 (87, 104), kadsurenone (28, 105), and SRI 63-441 (80) are reported effective against exogenous or endogenous PAF-induced hyperpermeability and hemoconcentration effects.

Similarly, various species develop a platelet-dependent bronchoconstriction following PAF administration, of which the guinea pig (38, 106, 107) and the rabbit (54, 108) are most sensitive. Bronchoconstriction induced by intravenous PAF injection is platelet dependent and develops rapidly, whereas the aerosol PAF administration appears to be independent of platelet involvement (46, 107), develops slowly, and is markedly tachyphylactic (17). The aerosol route brings PAF to an area of the lung where alveolar macrophages would normally generate PAF in response to airborne antigens (57, 109). Several PAF antagonists inhibit PAF-related pulmonary responses, including SRI 63-072 (102), BN 52021 (53, 110), L-652-731 (111), and ONO-6240 (112).

IDENTIFIED PAF ANTAGONISTS

PAF Analogues

The structures of many PAF antagonists discussed in this review are illustrated in Figure 2. The first PAF receptor antagonist to appear in the literature was CV-3988 (83), which contains an octadecyl carbamate in position 1, a methoxy group in position 2, and a thiazolium ethyl phosphate group in position 3. In rats CV-3988 inhibits hypotension induced by PAF (83) and endotoxin (84). CV-3988 also inhibits PAF-induced hemoconcentration in the rat (84), guinea pig (29, 98), and cebus primate (113), and in the hypertensive rat it counteracts the hypotension that occurs after unclipping the renal artery

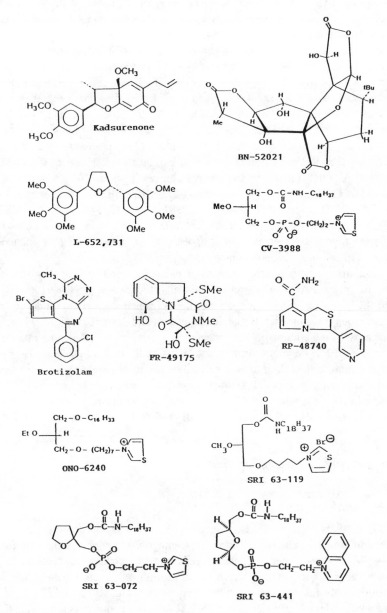

Figure 2   PAF antagonists structures.

in the one-kidney clip model (91). It also inhibits a variety of dermal inflammatory reactions (103) and endotoxin-induced gastrointestinal damage (114).

Substitution of the phosphoryl choline moiety of CV-3988 with a heptamethylene thiazolium results in a group of quaternary salt PAF antagonists, including ONO-6240. This compound inhibits several endotoxin-induced circulatory and pulmonary manifestations in unanesthetized sheep (112), PAF-induced hypotension in the rat (85), and dermal vascular permeability in the guinea pig (85).

Several PAF antagonists related to CV-3988 and ONO-6240 have recently been developed by Sandoz, including SRI 63-072, SRI 63-073, SRI 63-119, and SRI 63-441. These compounds inhibit PAF-, endotoxin-, and immune aggregate–induced hypotension in the rat (61, 80), PAF-induced hemoconcentration and bronchoconstriction in the guinea pig (21, 80, 99, 115), and PAF-induced hypotension and hemoconcentration in the dog (80). They also inhibit PAF-induced hemoconcentration and airway responses in the primate (80, 100, 102) and the reverse-passive arthus reaction in the guinea pig (116). However, unlike PAF, which loses a significant amount of activity when the chirality at carbon 2 changes from R to S (117), both enantiomeric forms of SRI 63-072 demonstrate similar PAF receptor binding inhibition (32) and similar inhibition of PAF-induced hemoconcentration in the guinea pig (D. A. Handley, unpublished observations). SRI 63-072 and SRI 63-119 inhibit PAF-induced ischemic bowel necrosis in the rat (118). The most potent of the series, SRI 63-441, inhibits all major physiological responses in rats, guinea pigs, dogs, and primates, indicating a broad intraspecies potency (80).

When the C-2 ester function of the PAF molecule is replaced with an amide and the phosphate ester, with a phosphonate ester, an amido phosphono analogue of PAF results (119) that moderately inhibits PAF-induced platelet aggregation (120). A series of PAF antagonists, having a heterocyclic group linked by an ester, have been developed. In this series RO 19-3704 is the most potent and inhibits PAF-induced platelet aggregation and in vivo platelet thrombi (121, 122).

RP-48740, a (3-pyridyl)-^{1}H,^{3}H-pyrrolo[1,2-C]-thiazole derivative, is a specific PAF antagonist that inhibits PAF-induced dermal extravasation (123, 124), hemoconcentration (123), bronchoconstriction (123), and hypotension (123, 124).

A number of substances exhibit PAF antagonistic properties, including triazolobenzodiazepines (125), calcium channel blockers (126), prostaglandins (17, 127), glucocorticoids (88), and thyrotropin-releasing hormones (89). Within the triazolobenzodiazepines, brotizolam inhibits PAF-induced platelet aggregation (128). When given orally, brotizolam inhibits PAF-induced bronchoconstriction and systemic hypotension. One of the calcium channel blockers, diltiazem, inhibits PAF receptor binding (126).

Natural Substances

Several naturally occurring PAF antagonists have been isolated. Kadsurenone, a terpene from the Chinese herbal plant *Piper futokadsurae*, is a competitive receptor antagonist to PAF (105). This neolignan is a specific and potent inhibitor of PAF-induced platelet aggregation and neutrophil degranulation (105). Kadsurenone also inhibits PAF-induced cutaneous permeability in the guinea pig (28, 105) and rat (28), as well as hematocrit changes (105), foot edema (129), and hypotension (86) in the rat. Other related structures isolated from the same plant demonstrated only weak PAF antagonist activity, however a synthetic derivative of kadsurenone is a potent PAF antagonist (130). This compound, L-652-731, inhibits ^{3}H-PAF receptor binding to rabbit platelets, PAF-induced platelet and PMN aggregation, and PAF-induced cutaneous vascular permeability (130) and hypotensive effects in the rat (131). It also inhibits immune complex–induced hypotension (131) and PAF-induced foot edema in the rat (129).

Several terpenoids isolated from the Chinese tree *Ginko biloba* L. were chemically characterized in the late 1960s (132, 133). Much later, these structures were determined to be PAF receptor antagonists (134). Three of these unique molecules (termed *Ginkgolides A, B,* and *C* or *BN 52020, BN 52021,* and *BN 52022*) are PAF receptor antagonists. BN 52021 is the most potent of the three. This compound is the most-evaluated PAF antagonist to date. BN 52021 inhibits PAF-induced responses including platelet aggregation (135), hypotension and extravasation in rats (87, 104), in vivo thrombus formation in injured arterial segments (41), and lung parenchymal strip contraction (53). BN 52021 is also effective in models involving endogenous PAF release such as immune aggregate–induced hypotension (87), endotoxin-induced lethality (104), antigen-induced pulmonary anaphylaxis (110), and cardiac allograft survival (136).

A fermentation broth product from *Streptomyces phaeofaciens*, FR-900452, has recently been described as a PAF antagonist (137). This cyclopentenopiperazinylindolinone blocks PAF-induced aggregation of rabbit platelets (138) and endotoxin-induced thrombocytopenia and leukopenia in rabbits (137). A second PAF antagonist isolated from the fermentation products of *Penicillium terlikowski* has been structurally characterized (139). This compound, FR-49175, inhibits PAF-induced platelet aggregation, bronchoconstriction, hypotension, and dermal vascular permeability (139). FR-49175, however, does not prevent systemic anaphylaxis in guinea pigs (139).

In a comparison of the leading PAF antagonists (SRI 63-441, BN 52021,

Table 1 Summary of PAF antagonist activity

Clinical condition	Animal model	Compound reference
Asthma/Pulmonary dysfunction	PAF-induced bronchoconstriction	BN 52021 (124), FR-49175 (139), L-652-731 (111), RP-48740 (123, 124), ONO-6240 (85), SRI 63-072 (102), SRI 63-119 (99), SRI 63-441 (80), brotizolam (128)
	Antigen-induced bronchoconstriction	BN 52021 (110)
	Endotoxin-induced pulmonary dysfunction	ONO-6240 (112)
Septic shock	PAF-induced hypotension	Kadsurenone (86), BN 52021 (87, 124), L-652-731 (131), RP-48740 (123, 124), CV-3988 (83, 84), ONO-6240 (85), SRI 63-072 (61), SRI 63-441 (80)
	Endotoxin-induced hypotension	Kadsurenone (86), CV-3988 (84), BN 52021 (104), SRI 63-072 (61)
	Immune complex–induced hypotension	BN 52021 (87), L-652-731 (131), SRI 63-072 (61)
Inflammation	PAF-induced vascular permeability	Kadsurenone (28, 105, 129), BN 52021 (87, 104), L-652,731 (100, 129, 130), CV-3988 (29, 98, 103), RP-48740 (123), ONO-6240 (85), SRI 63-072 (21, 46), SRI 63-119 (46, 99), SRI 63-441 (80)
	Carrageenin-induced edema	Kadsurenone (129), L-652-731 (129)
	Immune complex–induced vascular permeability	BN 52021 (87), L-652-731 (100, 131), SRI 63-072 (116), CV-3988 (103)
Ulcerogenic/ Enterocolitis	Endotoxin-induced	CV-3988 (114), ONO-6240 (118, 160), SRI 63-072 (118, 160), SRI 63-119 (118, 160)
Transplanted organ rejection	Cardiac allograft	BN 52021 (136)

RP-48740, L-652-731, SRI 63-072, CV-3988), L-652-731 exhibited the best oral activity against PAF-induced hypotension in the rat, followed by BN 52021, RP-48740, and SRI 63-072 (140). A similar order of oral potency was observed for inhibition of PAF-induced hemoconcentration and bronchoconstriction in the guinea pig (140). Recently, BN 52021 was found to be more potent in vitro than CV-3988 or kadsurenone (74).

CLINICAL INDICATIONS FOR PAF ANTAGONISTS

Animal Models

The variety of in vivo responses to PAF are consonant with involvement in respiratory diseases, inflammation, and anaphylactic shock (141). Although the role of PAF in human disease has yet to be determined, specific areas of suspected involvement include septic shock, hyperacute organ rejection, cardiac anaphylaxis, necrotizing enterocolitis, and asthma. Animal models developed to mimic these diseases generally involve endogenous PAF production through immunological and nonimmunological stimuli. Endotoxin is the biological provoker of endogenous PAF release that has most often been used to simulate disease states related to man. Endotoxin (84), and the related condition of gram-negative sepsis (90), stimulates PAF production resulting in hypotension and increased vascular permeability leading to extravasation. Endotoxin challenge is used in animal models of septic shock (97), necrotizing enterocolitis (142), adult respiratory distress syndrome (112, 143), intravascular thrombocytopenia and leukopenia (138), and lethality (104).

Immunologically, IgE-mediated responses are accompanied by endogenous PAF production, leading to lethal systemic anaphylaxis (144), severe alterations in pulmonary and cardiac function (78, 145), and immune complex deposition in acute serum sickness that leads to glomerulonephritis (146). These IgE-mediated models of PAF release suggest its potential involvement in pulmonary, cardiac, and renal failure during systemic anaphylaxis and serum sickness. The role of PAF in renal failure is further supported by observations that PAF can induce a loss of glomerular anionic charges (147), can cause fibrinogen accumulation in the perfused kidney (148), and is released from sensitized animals to participate in hyperacute renal allograft rejection (149).

IgG-mediated models of PAF release are not as severe as the IgE or endotoxin models in terms of the resulting pathology. IgG responses can be induced with soluble aggregates of IgG (79, 87), and by passive sensitization to nonspecific (110, 150) or pulmonary-specific (151) antigens. These models simulate affected pulmonary function and induced vascular leakage (79, 87, 103), and are related to the development of inflammatory lung disease and asthma (110, 150).

PAF in Humans

PAF has been identified in human blood (71), urine (70), amniotic fluid (152), and saliva (153). Release of PAF has been suggested to occur in systemic lupus erythematosus (154), cold urticaria (155), parturition (152), and psoriasis (156). The intradermal injection of PAF produces an immediate weal-and-flare response (157). A later (3–6 hr) response at the same site is characterized by erythema and algesia. Topical application of PAF to the nasal mucosa induced a dose-dependent vasoconstriction of the capacitance vessels and a reduction in mucosal blood flow (158). Two groups characterized the airway response to aerosolized PAF in man (44, 45). In these studies PAF induced bronchoconstriction in 11 of 12 subjects tested. Nonspecific bronchial reactivity, as measured by methacholine aerosol administration, was enhanced for as long as two weeks after a single PAF inhalation.

SUMMARY

Over the past decade platelet-activating factor has achieved the status of an important inflammatory mediator. The scientific enthusiasm and number of research investigators, publications, and meetings recently devoted to PAF suggest that this mediator will be the subject of continued study in the foreseeable future. The potential for the presence and involvement of PAF in human disease is easily concluded from the reports described in this review.

Both the need for low concentrations for cellular response and the rapid biological clearance mechanisms have made the proof of the involvement of PAF in human disease difficult. The discovery of PAF receptor antagonists and structure-activity relationships of such antagonists (159) will make this determination possible in the near future. The current PAF antagonists may be considered as first generation agents, since the most potent antagonist is still less than 1/100th as potent as PAF is as an agonist. The wide diversity of clinical applications from asthma to septic shock may also require antagonists with selective attributes such as delivery route (oral vs intravenous vs topical) or biological half-life (prolonged vs short). PAF may prove to be the key mediator of several poorly understood disease syndromes such as hyperacute organ transplant rejection, ischemic bowel necrosis (160), and adult respiratory distress syndrome. We must wait for clinical results to draw further conclusions.

Literature Cited

1. Barbaro, J. F., Zvaifler, N. J. 1966. Antigen-induced histamine release from platelets of rabbits producing homologous PCA antibody. *Proc. Soc. Exp. Biol. Med.* 122:1245–47
2. Siraganian, R. P., Oliveira, B. 1968. The allergic response of rabbit platelets and leukocytes. *Fed. Proc.* 27:315 (Abstr.)
3. Siraganian, R. P., Osler, A. G. 1969.

Histamine release from sensitized rabbit leukocytes and associated platelet involvement. *J. Allergy* 43:167 (Abstr.)
4. Henson, P. M. 1969. Role of complement and leukocytes in immunologic release of vasoactive amines from platelets. *Fed. Proc.* 28:1721 (Abstr.)
5. Henson, P. M. 1970. Release of vasoactive amines from rabbit platelets induced by sensitized mononuclear leu-

kocytes and antigen. *J. Exp. Med.* 131: 287–95

6. Benveniste, J., Henson, P. M., Cochrane, C. G. 1972. Leukocyte-dependent histamine release from rabbit platelets: The role of IgE-basophils and platelet-activating factor. *J. Exp. Med.* 136:1356–68

7. Benveniste, J. 1974. Platelet-activating factor, a new mediator of anaphylaxis and immune complex deposition from rabbit and human basophils. *Nature* 249:581–83

8. Henson, P. M., Pinckard, R. N. 1976. Platelet-activating factor (PAF) as a mediator in IgE anaphylaxis. *Fed. Proc.* 35:516 (Abstr.)

9. Henson, P. M., Pinckard, R. N. 1977. Platelet activating factor (PAF): A possible direct mediator of anaphylaxis in the rabbit and a trigger for the vascular deposition of circulating immune complexes. *Monogr. Allergy* 12:13–26

10. Benveniste, J., Le Couedic, J. P., Polonsky, J., Tencé, M. 1977. Structural analysis of purified platelet-activating factor by lipases. *Nature* 269:170–71

11. Benveniste, J., Camussi, G., Polonsky, J. 1977. Platelet-activating factor. *Monogr. Allergy* 12:138–42

12. Pinckard, R. N., Farr, R. S., Hanahan, D. J. 1979. Physicochemical and functional identity of platelet-activating factor (PAF) release *in vivo* during IgE anaphylaxis with PAF released *in vitro* from IgE sensitized basophils. *J. Immunol.* 123:1847–56

13. Demopoulus, C. A., Pinckard, R. N., Hanahan, D. J. 1979. Platelet-activating factor. Evidence for 1-O-alkyl-2-acetyl-*sn*-glycerol-3-phosphoryl-choline as the active component (a new class of lipid chemical mediators). *J. Biol. Chem.* 254:9355–58

14. Benveniste, J., Tencé, M., Varenne, P., Bidault, J., Boullet, C., Polonsky, J. 1979. Semisynthése et structure proposeé du facteur activant les plaquettes (P.A.F.): PAF-acether, un alkyl ether analogue de la lysophosphatidyl-choline. *C. R. Acad. Sci. Ser. D.* 289:1037–40

15. Prewitt, R. L., Leach, B. E., Byers, L. W., Brooks, B., Lands, W. E. M., Muirhead, E. E. 1979: Antihypertensive polar renomedullary lipid, a semisynthetic vasodilator. *Hypertension* 1:299–308

16. Pinckard, R. N., Jackson, E. M., Hoppens, C., Weintraub, S. T., Ludwig, J. C., et al. 1984. Molecular heterogeneity of platelet-activating factor produced by stimulated human polymorphonuclear leukocytes. *Biochem. Biophys. Res. Commun.* 122:325–32

17. Braquet, P., Touqui, L., Vargaftig, B. B., Shen, T. Y. 1987. Perspectives in platelet activating factor research. *J. Med. Chem.* In press

18. Farr, R. S., Cox, C. P., Wardlow, M. L., Jorgensen, R. 1980. Preliminary studies of an acid-labile factor (ALF) in human sera that inactivates platelet-activating factor (PAF). *Clin. Immunol. Immunopathol.* 15:318–30

19. Snyder, F. 1985. Chemical and biochemical aspects of platelet activating factor: a novel class of acetylated ether-linked choline-phospholipids. *Med. Res. Rev.* 5:107–40

20. Braquet, P., Godfroid, J. J. 1987. Conformational properties of the paf-acether receptor in platelets based on structural-activity studies. In *Platelet Activating Factor*, ed. F. Snyder. Plenum. In press

21. Handley, D. A., Saunders, R. N. 1986. Platelet activating factor and inflammation in atherosclerosis: Targets for drug development. *Drug Dev. Res.* 7:361–75

22. Henson, P. M., Cochrane, C. G. 1971. Acute immune complex disease in rabbits: the role of complement and of a leukocyte-dependent release of vasoactive amines from platelets. *J. Exp. Med.* 133:554–71

23. Wedmore, C. V., Williams, T. J. 1981. Platelet-activating factor (PAF), a secretory product of polymorphonuclear leukocytes, increases vascular permeability in rabbit skin. *Br. J. Pharmacol.* 74:916P–18P

24. Humphrey, D. M., McManus, L. M., Hanahan, D. J., Pinckard, R. N. 1984. Morphological basis of increased vascular permeability induced by acetyl glyceryl ether phosphorylcholine. *Lab. Invest.* 50:16–25

25. Handley, D. A., Arbeeny, C. M., Lee, M. L., Van Valen, R. G., Saunders, R. N. 1984. Effect of platelet-activating factor on endothelial permeability to plasma macromolecules. *Immunopharmacology* 8:137–42

26. Björk, J., Smedegard, G. 1983. Acute microvascular effects of paf-acether, as studied by intravital microscopy. *Eur. J. Pharmacol.* 96:87–94

27. Pirotzky, E., Page, C. P., Roubin, R., Pfister, A., Paul, W., et al. 1984. Paf-acether-induced plasma exudation in rat skin is independent of platelets and neutrophils. *Microcirc. Endothelium Lymphatics* 1:107–22

28. Hwang, S. B., Li, C.-H., Lam, M. H., Shen, T. Y. 1985. Characterization of

cutaneous vascular permeability induced by platelet-activating factor in guinea pigs and rats and its inhibition by a platelet-activating factor receptor antagonist. *Lab. Invest.* 52:617–30

29. Handley, D. A., Farley, C., Deacon, R. W., Saunders, R. N. 1986. Evidence for distinct systemic extravasation effects of platelet activating factor, leukotrienes B_4, C_4, D_4 and histamine in the guinea pig. *Prostaglandins Leukotrienes Med.* 21:269–77

30. Valone, F. H., Coles, E., Reinhold, V. R., Goetzl, E. J. 1982. Specific binding of phospholipid platelet-activating factor by human platelets. *J. Immunol.* 129: 1637–41

31. Hwang, S. B., Lee, C.-S. C., Cheah, M. J., Shen, T. Y. 1983. Specific receptor sites for 1-O-alkyl-2-O-acetyl-*sn*-glycero-3-phosphocholine (platelet activating factor) on rabbit platelet and guinea pig smooth muscle membranes. *Biochemistry* 22:4756–63

32. Winslow, C. M., Anderson, R. C., D'Aries, F. J., Frisch, G. E., DeLillo, A. K., et al. 1987. Toward understanding the mechanism of action of PAF receptor antagonists. In *New Horizons in Platelet Activating Factor Research*, ed. C. M. Winslow, M. L. Lee, pp. 153–64. New York: Wiley.

33. Saunders, R. N., Handley, D. A., Kowal-DeLillo, A. H., Van Valen, R. G., Winslow, C. M. 1985. Effects of platelet activating factor in primates. *Thromb. Haemostasis* 54:244 (Abstr.)

34. Handley, D. A., Van Valen, R. G., Saunders, R. N. 1987. Cebus apella primate responses to platelet activating factor and inhibition by PAF-antagonist SRI 63-072. See Ref. 32, pp. 335–42

35. Sanchez-Crespo, M., Alonso, F., Inarrea, P., Vlvarez, V., Egido, J. 1982. Vascular actions of synthetic PAF-acether (a synthetic platelet-activating factor) in the rat: evidence for a platelet independent mechanism. *Immunopharmacology* 4:173–85

36. Namm, I. H., Tadepalli, A. S., High, J. A. 1982. Species specificity of the platelet responses to 1-O-alkyl-2-acetyl-*sn*-glycero-3-phosphocholine. *Thromb. Res.* 25:341–50

37. Terashita, Z., Imura, Y., Nishikawa, K. 1985. Inhibition by CV-3988 of the binding of [^{3}H]-platelet activating factor (PAF) to the platelet. *Biochem. Pharmacol.* 34:1491–95

38. Vargaftig, B. B., Lefort, J., Chignard, M., Benveniste, J. 1980. Platelet-activating factor induces a platelet-dependent bronchoconstriction unrelated

to the formation of prostaglandin derivatives. *Eur. J. Pharmacol.* 65:185–92

39. McManus, L. M., Hanahan, D. M., Demopoulos, C. A., Pinckard, R. N. 1980. Pathobiology of the intravenous infusion of acetyl glyceryl ether phosphorylcholine (AGEPC), a synthetic platelet-activating factor (PAF), in the rabbit. *J. Immunol.* 124:2919–24

40. McManus, L. M., Pinckard, R. N., Fitzpatrick, F. A., O'Rourke, R. A., Crawford, M. H., Hanahan, D. J. 1981. Acetyl glyceryl ether phosphorylcholine (AGEPC): Intravascular alterations following intravenous infusion in the baboon. *Lab. Invest.* 45:303–7

41. Bourgain, R. H., Maes, L., Braquet, P., Andries, R., Touqui, L., Braquet, M. 1985. The effect of 1-O-alkyl-2-acetyl-*sn*-glycero-3-phosphocholine (PAF-acether) on the arterial wall. *Prostaglandins* 30:185–96

42. Yamada, G., Watanabe, S., Fukuda, T., Makino, S. 1986. *Effect of inhaled PAF-acether on responsiveness of the bronchi in normal subjects.* Presented at Symp. Platelet Activating Factor, Pulmonary Hyperreactivity and Asthma, L'Esterel, Quebec

43. Karlsson, G., Pipkorn, U. 1984. Effect of disodium chromoglycate on changes in nasal airway resistance induced by platelet activating factor. *Eur. J. Clin. Pharmacol.* 27:371–73

44. Cuss, R. M., Dixon, C. M., Barnes, P. J. 1986. Inhaled platelet-activating factor causes bronchoconstriction and increased bronchial reactivity in man. *Am. Rev. Respir. Dis.* 133:A212 (Abstr.)

45. Rubin, A. E., Smith, L. J., Patterson, R. 1986. Effect of platelet activating factor (PAF) on normal human airways. *Am. Rev. Respir. Dis.* 133:A91 (Abstr.)

46. Handley, D. A., Van Valen, R. G., Saunders, R. N. 1986. Vascular responses of platelet activating factor in the cebus apella primate and inhibitory profiles of antagonists SRI 63-072 and SRI 63-119. *Immunopharmacology* 11:175–82

47. Morley, J., Page, C. P., Sanjar, S. 1985. Platelets in asthma. *Lancet* 2:726–27

48. Morley, J., Page, C. P., Mazzoni, L., Sanjar, S. 1985. Anti-allergic drugs in asthma. *Triangle* 24:59–70

49. Lellouch-Tubiana, A., Lefort, J., Pirotzky, E., Vargaftig, B. B., Pfister, A. 1985. Ultrastructural evidence for extravascular platelet recruitment in the lung upon intravenous injection of

250   SAUNDERS & HANDLEY

platelet-activating factor (PAF-acether) to guinea-pigs. *Br. J. Exp. Pathol.* 66:345–55

50. McManus, L. M., Pinckard, R. N. 1985. Kinetics of acetyl glyceryl ether phosphorylcholine (AGEPC)-induced acute lung alterations in the rabbit. *Am. J. Pathol.* 121:55–68

51. Numao, T., Makino, S. 1986. Specific binding of AGEPC by human eosinophils. See Ref. 42

52. Valone, F. H., Goetzl, E. J. 1983. Specific binding by human polymorphonuclear leukocytes of the immunological mediator 1-O-hexadecyl/octadecyl-2-acetyl-*sn*-glycero-3-phosphorylcholine. *Immunology* 48:141–49

53. Touvay, C., Vilain, B., Etienne, A., Sirois, P., Braquet, P. 1987. Pharmacological control of the contraction of guinea-pig lung strips induced by platelet-activating factor (PAF-acether). *Prostaglandins Leukotrienes Med.* In press

54. Stimler, N. P., Bloor, C. M., Hugli, T. E., Wykle, R. L., McCall, C. E., O'Flaherty, J. T. 1981. Anaphylactic actions of platelet-activating factor. *Am. J. Pathol.* 105:64–69

55. Stimler, N. P., O'Flaherty, J. T. 1983. Spasmogenic properties of platelet-activating factor: Evidence for a direct mechanism in the contractile response of pulmonary tissue. *Am. J. Pathol.* 113:75–84

56. Doyle, V. M., Creba, J. A., Rüegg, U. T. 1986. Platelet-activating factor mobilizes intracellular calcium in vascular smooth muscle cells. *FEBS Lett.* 197:13–16

57. Patterson, R., Harris, K. E. 1983. The activity of aerosolized and intracutaneous synthetic platelet-activating factor (AGEPC) in rhesus monkeys with IgE-mediated airway responses and normal monkeys. *J. Lab. Clin. Med.* 102:933–38

58. Blank, M. L., Snyder, F., Byers, L. W., Brooks, B., Muirhead, E. E. 1979. Antihypertensive activity of an alkyl ether analog of phosphatidylcholine. *Biochem. Biophys. Res. Commun.* 90:1194–200

59. Tanaka, S., Kasuya, Y., Masuda, Y., Shigenobu, K. 1983. Studies on the hypotensive effects of platelet activating factor (PAF, 1-O-alkyl-2-acetyl-*sn*-glyceryl-3-phosphorylcholine) in rats, guinea pigs, rabbits and dogs. *J. Pharmacol. Dyn.* 6:866–73

60. Sanchez-Crespo, M., Alonso, F., Inarrea, P., Egido, J. 1981. Non-platelet-

mediated vascular actions of 1-O-alkyl-2-acetyl-*sn*-3-glycerol phosphorylcholine (a synthetic PAF). *Agents Actions* 11:566–67

61. Handley, D. A., Van Valen, R. G., Melden, M. K., Flury, S., Lee, M. L., Saunders, R. N. 1986. Inhibition and reversal of endotoxin-, aggregated IgG- and paf-induced hypotension in the rat by SRI 63-072, a paf receptor antagonist. *Immunopharmacology.* 12:11–17

62. Cervoni, P., Herzlinger, H. E., Lai, F. M., Tanikella, T. K. 1983. Aortic vascular and atrial responses to (±)-1-O-octadecyl-2-acetyl-glyceryl-3-phosphorylcholine. *Br. J. Pharmacol.* 79:667–71

63. Kasuya, Y., Masuda, Y., Shigenobu, K. 1984. Possible role of endothelium in the vasodilator response of rat thoracic aorta to platelet activating factor (PAF). *J. Pharmacol. Dyn.* 7:138–42

64. Lefer, D. J., Lefer, A. M. 1986. Failure of endothelium to mediate potential vasoactive action of platelet activating factor (PAF). *Int. Res. Commun. Syst. Med. Sci.* 14:356–57

65. Struyker-Boudier, H. A. J., Nievelstein, H. M. N. W., Tijssen, C. M., Smits, J. F. M. 1985. Regional hemodynamic actions of platelet activating factor (PAF) in conscious spontaneously hypertensive rats (SHR). *Prostaglandins* 30:726 (Abstr.)

66. Jackson, C. V., Schumacher, W. A., Kunkel, S. L., Driscoll, E. M., Lucchesi, B. R. 1986. Platelet-activating factor and the release of a platelet-derived coronary artery vasodilator substance in the canine. *Circ. Res.* 58:218–29

67. Sybertz, E. J., Watkins, R. W., Baum, T., Pula, K., Rivelli, M. 1985. Cardiac, coronary, and peripheral vascular effects of acetyl glyceryl ether phosphoryl choline in the anesthetized dog. *J. Pharmacol. Exp. Ther.* 232:156–62

68. Kamitani, T., Katamoto, M., Tatsumi, M., Katsuta, K., Ono, T., et al. 1984. Mechanism(s) of the hypotensive effect of synthetic 1-O-octadecyl-2-O-acetyl-glycero-3-phosphorylcholine. *Eur. J. Pharmacol.* 98:357–66

69. Pirotzky, E., Benveniste, J. 1981. Platelet-activating factor (PAF-acether) is released from isolated perfused rat kidney. *Int. Arch. Allergy Appl. Immunol.* 66:176–77

70. Sanchez-Crespo, M., Inarrea, P., Alvarez, V., Alonso, F., Egido, J., Hernando, L. 1983. Presence in normal human urine of a hypotensive and platelet-

activating phospholipid. *Am. J. Physiol.* 244:F706–11

71. Caramelo, C., Fernandez-Gallardo, S., Marin-Cao, D., Inarrea, P., Santos, J. C., et al. 1984. Presence of platelet-activating factor in blood from humans and experimental animals. Its absence in anephric individuals. *Biochem. Biophys. Res. Commun.* 120:789–96

72. Kloprogge, E., Akkerman, J. W. N. 1984. Binding kinetics of PAF-acether (1-O-alkyl-2-acetyl-*sn*-glycerol-3-phosphocholine) to intact human platelets. *Biochem. J.* 223:901–9

73. Winslow, C. M., Vallespir, S. R., Frisch, G. E., D'Aires, F. J., Kowal-DeLillo, A., et al. 1985. A novel platelet activating factor receptor antagonist. *Prostaglandins* 30:697 (Abstr.)

74. Nunez, D., Chignard, M., Korth, R., Le Courdic, J.-P., Novel, X., et al. 1986. Specific inhibition of PAF-acether-induced platelet activation by BN 52021 and comparison with PAF-acether inhibitors kadsurenone and CV-3988. *Eur. J. Pharmacol.* 123:197–205

75. Vargaftig, B. B., Benveniste, J. 1983. Platelet-activating factor today. *Trends Pharmacol. Sci.* 4:341–43

76. McManus, L. M., Hanahan, D. J., Pinckard, R. N. 1981. Human platelet stimulation by acetyl glyceryl ether phosphorylcholine. *J. Clin. Invest.* 67:903–6

77. Chesney, C. M., Pifer, D. D., Byers, L. W., Muirhead, E. E. 1982. Effect of platelet-activating factor (PAF) on human platelets. *Blood* 59:582–85

78. Halonen, M., Palmer, J. D., Lohman, I. C., McManus, L. M., Pinckard, R. N. 1981. Respiratory and circulatory alterations induced by acetyl glyceryl ether phosphorylcholine: a mediator of IgE anaphylaxis in the rabbit. *Am. Rev. Respir. Dis.* 122:915–22

79. Inarrea, P., Alonso, F., Sanchez-Crespo, M. 1983. Platelet-activating factor: an effector substance of the vasopermeability changes induced by the infusion of immuno aggregates in the mouse. *Immunopharmacology* 6:7–14

80. Handley, D. A., Tomesch, J. D., Saunders, R. N. 1986. Inhibition of PAF-induced responses in the rat, guinea pig, dog and primate by the receptor antagonist, SRI 63-441. *Thromb. Haemostasis* 56:40–44

81. Muirhead, E. E., Byers, L. W., Desiderio, D., Smith, K. A., Prewitt, R. L., Brooks, B. 1981. Alkyl ether analogs of phosphatidylcholine are orally active in hypertensive rabbits. *Hypertension* 3:107–13

82. Lewis, A. J., Dervinis, A., Chang, J. 1984. The effects of antiallergic and bronchodilator drugs on platelet-activating factor (PAF-acether) induced bronchospasm and platelet aggregation. *Agents Actions* 15:636–40

83. Terashita, Z., Taushima, S., Yoshioka, Y., Nomura, H., Inada, Y., Nishikawa, K. 1983. CV-3988—A specific antagonist of platelet-activating factor (PAF). *Life Sci.* 32:1975–81

84. Terashita, Z., Imura, Y., Nishikawa, K., Sumida, S. 1985. Is platelet activating factor (PAF) a mediator of endotoxin shock? *Eur. J. Pharmacol.* 109:257–63

85. Miyamoto, T., Ohno, H., Yano, T., Okada, T., Hamanaka, N., Kawasaki, A. 1985. ONO-6240: A new potent antagonist of platelet-activating factor. *Adv. Prostaglandins Thromb. Leukotriene Res.* 15:719–20

86. Doebber, T. W., Wu, M. S., Robbins, J. C., Choy, B. M., Chang, M. N., Shen, T. Y. 1985. Platelet-activating factor (PAF) involvement in endotoxin-induced hypotension in rats. Studies with PAF-receptor antagonist kadsurenone. *Biochem. Biophys. Res. Commun.* 127:799–808

87. Sanchez-Crespo, M., Fernandez-Gallardo, S., Nieto, M.-L., Braanes, J., Braquet, P. 1985. Inhibition of the vascular actions of IgG aggregates by BN 52021, a highly specific antagonist of PAF-acether. *Immunopharmacology* 10:69–75

88. Myers, A., Ramey, E., Ramwell, P. 1983. Glucocorticoid protection against PAF-acether toxicity in mice. *Br. J. Pharmacol.* 79:595–98

89. Feuerstein, G., Lux, W. E., Snyder, F., Ezra, D., Faden, A. I. 1984. Hypotension produced by platelet-activating factor is reversed by thyrotropin-releasing hormone. *Circ. Shock* 13:255–60

90. Inarrea, P., Gomez-Cambronero, J., Pascual, J., del Carmen Ponte, M., Hernando, L., Sanchez-Crespo, M. 1985. Synthesis of PAF-acether and blood volume changes in gram-negative sepsis. *Immunopharmacology* 9:45–53

91. Masugi, F., Ogihara, T., Otsuka, A., Saeki, S., Kumahara, Y. 1984. Effect of 1 - alkyl - 2 - acetyl - sn - glycero - 3 - phosphorylcholine inhibitor on the reduction of one-kidney, one clip hypertension after unclipping in the rat. *Life Sci.* 34:197–201

92. Gimbrone, M. A. 1982. Blood vessels

and the new mediators of inflammation. *Lab. Invest.* 46:454–55

93. Handley, D. A., Van Valen, R. G., Melden, M. K., Saunders, R. N. 1984. Evaluation of dose and route effects of platelet activating factor–induced extravasation in the guinea pig. *Thromb. Haemostasis* 52:34–36

94. Björk, J., Lindbom, L., Gerdin, B., Smedegard, G., Arfors, K. E., Benveniste, J. 1983. PAF-acether (platelet activating factor) increases microvascular permeability and affects endothelium-granulocyte interaction in microvascular beds. *Acta. Physiol. Scand.* 119:305–8

95. Bessin, P., Bonnet, J., Apffel, D., Soulard, C., Desgroux, L., et al. 1983. Acute circulatory collapse caused by platelet-activating factor (PAF-acether) in dogs. *Eur. J. Pharmacol.* 86:403–13

96. Heffner, J. E., Shoemaker, S. A., Canham, E. M., Patel, M., McMurtry, I. F., et al. 1983. Platelet-induced pulmonary hypertension and edema. A mechanism involving acetyl glyceryl ether phosphorylcholine and thromboxane A₂. *Chest* 83:78–85

97. Mojarad, M., Hamasaki, Y., Said, S. I. 1983. Platelet-activating factor increases pulmonary microvascular permeability and induces pulmonary edema. A preliminary report. *Bull. Eur. Physiopathol. Respir.* 19:253–56

98. Handley D. A., Lee, M. L., Saunders, R. N. 1985. Evidence for a direct effect on vascular permeability of platelet-activating factor induced hemoconcentration in the guinea pig. *Thromb. Haemostasis* 54:756–59

99. Farley, C., Melden, M. K., Van Valen, R. G., Deacon, R. W., Anderson, R. W., et al. 1986. In vivo inhibition by SRI 63-072 and SRI 63-119 of PAF-induced hemoconcentration and bronchoconstriction in the guinea pig. *Fed. Proc.* 45:855 (Abstr.)

100. Hellewell, P. G., Williams, T. J. 1986. A specific antagonist of platelet-activating factor suppresses oedema formation in an arthus reaction but not oedema induced by leukocyte chemoattractants in rabbit skin. *J. Immunol.* 137:302–7

101. Humphrey, D. M., Hanahan, D. J., Pinckard, R. N. 1982. Induction of leukocytic infiltrates in rabbit skin by acetyl glyceryl ether phosphorylcholine. *Lab. Invest.* 47:227–34

102. Patterson, R., Harris, K. E., Lee, M. L., Houlihan, W. J. 1986. Inhibition of rhesus monkey airway and cutaneous responses to platelet activating factor (PAF) (AGEPC) with the anti-PAF agent SRI 63-072. *Int. Arch Allergy Appl. Immunol.* 81:265–68

103. Issekutz, A. C., Szpejda, M. 1986. Evidence that platelet activation factor may mediate some acute inflammatory responses. *Lab. Invest.* 54:275–81

104. Etienne, A., Hecquet, F., Souland, C., Spinnewyn, B., Clostre, F., Braquet, P. 1985. In vivo inhibition of plasma protein leakage and *Salmonella enteritidis*–induced mortality in the rat by a specific PAF-acether antagonist, BN 52021. *Agents Actions* 17:368–70

105. Shen, T. Y., Hwang, S. B., Chang, M. N., Doebber, W., Lam, M. H. T., et al. 1985. Characterization of a platelet-activating factor receptor antagonist isolated from haifenteng (*Piper futokadsura*): specific inhibition of in vitro and in vivo platelet-activating factor–induced effects. *Proc. Natl. Acad. Sci. USA* 82:672–76

106. Vargaftig, B. B., Lefort, J., Prancan, A. V., Chignard, M., Benveniste, J. 1979. Platelet-lung in vivo interaction: an artifact of multi-purpose model. *Haemostasis* 8:171–76

107. Lefort, J., Wal, F., Chignard, M., Medeiros, M. C., Vargaftig, B. B. 1982. Pharmacological properties of PAF-acether in guinea pigs: platelet dependent and independent reactions. *Agents Actions* 12:723–25

108. McManus, L. M., Fitzpatrick, F. A., Hanahan, D. J., Pinckard, R. N. 1983. Thromboxane B₂ release following acetyl glyceryl ether phosphorylcholine (AGEPC) infusion in the rabbit. *Immunopharmacology* 5:125–30

109. Denjean, A., Arnoux, B., Masse, R., Lockhart, A., Benveniste, J. 1983. Acute effects of intratracheal administration of platelet-activating factor in baboons. *J. Appl. Physiol.* 55:799–804

110. Touvay, C., Etienne, A., Braquet, P. 1985. Inhibition of antigen-induced lung anaphylaxis in the guinea-pig by BN 52021 a new specific PAF-acether receptor antagonist isolated from Ginkgo biloba. *Agents Actions* 17:371–72

111. Cox, C. P., Sata, T., Liu, L. W., Said, S. I. 1986. L-652,731, a specific antagonist of platelet-activating factor (PAF), prevents PAF-induced lung injury in guinea pigs. *Am. Rev. Respir. Dis.* 133:A278 (Abstr.)

112. Toyofuku, T., Kubo, K., Kobayashi, T., Kusama, S. 1986. Effects of ONO-6240, a platelet-activating factor antagonist, on endotoxin shock in un-

anesthetized sheep. *Prostaglandins* 31: 271–80

113. Handley, D. A., Deacon, R. W., Farley, C., Saunders, R. N., Van Valen, R. G. 1985. Biological effects of PAF in the nonhuman primate Cebus apella. *Fed. Proc.* 44:1268 (Abstr.)

114. Wallace, J. L., Whittle, B. J. R. 1986. Prevention of endotoxin-induced gastrointestinal damage by CV-3988, an antagonist of platelet-activating factor. *Eur. J. Pharmacol.* 124:209–10

115. Lee, M. L., Winslow, C. M., Jaeggi, C., D'Aries, F., Frisch, G., et al. 1985. Inhibition of platelet activating factor: synthesis and biological activity of SRI 63-073, a new phospholipid PAF-acether antagonist. *Prostaglandins* 30:690 (Abstr.)

116. Deacon, R. W., Melden, M. K., Saunders, R. N., Handley, D. A. 1986. PAF involvement in dermal extravasation in the reverse passive arthus reaction. *Fed. Proc.* 45:995 (Abstr.)

117. Heymans, F., Michel, E., Borrel, M.-C., Wichrowski, B., Godfroid, J. J., et al. 1981. New total synthesis and high resolution ^{1}H-NMR spectrum of platelet-activating factor, its enantiomer and racemic mixtures. *Biochem. Biophys. Acta* 666:230–41

118. Gonzalez-Crussi, F., Hsueh, W., Anderson, R. C., Lee, M. L., Houlihan, W. J. 1986. Platelet activating factor (PAF) induced-ischemic bowel necrosis (IBN). The effect of PAF antagonists. *Fed. Proc.* 45:336 (Abstr.)

119. Moschidis, M. C., Demopoulos, C. A. Kritikou, L. G. 1983. Phosphono-platelet activating factor. I. Synthesis of 1-O-hexadecyl-2-O-acetyl-glyceryl-3-(2-trimethyl ammoniummethyl) phosphonate and its platelet activating potency. *Chem. Phys. Lipids* 33:87–92

120. Steiner, M., Landolfi, R., Motola, N. C., Turcotte, J. G. 1985. Biological activity of platelet activating factor–amido phosphonate (PAF-AP), a novel phospholipid selective inhibitor of platelet activating factor (PAF). *Biochem. Biophys. Res. Commun.* 133:851–55

121. Berri, K., Barner, R., Cassal, J.-M., Hadvary, P., Hirth, G., Muller, K. 1985. PAF: From agonists to antagonists by synthesis. *Prostaglandins* 30:691 (Abstr.)

122. Hadvary, P., Baumgartner, H. R. 1985. Interference of PAF-acether antagonists with platelet aggregation and with the formation of platelet thrombi. *Prostaglandins* 30:694 (Abstr.)

123. Sediry, P., Caillard, C. G., Floch, A., Folliard, F., Mondot, S., et al. 1985. 48740-R.P.: A specific PAF-acether antagonist. *Prostaglandins* 30:688 (Abstr.)

124. Coeffier, E., Borrel, M.-C., LeFort, J., Chignard, M., Broquet, C., et al. 1985. Effect of PAF-acether antagonists, RP 48740 and BN 52021, on platelet activating and bronchoconstriction induced by PAF-acether and structural analogous in guinea pig. *Prostaglandins* 30:699 (Abstr.)

125. Kornecki, E., Ehrlich, Y. M., Lemox, R. W. 1984. Platelet-activating factor induced aggregation of human platelets specifically inhibited by triazolobenzodiazepines. *Science* 226:1954–57

126. Westwick, J., Marks, G., Powling, M. J., Kakkar, V. V. 1983. Diltiazem, the cardiac channel calcium antagonist, is a potent, selective and competitive inhibitor of platelet activating factor on human platelets. *J. Pharmacol.* 14:62–68

127. Camussi, G., Tetta, C., Bussolino, F. 1983. Inhibitory effect of prostacyclin (PGI$_2$) on neutropenia induced by intravenous injection of platelet-activating factor (PAF) in the rabbit. *Prostaglandins* 25:343–49

128. Casals-Stenzel, J. 1987. The inhibitory activity of brotizolam and related compounds on platelet activating factor (PAF) induced effects in vitro and in vivo. See Ref. 32, pp. 277–84

129. Hwang, S. B., Lam, M. H., Li, C. L., Shen, T. Y. 1986. Release of platelet activating factor and its involvement in the first phase of carrageenin-induced rat foot edema. *Eur. J. Pharmacol.* 120:33–41

130. Hwang, S. B., Lam, M. H., Biftu, T., Beattie, T. R., Shen, T. Y. 1985. Trans-2-5-bis-(3,4,5-trimethoxyphenyl)tetrahydrofuran. *J. Biol. Chem.* 260:15639–45

131. Doebber, T. W., Wu, M. S., Biftu, T. 1986. Platelet-activating factor (PAF) mediation of rat anaphylactic responses to soluble immune complexes. Studies with PAF receptor antagonist L-652,731. *J. Immunol.* 136:4659–68

132. Maruyama, M., Terahara, A., Itagaki, Y., Nakanishi, K. 1967. The ginkgolides. II. Derivation of partial structures. *Tetrahedron Lett.* 4:303–8

133. Maruyama, M., Terahara, A., Nakadaira, Y., Woods, M. C., Nakanishi, K. 1967. The ginkgolides. III. The structure of the ginkgolides. *Tetrahedron Lett.* 4:309–13

134. Braquet, P., Etienne, A., Clostre, F.

1985. Down-regulation of B_2-adrenergic receptors by PAF-acether and its inhibition by the PAF-acether antagonist BN 52021. *Prostaglandins* 30:721 (Abstr.)

135. Braquet, P., Godfroid, J. J. 1986. PAF-acether specific binding sites: 2. Design of specific antagonists. *Trend Pharmacol. Sci.* 7:397–403

136. Foegh, M. L., Khirabadi, B. S., Braquet, P., Ramwell, P. W. 1985. Platelet-activating factor antagonist BN 52021 prolongs experimental cardiac allograft survival. *Prostaglandins* 30: 718 (Abstr.)

137. Okamoto, M., Yoshida, K., Nishikawa, M., Kotisaka, M., Aoki, H. 1986. Platelet activating factor (PAF) involvement in endotoxin-induced thrombocytopenia in rabbits: studies with FR-900452, a specific inhibitor of PAF. *Thromb. Res.* 42:661–71

138. Okamoto, M., Yoshida, K., Nishikawa, M., Ando, T., Iwami, M., et al. 1986. FR-900452, a specific antagonist of platelet activating factor (PAF) produced by *Streptomyces phalofaciens*. *J. Antibiot.* 39:198–204

139. Okamoto, M., Yoshida, K., Uchida, I., Kohsaka, M., Aoki, H. 1986. Studies of platelet activating factor (PAF) antagonists from microbial products II. Pharmacological studies of FR-49175 in animal models. *Chem. Pharm. Bull.* 34:345–48

140. Handley, D. A., Farley, C., Melden, M. K., Deacon, R. W., Van Valen, R. G., Saunders, R. N. 1986. *Comparative parenteral and oral activities of several PAF antagonists in the rat and guinea pig.* Presented at Platelet Activating Factor, 2nd Int. Conf., Gatlinburg, Tenn.

141. Pinckard, R. N. 1983. Platelet-activating factor. *Hosp. Pract.* 70:67–76

142. Gonzalez-Crussi, F., Hsueh, W. 1983. Experimental model of ischemic bowel necrosis. The role of platelet-activating factor and endotoxin. *Am. J. Pathol.* 112:127–35

143. Esbenhade, A. M., Neuman, J. H., Lams, P. M., Jolles, H., Brigham, K. L. 1982. Respiratory failure after endotoxin infusion in sheep: lung mechanics and lung fluid balance. *J. Appl. Physiol.* 53:967–78

144. Pinckard, N., Halonen, M., Palmer, J. D., Butler, C., Shaw, J. O., Hensen, P. M. 1977. Intravascular aggregation and pulmonary sequestration of platelets during IgE-induced systemic anaphylaxis in the rabbit: abrogation of lethal ana-

phylactic shock by platelet depletion. *J. Immunol.* 119:2185–93

145. Levi, R., Burke, J. A., Guo, Z.-G., Hattori, Y., Hoppens, C. M., et al. 1984. Acetyl glyceryl ether phosphorylcholine (AGEPC). A putative mediator of cardiac anaphylaxis in the guinea pig. *Circ. Res.* 54:117–24

146. Camussi, G., Tetta, C., Deregibus, C., Bussolino, F., Segoloni, G., Vercellone, A. 1982. Platelet-activating factor (PAF) in experimentally-induced rabbit acute serum sickness: role of basophil-derived PAF in immune complex deposition. *J. Immunol.* 128:86–94

147. Camussi, G., Tetta, C., Coda, R., Segoloni, G. P., Vercellone, A. 1984. Platelet-activating factor-induced loss of glomerular anionic charges. *Kidney Int.* 25:73–81

148. Pirotzky, E., Page, C., Morley, J., Bidault, J., Benveniste, J. 1985. Vascular permeability induced by paf-acether (platelet-activating factor) in the isolated perfused rat kidney. *Agents Actions* 16:17–18

149. Ito, S., Camussi, G., Tetta, C., Milgrom, F., and Andres, G. 1984. Hyperacute renal allograft rejection in the rabbit. *Lab. Invest.* 51:148–61

150. Page, C. P., Paul, W., Morley, J. 1984. Platelets and bronchospasm. *Int. Arch. Allergy Appl. Immunol.* 74:347–50

151. Camussi, G., Pawlowski, I., Bussolino, F., Caldwell, P. R. B., Brentjens, J., Andres, G. 1983. Release of platelet-activating factor in rabbits with antibody-mediated injury of the lung: role of leukocytes and of pulmonary injury. *J. Immunol.* 131:1802–7

152. Nishihira, J., Ishibashi, T., Imai, Y., Muramatsu, T. 1984. Mass spectrometric evidence for the presence of platelet-activating factor (1-0-alkyl-2-acetyl-*sn*-glycerol-3-phosphocholine) in human amniotic fluid during labor. *Lipids* 19:907–10

153. Cox, C. P., Wardlow, M. L., Jorgensen, R., Farr, R. S. 1981. The presence of platelet-activating factor (PAF) in normal human mixed saliva. *J. Immunol.* 127:46–50

154. Camussi, G., Tetta, C., Coda, R., Benveniste, J. 1981. Release of platelet-activating factor in human pathology. I. Evidence for the occurrence of basophil degranulation and release of platelet-activating factor in systemic lupus erythematous. *Lab. Invest.* 44:241–51

155. Grandel, K. E., Farr, R. S., Wanderer, A. A., Eisenstadt, T. C., Wasserman, S. I. 1985. Association of platelet-

activating factor with primary acquired cold urticaria. *N. Engl. J. Med.* 313:405–9
156. Mallet, A. I., Cunningham, F. M. 1985. Structural identification of platelet activating factor in psoriatic scale. *Biochem. Biophys. Res. Commun.* 126:192–98
157. Basran, G. S., Page, C. P., Paul, W., Morley, J. 1985. Platelet-activating factor: a possible mediator of the dual response to allergen? *Clin. Allergy* 14:75–79
158. Pipkorn, U., Goeran, K., Bake, B.

1984. Effect of platelet-activating factor on the human nasal mucosa. *Allergy* 32:141–45
159. Godfroid, J. J., Braquet, P. 1986. PAF-acether specific binding sites: 1. Quantitative SAR study of PAF-acether isoteres. *Trends Pharmacol. Sci.* 7:368–73
160. Hsueh, W., Gonzalez-Crussi, F., Arroyare, J. L., Anderson, R. C., Lee, M. L., Houlihan, W. J. 1986. Platelet activating factor–induced ischemic bowel necrosis: the effect of PAF antagonists. *Eur. J. Pharmacol.* 123:79–83

Ann. Rev. Pharmacol. Toxicol. 1987. 27:257–77

THE PHARMACOLOGY OF CARNITINE

Joseph J. Bahl and Rubin Bressler

University of Arizona Health Sciences Center, Department of Internal Medicine, Tucson, Arizona 85724

INTRODUCTION

Carnitine (3-hydroxy-4-N-trimethylaminobutyric acid; see Figure 1) was isolated from meat in 1905 (1). In 1959 Fritz (2) demonstrated that carnitine has an obligatory role in long-chain fatty acid (LCFA) oxidation. Cederblad & Lindstedt (3) developed a sensitive assay in 1972, which was later modified by McGarry & Foster (4). This assay catalyzed investigation into the biochemical role of L-carnitine. These studies led to the administration of carnitine as a pharmacological agent in various situations. This use of carnitine we view as derivative of its role in intermediary metabolism, generally related to fatty acid metabolism. We refer the reader to the primary literature, reviews, and books describing the physiological and biochemical role of carnitine (5–9).

BIOCHEMICAL ROLE

LCFA oxidation is of some importance in plants, especially in fruits and seeds, but in general carnitine levels are much higher in the fat-oxidizing cells of animals. No dietary requirement is established for carnitine in humans. Biosynthesis of carnitine requires a prior trimethylation of protein-bound lysine. The steps in carnitine biosynthesis are known, but the factors that regulate in vivo rates of biosynthesis are not well characterized (9). Inside the cell, carnitine acts as a cofactor, allowing acyl groups to be shuttled between intra- and extramitochondrial pools of coenzyme A (CoA) (Figure 2). A LCFA such as palmitate is activated by becoming an ester of CoA on the outer aspect of the inner mitochondrial matrix membrane. It is transesterified to

257

0362-1642/87/0415-0257$02.00

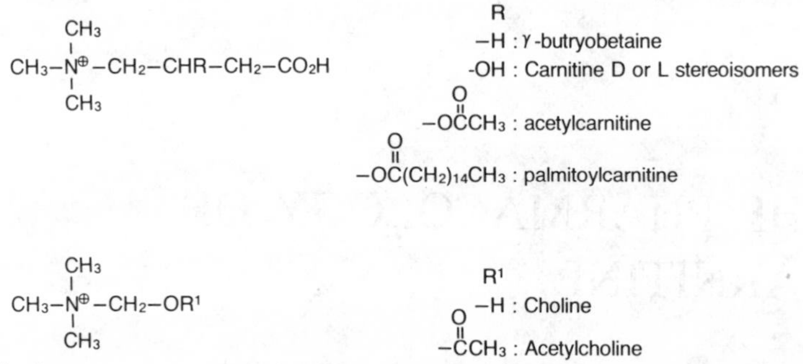

$$CH_3-\overset{\overset{\displaystyle CH_3}{|}}{\underset{\underset{\displaystyle CH_3}{|}}{N}}{}^{\oplus}-CH_2-CHR-CH_2-CO_2H$$

R

$-H : \gamma$-butryobetaine

-OH : Carnitine D or L stereoisomers

$-O\overset{\overset{\displaystyle O}{||}}{C}CH_3$: acetylcarnitine

$-O\overset{\overset{\displaystyle O}{||}}{C}(CH_2)_{14}CH_3$: palmitoylcarnitine

$$CH_3-\overset{\overset{\displaystyle CH_3}{|}}{\underset{\underset{\displaystyle CH_3}{|}}{N}}{}^{\oplus}-CH_2-OR^1$$

R^1

$-H$: Choline

$-\overset{\overset{\displaystyle O}{||}}{C}CH_3$: Acetylcholine

Figure 1 Structures of carnitine, its metabolic precursor gamma-butyrobetaine, and the acetyl and palmitoyl esters of carnitine. The structures of choline and acetyl choline are shown for comparison.

carnitine by the long-chain fatty acylcarnitine transferase enzyme, carnitine palmitoyltransferase I (CPT I). A specific translocase allows the palmitoylcarnitine to enter the mitochondrion and be exchanged for either acetylcarnitine or carnitine. The transesterification by the enzyme CPT II on the inner surface of the matrix membrane presents the enzymes of β-oxidation with the activated substrate palmitoyl-CoA. Short-chain fatty acids (such as propionate in the liver and acetate in all tissues) can enter mitochondria by routes not requiring the carnitine translocator. Medium-chain fatty acids may be activated by the liver peroxisomal medium-chain acyl-CoA synthetase and transesterified to carnitine for entry into mitochondria, or as with short-chain compounds, they may be activated inside of the mitochondrion. The substrate specificity of CPT II and the short-chain acyl transferase (SCAT) ensures that β-oxidation proceeds completely to acetyl-CoA. Medium-chain fatty acids may be able to enter mitochondria of extrahepatic tissue but may not be activated there.

The enzymes of β-oxidation produce acetyl-CoA. If acetyl-CoA is rapidly consumed by the tricarboxylic acid cycle for energy production, free CoA (nonesterified) is regenerated. Depending on the tissue and metabolic state other acetyl-CoA-consuming pathways may be available. Oxaloacetic acid may be used to produce citrate as part of a shuttle mechanism that allows acetate groups to travel to the cytosilic compartment and regenerate free intermitochondrial CoA. In the liver when the rate of acetyl-CoA production is high, ketone bodies are synthesized, again regenerating free CoA. The ratio of acyl-CoA to free CoA increases as the level of LCFA increases in the mitochondria. Without a mechanism to limit the delivery of LCFA as carnitine esters, the capacity of these acetate-consuming reactions would become overwhelmed, and production of LCFA-CoA esters would soon consume the remaining free CoA. The problem with filling the mitochondrial larder with

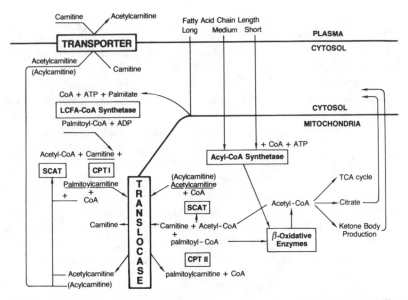

Figure 2   Pathway of intermediary metabolism featuring carnitine's role. Arrowheads indicate general direction of substrate pathway but are readily reversible for all reactions involving carnitine. Abbreviations: CPT, carnitine palmitoyltransferase, SCAT, short-chain acyl transferase.

LCFA groups is that acyl-CoAs inhibit the function of many enzymes. Pyruvate carboxylase and citrate synthetase are enzymes that might participate in pathways that consume acetyl-CoA. These enzymes are inhibited by long-chain acyl-CoAs. The adenine nucleotide translocase, which has similar susceptibility if inhibited by long-chain acyl-CoAs, would stop the translocation of ATP from the mitochondria to the cytoplasm and the intramitochondrial consumption of acetyl-CoA and regeneration of free CoA. As LCFA-CoA esters are good detergents in high concentration, they may damage the structure of the mitochondria. Many substrate pathways are regulated by LCFA-CoA esters or acetyl-CoA inhibiting or activating enzymes. This regulation often depends upon the availability of free CoA, as a high ratio of acyl-CoA to free CoA or high levels of long-chain acyl-CoAs may harm the mitochondria (10, 11).

The majority of the cell's CoA is contained within mitochondria. In the heart 95% and in the liver 60% of the CoA is intramitochondrial (12, 13). Carnitine is more uniformly dispersed in the cell than the CoA. The concentration of CoA and carnitine is similar inside the mitochondria. Transfer of the acetyl group from CoA to carnitine is catalyzed by the SCAT enzyme (see Figure 2, lower center). The equilibrium ratio for this transfer effectively ensures that carnitine and CoA in the mitochondrial pool have the same acyl

CoA to free CoA ratio. The carnitine translocator, while not always achieving a one-for-one exchange (13, 14), generally functions to rapidly exchange free carnitine (nonesterified) from the cytoplasm for acetyl- or other acylcarnitines from the mitochondria. This mechanism would soon exhaust the cytosolic free carnitine except that SCAT on the outer side of the mitochondria reverses the transesterification generating acetyl-CoA. Extramitochondrial LCFA activation decreases as the availability of free CoA becomes limiting to the LCFA-CoA synthetase. This observation provides a regulatory feedback loop for LCFA activation and other cytosolic CoA-dependent reactions that can quickly respond to changes in the mitochondria (10).

In this sequence of events carnitine has been a cofactor in four metabolic events without expending energy: (a) delivery of activated LCFA to the intramitochondrial enzymes of β-oxidation; (b) removal of intramitochondrial acyl groups, which prevents the mitochondrial acyl to free CoA ratio from rising (regenerating intramitochondrial free CoA); (c) regulation of the rate of extramitochondrial LCFA activation; (d) removal of acyl groups that are inhibitory and might be catastrophically disruptive (toxic) if left to accumulate in the mitochondrial pool of CoA esters.

The enzymes that utilize carnitine are all specific for the L-isomer. However, the transporter protein that maintains high intracellular levels of carnitine relative to the plasma does not discriminate between D and L isomers. Choline (see Figure 1) in nonphysiological concentrations can inhibit carnitine transport (15), but it is unclear how these two biologically important molecules affect the transport of each other in vivo or if they always share the same transport system. Injecting choline into a rat can result in the rapid efflux of carnitine from peripheral tissues (16). As this carnitine does not arise from biosynthesis it is likely the result of choline-carnitine exchange. Discrimination of acyl esters from free carnitine is achieved by the transporter, but is not absolute. Liver cells show a preference for the metabolic precursors of carnitine (e.g. γ-butyrobetaine over carnitine) for transport (17). Each tissue, and perhaps each separate cell type in a tissue, has individual kinetic descriptions for carnitine transport (15, 17, 18). The liver has a large capacity for transport and can double its pool size within a short period as plasma carnitine levels rise (16, 19). Skeletal muscle has high levels of carnitine but does not show rapid exchange of radioactive label or change in concentration. The carnitine present in high levels in the heart exchanges with plasma carnitine rapidly. If the level of carnitine in the heart is below the set point, as determined by the kinetic parameters, active carrier-mediated transport results in net accrual (15). Once the pool is filled, carrier-mediated exchange is observed. At this point it is difficult to increase the amount of carnitine above a certain level (20). Generally, rapid turnover indicates an extended period of elevated lipid use, and high levels (less subject to short-term fluctuations) indicate that fatty acid oxidation occurs in proportion to tissue levels of carnitine. Free carnitine is preferred over acyl carnitine in the kidney tubule's reabsorption of carnitine. Carnitine at elevated concentrations down-regulates its own transport across renal brush border membranes in vitro, although the physiological necessity for this mechanism is not clear (21). The preferential reuptake of free carnitine by the kidneys results in clearance of acyl compounds that might otherwise lower the rate of fatty acid oxidation and other CoA-dependent reactions. Each tissue, and the body as a whole, keeps a low acyl CoA to free CoA ratio by excreting acyl carnitines. Plasma levels typically reported for total carnitine are 50 ± 15 μM; males have higher levels than females (22, 23).

The function of the tissue and the availability of substrate determine the balance of carbohydrates and lipids used for energy. However, the level of carbohydrate and lipid oxidation is tightly regulated in each cell (24, 25). The overall rate of metabolic activity is regulated by ADP, which allows ATP translocation from the mitochondria. Carnitine, its esters, and the corresponding cytosolic and mitochondrial CoA esters partly ensure that fatty acid metabolism occurs to maintain homeostasis. Carnitine supplementation may show pharmacological activity, brought about by increasing pool size or increasing the rate of free carnitine and acyl carnitine exchange. We elaborate on this basic description as appropriate for each of the following sections.

CARNITINE DEFICIENCY SYNDROMES

Two reviews of the literature describing carnitine deficiency syndromes cover the period from the first reported human deficiency in 1973 until 1983 (26, 27). In one case a 3½-year old had systemic carnitine deficiency (SCD), which presented as Reye's Syndrome. The nonfatal 36-hour fast of this patient, with less than 5% of the normal liver and skeletal muscle carnitine levels shows that fatty acids can be delivered to mitochondria even with low levels of carnitine. When treated with carnitine, liver carnitine levels returned to normal and skeletal muscle carnitine was increased to 40% of normal. Neurological disturbances and hepatomegaly disappeared after two weeks of therapy, and the cardiomyopathy was largely resolved by three months (28). A recent review by Stumpf et al (29) defined carnitine deficiency with a focus on possibly the most important clinical role of carnitine yet established. These authors state that "Carnitine deficiency exists when there is insufficient carnitine to buffer toxic acyl-CoA compounds" (29). In eliminating such acyl compounds, a tissue may have a net efflux of carnitine and a syndrome of carnitine deficiency may result.

The term *primary carnitine deficiency*, as pointed out by Irias (30), should probably be restricted to carnitine deficiencies of idiopathic origin. Secondary deficiencies arise from defects in intermediary metabolism, from disease or pathophysiological states, and from normal physiological states that reflect metabolic stress such as starvation or pregnancy. These authors suggest that the term *primary* be omitted in cases relating to carnitine supply (biosynthesis, diet, absorption), transport (uptake, release, reabsorption), or degradation. This would eliminate the need to reclassify a reported deficiency in biosynthesis that is later shown to be due to a methionine or iron deficiency.

Any condition that causes liver carnitine to be lost from the body may eventually result in depletion of muscle carnitine. Periodic increases of carnitine levels may follow dietary supplementation or periods of intense lipid use by muscle (31). Skeletal muscle levels can fall without a decrease in liver or plasma levels. Loss of carnitine in muscles can result from chronic overuse of lipids by the mitochondria. This overuse may occur during extensive physical activity or may result from a defect in the intermediary metabolism of the muscle. The heart, with its high turnover of carnitine, is susceptible to tissue-specific depletion of L-carnitine by the D isomer (32). The depletion of carnitine caused by net efflux of carnitine as an acyl ester is distinct from the depletion that occurs because of transporter defects or renal loss. In interpreting plasma levels of carnitine, the researcher must recognize that values represent only one moment in time. Although the plasma level may reflect the carnitine level of liver and other tissues, the skeletal muscle pool cannot be estimated by the plasma level. Also, the investigator should know and report both free carnitine and acyl carnitine values. Without knowing the amount of acyl carnitine that accompanies free carnitine, it is impossible to know whether a hypercarnitine- or hypocarnitine-related metabolic state is present.

A redistribution of carnitine may result in increased plasma and liver levels, but also in decreased levels in the tissue supplying the carnitine. The increased level of plasma carnitine might result in a smaller fraction of carnitine being reabsorbed by the kidney, and the levels of carnitine would decrease more rapidly.

In SCD a renal leak occurs in some patients (33). Replacement therapy normalizes plasma and liver carnitine levels only as long as carnitine supplementation is continued. This renal leak is postulated to result from a genetic defect in the renal reuptake system that handles carnitine (34). Glucocorticoids [prednisone (35), dexamethasone (36)] and cholesterol (37) can result in increased tissue (nonliver) and plasma levels of carnitine. The effect of glucocorticoids and cholesterol on renal handling has not been investigated. Therefore, to conclude that all reabsorption defects are genetic may be premature.

Organic Acidemias

Organic acidemias (a fall in blood pH caused by high levels of specific organic acids) provide an example of a group of metabolic diseases that can be successfully treated by the pharmacological use of carnitine (26–29). Acyl CoA metabolites are generated by the oxidation of certain fats or organic acids that cannot be readily metabolized. This metabolic inability may be due to the inherent structure of the substrate or to a genetic defect. The acyl group becomes a carnitine ester and thus does not remain to retard the function of mitochondrial CoA-dependent metabolic pathways. The continued removal of acyl groups may lead to a depletion of carnitine stores. Patterns of specific tissue protection or depletion may arise because the liver has the enzymes necessary for activating medium-chain fatty acids, but muscle does not (29).

Propionate is only poorly converted to a CoA ester in muscle (38). It is, however, activated in liver, where it inhibits oxidative phosphorylation. Stumpf et al showed that carnitine could reverse the inhibition of oxidative phosphorylation in isolated hepatic mitochondria and suggested carnitine as a potentially effective treatment (39). Propionic acidemia shows clinically significant response to carnitine treatment (40, 41). Other acidemias that result from inborn errors of metabolism also respond to carnitine as does the ingestion of excessive quantities of nonphysiological fatty acids or organic acids that result in acyl CoA accumulation (29). Treatment for carnitine deficiency syndrome is 100 mg/kg/day of L-carnitine, administered orally in 3 or 4 doses (29).

Lipid deposits are found in muscle biopsy specimens of patients with carnitine deficiencies, and often nonketotic hypoglycemia occurs with fasting. After carnitine supplementation clinical improvement occurs (26, 27). Carnitine depletion can cause lower rates of LCFA oxidation, suggesting that carnitine has become limiting for CPT I (42). In addition, CPT I (24) and SCAT (43) are inhibited by malonyl CoA, the first step in fatty acid synthesis or chain elongation. Long et al demonstrated that malonyl-CoA, produced when carbohydrate is used as the main source of mitochondrial substrate, inhibits fatty acid oxidation and increases synthesis of fatty acids. When acetyl CoA is provided by the citrate shuttle for elongating a fatty acid chain, SCAT inhibition prevents the acetyl CoA from being consumed while generating acetyl carnitine. Carnitine-deficient cells become more dependent on carbohydrate, as depleted carnitine levels result in lower rates of fatty acid oxidation (42). With a greater dependence on carbohydrate and decreased fatty acid oxidation, the increase in triglyceride (TG) may represent synthesis of fatty acids in excess of oxidation and phospholipid synthesis. Carnitine supplementation increases plasma and usually liver stores at least to control levels but is less effective in replenishing skeletal muscle carnitine (44). Carnitine replacement results in a more efficient metabolism of both carbohydrates and lipids, with patients showing weight gain as tissue lipid stores decrease.

Cardiomyopathies

A number of reports indicate that cardiomyopathic patients with low levels of serum carnitine may benefit from L-carnitine supplementation (28, 45–47).

Following chronic carnitine supplementation, thickness of the left ventricle returns to normal as does cardiac performance, with EKG abnormalities disappearing. In one study of cardiomyopathic patients an unexpected inverse correlation between survival and plasma carnitine levels was observed (47). However, a recent abstract suggests that the elevated level of serum carnitines in cardiomyopathic patients results from decreased renal clearance (48). Not all of the patients with elevated levels of plasma carnitine had high amounts of plasma acyl carnitines, but it may be that acyl carnitines increased in the sequence of events that led to death.

Diphtheria results in low levels of cardiac carnitine. These levels have been increased by treatment with D,L-carnitine (49).

Reye's and Reye's-Like Syndromes

Several cases of Reye's-like syndromes (RLS) with associated carnitine deficiency have been reported (28, 33, 44, 50). The clinical description—hypoglycemia, hypoketonemia, and coma—that appears episodically may represent a failure of the carnitine and CoA acyl regulatory mechanism that normally functions to prevent accumulation of acyl CoA esters.

One group of RLS patients has a defect in their medium-chain acyl-CoA dehydrogenase (44, 50). For heuristic purposes let us assume that the defect is absolute and the LCFA is metabolized to the eight-carbon acid octanoate. For every palmitic acid (C16:O) taken into the mitochondria only four acetyl CoA and one octanoyl CoA would be generated instead of the normal eight acetyl CoAs. To provide the equivalent "acetate pressure" produced by five palmitates, eight would have to be used. The altered metabolic economy from using only half of the LCFA would suggest that ten palmitates be used rather than five. Thus, for any level of LCFA metabolic activity, the percentage of the acyl pool that would be nonacetyl CoA would increase. Chronically, carnitine could become depleted as the octanoyl CoA was continuously removed. SCAT and CPT II would remove the octanoyl CoA only as its concentration became elevated.

Decreased stores of carnitine lower the buffering capacity and increase the accumulation of nonacetyl medium- and long-chain acyl CoA's during intense lipid use. Episodic symptoms of RLS might occur even during fasting for a short duration. The hypoglycemia reflects the lack of acetyl CoA as a positive regulator of pyruvate carboxylase activity inhibiting gluconeogenesis. The lack of ketone body formation reflects the lack of acetyl CoA as substrate for ketone body production. The defect in medium-chain acyl CoA dehydrogenase observed clinically may not be absolute. Plasma levels of carnitine are approximately one half of normal, and a single dose of supplemental carnitine results in a large efflux of acyl carnitines, 63% of which are octanoyl carnitines (44). The management of this RLS includes a diet low in fat, avoidance of fasting, as well as administering L-carnitine supplementation (44, 50).

The anticonvulsant valproic acid induces RLS in a small percentage of patients. Fatty acid oxidation rates are depressed by valproic acid, and neither carnitine nor glycine causes rapid exit of valproyl CoA from mitochondria (51). After a single injection of valproic acid into infant mice acetyl CoA fell 71%, medium-chain acyl carnitine rose 650%, and long-chain esters increased 68% (52). These observations suggest that valproyl CoA inhibits the mitochondrial β-oxidative pathway in a similar manner to a deficiency in medium-chain acyl dehydrogenase. Hypoglycin, the active component of the unripe Ackee fruit that causes the vomiting sickness of Jamacia (53), also inhibits the mitochondrial β-oxidative pathway. Adult mice showed a similar response, only with higher doses of valproate, when starved (54). Increased acyl group flux (and accumulation) may be necessary in the adult animals that start with larger pools of tissue carnitine and may activate valproate at a different fractional rate. Becker & Harris reported that valproate does not accumulate in the brain (51). This finding suggests that valproate's action to deplete carnitine may be more closely related to its mechanism of action than previously appreciated. Carnitine deficiency might be linked in three ways: (a) by decreasing the rate of choline biosynthesis (55) (see "Carnitine in the Neonate"); (b) by effecting a redistribution of choline to the periphery, as carnitine no longer competes for peripheral transport into liver and muscle and/or increased phosphatidyl choline synthesis does not compete for choline; and (c) by altering the metabolism of neurotransmitter production secondary to the carnitine deficiency state, thereby causing a greater utilization of glucose by all tissues. Plasma levels of carnitine correlate inversely with the dose of valproic acid in patients (56). In that relatively short-term study D,L-carnitine did not alter the electroencephalogram or frequency of seizures; however, it did normalize the associated hyperammonemia and plasma L-carnitine concentration.

Thurston et al (54) suggest testing patients for susceptibility to valproate-induced Reye's Syndrome by measuring the capacity for normal ketogenesis during a fast to uncover unrecognized metabolic deficiencies. Roe et al (57) recently warned that fasting in patients who may have low plasma carnitine levels can result in induction of coma and death. Alternatively, administration of a bolus of L-carnitine with identification of abnormal distribution, type, or quantity of acyl esters appearing in the urine is suggested (52).

Patients with true Reye's Syndrome do not respond to carnitine therapy (58). Aspirin use in juveniles is associated with Reye's Syndrome. It would be analogous with the previous example if salicylic acid or acetyl-salicylic acid (the parent compound) were found to form a CoA ester that decreased the rate of LCFA oxidation. Induction of acyl transferases may contribute to a higher concentration of the intramitochondrial CoA ester than usually occurs. However, any defect in the enzymes of β-oxidation, or inhibition of their activity by any exogenous or endogenous compound with valproatelike activity, would set the stage for Reye's Syndrome. The uncoupling of oxidative phosphorylation by salicylate would create high flux rates that would amplify any problem in LCFA oxidation. Decreasing liver levels of carnitine following the metabolic stress associated with illness may also contribute to susceptibility to Reye's Syndrome. During recovery from an attack, carnitine could be restored, and tissue levels would appear normal (59). Until the acyl CoA responsible for altering fatty acid oxidation is cleared from the mitochondria, episodic attacks would be expected. Other diseases or conditions where long-chain esters of carnitine or CoA are increased might respond to carnitine supplementation. In limb girdle dystrophy and Duchenne muscular dystrophy, long-chain acyl CoA levels are elevated (60). Also, in Duchenne dystrophy, muscle and plasma levels of carnitine are decreased (61).

Carnitine in the Neonate

Carnitine levels are lower in newborns than in adults (62, 63). During fetal development glucose is the predominant energy source for most tissues. Around the time of birth many tissues begin to utilize fatty acids for energy and therefore are dependent on carnitine for this function. The brain is an important exception to this generalization; it never develops a reliance on LCFA use for energy although it does use medium-chain fatty acids (64). The brain uses sugars as the main energy source only at some time after birth (65, 66). Ketone bodies, initially from the mother and subsequently from other tissues that begin to switch to LCFA utilization, may be crucial for normal development (67, 68). Carnitine in milk is a major source of the carnitine that fills the neonate's body pool (69).

Orzali et al (70) reported that D,L-carnitine administration [and later L-carnitine (71)] did not significantly alter existing fatty acid metabolism; lipid loading occurred in neonates receiving total parental nutrition (TPN). These authors concluded that enough tissue carnitine was present to maintain good lipid utilization in the neonate receiving TPN. Schmidt-Sommerfeld et al (72) pointed out that the lipid bolus contained glucose, which might tend to mask potential differences in lipid use. They also indicated that the 6-hr i.v. administration of carnitine following a bolus loading dose may not have been long enough for the carnitine to enter a pool where it could be useful (72). Schmidt-Sommerfeld et al studied TPN-fed neonates with chronic carnitine supplementation. Only premature, and not full-term, neonates showed an augmented ability to use lipid with supplemental carnitine (73). Skeletal muscle carnitine levels correlate with gestational age (62, 63), although those of the liver or heart do not (63). Carnitine supplementation in premature neonates does increase carnitine tissue levels (62).

Exogenous carnitine supplementation in the premature neonate may be especially important in TPN-fed neonates (73, 74). Biosynthetic enzymatic activity may be greatly reduced in all neonates (75), but with TPN-fed neonates the overall biosynthetic rate may become substrate limited. Infusion of nutrient solutions into the superior vena cava for TPN-fed neonates bypasses the intestine and the first-pass effect of the liver. Methionine in peripheral tissue is largely consumed by reactions leading to sulfate rather than by those leading to methyl groups available for transmethylation (76). Limitation of active methyl groups may lead to diminished rates of synthesis of both carnitine and choline in TPN-fed patients (77). Ethanolamine levels doubled in the heart and increased fourfold in the brain of miniature piglets when carnitine was added to the TPN solution (78). This observation suggests that ethanolamine production stimulated by carnitine was probably not converted to choline because of the lack of methyl donors. Because of the competition for methyl donors a lack of dietary choline causes a functional deficit of carnitine in the liver (55).

Maternal human plasma carnitine levels gradually fall during the course of pregnancy, and acute postpartum crisis can result (79). Maternal carnitine levels correspond to levels in full-term neonates delivered by elective cesarean section following uncomplicated pregnancies (80). Carnitine is used to treat respiratory distress syndrome associated with premature births, a syndrome caused by inadequate synthesis of phosphatidyl choline necessary for surfactant production (81, 82). When injected into pregnant female rats, carnitine caused an increase in total phospholipid synthesis in the lungs of fetal pups (83). This finding suggests that the importance of carnitine extends beyond fatty acid oxidation, especially for the fetus and neonate. It also points out that regulation of carnitine and choline biosynthesis may be related.

PHARMACOLOGY OF CARNITINE IN NONDEFICIENCY SYNDROMES

Neuropharmacology of Carnitine

The actions of acetyl carnitine and carnitine on the central nervous system were previously reviewed (84). Similarities in structure between acetyl carnitine and acetylcholine are often cited as circumstantial evidence that these compounds interact at the same receptor, but direct evidence has not been forthcoming. Electrophysiological studies suggest that carnitine and its derivatives may have important interactions with neuronal metabolism; neurotransmitter uptake, reuptake, and/or turnover; and receptor coupling in a variety of neurons. Insightful studies combining multiple areas of neuropharmacology are needed to help clarify and interpret the existing data of this area.

As previously discussed, choline is taken up by peripheral tissues for phosphatidyl choline synthesis and may share a common transporter with carnitine. Choline competes with the carnitine biosynthetic pathway for methyl donors, and the rate of choline biosynthesis may be related to tissue carnitine levels.

Hemodialysis

Patients on hemodialysis have elevated levels of acyl carnitine esters in both plasma and tissue (85, 86). Unlike the functional kidney that excretes acyl carnitine and preferentially reabsorbs free carnitine, hemodialysis results in the preferential loss of free carnitine; therefore, acyl carnitines accumulate (87, 88). In this semiclosed system the absolute level of LCFA acyl esters of CoA and carnitine may be more important than the acyl to free ester ratio. During hemodialysis plasma carnitine levels fall, and concurrently the rate of spontaneous cardiac arrhythmias increases. Administration of L-carnitine prevents these arrhythmias from increasing (89). At the conclusion of hemodialysis plasma carnitine levels rebound (85, 86). However, chronic hemodialysis results in depletion of muscle stores of carnitine. Plasma triglyceride (TG) levels increase, possibly because of both decreased peripheral use of lipid and increased hepatic synthesis of fatty acids. In six separate studies in hemodialysis patients (90–95), two studies in noninsulin-dependent diabetics (96, 97), and two studies in rats chronically administered alcohol (98, 99), D,L-carnitine administration resulted in a decrease in the level of TG. In another study in uremic rats L-carnitine prevented the rise of TG that accompanied the establishment of uremia but did not decrease the TG level once the level was elevated (100). There was, however, no effect with L-carnitine on TG level in at least four studies of hemodialysis patients (89, 101–103), and a paradoxical increase in TG with an increase in platelet aggregation was reported in one study (104). Another study reported no clinical improvement (105). While not all studies agree with the summary of these findings (106, 107), they show that the effects of a dose of D,L-carnitine may not always be equivalent to those of half the dose of L-carnitine. D,L-Carnitine, but not L-carnitine, has been reported to cause a myasthenialike syndrome in hemodialysis patients (108–110).

The kinetics of D,L-carnitine should not be ignored in looking for a basis for this effect. While D,L-carnitine may eventually result in increased plasma and tissue levels of L-carnitine (the D isomer not measured by the enzymatic assay) for tissues containing low levels of carnitine, exchange with the 50% mixture of D and L isomers would result in a transient decrease in tissue L-carnitine. The uptake and half-life of D-carnitine are less than those of L-carnitine, with the time to peak plasma level following oral dosing occurring after that of L-carnitine (111). An additional possibility is that D-carnitine is metabolized to an active molecule, which does not happen with L-carnitine (112).

In nonhemodialysis patients the level of high-density lipoprotein (HDL) increases, and serum cholesterol decreases slightly following L-carnitine supplementation. In two patients normal except for low HDL levels, L-carnitine increased HDL levels and decreased TG and total plasma cholesterol levels in one, but not the other, patient (113). Supplementation of carnitine may help prevent the decrease in very low density lipoproteins (VLDL) apoprotein CII to apoprotein CIII ratio observed in hemodialysis patients with elevated TG levels (114).

Myocardial Protection

Carnitine protects or improves the performance of the heart under certain laboratory conditions. Although not proven, it is assumed that carnitine in the heart acts analogously to carnitine in other tissues.

ANGINA   Effort-induced angina pectoris improves with L-carnitine administration. In a study of patients with angiographically proven coronary artery disease, paced human hearts that were lactate producers extracted lactate from plasma following carnitine infusion (115). In patients with stable angina pectoris carnitine significantly increased the time of multistage-treadmill exercise over the placebo time during a 12-week study (116).

ISCHEMIA   During zero-flow ischemia (cessation of coronary flow) futile and excessive production of lactic acid occurs as the glycolytic pathway is utilized to prevent depletion of ATP and irreversible damage to the heart. L-Carnitine does not temper the decrease in performance and the cellular damage caused by this type of ischemia (117). During low-flow ischemia, ATP decreases as long-chain acyl-CoA levels increase and finally plateau. Long-chain acyl carnitines accumulate in the heart cell, bound loosely to membrane structures and protein, as less acetyl carnitine is produced and carnitine levels of the heart decrease.

Arrhythmias develop during ischemia, especially with increased levels of free fatty acids, as the ischemic area becomes electrically and mechanically uncoupled from the rest of the heart (117). Acetyl carnitine decreases the incidence of arrhythmias at a lower concentration than carnitine (118). These arrhythmias might be caused by the long-chain acyl carnitine esters that accumulate when their production is not limited by acetyl carnitine's sequestering CoA. The long-chain acyl carnitines are not passed to the blood in exchange for carnitine and cannot be readily consumed by the mitochondria.

Reperfusion with oxygen-containing solutions increases mitochondrial activity as the backlog of acyl carnitine and mitochondrial acyl-CoA levels decrease. By perfusing with carnitine during low-flow ischemia, acyl carnitine exchange for free carnitine is at least partially maintained (119).

In the dog-heart model of low-flow ischemia, levels of long-chain acyl-CoA's, ATP, and related compounds do not change with acetyl L-carnitine, but recovered performance earlier (117). Acetyl carnitine reduces the rate of fatty acid activation by sequestering the necessary cytosolic CoA. Long-chain acyl carnitine production is then limited by the cytosolic production of long-chain acyl-CoA. The amount of acyl carnitine accumulation may have a significant impact on both the time to recovery and the extent of recovery. Significantly, smaller infarct size has been reported when nicotinic acid and/or oxfenicine was added to the perfusion medium of dogs with a ligated branch of the coronary artery (120). Nicotinic acid decreases concentrations of free fatty acids in plasma. Oxfenicine decreases fatty acid oxidation at a step before CPT II. Both agents reduce long-chain acyl-CoAs, long-chain acyl carnitines, and infarct size in treated hearts in this model of low-flow ischemia. The level of long-chain acyl-CoAs was reduced to or reduced below normal control levels, but long-chain acyl carnitine levels were significantly higher (120). Although it appears that infarct size could correlate with levels of long-chain acyl carnitines, another study did not find any such correlation (121). The studies may not be comparable because of differences in the model of ischemia and in the species. Since both carnitine and acetyl carnitine may prevent accumulation of acyl carnitines, they may have an effect on infarct size for both the dog and the rat heart. Tetradecylglycidic acid inhibits the long-chain fatty acid transfer from CoA to carnitine in the cytosol (122). This agent was developed to decrease the inappropriately overaggressive gluconeogenesis of diabetes, but by preventing LCFA-carnitine formation its use might help clarify the mechanism of myocardial damage during ischemia.

Experimental animal models of diabetes show diabetic hearts have low levels of total carnitine, increased levels of long-chain acyl carnitine with long-chain acyl-CoA and ATP levels the same as in the ischemic heart (123). Chronic lower plasma levels of free carnitine and increased levels of acyl carnitine may contribute to these effects. In humans treated for diabetes these altered levels are less of a problem. During a period of relatively good control of blood glucose levels they do not show the altered level of plasma and tissue carnitine seen in the untreated experimental animal (124, 125).

Di Lisa et al (126) studied the molecular mechanism of carnitine stabilization of energy-linked processes in the rat liver mitochondria and concluded that it was caused by removal of membrane-bound long-chain acyl-CoAs. The effect may have been due to the removal of acyl carnitine ester rather than acyl-CoA ester. Also, carnitine itself may have had a direct stabilizing activity. Di Lisa et al pointed out that carnitine acted primarily as a stabilizing factor rather than as a specific antidote for a particular noxious factor or condition.

Adriamycin's effect as an anticancer drug is limited by its cardiac toxicity. When carnitine is coadministered with adriamycin there is no evidence of the acute cardiotoxicity in humans as measured by EKG (127). This finding may be another example of a circumstance in which carnitine acts as a stabilizing factor.

CONCLUSION

Carnitine, as an obligatory cofactor of LCFA oxidation, plays an important role in lipid metabolism. Carnitine and CoA esters generated in LCFA oxidation regulate multiple enzymes. A transport system maintains a gradient between low plasma levels and high cellular level. Acyl groups that are difficult to metabolize or that are only slowly metabolized are transferred from CoA to carnitine. The transporter exchanges these cytosolic acyl carnitines for free carnitine of the plasma before they are finally eliminated via the kidney. Carnitine deficiency states result in greater reliance on glucose for energy production. The basis for the pharmacological actions of carnitine is in large measure accounted for by the increased utilization of LCFA for energy production. Also, these pharmacological actions are effected by the elimination of acyl carnitine that could potentially interfere with the integrated regulatory system comprising the intermediary metabolism.

The development of a rapid assay for carnitine and the availability of significant quantities of L-carnitine help to accelerate the rate at which knowledge has been acquired. The relatively new tools of inhibitors of carnitine-related enzymes are also beneficial. These inhibitors include tetradecylglycidic acid (122); 2[5(4-chlorophenyl)pentyl] oxirane-2-carboxylic acid (128); CPT inhibitors, preventing transfer of LCFA from CoA to carnitine in the cytoplasm; 2–(3–methylcinnamyl) hydrazonal-propionic acid (129); translocase inhibitor, blocking carnitine esters from entering the mitochondria; and methoxycarbonyl-CoA disulfide (130), a substrate directed at the SCAT enzyme that transfers acetate between CoA and carnitine in the cytosol. Molecular biology, with its rapid advances in many aspects of cellular regulation, may be of assistance in explaining what factors regulate the production of the proteins found in the biosynthetic pathway and the one or more proteins that make up the transporter.

To date limited specific patient populations have been identified that benefit from carnitine supplementation. However, it is appropriate to ask and determine if chronic excessive elevation of carnitine might not result in chronic choline loss. Potentially, choline loss could induce the functional deficits both centrally and peripherally. Twenty years ago it was shown that a rat injected with carnitine had brain levels of acetylcholine that were only one-half those of control animals (131). On the other hand, if competition for methyl groups normally limits choline availability to the brain, low-dose supplementation of carnitine might result in the opposite, and potentially therapeutic, effect. No compound is more efficacious in the treatment of a patient with a carnitine deficiency. However, there is no evidence that carnitine in reasonable doses is of benefit or harm to a healthy individual.

Literature Cited

1. Gulewitsch, V. S., Krimberg, R. 1905. Zur Kenntnis der Extraktivstoffe der Muskeln. II. Mitteilung—Über das Carnitin. *Hoppe-Seylers Z. Physiol. Chem.* 45:326–30
2. Fritz, I. B. 1959. Action of carnitine on long chain fatty acid oxidation by liver. *Am. J. Physiol.* 197:297–304
3. Cederblad, G., Lindstedt, S. 1972. A method for the determination of carnitine in the picomole range. *Clin. Chim. Acta* 37:235–43
4. McGarry, J. D., Foster, D. W. 1976. An improved and simplified radio-isotopic assay for the determination of free and esterified carnitine. *J. Lipid Res.* 17:277–81
5. Borum, P. R., ed. 1986. *Clinical Aspects of Human Carnitine Deficiency.* New York: Pergamon. 280 pp.
6. Bremer, J. 1983. Carnitine—metabolism and functions. *Physiol. Rev.* 63:1420–80
7. Frenkel, R. A., McGarry, J. D. 1980. *Carnitine Biosynthesis, Metabolism, and Functions.* New York: Academic. 356 pp.
8. Borum, P. R. 1983. Carnitine. *Ann. Rev. Nutr.* 3:233–59
9. Broquist, H. P. 1981. Carnitine biosynthesis and function. *Fed. Proc.* 41:2840–62
10. Idell-Wenger, J. A., Grotyohann, L. W., Neely, J. R. 1982. Regulation of fatty-acid utilization in heart. Role of the carnitine-acetyl-CoA transferase and carnitine-acetyl carnitine translocase system. *J. Mol. Cell. Cardiol.* 14:413–17
11. Paulson, D. J., Shug, A. L. 1984. Inhibition of the adenine nucleotide translocator by matrix-localized palmityl-CoA in rat heart mitochondria. *Biochim. Biophys. Acta* 766:70–76
12. Oram, J. D., Wenger, J. I., Neely, J. R.

1975. Regulation of long chain fatty acid activation in heart muscle. *J. Biol. Chem.* 250(1):73–78
13. Murthy, M. S. R., Pande, S. V. 1984. Mechanism of carnitine acylcarnitine translocase-catalyzed import of acylcarnitines into mitochondria. *J. Biol. Chem.* 259:9082–89
14. Idell-Wenger, J. A., Grotyohann, L. W., Neely, J. R. 1978. Coenzyme A and carnitine distribution in normal and ischemic hearts. *J. Biol. Chem.* 253:4310–18
15. Bahl, J., Navin, T., Manian, A. A., Bressler, R. 1981. Carnitine transport in isolated adult rat heart myocytes and the effect of 7,8 diOH chlorpromazine. *Circ. Res.* 48:378–85
16. Carter, A. L., Frenkel, R. 1978. The relationship of choline and carnitine in the choline deficient rat. *J. Nutr.* 108:1748–54
17. Christiansen, R. Z., Bremer, J. 1976. Active transport of butyrobetaine and carnitine into isolated liver cells. *Biochim. Biophys. Acta* 448:562–77
18. Avigan, J., Askansas, V., Engel, W. K. 1983. Muscle carnitine deficiency: fatty acid metabolism in cultured fibroblasts and muscle cells. *Neurology* 33:1021–26
19. Gudjonsson, H., Li, B. U. K., Shug, A. L., Olsen, W. A. 1985. Studies of carnitine metabolism in relation to intestinal absorption. *Am. J. Physiol.* 248:G313–19
20. Vary, T. C., Neely, J. R. 1983. Sodium dependence of carnitine transport in isolated perfused adult rat hearts. *Am. J. Physiol.* 244:H247–52
21. Rebouche, C. J., Mack, D. L. 1984. Sodium gradient–stimulated transport of L-carnitine into renal brush border membrane vesicles: Kinetics, specificity, and regulation by dietary carnitine. *Arch. Biochem. Biophys.* 235:393–402

22. Rössle, C., Kohse, K. P., Franz, H.-E., Fürst, P. 1985. An improved method for the determination of free and esterified carnitine. *Clin. Chim. Acta* 149:263–68

23. Maebashi, M., Kawamura, N., Sato, M., Yoshinaga, K., Suzuki, M. 1976. Urinary excretion of carnitine in man. *J. Lab. Clin. Med.* 87:760–66

24. McGarry, J. D., Foster, D. W. 1979. In support of the roles of malonyl-CoA and carnitine acyl-transferase I in the regulation of hepatic fatty acid oxidation and ketogenesis. *J. Biol. Chem.* 254:8163–68

25. Olson, R. E. 1979. Hormonal regulation of hepatic ketogenesis—pivotal role of malonyl-CoA. *Nutr. Rev.* 37:236–37

26. Rebouche, C. J., Engel, A. G. 1983. Carnitine metabolism and deficiency syndromes. *Mayo Clin. Proc.* 58:533–40

27. Gilbert, E. F. 1985. Carnitine deficiency. *Pathology* 17:161–71

28. Chapoy, P. R., Angelini, C., Brown, W. J., Stiff, J. E., Shug, A. L., et al. 1980. Systemic carnitine deficiency—a treatable inherited lipid-storage disease presenting as Reye's syndrome. *N. Engl. J. Med.* 303:1389–94

29. Stumpf, D. A., Parker, W. D., Angelini, C. 1985. Carnitine deficiency, organic acidemias, and Reye's syndrome. *Neurology* 35:1041–45

30. Irias, J. 1986. Genetic primary carnitine deficiency? See Ref. 5, pp. 117–28

31. Lennon, D. L. F., Stratman, F. W., Shrago, E., Nagle, F. J., Madden, M., et al. 1983. Effects of acute moderate-intensity exercise on carnitine metabolism in men and women. *J. Appl. Physiol.* 55:489–95

32. Paulson, D. J., Shug, A. L. 1981. Tissue specific depletion of L-carnitine in rat heart and skeletal muscle by D-carnitine. *Life Sci.* 28:2931–38

33. Engel, A. G., Rebouche, C. J., Wilson, D. M., Glasgow, A. M., Romshe, C. A. 1981. Primary systemic carnitine deficiency. II. Renal handling of carnitine. *Neurology* 31:819–25

34. Waber, L. J., Valle, D., Neill, C., DiMauro, S., Shug, A. L. 1982. Carnitine deficiency presenting as familial cardiomyopathy: A treatable defect in carnitine transport. *J. Pediatr.* 101:700–5

35. Mølstad, P., Bøhmer, T. 1979. Transport of L-carnitine induced by prednisolone in an established cell line (CCL 27): A possible explanation of the therapeutic effect of glucocorticoids in muscular carnitine deficiency syndrome. *Biochim. Biophys. Acta* 585:94–99

36. French, T. J., Good, A. W., Palmer, T. N., Sugden, M. C. 1985. Effects of dexamethasone on carnitine metabolism in liver and extrahepatic tissues. *Biosci. Rep.* 5:729–34

37. Bell, F. P., Armstrong, M. L., Megan, M. B., Patt, C. S. 1983. The effect of diet on plasma carnitine, triglyceride, cholesterol and arterial carnitine levels in cynomolgus monkeys. *Biochem. Physiol.* 75B:211–15

38. Trevisan, C., DiMauro, S. 1983. Activation of free fatty acids in subcellular fractions of human skeletal muscle. *Neurochem. Res.* 8:551–61

39. Stumpf, D. A., McAfee, J., Parks, J. K., Eguren, L. 1980. Propionate inhibition of succinate: CoA ligase (GDP) and the citric acid cycle in mitochondria. *Pediatr. Res.* 14:1127–31

40. Bohles, H., Lehnert, W. 1984. The effect of intravenous L-carnitine on propionic acid excretion in acute propionic acidaemia. *Eur. J. Pediatr.* 143:61–63

41. Roe, C. R., Bohan, T. P. 1982. L-Carnitine therapy in propionic acidaemia. *Lancet* 1:1411–12

42. Long, C. S., Haller, R. G., Foster, D. W., McGarry, J. D. 1982. Kinetics of carnitine-dependent fatty acid oxidation: Implications for human carnitine deficiency. *Neurology* 32:663–66

43. Lund, H., Bremer, J. 1983. Carnitine acetyltransferase: effect of malonyl-CoA, fasting and cloribrate feeding in mitochondria from different tissues. *Biochim. Biophys. Acta* 750:164–70

44. Roe, C. R., Millington, S., Maltby, A., Bohan, T. P., Kahler, S. G., et al. 1985. Diagnostic and therapeutic implications of medium-chain acylcarnitines in the medium-chain acyl-CoA dehydrogenase deficiency. *Pediatr. Res.* 19:459–66

45. Tripp, M. E., Katcher, M. L., Peters, H. A., Gilbert, E. F., Arya, S., et al. 1981. Systemic carnitine deficiency presenting as familial endocardial fibroelastosis: A treatable cardiomyopathy. *N. Engl. J. Med.* 305:385–90

46. Matsuichi, T., Hirata, K., Terasawa, K., Kato, H., Yoshino, M. 1985. Successful carnitine treatment in two siblings having lipid storage myopathy with hypertrophic cardiomyopathy. *Neuropediatrics* 16:6–12

47. Tripp, M. E., Shug, A. L. 1984. Plasma carnitine concentrations in cardiomyopathy patients. *Biochem. Med.* 32:199–206

48. Waber, L. J., Feldman, A. M., Baughman, K. L. 1985. Elevated plasma car-

nitine (C) in patients with idiopathic cardiomyopathy. *Pediatr. Res.* 19:135A
49. Ramos, A. C. M. F., Elias, P. R. P., Barrucand, L., Da Silva, J. A. F. 1984. The protective effect of carnitine in human diphtheric myocarditis. *Pediatr. Res.* 18(9):815–19
50. Coates, P. M., Hale, D. E., Stanley, C. A., Corkey, B. E., Cortner, J. A. 1985. Genetic deficiency of medium-chain acyl coenzyme A dehydrogenase: Studies in cultured skin fibroblasts and peripheral mononuclear leukocytes. *Pediatr. Res.* 19:671–76
51. Becker, C.-M., Harris, R. A. 1983. Influence of valproic acid on hepatic carbohydrate and lipid metabolism. *Arch. Biochem. Biophys.* 223:381–92
52. Thurston, J. H., Carroll, J. E., Hauhart, R. E., Schiro, J. A. 1984. Valproate treatment and carnitine deficiency. *Neurology* 34:1129
53. Entman, M., Bressler, R. 1967. The mechanism of action of hypoglycin on long-chain fatty acid oxidation. *Mol. Pharmacol.* 3:333–40
54. Thurston, J. H., Carroll, J. E., Hauhart, R. E., Schiro, J. A. 1985. A single therapeutic dose of valproate affects liver carbohydrate, fat, adenylate, amino acid, coenzyme A, and carnitine metabolism in infant mice: possible clinical significance. *Life Sci.* 36:1643–51
55. Corredor, C., Mansbach, C., Bressler, R. 1967. Carnitine depletion in the choline-deficient state. *Biochim. Biophys. Acta* 144:366–74
56. Ohtani, Y., Endo, F., Matsuda, I. 1982. Carnitine deficiency and hyperammonemia associated with valproic acid therapy. *J. Pediatr.* 101:782–85
57. Roe, C. R., Millington, D. S., Maltby, D. A., Kahler, S. G., Bohan, T. P. 1984. L-Carnitine therapy in isovaleric acidemia. *J. Clin. Invest.* 74:2290–95
58. Roe, C. R., Millington, D. S., Maltby, D., Bohan, T. P. 1983. Status and function of L-carnitine in Reye's syndrome (RS) and related metabolic disorders. *J. Natl. Reyes Syndrome Found.* 4:58–59
59. Willner, J. H., Chutorian, A. M., DiMauro, S. 1978. Tissue carnitine in Reye syndrome. *Ann. Neurol.* 4:468–69
60. Carroll, J. E., Villadiego, A., Brook, M. H. 1983. Increased long chain acyl CoA in Duchenne muscular dystrophy. *Neurology* 33:1507–10
61. Berthillier, G., Eichenberger, D., Carrier, H. N., Guibaud, P., Grot, R. 1982. Carnitine metabolism in early stages of Duchenne muscular dystrophy. *Clin. Chim. Acta* 122:369–75

62. Penn, D., Ludwigs, B., Schmidt-Sommerfeld, E., Pacu, F. 1985. Effect of nutrition on tissue carnitine concentrations in infants of different gestational ages. *Biol. Neonate* 47:130–35
63. Shenai, J. P., Borum, P. R. 1984. Tissue carnitine reserves of newborn infants. *Pediatr. Res.* 18:679–81
64. Wells, M. A. 1985. Fatty acid metabolism and ketone formation in suckling rat. *Fed. Proc.* 44:2365–68
65. Yeh, Y. Y., Sheehan, P. M. 1985. Preferential utilization of ketone bodies in the brain and lung of newborn rats. *Fed. Proc.* 44:2352–58
66. Edmond, J., Auestad, N., Robbins, R. A., Bergstrom, J. D. 1985. Ketone body metabolism in the neonate: development and the effect of diet. *Fed. Proc.* 44:2359–64
67. Shambaugh, G. E. III. 1985. Ketone body metabolism in the mother and fetus. *Fed. Proc.* 44:2347–51
68. Hahn, P. 1985. Ketone body and carnitine metabolism in newborns. *Fed. Proc.* 44:2339–41
69. Hahn, P., Novak, M. 1985. How important are carnitine and ketones for the newborn infant? *Fed. Proc.* 44:2369–2373
70. Orzali, A., Donzelli, F., Enzi, G., Rubaltelli, F. F. 1983. Effect of carnitine on lipid metabolism in the newborn—I. Carnitine supplementation during total parenteral nutrition in the first 48 hours of life. *Biol. Neonate* 43:186–90
71. Orzali, A., Maetzke, G., Donzelli, F., Rubaltelli, F. 1984. Effect of carnitine on lipid metabolism in the neonate. II. Carnitine addition to lipid infusion during prolonged total parenteral nutrition. *J. Pediatr.* 104:436–40
72. Schmidt-Sommerfeld, E., Penn, D. 1984. Carnitine and neonatal lipid metabolism. *J. Pediatr.* 105:848–49
73. Schmidt-Sommerfeld, E., Penn, D., Wolf, H. 1983. Carnitine deficiency in premature infants receiving total parenteral nutrition: Effect of L-carnitine supplementation. *J. Pediatr.* 102:931–35
74. Borum, P. R. 1985. Role of carnitine during development. *Can. J. Physiol. Pharmacol.* 63:571–76
75. Hahn, P. 1981. The development of carnitine synthesis from γ-butyrobetaine in the rat. *Life Sci.* 29:1057–60
76. Everett, G. B., Mitchell, A. D., Benevenga, N. J. 1979. Methionine transamination and catabolism in vita-

min B-6 deficient rats. *J. Nutr.* 109:597–605

77. Rudman, D., Williams, P. J. 1985. Nutrient deficiencies during total parenteral nutrition. *Nutr. Rev.* 43:1–13

78. Böhles, H., Michalk, D., Brandl, U., Fekl, W., Börresen, H., et al. 1984. The effect of L-carnitine-supplemented total parenteral nutrition on tissue amino acid concentrations in piglets. *J. Nutr.* 114:671–76

79. Angelini, C., Govoni, E., Bragaglia, M. M., Vergani, L. 1978. Carnitine deficiency: acute postpartum crisis. *Ann. Neurol.* 4:558–61

80. Cederblad, G., Niklasson, A., Rydgren, B., Albertsson-Wikland, K., Olegard, R. 1985. Carnitine in maternal and neonatal plasma. *Acta Paediatr. Scand.* 74:500–4

81. Salzer, H., Husslein, P., Lohninger, A., Binstorfer, E., Langer, M., et al. 1983. Erste Mitteilung: Alternativen zur Cortisontherapie. Erste klinische Erfahrungen mit einer Carnitin-Betamethason-Kombination zur Stimulation der fetalen Lungenreife. *Wien. Klin. Wochenschr.* 95:724–28

82. Salzer, H. 1982. Neue Aspekte in Diagnose und Therapie der fetalen Lungenunreife. *Wien. Klin. Wochenschr.* 94:3–30 (Suppl. 136)

83. Lohninger, A., Krieglsteiner, P., Nikiforov, A., Ehrhardt, W., Specker, M., et al. 1984. Comparison of the effects of betamethasone and L-carnitine on dipalmitoylphosphatidylcholine content and phosphatidycholine species composition in fetal rat lungs. *Pediatr. Res.* 18:1246–52

84. Janiri, L., Tempesta, E. 1983. A pharmacological profile of the effects of carnitine and acetyl carnitine on the central nervous system. *Int. J. Clin. Pharmacol. Res.* 3:295–306

85. Savica, V., Bellinghieri, G., Di Stephano, C., Corvaja, E., Consolo, F., et al. 1983. Plasma and muscle carnitine levels in haemodialysis patients with morphological-ultrastructural examination of muscle samples. *Nephron* 35:232–36

86. Vacha, G. M., Corsi, M., Giorcelli, G., Iddio, S. D., Maccari, F. 1985. Serum and muscle L-carnitine levels in hemodialyzed patients, during and after long-term L-carnitine treatment. *Curr. Ther. Res.* 37:505–16

87. Penn, D., Schmidt-Sommerfeld, E. 1983. Carnitine and carnitine esters in plasma and adipose tissue of chronic

uremic patients undergoing hemodialysis. *Metabolism* 32:806–9

88. Moorthy, A. V., Shug, A. L. 1985. Elevated plasma carnitine levels in patients on CAPD. *Peritoneal Dialysis Bull.* 5:175–79

89. Suzuki, Y., Narita, M., Yamazaki, N. 1982. Effects of L-carnitine on arrhythmias during hemodialysis. *Jpn. Heart J.* 349–59

90. Bartoli, M., Battistella, P. A., Vergani, L., Naso, A., Gasparotto, M. L. et al. 1981. Carnitine deficiency induced during hemodialysis and hyperlipidemia: effect of replacement therapy. *Am. J. Clin. Nutr.* 34:1496–500

91. Maebashi, M., Kawamura, N., Sato, M., Imamura, A., Yoshinaga, K. 1978. Lipid-lowering effect of carnitine in patients with type-IV hyperlipoproteinaemia. *Lancet* 2:805–7

92. Maebashi, M., Imamura, A., Yoshinaga, K., Sato, T., Funyu, T., et al. 1983. Carnitine depletion as a probable cause of hyperlipidemia in uremic patients on maintenance hemodialysis. *Tohoku J. Exp. Med.* 139:33–42

93. Chan, M. K., Persaud, J. W., Varghese, Z., Baillod, R. A., Moorhead, J. F. 1982. Response patterns to DL-carnitine in patients on maintenance haemodialysis. *Nephron* 30:240–43

94. Guarnieri, G. F., Ranieri, F., Toigo, G., Vasile, A., Ciman, M., et al. 1980. Lipid-lowering effect of carnitine in chronically uremic patients treated with maintenance hemodialysis. *Am. J. Clin. Nutr.* 33:1489–92

95. Bougneres, P. F., Lacour, B., Di Guilio, S., Assan, R. 1979. Hypolipaemic effect of carnitine in uraemic patients. *Lancet* 1:1401–2

96. Bekaert, J., Deltour, G. 1960. Effet de la carnitine sur l'hyperlipidémie diabétique. *Clin. Chim. Acta* 5:177–80

97. Abdel-Aziz, M. T., Abdou, M. S., Soliman, K., Shawky, M. A., Tawadrous, G. A., et al. 1984. Effect of carnitine on blood lipid pattern in diabetic patients. *Nutr. Rep. Int.* 29:1071–79

98. Sachan, D. S., Rhew, T. H., Ruark, R. A. 1984. Ameliorating effects of carnitine and its precursors on alcohol-induced fatty liver. *Am. J. Clin. Nutr.* 39:738–44

99. Hosein, E. A., Bexton, B. 1975. Protective action of carnitine on liver lipid metabolism after ethonal administration to rats. *Biochem. Pharmacol.* 24:1859–63

100. Basile, C., Lacour, B., Di Giulio, S., Drüeke, T. 1985. Effect of oral carnitine

supplementation on disturbances of lipid metabolism in the uremic rat. *Nephron* 39:50–54

101. Caruso, U., Cravotto, E., Tisone, G., Elli, M., Stortoni, F., et al. 1983. Long-term treatment with L-carnitine in uremic patients undergoing chronic hemodialysis: effects on the lipid pattern. *Curr. Ther. Res.* 33:1098–104

102. Bellinghieri, G., Savica, V., Mallamace, A., Di Stefano, C., Consolo, F., et al. 1983. Correlation between increased serum and tissue L-carnitine levels and improved muscle symptoms in hemodialized patients. *Am. J. Clin. Nutr.* 38:523–31

103. Casciani, C. U., Caruso, U., Cravotto, E., D'Iddio, S., Corsi, M., et al. 1982. L-Carnitine in haemodialysed patients. *Arzneim. Forsch.* 32:293–97

104. Weschler, A., Aviram, M., Levin, M., Better, O. S., Brook, J. G. 1984. High dose of L-carnitine increases platelet aggregation and plasma triglyceride levels in uremic patients on hemodialysis. *Nephron* 38:120–24

105. Fagher, B., Cederblad, G., Eriksson, M., Monti, M., Moritz, U., et al. 1985. L-Carnitine and haemodialysis: Double blind study on muscle function and metabolism and peripheral nerve function. *Scand. J. Clin. Lab. Invest.* 45:169–78

106. Fagher, B., Thysell, H., Nilsson-Ehle, P., Monti, M., Olsson, L., et al. 1982. The effect of D,L-carnitine supplementation on muscle metabolism, neuropathy, cardiac and hepatic function in hemodialysis patients. *Acta Med. Scand.* 212:115–20

107. Bazzato, G., Lucatello, S., Landini, S., Coli, U., Fracasso, A., et al. 1981. Intraperitoneal (IP) L-carnitine administration: successful therapeutic approach of hypertriglyceridaemia in patients on double-bag system CAPD. *Artif. Organs.* 5:429

108. Bazzato, G., Mezzina, C., Ciman, M., Guarnieri, G. 1979. Myasthenia-like syndrome associated with carnitine in patients on long-term haemodialysis. *Lancet* 1:1041–42

109. Bazzato, G., Coli, U., Landini, S., Mezzina, C., Ciman, M. 1981. Myasthenia-like syndrome after D,L- but not L-carnitine. *Lancet* 1:1209

110. DeGrandi, D., Mezzina, C., Fiaschi, A., Pinelli, P., Bazzato, G., et al. 1980. Myasthenia due to carnitine treatment. *J. Neurol. Sci.* 46:365–71

111. Gross, C. J., Henderson, L. M. 1984. Absorption of D- and L-carnitine by the intestine and kidney tubule in the rat. *Biochim. Biophys. Acta* 772:209–19

112. Seim, H., Löster, H., Strack, E. 1980. Kataboler Carnitinstoffwechsel: Reaktionsprodukte der Carnitin-Decarboxylase und der Carnitin-Dehydrogenase in vivo. *Hoppe-Seylers Z. Physiol. Chem.* 361:1427–35

113. Rossi, C. S., Siliprandi, N. 1982. Effect of carnitine on serum HDL-cholesterol: Report of two cases. *Johns Hopkins Med. J.* 150:51–54

114. Wakabayashi, Y., Okubo, M., Shimada, H., Sato, N., Marumo, F. 1986. Decreased VLDL apoprotein CII/ apoprotein CIII ratio with superimposed carnitine deficiency may be pathogenic factors of hypertriglyceridemia in patients on chronic hemodialysis treatment. *Kidney Int.* 29:327

115. Ferrari, R., Cucchini, F., Visioli, O. 1984. The metabolic effects of L-carnitine in angina pectoris. *Int. J. Cardiol.* 5:213–16

116. Kamikawa, T., Yoshikazu, S., Kobayashi, A., Hayashi, H., Masumura, Y., et al. 1984. Effects of L-carnitine on exercise tolerance in patients with stable angina pectoris. *Jpn. Heart J.* 25:587–97

117. Paulson, D. J., Schmidt, M. J., Romens, J., Shug, A. L. 1984. Metabolic and physiological differences between zero-flow and low-flow myocardial ischemia: effects of L-acetylcarnitine. *Basic Res. Cardiol.* 79:551–61

118. Imai, S., Matsui, K., Nakazawa, M., Takatsuka, N., Takeda, K., et al. 1984. Anti-arrhythmic effects of (–)-carnitine chloride and its acetyl analogue on canine late ventricular arrhythmia induced by ligation of the coronary artery as related to improvement of mitochondrial function. *Br. J. Pharmacol.* 82:533–42

119. Liedtke, A. J., Nellis, S. H. 1979. Effects of carnitine in ischemic and fatty acid supplemented swine hearts. *J. Clin. Invest.* 64:440–47

120. Vik-Mo, H., Mjos, O. D., Neely, J. R., Maroko, P. R., Ribeiro, G. T., et al. 1986. Limitation of myocardial infarct size by metabolic interventions that reduce accumulation of fatty acid metabolites in ischemic myocardium. *Am. Heart J.* 111:1048–54

121. Ichihara, K., Neely, J. R. 1985. Recovery of ventricular function in reperfused ischemic rat hearts exposed to fatty acids. *Am. J. Physiol.* 249:H492–97

122. Kiorpes, T. C., Hoerr, D., Ho, W., Weaner, L. E., Inman, M. G., et al.

1984. Identification of 2-tetra-decylglycidyl coenzyme A as the active form of methyl 2-tetradecylglycidate (methyl palmoxirate) and its characterization as an irreversible, active site-directed inhibitor of carnitine palmitoyltransferase A in isolated rat liver mitochondria. *J. Biol. Chem.* 259:9750–55

123. Pieper, G. M., Salhany, J. M., Murray, W. J., Shao, T. W., Eliot, R. S. 1984. Lipid-mediated impairment of normal energy metabolism in the isolated perfused diabetic rat heart studied by phosphorus-31 NMR and chemical extraction. *Biochim. Biophys. Acta* 803:229–40

124. DePalo, E., Gatti, R., Sicolo, N., Padovan, D., Vettor, R., et al. 1981. Plasma and urine free L-carnitine in human diabetes mellitus. *Acta Diabetol. Lat.* 18:91–95

125. Cederblad, G., Lundholm, K., Scherstén, T. 1977. Carnitine concentration in skeletal muscle tissue from patients with diabetes mellitus. *Acta Med. Scand.* 202:305–6

126. Di Lisa, F., Bobyleva-Guarriero, V., Jocelyn, P., Toninello, A., Siliprandi, N. 1985. Stabilising action of carnitine on energy linked processes in rat liver

mitochondria. *Biochem. Biophys. Res. Commun.* 131:968–73

127. Furitano, G., Paterna, S., Perricone, R., Barbarino, C., Palumbo, F. P., et al. 1984. Polygraphic evaluation of effects of carnitine in patients on adriamycin treatment. *Drugs Exp. Clin. Res.* 10:107–11

128. Bartlett, K., Bone, A. J., Koundakjian, P. P., Meredith, E., Turnbull, D. M., et al. 1981. Inhibition of mitochondrial β-oxidation at the stage of carnitine palmitoyltransferase I by the coenzyme A esters of some substituted hypoglycemic oxirane-2-carboxylic acids. *Biochem. Soc. Trans.* 9:574–75

129. Schmidt, F. H., Deaciuc, I. V., Kuhnle, H. F. 1985. A new inhibitor of the long-chain fatty acid transfer across the mitochondrial membrane: 2-(3-methylcinnamylhydrazono)-propionate (BM 42.304). *Life Sci.* 36:63–67

130. Venkatraghavan, V., Smith, D. J. 1983. Active-site-directed inhibition of carnitine acetyltransferase. *Arch. Biochem. Biophys.* 220:193–99

131. Thomitzek, W. D., Winter, H., Strack, E. 1966. Über den Einfluss von Carnitin auf den Azetylcholingehalt in Gehirn und Herzmuskel in vivo und auf die Azetylierung von Sulfanilamid in der Leber. *Acta Biol. Med. Ger.* 16:350–58

Ann. Rev. Pharmacol. Toxicol. 1987. 27:279–300

HEALTH EFFECTS OF EXPOSURE TO DIESEL EXHAUST PARTICLES[1]

Roger O. McClellan

Inhalation Toxicology Research Institute, Lovelace Biomedical and Environmental Research Institute, P. O. Box 5890, Albuquerque, New Mexico 87185

INTRODUCTION

The health effects of diesel exhaust (DE) have been a focus of intensive research during the last decade. Increased use of diesel engines in light-duty passenger cars and vans stimulated this research. These vehicles are used extensively in populated areas and thus could increase the exposure of urban residents to DE.

Diesel engine–powered vehicles emit more oxides of nitrogen and some 30 to 100 times more particles than do gasoline engines with contemporary emission-control devices. The small size of diesel exhaust particles (DEP) makes them readily respirable, which raises concern for their health effects. As early as 1955, Kotin et al (1) evaluated the chemical composition of diesel exhaust particle extracts (DEPE) and demonstrated their carcinogenicity in mouse-skin-painting studies. However, little additional research was done on DE until the mid-1970s, when advances in biology provided improved methods such as the Ames *Salmonella typhimurium* assay (2) for detecting mutagenicity and, potentially, carcinogenicity. In 1977 the US Environmental Protection Agency issued a precautionary notice (3) reporting that DEPE were mutagenic in bacterial assays. These findings were subsequently published by Huisingh et al (4). This observed mutagenicity triggered a major research effort on the health effects of DE. The results of this research have been the topic of several symposia and reviews (5–11), and are briefly reviewed in this article.

[1]The US Government has the right to retain a nonexclusive, royalty-free license in and to any copyright covering this paper.

279

PHYSICAL AND CHEMICAL CHARACTERISTICS

Shape, Size, and Surface Area

DEP are chain aggregates of very small, spherical primary particles. Under the microscope they appear as chains of beads or clusters of grapes. The aggregates have a mass median diameter of a few tenths of a micrometer, and the primary particles have a diameter of 10–80 nm (12, 13). The specific surface area of DEP is high and strongly dependent on the outgassing temperature, ranging from $\cong$ 10 m^2 per g at 25°C to $\cong$ 100 m^3 per g at 450°C (14). The high surface area indicates the potential for DEP to absorb large amounts of vapor-phase organic compounds.

Chemical Composition

The DEP consist primarily of carbon, hydrogen, oxygen, and nitrogen. They also contain trace quantities of sulfur, zinc, phosphorus, calcium, iron, silicon, and chromium, with nonextractable and extractable fractions (15). The nonextractable, or dry soot, fraction resembles carbon black. The extractable fraction (5–50%) is removed with solvents, such as dichloromethane or benzene ethanol, using ultrasonication or continuous (Soxhlet) extraction of DEP collected on filters. The relative amount of extractable vs nonextractable material depends upon factors including engine type and condition, fuel composition, and load (16). For some engines the carbon in DEPE originates primarily from the fuel, whereas in other cases the lubricating oil is a major source of the carbon (17).

The chemical composition of DEPE has been extensively investigated (18–20). Because of interest in the biological activity of DEPE, much of the characterization work has involved bioassay-directed chemical analysis aimed to identify specific chemical classes and compounds responsible for biological activity. This approach uses liquid chromatography or liquid–liquid separation procedures to fractionate the compounds according to chemical functional groups. High-pressure liquid chromatography may be used to separate the DEPE into nonpolar, moderately polar, and polar fractions. Most of the mass is in the nonpolar fraction, which includes aliphatic hydrocarbons, polycyclic aromatic hydrocarbons (PAH), and higher molecular weight, bridged, and methylated PAH. The moderately polar fraction contains PAH ketones, aldehydes, quinones, and acid anhydrides as well as hydroxy- and nitro-PAH. The polar fraction contains PAH carboxylic acids and other oxygenated PAH.

When assayed with *S. typhimurium* strain 98, most of the mutagenic activity is found in the moderately polar fraction, less in the polar fraction, and very little in the nonpolar fraction. DEP probably contains over 1000 compounds, more than 100 of which have been specifically identified. Nitroaromatic compounds, for example, are major contributors to the mutagenicity observed in the *S. typhimurium* assay in the absence of S-9, the liver enzyme fraction (21, 22). This observation has given impetus to their identification. Paputa-Peck et al (23) reported positive identification of 15, and tentative identification of 45, nitro-PAH, including naphthalenes, biphenyls, fluorenes, anthracenes, and pyrenes. Some investigators have suggested that a few individual compounds be considered "model compounds" to facilitate the study of exhaust and the development of quantitative measures of exposure and risk (19).

Pitts et al (24) observed that nitro-PAH could be formed during sampling of ambient air. This finding, and subsequent observations by Lee et al (25), triggered debate over the role of sampling artifacts in forming nitroaromatics during collection of DEP. Schuetzle (18) and Schuetzle & Perez (26) presented convincing evidence that little of the 1-nitropyrene measured in DEPE is formed during sampling; the majority of the nitro-PAH is formed in the engine and/or tailpipe.

SHORT-TERM IN VITRO AND ANIMAL STUDIES

Activity in Short-Term Bioassays

A number of papers on the effects of DEPE in short-term bioassays are included in recent symposia (7, 8, 11, 27). The review of Lewtas & Williams (27) is especially notable. It details the utility of a battery of assays in predicting carcinogenic potency. Assays in several strains of *S. typhimurium* suggest that the mutagens cause frameshift, but not base-substitution, mutations in the bacteria (4). The response occurred without an S-9 fraction, indicating that an exogenous source of promutagen activation was unnecessary. Indeed, with the exception of strain TA-1538 the response to DEPE was usually decreased by adding S-9 (28). Clark & Vigil (29) demonstrated that enzyme preparations from lung also decreased the mutagenicity of DEPE. They observed a similar decrease with serum and albumin, which suggested that the reduced effect might be due to nonspecific binding of direct mutagens. In some instances addition of liver S-9 increases the mutagenicity of DEPE, indicating the presence of compounds that act as promutagens. Pederson & Siak (30) found they could optimize culture conditions to observe mutagens requiring activation.

Lewtas (31) suggested using "revertants per mile" to compare mutagenic emission rates for vehicles. This approach led to the finding that diesel vehicles emit 45–800 times more mutagenic activity per mile than gasoline catalyst vehicles (32). Clark (16) summarized data obtained in a single laboratory for a number of vehicles, fuels, environmental conditions, and driving cycles, and found a range of between 2.4×10^5 and 19×10^5 revertants per mile. These data indicate the general similarity of mutagenic emission rates for different light-duty diesel vehicles. Schuetzle & Perez (26) have observed that as a class, heavy-duty diesels emit only slightly more solvent-extractable material than do light-duty engines.

In studies using nitroreductase-deficient bacteria, DEPE was less mutagenic than in customary tester strains such as TA-98 (33, 34). These results and chemical analyses provide strong evidence that reduced nitro-PAH compounds cause much of the mutagenicity observed in strain TA-98. Rosenkranz et al (35) and Mermelstein et al (36) reported the extraordinary responsiveness of some strains to the nitroarenes and noted both the utility and the need for caution in using nitroreductase-deficient strains to assay complex mixtures. Rosenkranz & Howard (37) reviewed the structural basis of the activity of nitrated PAH.

Mammalian cell mutagenicity assays can also be used to evaluate DEPE. Positive dose-related effects have been found using the L5178Y mouse lymphoma assay without adding liver S-9. The mutagenicity was variable when liver S-9 was added (38). Li (39) observed most cytotoxicity in Chinese hamster ovary (CHO) cells when the concentrations of sera in the media were lowest. Addition of sera, lung S-9, lung S-9 plus cofactors, liver S-9, or liver S-9 plus cofactors had a protective effect. Li & Royer (40) reported a small, but dose-dependent, mutagenic response in CHO cells that was enhanced with the addition of liver S-9. They also found a greater than additive effect on mutagenicity of benzo(a)pyrene [B(a)P] plus DEPE over that observed with either B(a)P or DEPE alone. A mutagenic response was also observed in CHO cells that had phagocytized DEP (41).

Thilly et al (42) reported positive mutagenic responses for DEPE evaluated in a human lymphoblast gene mutation assay. However, DEPE was mutagenic only when tested with metabolic activation. These authors calculated that a substantial portion of the observed mutagenicity could be caused by fluoranthene, 1-methylphenanthrene, and 9-methylphenanthrene. The cell-transforming capacity of DEPE was assayed in BALB/c 3T3 mouse embryo cells with variable results (43). The lack of a clear dose-response relationship may have been related to the solubility of the extracts in the test system.

Chromosomal damage has occurred in animals exposed to DEP or DEPE. Pereira (44) reported that exposure of Syrian hamsters to high levels of DEP for several months increased the frequency of sister-chromatid exchanges in primary cultures of lungs from exposed animals. Intratracheal instillation of either DEP or DEPE also caused more sister-chromatid exchanges. An increase in the sister-chromatid exchange frequency occurred in CHO cells exposed in vitro to DEPE (45). A clear dose-response relationship for induction of chromosome aberrations was noted in CHO cells exposed to a potent DEP extract.

Mouse-Skin Tumor Bioassay

Nesnow et al (46) reviewed the results of extensive tests measuring the tumorigenic and carcinogenic potentials of DEPE applied to the skin of SENCAR mice. These studies compared the mutagenicity of DEPE to that of gasoline engine exhaust, coke oven emissions, and roofing tar, and extended the early observations of Kotin et al (1) that DEPE caused skin tumors in Strain A mice. A spectrum of tumor-initiating capacities was observed for DEPE from different engines, ranging from an inactive sample from one heavy-duty engine to a highly active sample from one light-duty engine. Using a log probit model with correction for background, the samples were ranked: B(a)P > coke oven mains ≥ the most active DEPE samples = roofing tar. A nonlinear Poisson model with background correction for tumor multiplicity provided the following ranking: topside coke oven > most active DEPE ≥ roofing tar ≥ intermediate DEPE sample = gasoline exhaust sample. The roofing tar– and coke oven–derived materials were effective promoters, but the DEPE samples were not. Data from complete carcinogenesis experiments after one year did not show DEPE to be complete carcinogens. In contrast, the coke oven– and roofing tar–derived samples and B(a)P were effective, complete carcinogens.

Disposition of Inhaled Particles

McClellan et al (47) emphasized the importance of complementing the results of in vitro studies with data from studies of the intact animal. A first step in this direction is to determine where inhaled DEP and their constituents are deposited in the body. Wolff et al (48) determined the deposition of radiolabeled particles, similar in size to DEP, in dogs. For particles with a mass median diameter of 0.02 or 0.1 μm, they observed pulmonary deposition of 32% and 25%, respectively. These results are in general agreement with those of Chan & Lippmann (49), who observed that approximately 18% of inhaled 0.2-μm particles landed in the pulmonary region of human volunteers. For risk assessment purposes, one could consider that 25–35% of inhaled DEP will be deposited in the pulmonary region.

Data are not available on long-term retention of very small particles in humans. This lack is of concern, since relatively insoluble particles larger in size than DEP have a long residence time in the pulmonary region (50). In the absence of data on DEP in people, this article reviews the data obtained in laboratory animals, from which estimates of human retention can be made.

Chan et al (51) and Lee et al (52) reported that rats exposed briefly to ^{14}C-DEP clear some of the DEP within hours or days. A smaller fraction is cleared with a half-life of 60 to 80 days. Strom & Chan (53), using these data, developed a model to predict the long-term retention of DEP in the chronically exposed rat. The model under-predicted the retention of DEP beyond 20 weeks of exposure when the exposure concentration exceeded 250 μg DEP/ m^3 for 20 hr per day, 5.5 days per week. The lung burdens of DEP did not plateau as expected, but continued to increase as a function of exposure time and concentration. The authors interpreted the buildup of DEP as evidence of impaired clearance and sequestering of DEP in aggregates.

Wolff et al (54) reported similar findings. Rats exposed to 3500 or 7000 μg/m^3 of diesel soot particles for 7 hr per day, 5 days per wk for 2 years accumulated more particles than did rats exposed to 350 μg/m^3. When administered a radiolabeled test aerosol after 2 years of exposure to DE, the control and 350-μg/m^3 rats had long-term clearance half-lives of 80 days, whereas those of the rats receiving 3500 and 7000 μg/m^3 were extended to 280 and 260 days, respectively. In considering these results, the investigator should recognize that the rat normally clears particles faster than man (55). In the guinea pig, as a further example, most of the inhaled DEP are very tenaciously retained, with little clearance between 10 and 432 days (52). The impaired clearance in the rat actually results in retention half-lives approximating those normally seen in man. It is not known if chronic exposure of people to high levels of DEP would increase retention times of particulate material in man. Our present data indicate that inhaled DEP in people have a half-life of several hundred days or more.

Disposition of Organic Constituents

This article has focused on the retention of the carbonaceous core of DEP. Of equal interest is the fate of the organic constituents of the DEP in view of their chemical identity and the established biological activity of DEPE. In attempting to relate in vitro data to studies more relevant to the mammalian body, several investigators (56–59) extracted DEP with many biological fluids and found, in general, that the mutagenic activity of DEP was reduced. Studies with macrophages and DEP suggest that macrophages can decrease the mutagenic activity of DEP, an observation consistent with other studies demonstrating that macrophages can metabolize particle-associated PAH to nonmutagenic metabolites (60). These data suggest the macrophages and biological fluids have a protective effect that reduces the mutagenicity of DEP constituents.

Another approach to obtaining information on the interaction of DEP constituents with tissues is to study the fate of radiolabeled constituents of DEP such as B(a)P and nitropyrene. Sun et al (61) reviewed the literature on the disposition of inhaled particle–associated organic compounds. Sun et al (62) studied the retention of inhaled B(a)P adsorbed on the surface of DEP. There was an initial phase of rapid clearance from the respiratory tract, followed by a second phase of slower clearance. A substantial portion of the B(a)P and its metabolites were retained, with a long-term clearance half-life of 18 days. These investigators demonstrated that up to 20 days after inhalation, approximately two-thirds of the retained radiolabel was B(a)P, with the remainder identified as phenol and quinone metabolites. These results are similar to those previously reported by Henry and coworkers (63), who observed that following intratracheal instillation into Syrian hamster lungs, B(a)P coated on carbon particles was retained much longer in the lung than when it was coated on aluminum or ferric oxide particles or given as a pure compound. Different types of carrier particles, including carbon black, effectively enhance respiratory tract carcinogenesis by B(a)P (64).

The fate of 1-nitropyrene inhaled as a coating on DEP or as a homogeneous ultrafine aerosol of the pure compound has been studied (65, 66). The 1-nitropyrene associated with particles, and especially with DEP, enhanced the long-term retention of 1-nitropyrene in the respiratory tract. Substantially more nitropyrene was found in the liver and kidneys when the nitropyrenes were inhaled with DEP.

Effects of Chronic Exposure

RESPIRATORY TRACT CANCER   One of the ultimate concerns for exposure to DE is that it may result in lung cancer. The positive mutagenicity results in several assays and tumorigenicity in the mouse-skin assay with DEPE indicate the potential carcinogenicity of inhaled DEP. However, the positive results in these assays have generally been obtained under extraordinary conditions, i.e. with high concentrations of extracts obtained by treating DEP with strong organic solvents. This approach presents the biological system with a large quantity of test material in a very short period of time and bypasses many of the protective mechanisms encountered by inhaled DEP. To directly assay for carcinogenicity, Syrian hamsters, mice, and rats have been exposed to various dilutions of whole DE (11). In several studies, animals were also exposed to exhaust from which the particles had been removed, whereas in other studies, animals were administered known carcinogens and exposed to DE.

Studies with Syrian hamsters exposed to whole DE or particle-free DE have shown no tumor production (67–69). Recognizing the difficulty of detecting a potential small increase in neoplasia, Heinrich (68) pretreated some of the hamsters with a known carcinogen, diethylnitrosamine (DEN), and then exposed them to DE. Exposure to whole or particle-free DE did not produce respiratory tract tumors. With a high dose of DEN (4.5 mg/kg), a 45% baseline incidence of papillomas of larynx and trachea was observed, which increased to 66% and 70% with inhalation of particle-free and whole DE, respectively. The similarity of the response in both groups suggests that it may have been promoted by irritant gases in the exhaust. Takemoto et al (70) observed a greater than additive effect on lung tumor induction in F344 rats exposed to DE and treated with a known carcinogen, di-isopropanol-nitrosamine (DIPN), compared to those exposed only to DIPN or DE.

Studies with mice exposed to DE have given variable results. Kaplan et al (71) and Orthoefer et al (72) exposed Strain A mice, which normally have a high spontaneous incidence of lung adenomas, to DE. The lung tumor incidence in the DE-exposed mice was not increased above that of controls. Indeed, Orthoefer et al (72) reported a decreased incidence in the DE-exposed mice. Stoeber (69) exposed female NMRI mice to DE at a concentration of 4.0 mg/m^3 for up to 120 weeks (19 hr per day, 5 days per week), and found the incidence of adenocarcinomas in both whole-exhaust and particle-free exposed groups was significantly higher than that in controls. The incidence of adenomas was not affected. Takemoto et al (70) exposed C57BL/6N mice to DE at 2–4 mg/m^3 for 4 hr per day, 4 days per week, and observed an increased incidence of both adenomas and adenocarcinomas at 19–28 months.

In contrast to the negative or variable results observed in Syrian hamsters and mice, five laboratories have found a statistically significant increase in lung tumor incidence in rats chronically exposed to DE. Figure 1 is a compilation of the results of six major studies (69, 73–77) in which rats were exposed to DE. To aid in comparing the results of the several studies, the exposure conditions have been normalized and expressed as mg · hr/m^3 · week. For example, an exposure of 7.0 mg/m^3 for 7 hr per day, 5 days per week would be recorded as a 245 mg · hr/m^3 · week exposure. The studies used F344 rats, except for the study reported by Stoeber (69), which used Wistar rats. The investigators exposed the rats to DE for 24–30 months and typically observed them for 30 months. The exception was the study reported by White et al (73), which involved only 15 months of exposure and 8 months of recovery. The studies varied in other experimental details, i.e. engine type and operating conditions, fuel, and exposure duration. Nonetheless, the similarity of the results is striking. Lung tumor incidence clearly increased with exposures at high levels (> 100 mg · hr/m^3 · week) for 2 years or more.

The tumors were observed late in the studies. For example, Mauderly et al (75) identified 81% of their tumors after 24 months of exposure. The late occurrence of the tumors may account for Lewis et al (78) not observing an increase in lung tumors in rats exposed for 2 years to DE alone or in combination with coal dust. Likewise, this delayed incidence may explain the lack of a statistically significant increase in lung tumor incidence in the study reported by White et al (73).

Four types of tumors have been observed, all of which appear to have derived from epithelial cells (75–79). Bronchoalveolar adenomas were typi-cally small in size, were composed of cuboidal cells resembling Type II or Clara epithelial cells, and were not invasive. The adenocarcinomas observed

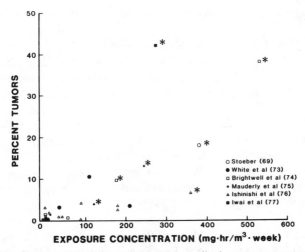

Figure 1 Lung tumor incidence in rats related to normalized exposure concentration of DE. Values marked with * differed from controls by statistical test.

were similar to the adenomas, but had central areas with hyperchromatic cells of nonuniform size arranged in irregular patterns. There were increased numbers of mitoses and invasion of adjacent vessels or interstitial connective tissue. Squamous cysts, composed of large keratin cores surrounded by well-differentiated uniform squamous epithelium, were frequently observed. Their malignant counterpart, squamous cell carcinomas, were similarly observed. The cells at the periphery of these carcinomas were less differentiated and the tumors were locally invasive. Metastasis to pulmonary lymph nodes or other organs was rare. The classification of the squamous lesions has been discussed by Mohr et al (79).

The pathogenesis of the tumors is not known at this time. It is tempting to speculate, based on the known mutagenicity of DEPE, that the tumors result from the organic compounds associated with the inhaled DEP. With rats from the Mauderly et al (75) study, Wong et al (80) observed increased numbers of adducts in DNA extracted from lungs of DE-exposed, as compared to control, rats. This observation lends support to a genetic mechanism for induction of the tumors.

Alternatively, Vostal (81) has suggested that the lung tumors in rats exposed to high levels of DE may be due to the overloading of the normal clearance mechanisms, accumulation of DEP, and nonmutational, epigenetic mechanisms of cancer induction. He further suggests a threshold relationship between administered or retained dose of DEP and lung tumor incidence. He notes that increased incidences of lung tumors also occur in rats exposed to high levels of shale dust, solvent-refined coal solids, titanium dioxide, titanium tetrachloride, and coal dusts, which are generally viewed as "nuisance" dusts.

At this time it is not possible to determine the relative role of genetic vs epignetic mechanisms in the initiation or promotion of lung tumors in the DE-exposed rats. Quite possibly, both mechanisms are involved in some complex interactive manner. Additional research should help clarify the situation. For example, it would be useful to assess the carcinogenicity of carbon black particles devoid of organic compounds and with various added amounts of selected organic compounds typically present in DEP. The rate of formation and repair of DNA adducts in DE-exposed animals should be determined both during the exposure period and following cessation of exposure. Finally, lung tumors in diesel-exposed animals should be evaluated for the presence of oncogenes.

NONCANCER ENDPOINTS   Many of the chronic exposure studies were designed to detect noncarcinogenic functional disorders as well as to assess the carcinogenicity of DE. The specific studies evaluated the deposition and clearance of DEP (as already noted), the pathological changes in lungs and associated lymph nodes, pulmonary function, clearance of particles, susceptibility to infectious agents, biochemical changes, and immunological alterations.

The pathological changes observed in the respiratory tracts of several laboratory animal species exposed to DE have been described (10, 59, 82). The major gross finding is an exposure concentration–related dark discoloration of the lungs and thoracic lymph nodes. Histologically, the number and size of alveolar macrophages increase. DEP are found in macrophages in alveoli, alveolar interstititium, peribronchial and perivascular interstititium, and lymphatic channels, in histocytes in the sinusoids of thoracic lymph nodes, in Type 1 epithelial cells, and in eosinphils. The Type 2 pneumocytes are increased in number and size in the alveoli that contain DEP-laden macrophages. At the highest levels, numbers of polymorphonuclear leukocytes also increase. The tissue response to DEP varies from no detectable changes to partial or complete obliteration of alveoli and replacement of them with fibrous connective tissue, which sometimes incorporates aggregates of DEP. There were foci of metaplastic epithelium in alveoli and terminal bronchioles.

Mauderly et al (83) reported a restrictive disorder of pulmonary function at the high levels of exposure to DE. This disorder included increased stiffness of the lung parenchyma and lower lung volumes, with reductions in total lung capacity and vital capacity per kg body weight. Intrapulmonary gas was distributed less uniformly, and alveolar gas exchange was impaired. Gross (84) reported similar trends in rats exposed to moderate levels of DE, although the changes were not statistically significant through 612 days of exposure. Pepelko (85) reported similar statistically significant functional changes in rats and Chinese hamsters exposed to high levels of DE for 6 months.

Campbell et al (86) observed that DE-exposed mice were more susceptible to experimentally induced infection with *Streptococcus pyogenes*. They suggested that this enhanced susceptibility may be caused by the NO_2 and acrolein vapor in the DE. The DE exposure did not enhance the mortality in response to influenza virus A/PR8-34 or *Salmonella typhimurium*.

Bice et al (87) reported exposure to DE affected pulmonary immunological function. They observed exposure concentration– and exposure time–related increases in the total number of cells in thoracic lymph nodes of rats and mice. These authors also noticed a trend toward increased numbers of IgM antibody–forming cells per 10^6 lymphoid cells after intratracheal instillation of particulate antigen in rats.

Henderson et al (88) reported alterations in the biochemical and cellular constituents recovered by lavage from airways of DE-exposed rats. The changes were consistent with an inflammatory response after 6 months of exposure to either 3.5 or 7.0 mg/m^3, but not with 0.35 mg/m^3, of DE. The changes persisted throughout the 30-month study.

EPIDEMIOLOGICAL STUDIES

A number of epidemiological studies have been conducted on DE-exposed populations. Although diesel engines have been used for many decades, their emissions are rapidly diluted, and relatively few individuals have been exposed to high concentrations of DE. Thus, populations with sufficient exposure and of appropriate size to warrant study are difficult to identify. In addition, because respiratory disease is of particular interest, the complications of exposure to other inhaled pollutants, and especially cigarette smoke, are important confounding variables (89). If the disease, or diseases, resulting from exposure to DE were unique, which they are not, the task would be much easier.

Four major populations exposed to DE have been studied: transportation workers, operators of heavy construction equipment, railroad workers, and miners. The most thoroughly evaluated set of data is that collected on the London Transit Authority Workers (90, 91). The overall annual lung cancer rate for the London Transit Authority Workers exposed to DE was 159 per 10^5, which was significantly lower than the corresponding rate of 202 per 10^5 for males in Greater London during the period of the study, 1950–1974. Harris (92, 93) analyzed these data using a linear exposure-effect relative risk model. This model assumes that the increased risk from exposure to DE is proportional to the average lifetime exposure to the concentration of DE in the air multiplied by the worker's normal risk. In his first analysis (92), he placed a quantitative limit on the probability that a carcinogenic risk had gone undetected. With this approach, he calculated the 95% upper confidence limit to be on the order of a 5×10^{-4} proportional increase in lung cancer incidence per unit of cumulative lifetime exposure, where one unit of exposure is equivalent to inhaling a concentration of 1 μg DEP/m^3 for one year. In his second analysis, Harris (93) compared the ratios of the observed cases to age-standardized expected cases for three job-grouping subpopulations. The observed-to-expected ratios for lung cancer for the three job groupings were ordered in relation to the degree of presumed exposure to DE. This order allowed the estimation of the maximum lung cancer risk to be 1.23×10^{-4} per unit of cumulative exposure. The original data set failed to show an effect of DE exposure on lung cancer incidence; however, the calculations serve to indicate the magnitude of a potential effect.

Wong et al (94) studied members of a heavy-construction-equipment operators union to evaluate the mortality of 34,156 male members between January 1, 1964 and December 31, 1978 for comparison with that of all white males in the United States. They observed that the standardized mortality ratio (SMR) for all causes of death was 81, which was significantly lower than the comparison population. The SMR for lung cancer was 99, with risk increasing with the interval between first exposure and death. The SMR for lung cancer was significantly increased for retirees; however, there was no association demonstrated between DE and lung cancer. Indeed, the SMR for lung cancer was lower for occupations believed to result in high DE exposures.

Hall & Wynder (95) reported a case-control study of lung cancer in which DE exposure was considered. They observed a strong association of lung cancer with cigarette smoking and a twofold increase in lung cancer for those exposed to DE when cigarette smoking was eliminated as a factor. When allowance was made for smoking, the difference for the DE-exposed cases was eliminated.

There have been three reports of case-control studies of bladder cancer that have considered DE exposure. These studies appear logical, considering the potential for urinary excretion of organic constituents of inhaled DE. Silverman et al (96) noted an increased risk of lower urinary tract cancer in truck drivers, with risk increasing with duration of employment. The relative risk for operators of diesel trucks was 11.9 times that of people who did not drive trucks. Some allowance was made for smoking in nontruck drivers, but not for the diesel drivers. In a second report, Silverman et al (97) noted truck drivers or delivery men had a 50% increase in risk of bladder cancer. Higher risks were also reported for bus and taxi cab drivers. Hoar & Hoover (98) reported a 50% increased risk of bladder cancers in truck drivers, which was inconsistently associated with duration of driving and was higher in drivers reported to have been exposed to DE. Hoar & Hoover (98) reported taking allowance for cigarette smoking and coffee drinking. Wynder et al (99) found an increased risk of bladder cancer in individuals having high exposure to DE in the absence of allowance for cigarette smoking, which was independently shown to result in an excess risk of bladder cancer. When allowance was made for smoking in the DE-exposed cases, the excess of lung cancer was eliminated.

The importance of considering multiple confounding factors in interpreting cancer epidemiology studies has been emphasized by Wynder & Higgins (89). They documented the unusual cigarette smoking and dietary fat intake of truck drivers. They are not convinced that the excess risk of bladder cancer reported by others is due to DE exposure or, indeed, even to occupation.

Kaplan (100), studying the cause of death of 6,506 US railroad workers, found no association between exposures to DE and lung cancer deaths. However, only 154 cases of lung cancer were recorded in the population, and diesel locomotives did not exceed 50% of all Class I locomotives in the United States until 1952 (101). Thus, Kaplan's population had been exposed to DE for a relatively short time. Howe et al (102) reported on a cohort study of 43,826 male pensioners of the Canadian National Railway Company. They observed highly significant exposure-response relationships for elevated risk of lung cancer in individuals employed in occupations involving exposure to DE and coal dust. The relative risk of those possibly exposed or probably exposed to DE were 1.20 and 1.35, respectively. Almost identical values were observed for coal dust exposures. The authors were not able to determine the role of the possible confounding effects of coal dust and asbestos exposure and of smoking. The study did not report quantitative information on duration or levels of exposure to DE. Such information is essential for deriving quantitative risk estimates for exposure to DE.

Schenker & Speizer (101) are making a large retrospective cohort study of approximately 80,000 railroad workers in the United States. In addition, they are conducting a case-control study of 300 incident lung cancer cases and matched controls in railroad workers and monitoring the environment in an attempt to quantitate exposures to DE. In a preliminary report Schenker et al (103) noted the SMR for the railroad workers compared to the US national rates was 87 for all causes of death and 85 for lung cancer. The relative risk of those exposed to DE compared to those not exposed was 1.42 ± 0.50. The low and high risk of lung cancer for DE exposure was 1.50 and 2.77, respectively. These data are suggestive of a DE exposure effect, however, they were not corrected for cigarette smoking. Garschick et al (104), studying the same population, has reported an exposure time-related increase in the relative risk for lung cancer among workers exposed to DE as compared to cohorts with little exposure.

Waxweiler et al (105) studied potash workers and found no significant mortality differences between DE-exposed and nonexposed miners. The population size was not large, and the 24 years of maximum diesel exposure was not great. Wheeler et al (106) reported on exposure data obtained in dieselized coal mines as part of a five-year effort initiated by the US National Institute of Occupational Safety and Health to study health implications of diesel engine use in coal mines.

ESTIMATING RISK OF LUNG CANCER

A major objective of the research on DE emissions has been to establish quantitative estimates of the potential health risks of exposure of people to DE. Three approaches (Table 1) have been taken based on (a) epidemiological observations of persons exposed to DE, (b) comparative potency studies, and (c) observations of lung tumors in rats. The approach using epidemiological data was reviewed earlier (107). The comparative potency approach uses information from epidemiological studies of known human respiratory tract carcinogens (coke oven emissions, roofing tar, and cigarette smoke) in combination with bioassay data on these same materials and DEPE (27, 108, 109). This approach assumes that the materials have the same basic mechanisms of action. The third approach, which uses data on lung tumor induction in rats, assumes that the mechanisms by which the lung tumors were produced in rats exposed to high levels of DE are operative in people exposed to low levels of DE. The value reported (109) was derived using the rat tumor data of Mauderly et al (75). To facilitate comparisons among the risk estimators (Table 1), these studies have all been applied to a common base, namely a population of 230×10^6 persons with an average life span of 70 years, annual deaths from lung cancer of 1×10^5, and continuous exposure to 1 μg of DEP/m^3.

The 1 μg/m^3 level of exposure approximates the average calculated to occur if 20% of the light-duty vehicles in the United States in 1995 were diesel powered and emitted 0.12 g DEP/km (107). In aggregate, this emission would represent 60,000 metric tons of DEP per year. Although the average exposure would approach 1 μg/m^3 in the projected scenario, individual exposures would vary greatly, e.g. parking garages would contain a DE concentration of 80 μg/m^3; typical metropolitan street canyons, 10 μg/m^3; cities, 0.5 μg/m^3; and rural areas, 0.05 μg/m^3. It now appears very unlikely that the use of light-duty diesel vehicles will even approach the 20% level in the United States. Nonetheless, the approach used is illustrative of the use of

Table 1 Comparison of lung cancer risk estimates for DE exposure[a]

Approach	Reference	Risk model	Risk estimator	Lung cancer (cases/yr)
Epidemiological data on diesel exhaust exposure	(92)	Proportional	$\dfrac{5 \times 10^{-4} \text{ increased lifetime risk}}{\mu g/m^3 \text{ for 1 yr}}$	3500
Epidemiological data on diesel exhaust exposure	(93)	Proportional	$\dfrac{1.23 \times 10^{-4} \text{ increased lifetime risk}}{\mu g/m^3 \text{ for 1 yr}}$	860
Comparative Potency	(93)	Proportional	$\dfrac{0.35 \times 10^{-4} \text{ increased lifetime risk}}{\mu g/m^3 \text{ for 1 yr}}$	245
Comparative Potency	(107)	Absolute	$\dfrac{0.3 \times 10^{-4} \text{ lifetime risk}}{\mu g/m^3}$	100
Comparative Potency	(108)	Absolute	$\dfrac{0.1 \text{ case/yr}/10^5 \text{ person}}{\mu g/m^3}$	230
Rat lung tumor data	(109)	Absolute	$\dfrac{0.12 \times 10^{-4} \text{ lifetime risk}}{\mu g/m^3}$	40

[a]See text for underlying assumptions.

risk assessment methodology combining quantitative risk estimators with estimates of exposure to assess risk to a population (9, 107).

In considering the calculated risks, it is appropriate to keep several points in mind. First, the range of the risk estimates is indicative of our current lack of certainty regarding human carcinogenic risks of DE exposure. Second, this range includes recognition that our current level of knowledge does not exclude the possibility that no cancers are attributable to low-level exposures to DE. Third, several of the estimates are based on proportional risk models. These models assume that the added risks occur primarily in the population with the highest base incidence, i.e. cigarette smokers. Fourth, to place the potential risks in perspective, it is currently estimated that in the United States approximately 100,000 lung cancer deaths occur per year in smokers and an additional 10,000 lung cancer deaths occur per year in nonsmokers.

SUMMARY

Diesel-powered vehicles emit substantially more particles than do gasoline-powered vehicles with contemporary emission control systems. The DEP are submicron in size and readily inhaled. Approximately one-fourth of the particle mass inhaled by people is deposited in the pulmonary region, some of which is retained with a half-life of several hundred days. In animal studies, exposure to high levels of DEP overwhelms the normal clearance mechanisms and results in lung burdens of DEP that exceed those predicted from observations at lower exposure concentrations.

A variable amount of the mass of DEP is extractable with strong organic solvents. The extracted material contains more than a thousand individual compounds and is mutagenic in a number of bacterial and mammalian cell assays. Bioassay-directed chemical analysis of DEP has identified several hundred compounds. Many are PAHs, some of which are considered to have human carcinogenic potential. A number of nitrated compounds have been identified that account for a significant portion of the mutagenicity assayed in bacteria. The mutagenicity of the DEPE is generally reduced by addition of an S-9 cellular fraction or of serum proteins. Macrophages rapidly reduce the recoverable mutagenic activity associated with DEP. These findings support a hypothesis that detoxification of DEP-associated organics occurs rapidly in vivo. The association of benzo(a)pyrene and nitropyrene with DEP prolongs their retention in the lungs. This increased retention suggests the need to clarify the relative importance of competing mechanisms that detoxify particle-associated compounds and those that serve to enhance the retention of toxicologically important compounds.

Some extracts of DEP evoke tumorigenic responses in skin-tumor bioassays, suggesting their carcinogenic potential in mammals. A number of large-scale studies have been conducted with laboratory rodents to evaluate the effects of chronic inhalation exposure to DE. An increased incidence of lung tumors, some of which were diagnosed as malignant, was observed in 5 studies with rats following exposure for 2 or more years to high levels of DE. Most of the lung tumors were observed after 2 years. Similar studies in Syrian hamsters have yielded negative results. Studies with mice have given mixed results. The results of some studies with laboratory animals exposed to DE and known carcinogens suggest that exposure to DE enhances the effect of the known carcinogens. The specific mechanisms of tumor induction in the DE-exposed rats are unknown. Hypotheses and experimental data have been advanced in support of both genetic and epigenetic mechanisms of action of the DE. Clarification of this issue has important implications in considering the use of the rat data for estimating the risk to people of low-level exposure to DE.

A number of epidemiological studies have been conducted to evaluate the risk of lung or bladder cancer in people exposed to DE. Analyzing these studies has been made difficult by the relatively low DE exposure of people and the substantial impact of confounding factors such as cigarette smoking. Taken in aggregate, the epidemiological evidence for DE exposure inducing lung or bladder cancer is negative or, at most, only suggestive of an effect.

The risk of lung cancer in humans from chronic exposure to DE has been estimated using (a) epidemiological data, (b) a comparative potency approach, and (c) tumor data from rats chronically exposed to DE. Applying the various risk estimators to the US population of 230×10^6 persons, and assuming exposure to 1 μg of DEP/m^3 of air for 70 year yields, estimates 40, 100, 230, 245, 860, or 3500 lung cancers per year in excess of the more than 10^5 lung cancer cases per year expected from other causes, principally smoking.

If 20% of the light-duty vehicles in the United States were to be diesel powered and to emit 0.12 g/km, total DEP emissions would be 60,000 metric tons per year. This amount would result in average rural exposures of 0.05 μg/m^3, urban exposures of 0.5 μg/m^3, and some situations with exposure of > 5 μg/m^3. The corresponding excess lung cancer risk is estimated to be fewer than 200 deaths per year; however, our current knowledge does not exclude the possibility that no lung cancer deaths could be attributed to low-level DE exposure.

ACKNOWLEDGMENTS

This work was performed for the Office of Health and Environmental Research, US Department of Energy, under Contract No. DE-AC0476EV01013. Grateful acknowledgment is made of the contributions of the many individuals whose research has resulted in a major increase in our knowledge of the health effects of DE in a remarkably short period of time. I especially appreciate the assistance given by my colleagues at the Inhalation Toxicology Research Institute in conducting portions of the work reported herein and in offering helpful suggestions.

Literature Cited

1. Kotin, P., Falk, H. L., Thomas, M. 1955. Aromatic hydrocarbons III. Presence in the particulate phase of diesel-engine exhausts and the carcinogenicity of exhaust extracts. *Arch. Ind. Health* 11:113–20
2. Ames, B. N., McCann, J., Yamaseki, E. 1975. Methods for detecting carcinogens as mutagens with the *Salmonella*/mammalian microsome mutagenicity test, *Mutat. Res.* 31:347–64
3. US Environmental Protection Agency. 1977. Precautionary notice on laboratory handling of exhaust products from diesel engines, USEPA Office Res. Dev., Washington, DC
4. Huisingh, J., Bradow, R., Jungers, R., Claxton, L., Zweidinger, R. 1978. Application of bioassay to the characterization of diesel particle emissions. In *Application of Short-Term Bioassay in the Fractionation and Analysis of Complex Environmental Mixtures* ed. M. D. Waters, S. Nesnow, J. L. Huisingh, S. S. Sandhu, L. Claxton, pp. 381–418. New York: Plenum
5. Pepelko, W. E., Danner, R. M., Clarke, N. A., eds. 1980. *Health Effects of Diesel Engine Emissions,* Vols. 1 and 2, Cincinnati, Ohio: US Environ. Protection Agency
6. National Research Council, National Academy of Science Health. *Effects of Exposure to Diesel Exhaust.* 1981. *Rep. Health Effects Panel Diesel Impacts Study Committee,* Washington, DC: Natl. Acad. Press
7. Lewtas, J., ed. 1982. *Toxicological Effects of Emissions from Diesel Engines,* New York: Elsevier Biomedical. 380 pp.
8. Holmberg, B., Ahlborg, U., eds. 1983. Symposium on biological tests in the evaluation of mutagenicity and carcinogenicity of air pollutants with special reference to motor exhausts and coal combustion products, *Environ. Health Perspect.* 47:1–341
9. McClellan, R. O. 1986. Health effects of diesel exhaust: A case study in risk assessment. *Am. Ind. Hyg. Assoc.* 47:1–13
10. McClellan, R. O., Bice, D. E., Cud-
dihy, R. G., Gillett, N. A., Henderson, R. F., et al. 1987. Health effects of diesel exhaust. In *Aerosols,* ed. S. D. Lee, T. Schneider, L. D. Grant, P. J. Verkerk, Chelsea, Mich: Lewis. In press
11. Ishinishi, N., Koizumi, A., McClellan, R. O., Stoeber, W., eds. 1986. *Carcinogenicity and Mutagenicity of Diesel Engine Exhaust* Amsterdam: Elsevier.
12. Carpenter, K., Johnson, J. H. 1979. Analysis of the physical characteristics of diesel particulate matter using transmission electron microscope techniques, *SAE Trans.* 88:2743
13. Cheng, Y. S., Yeh, H. C., Mauderly, J. L., Mokler, B. V. 1984. Characterization of diesel exhaust in a chronic inhalation study. *Am. Ind. Hyg. Assoc. J.* 45:547–55
14. Rothenberg, S., Kittelson, D. B., Cheng, Y. S., McClellan, R. O. 1985. Adsorption of nitrogen and xylene by light duty diesel exhaust samples. *Aerosol Sci. Technol.* 4:383–400
15. Williams, R. L., Chock, D. P. 1980. Characterization of diesel particulate exposure, See Ref. 5, pp. 3–33
16. Clark, C. R. 1982. Mutagenicity of diesel exhaust particle extracts, *DOE Research and Development Report, LMF-96.* Springfield: Natl. Tech. Inf. Service
17. Black, F., High, L. 1979. Methodology for determining particulate and gaseous diesel hydrocarbon emissions, *SAE Paper 790422*
18. Schuetzle, D. 1983. Sampling of vehicle emissions for chemical analysis and biological testing. *Environ. Health Perspect.* 47:65–80
19. Schuetzle, D., Frazier, J. A. 1986. Factors influencing the emission of vapor and particulate phase components from diesel engines, See Ref. 11, pp. 41–64
20. Schuetzle, D., Lewtas, J. 1987. Bioassay directed chemical analysis in environmental research. *Anal. Chem.* In press
21. Pederson, T. C., Siak, J.-S. 1981. The role of nitroaromatic compounds in the direct-acting mutagenicity of diesel par-

ticulate extracts. *J. Appl. Toxicol.* 1:54–60

22. Schuetzle, D., Lee, F. S. C., Prater, T. J., Tejada, S. B. 1981. The identification of polynuclear aromatic (PAH) derivatives in mutagenic fractions of diesel particulate extracts. *Int. J. Environ. Anal. Chem.* 9:93–144

23. Paputa-Peck, M. C., Marano, R. S., Schuetzle, D., Riley, T. L., Hampton, C. V., et al. 1983. Determination of nitrated polynuclear aromatic hydrocarbons (Nitro-PAH) in particulate extracts using capillary column GC/nitrogen selective detection. *Anal. Chem.* 55:1946–54

24. Pitts, J. N. Jr., van Cauwenberghe, K. A., Grosjean, D., Schmid, J. P., Fitz, D. R., et al. 1978. Atmospheric reactions of polycyclic aromatic hydrocarbons: Facile formation of mutagenic nitro Derivatives, *Science* 202:515–19

25. Lee, F. S. C., Harvey, T. M., Prater, T. J., Paputa, M. C., Schuetzle, D. 1981. Chemical analysis of diesel particulate matter and an evaluation of artifact formation. In *Proc. ASTM Symp. Sampling and Analysis of Toxic Organics in Source-Related Atmospheres,* pp. 92–110. Am. Soc. Test. Mat.

26. Schuetzle, D., Perez, J. 1983. Factors influencing the emissions of nitrated polynuclear aromatic hydrocarbons (nitro-PAH) from diesel engines. *J. Air Pollution Control Assoc.* 33:751–55

27. Lewtas, J., Williams, K. 1986. A retrospective view of the value of short-term genetic bioassays in predicting the chronic effects of diesel soot. See Ref. 11, pp. 119–40

28. Claxton, L. D. 1983. Characterization of automotive emissions by bacterial mutagenesis bioassay: A review. *Environ. Mutagen* 5:609–31

29. Clark, C. R., Vigil, C. L. 1980. Influence of rat lung and liver homogenates in the mutagenicity of diesel exhaust particulate extracts. *Toxicol. Appl. Pharmacol.* 56:110–15

30. Pederson, T. C., Siak, J.-S. 1981. The activation of mutagens in diesel particle extract with rat liver S-9 enzymes, *J. Appl. Toxicol.* 1:61–66

31. Lewtas, J. 1983. Evaluation of the mutagenicity and carcinogenicity of motor vehicle emissions by use of short-term assays, *Environ. Health Perspect.* 47:141–52

32. Claxton, L. D., Kohan, M. 1981. Bacterial mutagenesis and the evaluation of mobile-source emissions. In *Short-Term Bioassays in the Analysis of Complex Environmental Mixtures,* ed. M. D. Waters, S. Sandhu, J. L. Huisingh, L. Claxton, S. Nesnow, pp. 299–318. New York: Plenum

33. Salmeen, I., Durisin, A. M., Prater, T. J., Riley, T., Schuetzle, D. 1982. Contributions of 1-nitropyrene to direct acting Ames mutagenicity of diesel particulate extracts. *Mutat. Res.* 104:17–23

34. Claxton, L. D. 1982. The utility of bacterial mutagenesis testing in the characterization of mobile source emissions: A review. See Ref. 7, pp. 69–82

35. Rosenkranz, H. S., McCoy, E. C., Mermelstein, R., Speck, W. T. 1981. A cautionary note on the use of nitroreductase-deficient strains of *Salmonella typhimurium* for the detection of nitroarenes as mutagens in complex mixtures including diesel exhausts. *Mutat. Res.* 91:102–5

36. Mermelstein, R., Kiriazides, D. K., Butler, M., McCoy, E. C., Rosenkranz, H. S. 1981. The extraordinary mutagenicity of nitropyrenes in bacteria. *Mutat. Res.* 89:187–96

37. Rosenkranz, H. A., Howard, P. C. 1986. Structural basis of the activity of nitrated polycyclic aromatic hydrocarbons. See Ref. 11, pp. 141–70

38. Mitchell, A. D., Evans, E. L., Jotz, M. M., Riccio, E. S., Mortelmans, K. E., Simmon, V. 1980. Mutagenic and carcinogenic potency of extracts of diesel and related environmental emissions: in vitro mutagenesis and DNA damage, See Ref. 5, pp. 810–42

39. Li, A. P. 1981. Antagonistic effects of animal sera, lung and liver cytosols and sulfhydryl compounds on the cytotoxicity of diesel exhaust particle extracts. *Toxicol. Appl. Pharmacol.* 57:55–62

40. Li, A. P., Royer, R. E. 1982. Diesel exhaust particle extract enhancement of chemical-induced mutagenesis in cultured chinese hamster ovary cells: Possible interaction of diesel exhaust with environmental carcinogens. *Mutat. Res.* 103:349–55

41. Chescheir, G. M., Garrett, N. E., Shelburne, J. D., Lewtas, J., Huisingh, J., Waters, M. D. 1981. Mutagenic effects of environmental particulates in the CHO/HGPRT system. See Ref. 32, pp. 337–50

42. Thilly, W. G., Longwell, J., Andon, B. M. 1983. A general approach to the biological analysis of complex mixtures in combustion effluents. *Environ. Health Perspect.* 48:129–36

43. Curren, R. D., Kouri, R. E., Kim, C. M., Schechtman, L. M. 1980. Mutagen-

ic and carcinogenic potency of extracts from diesel related environmental emissions: Simultaneous morphological transformation and mutagenesis in BALB/c 3T3 Cells. See Ref. 5, pp. 861–73

44. Pereira, M. A. 1982. Genotoxicity of diesel exhaust emissions in laboratory animals. See Ref. 7, pp. 265–76

45. Li, A. P., Brooks, A. L., Clark, C. R., Shimizu, R. W., Hanson, R. L., Dutcher, J. S. 1983. Mutagenicity testing of complex environmental mixtures with Chinese hamster ovary cells. In *Short-Term Bioassays in the Analysis of Complex Environmental Mixtures III,* ed. M. D. Waters, S. Sandhu, J. Lewtas, L. Claxton, N. Chernoff, S. Nesnow, pp. 183–96. New York: Plenum

46. Nesnow, S., Triplett, L. L., Slaga, T. J. 1983. Mouse skin tumor initiation—promotion and complete carcinogenesis bioassays: Mechanisms and biological activities of emission samples. *Environ. Health Perspect.* 47:255–68

47. McClellan, R. O., Brooks, A. L., Cuddihy, R. G., Jones, R. K., Mauderly, J. L., Wolff, R. K. 1982. Inhalation toxicology of diesel exhaust particles. See Ref. 7, pp 99–120

48. Wolff, R. K., Kanapilly, G. M., DeNee, P. B., McClellan, R. O. 1981. Deposition of 0.1 μm chain aggregate aerosols in beagle dogs. *J. Aerosol Sci.* 12:119–29

49. Chan, T. L., Lippmann, M. 1980. Experimental measurements and empirical modelling of the regional deposition of inhaled particles in humans. *Am. Ind. Hyg. Assoc. J.* 41:399–409

50. Bailey, M. R., Fry, F. A., James, A. C. 1982. The long-term clearance kinetics of insoluble particles from the human lung. *Ann. Occup. Hyg.* 26:273–90

51. Chan, T. L., Lee, P. S., Hering, W. E. 1981. Deposition and clearance of inhaled diesel exhaust particles in the respiratory tract of Fischer rats. *J. Appl. Toxicol.* 1:77–82

52. Lee, P. S., Chan, T. L., Hering, W. E. 1983. Long-term clearance of inhaled diesel exhaust particles in rodents. *J. Toxicol. Environ. Health* 12:801–13

53. Strom, K. A., Chan, T. L. 1987. Pulmonary retention of inhaled submicron particles in rats: Diesel exhaust exposures and lung retention model. In *Proc. 6th Int. Symp. Inhaled Particles,* ed. W. Walton, Oxford: Pergamon. In press

54. Wolff, R. K., Henderson, R. F., Snipes, M. B., Sun, J. D., Bond, J. A., et al. 1986. See Ref. 11, pp. 199–212

55. Snipes, M. G., Boecker, B. B., McClellan, R. O. 1983. Retention of monodisperse or polydisperse aluminosilicate particles inhaled by dogs, rats and mice. *Toxicol. Appl. Pharmacol.* 69:345–62

56. Brooks, A. L., Wolff, R. K., Royer, R. E., Clark, C. R., Sanchez, A., McClellan, R. O. 1981. Deposition and biological availability of diesel particles and their associated mutagenic chemicals. *Environ. Int.* 5:263–67

57. Siak, J.-S., Chan, T. L., Lee, P. S. 1980. Diesel particle extracts in bacterial test systems. See Ref. 5, pp. 245–62

58. King, L. C., Kohan, M. J., Austin, A. C., Claxton, L. D., Huisingh, J. L. 1981. Evaluation of the release of mutagens from diesel particles in the presence of physiological fluids. *Environ. Mutagen* 3:109–21

59. Vostal, J. J., White, H. J., Strom, K. A., Siak, J. S., Chen, K. C., Dziedzic, D. 1982. Response of the pulmonary defense system to diesel particulate exposure. See Ref. 7, pp. 201–24

60. Bond, J. A., Butler, M. M., Medinsky, M. A., Muggenburg, B. A., McClellan, R. O. 1984. Dog pulmonary macrophage metabolism of free and particle-associated [^{14}C]benzo[a]pyrene. *J. Toxicol. Environ. Health* 14:181–89

61. Sun, J. D., Bond, J. A., Dahl, A. R. 1987. Particle-associated organic constituents. In *Air Pollution and Health,* ed. R. R. Bates, A. Y. Watson, D. Kennedy. In press

62. Sun, J. D., Wolff, R. K., Kanapilly, G. M., McClellan, R. O. 1983. Lung retention and metabolic fate of inhaled benzo(a)pyrene associated with diesel exhaust particles. *Toxicol. Appl. Pharmacol.* 73:48–59

63. Henry, M. C., Port, C. D., Kaufman, D. G. 1975. Importance of physical properties of benzo(a)pyrene—Ferric oxide mixture in lung tumor induction. *Cancer Res.* 35:207–17

64. Stenbäck, F., Rowland, J., Sellakumar, A. 1976. Carcinogenicity of benzo(a)pyrene and dusts in the hamster lung instilled intratracheally with titanium oxide, aluminum oxide, carbon and ferric oxide. *Oncology* 33:29–34

65. Sun, J. D., Wolff, R. K., Aberman, H. M., McClellan, R. O. 1983. Inhalation of 1-nitropyrene associated with ultrafine insoluble particles and as a pure aerosol: A comparison of deposition and biological fate. *Toxicol. Appl. Pharmacol.* 69:185–98

66. Bond, J. A., Sun, J. D., Medinsky, M. A., Jones, R. K., Yeh, H. C. 1986.

Deposition, metabolism and excretion of ^{14}C-1-nitropyrene and ^{14}C-1-nitropyrene coated on diesel exhaust particles as influenced by exposure concentration. *Toxicol. Appl. Pharmacol.* 85:102–17

67. Cross, F. T., Palmer, R. K., Filipy, R. E., Busch, R. H., Stuart, B. O. 1978. Study of the combined effects of smoking and inhalation of uranium ore dust, radon daughters and diesel oil exhaust fumes in hamsters and dogs. *Pac. Northwest Lab. Rep. 2744*

68. Heinrich, U., Peters, L., Funcke, W., Pott, F., Mohr, U., Stober, W. 1982. Investigation of toxic and carcinogenic effects of diesel exhaust in long-term inhalation exposure of rodents. See Ref. 7, pp. 225–42

69. Stoeber, W. 1986. Experimental induction of tumors in hamsters, mice and rats after long-term inhalation of filtered and unfiltered diesel engine exhaust. See Ref. 11, pp. 421–40

70. Takemoto, K., Yoshimura, H., Katayama, H. 1987. Effects of chronic inhalation exposure to diesel exhaust on the development of lung tumors in diisopropaneol-nitrosamine-treated F344 rats and newborn C57BL and ICR mice, See Ref. 11. In press

71. Kaplan, H. L., Springer, K. J., MacKenzie, W. F. 1983. Studies of potential health effects of long-term exposure to diesel exhaust emissions. *Final Rep. No. 01-0750-103 (SWRI) and No. 1239 (SFRE)*, pp. 1–59. San Antonio, Texas: Southw. Res. Inst.

72. Orthoefer, J. G., Moore, W., Kraemer, D., Truman, F., Crocker, W., Yang, Y. Y. 1980. Carcinogenicity of diesel exhaust as tested in strain "A" mice. See Ref. 5, pp. 1048–72

73. White, H., Vostal, J. J., Kaplan, H. L., MacKenzie, W. F. 1983. A long-term inhalation study evaluates the pulmonary effects of diesel emissions. *J. Appl. Toxicol.* 3:332

74. Brightwell, J., Fouillet, X., Cassano-Zoppi, A.-L., Gatz, R., Duchosal, F. 1986. Neoplastic and functional changes in rodents after chronic inhalation of engine exhaust emissions. See Ref. 11, pp. 471–88

75. Mauderly, J. L., Jones, R. K., McClellan, R. O., Henderson, R. F., Griffith, W. C. 1986. Carcinogenicity of diesel exhaust inhaled chronically by rats. See Ref. 11, pp. 397–410

76. Ishinishi, N., Kuwabara, N., Nagase, S., Suzuki, T., Ishiwata, S., Kohno, T. 1986. Long-term inhalation studies on effects of exhaust from heavy and light

duty diesel engines on F344 rats. See Ref. 11, pp. 329–48

77. Iwai, K., Udagawa, T., Yamagishi, M., Yamada, H. 1986. Long-term inhalation studies of diesel exhaust on F344 SFP rats: Incidence of lung cancer and lymphoma. See Ref. 11, pp. 349–60

78. Lewis, T. R., Green, F. H. Y., Moorman, W. J., Burg, J. A. R., Lynch, D. W. 1986. A chronic inhalation toxicity study of diesel engine emissions and coal dust, alone and combined. See Ref. 11, pp. 361–80

79. Mohr, U., Takenaka, S., Dungworth, D. L. 1986. Morphologic effects of inhaled diesel engine exhaust on lungs of rats: Comparison with effects of coal oven flue gas mixed with pyrolyzed pitch. See Ref. 11, pp. 459–70

80. Wong, D., Mitchell, C. E., Wolff, R. K., Mauderly, J. L., Jeffrey, A. M. 1987. Identification of DNA damage as a result of exposure of rats to diesel engine exhaust. *Carcinogenesis* In press

81. Vostal, J. J. 1986. Factors limiting the evidence for chemical carcinogenicity of diesel emissions in long-term inhalation experiments. See Ref. 11, pp. 381–96

82. White, H. J., Garg, B. D. 1981. Early pulmonary response of the rat lung to inhalation of high concentration of diesel particles. *J. Appl. Toxicol.* 1:104–10

83. Mauderly, J. L., Gillett, N. A., Henderson, R. F., Jones, R. K., McClellan, R. O. 1987. Relationship of lung structural and functional changes to accumulation of diesel exhaust particles. See Ref. 53. In press

84. Gross, K. B. 1981. Pulmonary function testing of animals chronically exposed to diluted diesel exhaust. *J. Appl. Toxicol.* 1:116–23

85. Pepelko, W. E. 1982. EPA studies on the toxicological effects of inhaled diesel engine emissions. See Ref. 7, pp. 121–42

86. Campbell, K. I., George, E. L., Washington, I. S. Jr. 1980. Enhanced susceptibility to infection in mice after exposure to dilute exhaust from light-duty diesel engines. See Ref. 5, pp. 772–85

87. Bice, D. E., Mauderly, J. L., Jones, R. K., McClellan, R. O. 1985. Effect of inhaled diesel exhaust on immune response after lung immunization. *Fund. Appl. Toxicol.* 5:1075–86

88. Henderson, R. F., Sun, J. D., Jones, R. K., Mauderly, J. L., McClellan, R. O. 1983. Biochemical and cytological response in airways of rodents exposed in life span studies to diesel exhaust. *Am. Rev. Resp. Dis.* 127:164 (Suppl.)

300   McCLELLAN

89. Wynder, E. L., Higgins, I. T. T. 1986. Exposure to diesel exhaust emissions and the risk of lung and bladder cancer. See Ref. 11, pp. 489–504
90. Raffle, P. 1957. The health of the worker. *Br. J. Ind. Med.* 14:73–80
91. Waller, R. 1980. Trends in lung cancer in London in relation to exposure to diesel fumes. See Ref. 5, pp 1085–97
92. Harris, J. E. 1981. Potential risk of lung cancer from diesel engine emissions. Washington, DC: Natl. Acad. Press. 62 pp.
93. Harris, J. E. 1983. Diesel emissions and lung cancer. *Risk Anal.* 3:83–100
94. Wong, O., Morgan, R. W., Keifets, L., Larson, S. R., Whorton, M. D. 1985. Mortality among members of a construction equipment operators union with potential exposure to diesel exhaust emissions. *Br. J. Ind. Med.* 42:435–48
95. Hall, N. E. L., Wynder, E. L. 1984. Diesel exhaust exposure and lung cancer: A case-control study. *Environ. Res.* 34:77–86
96. Silverman, D. T., Hoover, R. N., Albert, S., Graff, K. M. 1983. Occupation and cancer of the lower urinary tract in Detroit. *J. Natl. Cancer Inst.* 70:237–45
97. Silverman, D. T., Hoover, R. N., Mason, T. J., Swanson, G. M. 1986. Motor exhaust-related occupations and bladder cancer. *Cancer Res.* 46:2113–16
98. Hoar, S. K., Hoover, R. 1985. Truck driving and bladder cancer mortality in rural New England. *J. Natl. Cancer Inst.* 74:771–74
99. Wynder, E. L., Dieck, G. S., Hall, N. E. L., Lahti, H. 1985. A case-control study of diesel exhaust exposure and bladder cancer. *Environ. Res.* 37:475–89
100. Kaplan, I. 1959. Relationships of noxious gases to carcinoma of the lung in railroad workers. *J. Am. Med. Assoc.* 171:2039–43
101. Schenker, M. B., Speizer, F. E. 1980. A retrospective cohort study of diesel exhaust in railroad workers: Study design and methodological issues. See Ref. 5, pp. 1085–97
102. Howe, G. R., Fraser, D., Lindsay, J., Presnal, B., Yu, S. Z. 1983. Cancer mortality (1965–1977) in relation to diesel fume and coal exposure in a cohort of retired railway workers. *J. Natl. Cancer Inst.* 70:1015–20
103. Schenker, M. B., Smith, T., Munos, A., Woske, S., Speizer, F. E. 1984. Diesel exposure and mortality among railway workers: Results of a pilot study. *Br. J. Ind. Med.* 41:320–27
104. Garshick, E., Muñoz, A., Schenker, M. B., Woskie, S., Smith, T., Spiezer, F. E. 1986. A retrospective cohort study of lung cancer and diesel exhaust exposure in railroad workers. *Am. Rev. Respir. Dis.* 133:A264
105. Waxweiler, R., Wagoner, J., Archer, V. 1973. Mortality of potash workers. *J. Occup. Med.* 15:486–89
106. Wheeler, R. W., Hearl, F. J., McCawley, M. 1980. An industrial hygiene characterization of exposure to diesel emissions in an underground coal mine. See Ref. 5, pp. 1085–97
107. Cuddihy, R. G., Griffith, W. C., McClellan, R. O. 1984. Health risks from light duty diesel vehicles. *Environ. Sci. Technol.* 18:14A–21A
108. Albert, R. E., Lewtas, J., Nesnow, S., Thorslund, T. W., Anderson, E. A. 1983. Comparative potency method for cancer risk assessment: Application to diesel particulate emissions. *Risk Anal.* 3:101–117
109. Albert, R. E., Chen, C. 1986. U.S. EPA diesel studies on inhalation hazards. See Ref. 11, pp. 411–20

Ann. Rev. Pharmacol. Toxicol. 1987. 27:301–13

PROSTAGLANDINS, LEUKOTRIENES, AND PLATELET-ACTIVATING FACTOR IN SHOCK[1]

Giora Feuerstein and John M. Hallenbeck

Neurobiology Research Division, Department of Neurology, Uniformed Services University of the Health Sciences, 4301 Jones Bridge Road, Bethesda, Maryland 20814-4799

INTRODUCTION

Shock is commonly defined as acute circulatory collapse due to dramatic decrease in blood volume, failure of cardiac or vascular circulation or of neurogenic control of the circulation. In essence, shock is inadequate tissue perfusion that impairs normal organ functions. As such, shock may be reversible (i.e. correction of the impaired organ perfusion leads to restoration of organ functions) or nonreversible (where noncorrectable damage was already produced during the low blood flow state). Irreversible shock leads to organ death and, if essential organs are involved, to death of the animal.

This review compiles the available evidence on the potential role of several vasoactive lipids in the pathophysiology of shock and provides an analysis of the potential interactions of these vasoactive lipids during various shock paradigms. We emphasize the role of the more recently discovered vasoactive lipids, leukotrienes (LTs), and platelet-activating factor (PAF) in shock and trauma and refer briefly to prostaglandins (PGs) and thromboxane A_2 (TXA_2), which have been extensively studied and reviewed in the past decade (1, 2).

PROSTAGLANDIN (PG) E_2, D_2, $F_{2\alpha}$ AND PGI_2 IN SHOCK

Numerous studies conducted in a variety of shock models show that circulating levels of the classical prostaglandins (e.g. PGE_2, $PGF_{2\alpha}$) are elevated in several shock states (1–3). Although bioassy techniques were used for much of the original work, confirmation has largely been obtained using radioimmunoassay procedures (1). Recent studies also demonstrate high levels of 6-keto-$PGF_{1\alpha}$ (a stable metabolite of PGI_2; Figure 1) in the circulation of animals subjected to various shock situations, including endotoxic (1, 4, 5), hemorrhagic (6), mycotoxic (7), and traumatic (8). Elevated levels of 6-keto-$PGF_{1\alpha}$ also occur in patients with septic shock (9). However, the significance of PG production in the various shock models is still unknown.

The recuperation of hemodynamic, endocrine, and metabolic functions was enhanced in endotoxic, traumatic, or hemorrhagic shock in which PGEs or PGI_2 was administered before or after the shock (1, 10–13). Furthermore, survival of dogs treated with PGD_2 during endotoxemia (14) was increased, as was survival of rats exposed to hemorrhage and treated with PGI_2 (12) or 16,16-dimethyl PGE_1 (10). However, the protective capacity of the vasodilator PGs (PGEs, PGI_2) across species and shock paradigms is controversial (1).

While selected prostanoids (primarily PGEs, PGI_2) are beneficial in several shock models, inhibition of eicosanoid production also provides protection in

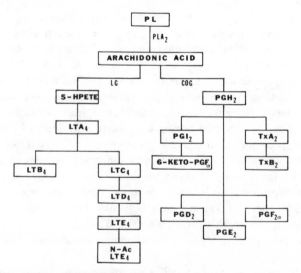

Figure 1 The cascade of arachidonate metabolism. Abbreviations: COG, cyclooxygenase pathway; LG, 5-lipoxygenase pathway; PLA_2, phospholipase A_2; PL, phospholipids.

various shock models. This phenomenon was first described by Northover & Subramanian. These investigators used acetyl-salicylic acid in endotoxic shock (15), and this inhibition was confirmed with several other nonsteroidal antiinflammatory drugs (NSAID) (1, 2). However, the beneficial effects of drugs that inhibit prostanoid synthesis occur primarily in endotoxic shock; in hemorrhagic shock, limited information indicates that inhibition of eicosanoid production exacerbates the hemodynamic derangements and decreases the incidence of survival from acute hypovolemic hypotension (6, 16, 17). Furthermore, some investigators have raised doubts about the detrimental role of eicosanoids even in endotoxic shock. Effective blockade of eicosanoid production by BW 755c (a dual lipoxygenase and cyclooxygenase inhibitor) in endotoxemia failed to improve survival or reduce detrimental outcomes of the endotoxin (5). Thus, although earlier views favored a pathological role for prostanoids in endotoxemia and the use of drugs that inhibit PG synthesis to improve survival in such syndromes (2), it is still unclear whether the beneficial actions demonstrated by NSAID are actually due to inhibition of eicosanoid production or, instead, to other pharmacologic properties of such agents.

THROMBOXANE A_2 IN SHOCK AND TRAUMA

Thromboxane A_2 (TXA_2) is one of the most potent arachidonic acid (AA) metabolites. It is produced by the cyclooxygenase and TXA_2-synthetase enzyme complexes (Figure 1). TXA_2 has an extremely short half-life (~ 30 sec) under normal biological conditions (pH = 7.4; 37°C); therefore, TXB_2, a stable and virtually nonactive metabolite of TXA_2 (Figure 1), is used to monitor levels of TXA_2. Several lines of evidence support a role for TXA_2 as a mediator of shock. Elevated plasma and lymph levels of TXB_2 are consistently found in a variety of experimental shock models, such as endotoxemic (18), traumatic (19), or hemorrhagic (6). Moreover, increased plasma levels of TXB_2 in humans suffering from severe septic shock were also reported (20).

Two major pathophysiological processes can be attributed to TXA_2. First, TXA_2 is a potent vasoconstrictor of small and large blood vessels; second, TXA_2 is an extremely potent platelet-aggregating factor. These effects have been demonstrated across all species (for review see 21). These two primary actions of TXA_2 are believed to act together to interfere with organ blood flow and promote ischemia in several shock states. Excessive TXA_2 production is considered to play a primary role in massive pulmonary thrombosis following AA or heterologous blood administration in various species (21, 22).

The role of TXA_2 and its endoperoxide precursor (PGH_2; Figure 1) in the pathophysiology of various shock states is also suggested by experiments demonstrating the therapeutic value of TXA_2 antagonists or synthesis inhibitors in such situations. Thus, the TXA_2 receptor antagonist EP 092 blocks the development of pulmonary hypertension in endotoxemia (23), and structurally different TXA_2 antagonists such as pinane-TXA_2 have a similar protective effect (24). However, all the TXA_2 antagonists are also PGH_2 antagonists. Therefore, it is not yet possible to evaluate the relative roles of PGH_2 and TXA_2 in shock. Furthermore, TXA_2 synthesis inhibitors have therapeutic efficacy in several shock and trauma models. UK 37248 and other TXA_2-synthetase inhibitors are effective in rat endotoxic shock (25, 26) and arachidonate-induced sudden death in rabbits (27), and U 63,557A has a protective effect in rat trauma (19). However, TXA_2 inhibition fails to modify the outcome of gram-negative septic shock (28).

Interestingly, TXA_2 synthesis inhibitors might not act only by inhibiting TXA_2 synthesis. They might also increase the availability of endoperoxides for the PGI_2 synthetase pathway by producing more PGI_2 (29).

LEUKOTRIENES IN SHOCK AND TRAUMA

Production of leukotrienes (LTs; Figure 1) in acute anaphylaxis is considered to play a major role in the cardiorespiratory derangements that lead to shock and death (30–33). The role of LTs in other forms of shock such as sepsis, trauma, or hemorrhage is still unclear, primarily owing to difficulties in assaying leukotrienes in biological tissues and fluids. Some recent evidence supports the generation of LTs in nonimmune pathophysiological processes (e.g. burns, trauma) by following the levels of LTs in the bile. Large increments of LTE_4 and N-acetyl-LTE_4 (Figure 1) are found in the plasma and bile of rats exposed to various traumatic injuries such as burns, bone fracture, abdominal surgery (34), and endotoxemia (35). This new evidence confirms earlier suggestions that were based on increases in 5-HETE derivative of 5-HPETE (Figure 1) in the lymph during endotoxemia (36) and the enhanced release of LTC_4 from mouse peritoneal macrophages exposed to endotoxin in vitro (37).

Although LTs have been argued to be rapidly cleared from the blood, metabolized by the liver, and excreted in the bile as nonactive metabolites, recent experiments indicate LTs have an enterohepatic cycle (38). In species where N-acetyl-LTE_4 is the major LT metabolite to reenter the circulation from the gut, little biological action can be anticipated since N-acetyl-LTE_4, is less than 1% as effective as LTE_4 (39). However, in species where LTE_4 is the major metabolite to reenter the circulation (e.g. the cynomolgus monkey) substantial potentiation and prolongation of the LT effects can be anticipated, since LTE_4 duplicates many of the biological activities of LTC_4/LTD_4 (40).

Numerous articles have described the effects of LTs on the various com-

ponents of the cardiorespiratory system, blood vessels, and the microcirculation (31–34). The key pathophysiological consequences include: (a) reduction
in cardiac output; (b) constriction of blood vessels and reduction in organ
blood flow (31, 32) [exceptions to (b) are the rabbit cerebral arterioles (41),
the canine renal and mesenteric arteries in vitro (42), and the differential
vascular responses to LTs that may occur in various segments of blood vessels
(43)]; (c) bronchoconstriction, reduced lung compliance, and increases in
pulmonary vascular resistance (31, 32); (d) increases in postcapillary venular
permeability and venoconstriction that lead to pronounced plasma extravasation and reduction in blood volume (31, 32, 44); and (e) aggregation and
activation of platelets and white blood cells contributing to circulatory shock.
Formation of microthrombi in the lung and release of multiple secondary
mediators from activated white blood cells and macrophages such as TXA_2,
PGs, kinins, oxygen radicals, and histamine amplify and confound the direct
effects of the LTs. The multiple sites of LT actions on the cardiovascular
system and the summation of these effects to produce shock are summarized
in Figure 2.

A third line of evidence that supports the role of LTs in the pathophysiological events of shock and trauma is derived from experiments utilizing LT
antagonists in treatment of various shock states. Two LT antagonists have
been evaluated so far: (a) FPL-55712, a short-acting LTC_4/D_4 antagonist,
protects mice from lethal endotoxemia (45) and (b) LY 171,883, a longer and
more potent LTD_4/E_4 antagonist, also provides some protection against endotoxemia (46) and traumatic shock (47) in rats. Furthermore, several inhibitors of the lipoxygenase pathway of arachidonate metabolism (e.g. CGS-
5391B, U-60,257, diethylcarbamazine, propylgallate) have protective effects
in traumatic and endotoxic shock (21). However, these data must be interpreted with caution, since none of the available lipoxygenase inhibitors is
highly specific for the 5-lipoxygenase enzyme complex; at high concentrations these compounds also inhibit the cyclooxygenase pathway (48).
Interestingly, the tripeptide thyrotropin-releasing hormone (TRH) also reverses the hypotension produced by LTD_4 in several species through a central
mechanism of action (49). More potent and specific LT antagonists and
synthesis inhibitors with clearly delineated actions are necessary to further
elucidate the role of LTs in selective pathophysiological processes.

PLATELET-ACTIVATING FACTOR IN SHOCK AND TRAUMA

The term *platelet-activating factor* (PAF) proposed by Benveniste et al (50)
originally defined the most prominent biological activity of a new class of
phospholipids released from basophils by immune (IgE) stimuli. The chemi-

cal nature of these phospholipids is 1-O-alkyl-2-acetyl-*sn*-glycero-3-phosphorylcholine (51, 52). This novel group of compounds has diverse biological action and is released from a variety of cell types, e.g. polymorphonuclear and endothelial cells and by immune and nonimmune stimuli (53, 54).

Understanding of the role of PAF in shock states was based on the demonstration that administration of PAF to several species (guinea pig, rat, rabbit, dog, pig) produced severe hypotension, shock, and death (56–59). In fact, PAF is the single most potent agent to cause shock when administered systemically (Figure 3). The shock syndrome produced by PAF involves

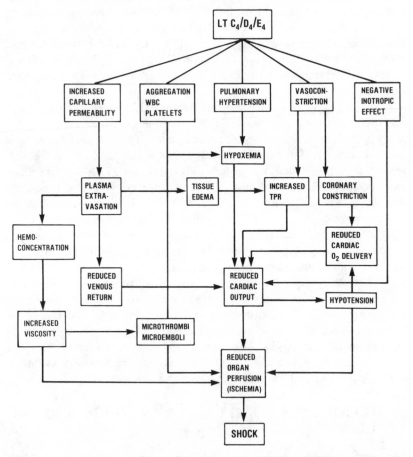

Figure 2 Schematic presentation of the cardiovascular effects of peptide leukotrienes, which lead to shock. TPR = total peripheral resistance. See text for detailed discussion of the multiple sites of the LT actions on the cardiovascular system.

several mechanisms and sites of action: First, pulmonary circulation is affected by an increase in pulmonary vascular resistance (PVR) (55, 59) and bronchoconstriction, both of which contribute to hypoxemia; the increase in PVR contributes to right heart failure (59). Also, the heart is affected by reduction in cardiac output due to coronary constriction (59–61), reduction in myocardial contractility (62–64), and reduced cardiac preload (58). However, some controversy exists as to whether PAF directly affects the myocardium (65) or whether reduction in O_2 leads to a secondary effect stemming from coronary vasoconstriction (60). Also, the PAF-induced coronary constriction and cardiac failure seem to be mediated, at least in part, by TXA_2, since much of the cardiac effect of PAF can be blocked by indomethacin (a potent inhibitor of prostaglandin synthesis) (60). Third, peripheral circulation is affected by vasodilation, which might also contribute to the hypotensive effect of PAF; the vasodilation produced by PAF is not mediated by eicosanoids (60, 61). Fourth, vascular permeability is altered. PAF increases vascular permeability and extravasates plasma to the tissue. This action ultimately results in contraction of blood and plasma volume, which contributes to the reduction in cardiac output (58). Finally, regarding activation of blood cells: activation and aggregation of white blood cells and platelets primarily in the pulmonary circulation contributes to elevation of PVR and reduces lung perfusion. Moreover, these activated blood cells release secondary mediators such as serotonin, TXA_2, leukotrienes, prostaglandins, vasoactive peptides, and oxygen radicals. These secondary mediators promote cell membrane damage, increase vascular permeability, and initiate proinflammatory processes. No other vasoactive lipid known to date produces sustained derangements in organ blood flow at doses as low as those shown in Figure 3.

Although many articles reported that PAF can cause circulatory collapse and death in several species, only a few reports documented the presence of PAF in organs or in the circulation during shock states. Elevated plasma levels of PAF were found in *E. coli* endotoxemia (66). Also, release of PAF from macrophages and spleen lymphocytes was enhanced in rats exposed to bacterial peritonitis (67).

Recent studies using selective and potent PAF antagonists provide additional support for the role of PAF in the pathophysiology of various shock syndromes. Such compounds (e.g. kadsurenone, CV 3988, BN 52021) have recently been described and examined in a variety of immune and nonimmune shock models. Kadsurenone reverses the lipopolysaccharide (LPS)-induced hypotension (66), whereas CV 3988 increases survival of rats exposed to LPS endotoxemia (68). BN 52021 reverses and prevents the effects of *Salmonella typhimurium* endotoxin (69, 70). Kadsurenone also provides additional protection in acute antigen anaphylaxis (71).

In summary, PAF can produce hypotension and shock through direct and

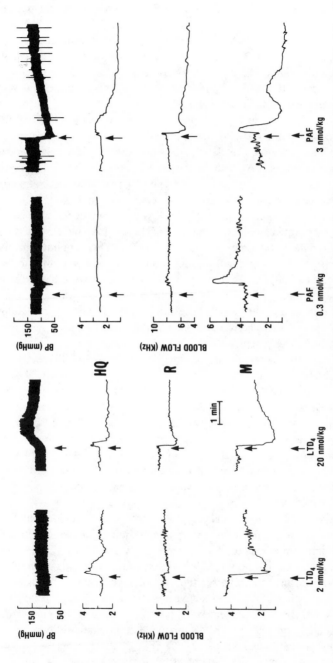

Figure 3 Comparison of LT and PAF effects on blood pressure and organ blood flow in the conscious rat. Abbreviations: HQ, hindquarters blood flow; R, renal blood flow; M, mesenteric blood flow. Time scale of 1 min is given in the figure. Vasodilator effect of PAF at low doses (0.3 nmol/kg) in the M is in marked contrast to the effect of LTD$_4$; a larger dose of PAF severely reduces HQ, R, and M blood flow in spite of recovery of the systemic blood pressure. Therefore, inadequate organ blood flow leads to shock while the systemic hemodynamic induces (e.g. BP) are still within a normal range.

indirect (e.g. TXA_2 of LT-mediated) actions on the heart, pulmonary system, blood vessels, and the microcirculation. Evidence supporting the role of PAF in shock states includes direct biochemical evidence as well as pharmacological studies using PAF antagonists. No specific PAF-acether synthesis inhibitor has been described to date.

SUMMARY AND CONCLUSION

Three major lines of evidence support a role of eicosanoids and PAF in shock. Formation of each of the cyclooxygenase metabolites of arachidonate is enhanced at some point during the shock; these metabolites include PGE_2, $PGF_{2\alpha}$, PGI_2, and TXA_2. Enhanced formation of 5-HETE and the cysteinyl-LTs provides evidence for activation of the 5-lipoxygenase pathway of arachidonate metabolism, and preliminary biochemical evidence suggests that formation of PAF in anaphylactic and endotoxic shock is also enhanced. Second, TXA_2, cysteinyl-leukotrienes, and, to an even greater extent, PAF are able to produce shock and death in intact animals. Third, pharmacological studies show that selective antagonists or synthesis inhibitors modify the course of the shock.

While any of these lines of evidence may not by itself provide proof for a cause–effect relationship, the data taken together strongly suggest that vasoactive lipids might be involved in fundamental processes in the pathophysiology of shock. However, the role of vasoactive lipids might vary in different shock paradigms, change at various time points during the evolution of the shock, and depend on the species studied. Moreover, while the majority of the reports tend to focus on a specific substance, the metabolism of all of the eicosanoids mentioned, as well as PAF and probably other arachidonate metabolites (e.g. 15-lipoxygenase products such as lipoxins), changes during shock states. This fact probably causes most of the discrepancies in studies using specific antagonists or synthesis inhibitors to modify the state of shock. Thus, while blockade of one mediator might provide some protection, it might not be sufficient to halt or reverse the main course of the pathophysiological process. For example, the increase in vascular permeability, a fundamental phenomenon in trauma, anaphylaxis, or endotoxemia, might be mediated by PAF, LTs, PGs, peptides (e.g. kinins, substance P, CGRP) and amines (e.g. histamine in some species). Attempting to reverse such a complex phenomenon by blocking one specific factor might not be productive unless the specific substance played a key role in generation of the other factors. It seems, however, that while interactions between PGs, LTs, and PAF do occur (31, 32, 70), none of the shock states are crucially dependent on one class of the vasoactive lipids. Therefore, the therapeutic strategy should be based on multiple sites of action, either by drug combinations or multiple actions of a specific drug. Such therapy will ultimately provide better protection in the complex situation of shock and trauma, where multiple vasoactive lipids, peptides, and amines act in concert to result ultimately in shock.

Finally, we must remember that none of the synthetic pathways for any of the vasoactive lipids (PGs, TXA_2, or PAF) can be blocked by a specific inhibitor; none of these vasoactive lipids has a highly potent and selective antagonist. The available receptor antagonists or synthesis inhibitors possess multiple sites of action along the arachidonate cascade or pathways of phospholipid metabolism. They also have various pharmacological actions unrelated to the arachidonate cascade. Until potent and selective antagonists and synthesis inhibitors are developed, the interpretation of results obtained by less selective compounds may be misleading.

Literature Cited

1. Bult, A., Herman, A. G. 1982. Prostaglandins and circulating shock. In *Cardiovascular Pharmacology of the Prostaglandins,* ed. P. M. Vanhoutte, H. Denolin, A. Goosens, A. G. Herman, pp. 327–45. New York: Raven

2. Fletcher, J. R., Ramwell, P. W. 1980. Prostaglandins in shock: to give or to block. *Adv. Shock Res.* 3:57–66

3. Anderson, F. L., Jubitz, W., Tsagarics, T. J., Kuida, H. 1975. Endotoxin induced prostaglandin E and F release in dogs. *Am. J. Physiol.* 228:410–14

4. Feuerstein, G., DiMicco, J. A., Kopin, I. J. 1981. Effect of indomethacin on blood pressure and plasma catecholamines response to acute endotoxemia. *J. Pharm. Pharmacol.* 33:576–79

5. McKenchnie, K., Furman, B. L., Parratt, J. R. 1985. Metabolic and cardiovascular effects of endotoxin infusion in conscious unrestrained rats: effects of methylprednidolone and BW 755c. *Circ. Shock* 15:205–15

6. Feuerstein, G., Bayorh, M. A., Stull, R., Goldstein, D. S., Zerbe, R. L., et al. 1985. Effects of nafazatrom on cardiovascular sympathetic and endocrine responses to hemorrhagic shock in conscious rats. *Circ. Shock* 17:223–32

7. Feuerstein, G., Golstein, D., Ramwell, P. W., Zerbe, R. L., Lux, W. E., et al. 1985. Cardiorespiratory, sympathetic and biochemical responses to T-2 toxin in the conscious guinea pig and rat. *J. Pharmacol. Exp. Ther.* 232:786–94

8. Lefer, A. M., Araki, H. 1983. Analysis of potential beneficial actions of prostaglandins in traumatic shock.

In *Molecular and Cellular Aspects of Shock and Trauma,* ed. A. M. Lefer, W. Schumer, pp. 199–210. New York: Liss

9. Halushka, P. V., Reines, D., Barrow, S. E., Blair, I. A., Dollery, C. T., et al. 1985. Elevated plasma 6-keto-prostaglandin $F_{1\alpha}$ in patients in septic shock. *Crit. Care Med.* 13:451–53

10. Feuerstein, G., Jimerson, D. C., Kopin, I. J. 1981. Prostaglandins, catecholamines and cardiovascular responses to hemorrhage. *Am. J. Physiol.* 240:R166–74

11. Krausz, M. M., Utsunomuija, T., Feuerstein, G., Wolfe, J. H. N., Shepro, D., et al. 1981. Prostacyclin reversal of lethal endotoxemia in dogs. *J. Clin. Invest.* 67:1118–25

12. Feuerstein, G., Zerbe, R. L., Meyer, D. K., Kopin, I. J. 1982. Alteration of cardiovascular, neurogenic and humoral responses to acute hypovolemic hypotension by administered prostacyclin. *J. Cardiovasc. Pharmacol.* 4:246–53

13. Machiedo, G. W., Warden, M. J., LoVerme, P. J., Rush, B. F. Jr. 1982. Hemodynamic effects of prolonged infusion of prostaglandin E_1 (PGE$_1$) after hemorrhagic shock. *Adv. Shock Res.* 8:171–76

14. Rao, P. S., Cavanagh, D., Mardsen, K. A., Knuppel, R. A., Spaziani, E. 1984. Prostaglandin D_2 in canine endotoxic shock. Hemodynamic, hematologic, biochemical and blood gas analysis. *Am. J. Obstet. Gynecol.* 148:964–72

15. Northover, B. J., Subramanian, G. 1962. Analgesic antipyretic drugs as an-

tagonists of endotoxin shock in dogs. *J. Pathol. Bacteriol.* 83:463–68

16. Feuerstein, G., Feuerstein, N., Gimmon, Z. 1980. The effect of indomethacin on blood pressure, catecholamines and renin response to acute hemorrhage. In *Advances in Prostaglandins, Thromboxane and Leukotriene Research*, ed. B. Samuelsson, P. W. Ramwell, R. Paoletti, 7:829–33. New York: Raven

17. Perbeck, L., Hedgvist, P. 1980. Prostaglandin E_1 and E_2 antagonize indomethacin induced decrease in survival rate of hemorrhagically shocked rats. *Acta Clin. Scand.* 500:91–94

18. Cook, J. A., Wise, W. C., Halushka, P. V. 1980. Elevated thromboxane levels in the rat during endotoxic shock. *J. Clin. Invest.* 65:227–30

19. Hock, C. E., Lefer, A. M. 1984. Beneficial effect of thromboxane synthetase inhibitor in traumatic shock. *Circ. Shock* 14:159–68

20. Reines, H. D., Halushka, P. V., Cook, J. A., Wise, W. C., Rambo, W. 1982. Plasma thromboxane concentrations are raised in patients dying with septic shock. *Lancet* 2:174–75

21. Lefer, A. M. 1985. Eicosanoid as mediators of ischemia and shock. *Fed. Proc.* 44:275–80

22. Bunting, S., Castro, S., Salmon, J. A., Moncada, S. 1983. The effect of cyclooxygenase and thromboxane synthetase inhibitors on shock induced by injection of heterologous blood in cats. *Thromb. Res.* 30:609–17

23. Armstrong, R. A., Jones, R. L., Wilson, N. H. 1985. Effect of the thromboxane receptor antagonist EP 092 on endotoxin shock in the sheep. *Prostaglandins* 29:703–13

24. Araki, H., Lefer, A. M., Smith, J. B., Nicolau, K. C., Magda, R. I. 1980. Beneficial actions of a new thromboxane analog in traumatic shock. See Ref. 16, pp. 835–38

25. Anderegg, K., Anzeveno, P., Cook, J. A., Halushka, P. V., McCarthy, J., et al. 1983. Effect of a pyridine derivative thromboxane synthetase inhibitor and its inactive isomer in endotoxic shock in the rat. *Br. J. Pharmacol.* 18:725–32

26. Halushka, P. V., Cook, J. A., Wise, W. C. 1983. Beneficial effects of UK 32748, a thromboxane synthetase inhibitor in experimental endotoxic shock in the rat. *Br. J. Clin. Pharmacol.* 15:1335–95

27. Lefer, A. M., Okamutsu, S., Smith, E. F., Smith, B. 1981. Beneficial effects of

a new thromboxane synthase inhibitor in arachidonate-induced sudden death. *Thromb. Res.* 23:265–73

28. Fletcher, J. R., Short, B. L., Casey, L. C., Walker, R. I., Gardiner, H., et al. 1983. Thromboxane inhibition in gram negative sepsis fails to improve survival. In *Advances in Prostaglandins, Thromboxane and Leukotriene Research*, ed. B. Samuelsson, R. Paoletti, P. W. Ramwell, 12:117–30. New York: Raven

29. Casey, L. C., Fletcher, J. R., Zmudea, M. I., Ramwell, P. W. 1982. Prevention of endotoxin induced pulmonary hypertension in primates by use of a selective thromboxane inhibitor OKY 1581. *J. Pharmacol. Exp. Ther.* 222: 441–46

30. Samuelsson, B. 1983. Leukotrienes: mediators of immediate hypersensitivity reactions and inflammation. *Science* 220:568–78

31. Piper, P. J. 1982. Pharmacology and biochemistry of leukotrienes. *Eur. J. Respir. Dis.* 122(63):54–61

32. Feuerstein, G. 1985. Autonomic pharmacology of leukotrienes. *J. Auton. Pharmacol.* 5:149–68

33. Hammarstrom, S. 1983. Leukotrienes. *Ann. Rev. Biochem.* 52:355–77

34. Denzlinger, C., Rapp, S., Hagmann, W., Keppler, D. 1985. Leukotrienes as mediators in tissue trauma. *Science* 230:330–32

35. Hagmann, W., Denzlinger, C., Keppler, D. 1985. Production of peptide leukotrienes in endotoxic shock. *FEBS Lett.* 180:309–13

36. Ogletree, M. L., Brigham, K. L., Oates, J. A., Hubbard, W. C. 1982. Increased flux of 5-HETE production in sheep lung lymph during pulmonary leukostasis after endotoxin. *Fed. Proc.* 40:767 (Abstr.)

37. Luderitz, T. H., Rietchel, E. T., Schade, U. 1983. Release of leukotrienes from macrophages stimulated by lipopolysaccharide endotoxin. *Immunology* 165:213–313

38. Denzlinger, C., Guhlman, A., Hagmann, W., Scheuber, P. H., Scheyerl, F., et al. 1986. Cysteinyl leukotrienes undergo enterohepatic circulation. *Prostaglandin Leukotriene Med.* 21:321–22

39. Foster, A., Fitzsimmons, B., Letts, C. G. 1986. The synthesis of N-acetyl-leukotriene E_4 and its effects on cardiovascular and respiratory function of the anesthetized pig. *Prostaglandins* 31:1077–86

40. Eimerl, J., Siren, A.-L., Feuerstein, G. 1986. Regional vascular effects of cys-

teinyl leukotrienes. *Am. J. Physiol.* In press

41. Kamitani, T., Little, M. H., Ellis, F. F. 1985. Effect of leukotrienes, 12-HETE, histamine, bradykinin and 5-hydroxy-tryptamine on in vivo rabbit cerebral arteriolar diameter. *J. Cereb. Blood Flow Metab.* 5:554–59

42. Secrest, R. J., Olsen, E. J., Chapnick, B. M. 1985. Leukotriene D_4 relaxes canine renal and superior mesenteric arteries. *Circ. Res.* 57:323–29

43. Berkowitz, B. A., Zabko Potapovich, B., Valocik, R., Gleason, J. G. 1984. Effect of leukotrienes on the vasculature and blood pressure of different species. *J. Pharmacol. Exp. Ther.* 229:105–12

44. Zukowska-Grojec, Z., Feuerstein, G. 1985. Leukotrienes and shock. In *Leukotrienes in Cardiovascular and Pulmonary Function,* ed. A. M. Lefer, pp. 101–13. New York: Liss

45. Hagmann, W., Denzlinger, C., Keppler, D. 1984. Role of peptide leukotrienes and their hepatobiliary elimination in endotoxin action. *Circ. Shock* 14:223–35

46. Cook, J. A., Wise, W. C., Halushka, P. V. 1985. Protective effect of a selective leukotriene antagonist in endotoxemia in the rat. *J. Pharmacol. Exp. Ther.* 235:470–74

47. Hock, C. E., Lefer, A. M. 1985. Protective effects of a new LTD_4 antagonist (LY-171,883) in traumatic shock. *Circ. Shock* 17:263–72

48. Levine, L. 1983. Inhibition of the A-23187 stimulated leukotriene and prostaglandin biosynthesis of rat basophil leukemia (RBL-1) cells by non-steroid anti-inflammatory drugs, antioxidants and calcium channel blockers. *Biochem. Pharmacol.* 32:3023–26

49. Lux, W. E., Feuerstein, G., Faden, A. I. 1983. Alteration of leukotriene D_4 hypotension by thyrotropin-releasing hormone. *Nature* 302:822–24

50. Benveniste, J., Henson, P. M., Cochrane, C. G. 1972. Leukocyte-dependent histamine release from rabbit platelets: the role of IgE, basophils and a platelet activating factor. *J. Exp. Med.* 136:1356–77

51. Demopoulos, C. A., Pickard, R. N., Hanahan, D. J. 1979. Platelet activating factor: evidence for 1-O-alkyl-2-acetyl-sn-glyceryl-3-phosphocholine as the active component (a new class of lipid chemical mediator). *J. Biol. Chem.* 254:9355–58

52. Blank, M. L., Snyder, F., Byers, L. W., Brooks, B., Muirhead, E. E. 1979.

Antihypertensive activity of an alkyl ether analog of phospholidylcholine. *Biochem. Biophys. Res. Commun.* 90:1194–1200

53. Snyder, F. 1985. Chemical and biochemical aspects of platelet activating factor: a novel class of acetylated ether linked choline phospholipids. *Med. Res. Rev.* 5:107–40

54. Benveniste, J. 1985. PAF-acether (platelet activating factor). *Advances in Prostaglandin, Thromboxane and Leukotriene Research* 13:11–18. New York: Raven

55. Voelkel, N. F., Worten, S., Reeves, J. T., Henson, P. M., Murphy, R. C. 1982. Nonimmunological production of leukotrienes induced by platelet activating factor. *Science* 218:286–89

56. Feuerstein, G., Zukowska-Grojec, Z., Krausz, M. M., Blank, M. L., Snyder, F., et al. 1982. Cardiovascular and sympathetic effects of 1-O-hexadecyl-2-acetyl-sn-glycero-3-phosphorylcholine in conscious SHR and WKY rats. *Clin. Exp. Hypertension* A4:1335–50

57. Feuerstein, G., Lux, W. E. Jr., Ezra, D., Hayes, E. C., Snyder, F., et al. 1985. Thyrotropin releasing hormone blocks the hypotensive effect of platelet activating factor in unanesthetized guinea pig. *J. Cardiovasc. Pharmacol.* 7:335–40

58. Bessin, P., Bonnet, J., Apffel, D., Soulard, C., Desgroux, L., et al. 1983. Acute circulating collapse caused by platelet activating factor (PAF acether) in dogs. *Eur. J. Pharmacol.* 86:403–13

59. Goldstein, R. E., Laurindo, F. R. M., Ezra, D., Feuerstein, G. 1987. Mechanism of circulating collapse induced by PAF-acether. In *Lipid Mediators in Immunology of Burn and Sepsis,* ed. M. Braquet. New York: Plenum. In press

60. Feuerstein, G., Boyd, L. M., Ezra, D., Goldstein, R. E. 1983. Effect of platelet activating factor on coronary circulation of the domestic pig. *Am. J. Physiol.* 246:H466–71

61. Sybertz, E. J., Watkins, R. W., Baum, T., Pula, K., Rivelli, M. 1984. Cardiac, coronary and peripheral vascular effects of acetyl ether phosphoryl choline in the anesthetized dog. *J. Pharmacol. Exp. Ther.* 232:156–62

62. Levi, R., Burke, J. A., Guo, Z. G., Hattori, Y., Hoppens, C. M., et al. 1984. Acetyl glyceryl ether phosphorylcholine (AGEPC) a putative mediator of cardiac anaphylaxis. *Circ. Res.* 54:117–24

63. Camussi, G., Aglietta, M., Malavasi, F., Tetta, C., Piacibelo, W., et al. 1983. The release of platelet activating factor from human endothelial cells in culture. *J. Immunol.* 131:2397–403

64. Benveniste, J., Boullet, C., Brink, C., Labat, C. 1983. The actions of PAF acether (platelet activating factor) on guinea pig isolated heart preparation. *Br. J. Pharmacol.* 80:81–83

65. Cervoni, P., Herzlinger, H. E., Lai, F. M., Tanikella, T. K. 1983. Aortic vascular and atrial responses to (±) 1 - O - octa - decyl - 2 - acetyl - glycero - 3 - phosphocholine. *Br. J. Pharmacol.* 79: 667–71

66. Doebber, T. W., Wu, M. S., Robbins, J. C., Choy, B. M., Chang, M. N., et al. 1985. Platelet activating factor (PAF) involvement in endotoxin induced hypotension in rats; studies with PAF-receptor antagonist kadsurenone. *Biochem. Biophys. Res. Commun.* 127: 799–808

67. Inarrea, P., Gomez-Cambronero, J.,

Pascual, J., del Carmen-Ponte, M., Hernando, L., et al. 1985. Synthesis of PAF acether and blood volume changes in gram negative sepsis. *Immunopharmacology* 9:45–52

68. Terashita, Z., Imura, Y., Nishikawa, K., Sumida, S. 1985. Is platelet activating factor (PAF) a mediator of endotoxin shock? *Eur. J. Pharmacol.* 109:257–61

69. Etienne, A., Hecquet, F., Soulard, C., Spinnewy, B., Clostre, F., et al. 1985. In vivo inhibition of plasma protein leakage and *Salmonella enteritidis*–induced mortality in the rat by specific PAF acether antagonist BN 52021. *Agents Actions* 17:368–70

70. Braquet, P., Touqui, L., Varagaftig, B. B., Sheh, T. Y. 1986. Perspectives in platelet activating factor research. *Pharmacol. Rev.* In press

71. Darius, H., Lefer, D. J., Smith, B., Lefer, A. M. 1986. Role of platelet activating factor-acether in mediating guinea pig anaphylaxis. *Science* 232:58–60

Ann. Rev. Pharmacol. Toxicol. 1987. 27:315–45
Copyright © 1987 by Annual Reviews Inc. All rights reserved

PURINE RECEPTORS IN MAMMALIAN TISSUES: PHARMACOLOGY AND FUNCTIONAL SIGNIFICANCE

Michael Williams

Drug Discovery Division, Research Department, Pharmaceuticals Division, CIBA-GEIGY Corporation, Summit, New Jersey 07901

ADENOSINE AND ADENINE NUCLEOTIDES IN CELL FUNCTION

Purine nucleosides and nucleotides are major factors in cell function. They are intermediates in energy pathways, in cellular metabolic processes and are constituents of the cofactors necessary for enzymatic reactions (1) and cell replication (2). It has therefore been difficult to visualize that such chemicals also act in cellular communication.

The criteria used for evaluating whether a given compound is a neurotransmitter have been developed by historical precedent (3). They are based on knowledge of the prototypic neurotransmitter, acetylcholine (4). Adenosine has been identified as a neuromodulator using such classical criteria. This evaluation has lessened the enthusiasm for purine-related processes as targets for therapeutic agents for malfunctions of mammalian homeostatis. There is no evidence that specific anabolic processes form adenosine, distinct from those involved in its general metabolic functions. Also, the physiological factors regulating the extracellular availability of the nucleoside and its distribution make the development of a "purinergic" hypothesis of neuromodulation difficult (5). These issues are compounded by the paucity of dissimilar chemical entities that interact with adenosine receptors. Agonists are almost exclusively purine nucleosides (6), whereas with few exceptions, most antagonists are imidazopyrimidines (7–10). Studies of adenosine receptor–mediated events are thus limited, comparable to in-

315

0362-1642/87/0415-0315$02.00

vestigations on adrenoceptors in which neither phentolamine, phenoxybenzamine, nor propranolol would be available as a selective receptor probe.

These caveats can also be applied to many of the recently discovered peptides thought to function as neuromodulators (11, 12). Potential physiological or pharmacological functions of the neuropeptides may result from optimistic conjecturing and may reflect, in part, a high technology bias, whereas the more negative view, in the case of adenosine, may reflect a "devil already known" component. The purine has marked effects on cardiovascular function, as was shown nearly 60 years ago (13). This fact, coupled with the limited usefulness of agonists as selective therapeutic agents, may lead to the conclusion that this neuromodulator has been judged and rejected. This review attempts to show that the therapeutic potential of adenosine-related compounds has yet to be objectively evaluated.

HISTORICAL PERSPECTIVE

Purine nucleosides and nucleotides are intercellular messengers. They function as chemoattractants in a variety of organisms and mammalian tissues (14). In 1929 Drury & Szent-Gyorgi (13) demonstrated the effects of purines in mammalian species. They discovered that adenosine caused bradycardia, coronary vasodilation, and blood pressure decreases. The short half-life of the nucleoside (16) confounded attempts to use adenosine as an antihypertensive agent (15). For the next three decades, basic research on "purinergic neurotransmission" concentrated on the physiological rather than the pharmacological. The purine has general vasodilatory actions (17, 18). In fact, it is a vasodilator in all vascular beds thus far studied, with the exception of the kidney (19) where it is a potent vasoconstrictor. Central administration of either adenosine or its nucleotide, ATP, can produce sedative and hypnotic effects (20, 21). The discovery of the second messenger cyclic AMP and the seminal biochemical studies of Sattin & Rall (22) gave further importance to adenosine as a neuromodulator. Adenosine is a potent activator of adenylate cyclase activity (6). However, the xanthines, theophylline, and caffeine (Figure 2), rather than potentiating the actions of adenosine, as their activity as phosphodiesterase (PDE) inhibitors would indicate, inhibited cyclic AMP formation (22). At this time Sattin & Rall (22) observed that the xanthines were acting as adenosine antagonists. Shortly after this observation, discrete cell-surface recognition sites, or receptors, were reported for the purine (23–25).

Modification of the xanthines also led to compounds such as 8-phenyltheophylline (8-PT; Figure 2) that were selective adenosine antagonists rather than PDE inhibitors (6, 9, 26). In 1980 the first of several radio-ligand-binding assays was reported (27), which increased interest (3, 6, 8, 28–30) in the pharmacological role of adenosine. Concomitantly, the search for the chemical mediator of the phenomenon described by Burnstock and his coworkers (31, 32) as "non-adrenergic, non-cholinergic" neurotransmission led to the identification of ATP as a likely candidate. It was considered unlikely that a chemical even more essential to cellular function in terms of its energy-charge characteristics than adenosine (33) would serve a role as an intercellular mediator and would participate in, to some extent, a process wasteful of intracellular energy charge. However, continued efforts have led to the identification of two separate receptors sensitive to the nucleotide (32).

ADENOSINE RECEPTORS

Adenosine-mediated increases in cyclic AMP formation (22) were ascribed to the existence of a single receptor class susceptible to blockade by the xanthines. In the initial nomenclature for purinoceptors (31), those receptors sensitive to adenosine were termed P_1 and those sensitive to ATP were termed P_2 (Table 1). Additional studies indicated that the P_1 receptors could be further subdivided using appropriate concentrations of adenosine to modulate adenylate cyclase activity. Because an intact ribose group must be present on the purine molecule (Figure 1) to produce agonist activity, Londos & Wolff (23) termed these receptors R_i and R_a (Table 1), the subscripts of which refer to the inhibition (i) and activation (a) of adenylate cyclase activity. Independently, Van Calker et al (25) termed these same two adenosine receptors A_1 and A_2. A third adenosine recognition site, termed the P site, was also described (34; Table 1). The P site is located on the catalytic subunit of adenylate cyclase. It shows a preference for purines that have intact purine rings (hence the P designation) such as 2',5'-dideoxyadenosine (DDA; Figure 1) and is activated by relatively high concentrations of adenosine (6). However, the physiological significance of the P site is unknown. A_1 and A_2 receptors are linked to the catalytic subunit of adenylate cyclase by coupling proteins N_i and N_s, respectively (24).

Changes in cyclic AMP formation cannot always be related to events modulated by adenosine (5, 35, 36). The nucleoside probably influences cellular function by its actions on other second messenger systems such as calcium (37). Adenosine can also indirectly modulate phosphatidyl inositol turnover (38). Because of these findings, A_1 and A_2 receptors are currently classified based on their agonist pharmacology (39) rather than on their effects on cyclic AMP formation. Receptors of the A_1 subtype are preferentially activated by adenosine agonists (Figure 1) with substitutions in the N^6 position, such as cyclopentyladenosine (CPA; 40, 41), cyclohexyladenosine (CHA; 6), and phenylisopropyladenosine (PIA; 6). Analogs substituted in the 5'-position, most notably 5'N-ethylcarboxamido adenosine (NECA; 6, 40),

Table 1 Purinergic receptor classification criteria[a]

Receptor class	Subclasses	Agonist pharmacology	
P$_1$	A$_1$(R$_i$)	CPA $\geq$ CHA $>$ R-PIA $\geq$ 2-CADO $\geq$ NECA $>$ S-PIA $>$ CV-1808	Receptor subtypes may exist
	A$_2$(R$_a$)	NECA $>$ MECA $=$ 2-CADO $>$ CV1808 $=$ R-PIA $>$ CPA $\geq$ S-PIA	A$_{2a}$ = high affinity sub-class A$_{2b}$ = lower affinity sub-class
P$_2$		ATP $>$ ADP $>$ AMP $\geq$ Ado	
	P$_{2x}$	α-β-MeATP $=$ β-α-MeATP $>$ ATP $=$ 2 MeSATP	
	P$_{2y}$	2 MeSATP $>>$ ATP $>$ α-β-MeATP $=$ β-α-MeATP	
P		2'5' DDA $>>$ Ado	

[a]For abbreviations see Figure 1 and text.

do show activity at A$_2$ receptors. NECA is not, however, A$_2$ selective (40). Rather, it is nonselective for either receptor subtype and may be considered to have A$_2$ activity solely because the A$_1$-selective compounds are inactive at A$_2$ receptors. A given biochemical or pharmacological event cannot be ascribed to A$_2$ activity merely because it is evoked by NECA. However, if both CHA and NECA are used and an additional response occurs with NECA, the event can probably be ascribed to A$_2$-receptor activation. Similarly, 2-chloroadenosine (2-CADO) is a relatively nonselective agonist (40), whereas 2-phenylaminoadenosine (CV 1808; Figure 1), the methyl analog of NECA, MECA, and aristeromycin (Figure 1), show A$_2$ selectivity with varying activity (40; M. Pankaskie, G. A. Stone & M. Williams, submitted for publication).

Both receptor subtypes can be blocked by the xanthine adenosine antagonists (6). 1,3-Dipropyl-8-(2-amino-4-chloro)phenylxanthine (PACPX; 7, 43; Figure 2) and the xanthine-peptide congener, XAC (10; Figure 2) are A$_1$ selective (9), whereas the triazoloquinazoline, CGS 15943A (Figure 3), is A$_2$ selective (44).

Both subclasses of adenosine receptor show stereoselectivity for the R- and

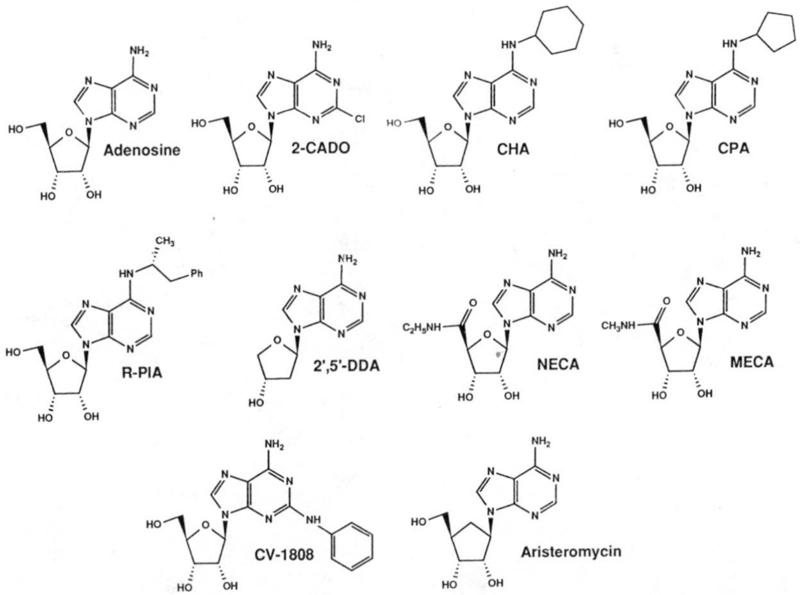

Figure 1   Adenosine agonists.

S-diastereomers of the amphetamine-derived adenosine analog, PIA (6). At the A_1 receptor, the R isomer has been reported to be up to 45-times more active than the S isomer. At the A_2 receptor the ratio of S-PIA to R-PIA is 10 or less. This ratio has been used as a criterion for the involvement of either receptor subclass (6, 28), but its magnitude appears to be dependent on the species used (45). Subclasses of both A_1 and A_2 receptors have been described, which are divided on the basis of a lack of interaction with adenylate cyclase (46, 47) or of agonist affinity (40, 47, 48). The designation A_3 has been used for an adenosine receptor present in cardiac tissue and nerve endings that is not cyclase linked (49).

Adenosine Receptor Ligands

CHA (27), CPA (41), and R-PIA (50) are routinely used to label A_1 receptors in CNS tissue, where dissociation constants (K_d) of 0.5–4.0 nM have been derived. Corresponding receptor densities (apparent B_{max} values) of 0.2–1.5 pmoles/mg protein have been observed (30; Table 2). High-affinity binding sites can only be demonstrated, however, when endogenous adenosine is removed using adenosine deaminase (ADA). These radioligands are less useful in peripheral tissues because of their relatively low specific activity (20–50 Ci/mmole) and because there are few such receptors in these tissues (8; Table 2). This problem has been circumvented by the use of iodinated

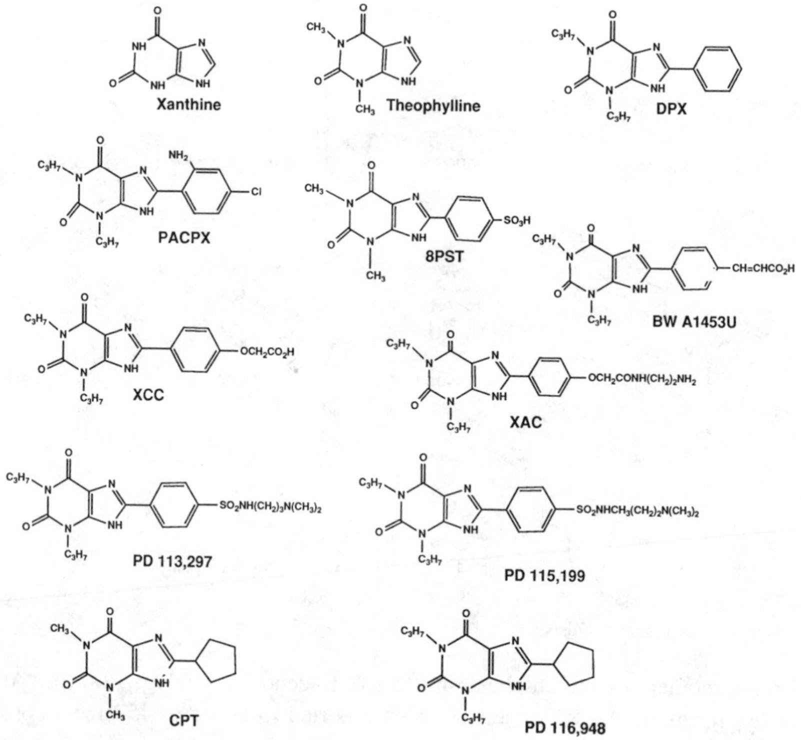

Figure 2   Xanthine adenosine antagonists.

forms of PIA (51), which have specific activities of up to 2200 Ci/mmole. 2-CADO has been used to label the A_1 (29) receptor; however, it is an unreliable ligand.

[^{3}H]NECA can be used to label A_2 receptors in striatal tissue from brain, after blocking binding to A_1 receptors using the alkylating agent *N*-ethylmaleimide (NEM; 52), NEM can uncouple the N_i protein from the receptor and dramatically reduce the affinity of the receptor for the ligand (53, 54) when cyclic AMP is the second messenger for the receptor. This approach lacks specificity, as NEM can also affect A_2-receptor affinity (40). An alternative method is to block the A_1 component of striatal NECA binding by adding low concentrations (50 nM) of the A_1-selective agonist, CPA (40). When this last method is used, NECA can bind selectively to A_2 receptors (40). Two of these sites have been identified. The first is a high-affinity site termed A_{2a} (40). It has a K_d value of approximately 4 nM (40, 45) and an apparent B_{max} value of 0.4–0.9 pmole/mg protein, depending on the species (45). A_{2b} (40) is a lower affinity site with K_d values of 13–245 nM and B_{max} values of 0.8–3.2 pmoles/mg protein, again dependent on the species (45).

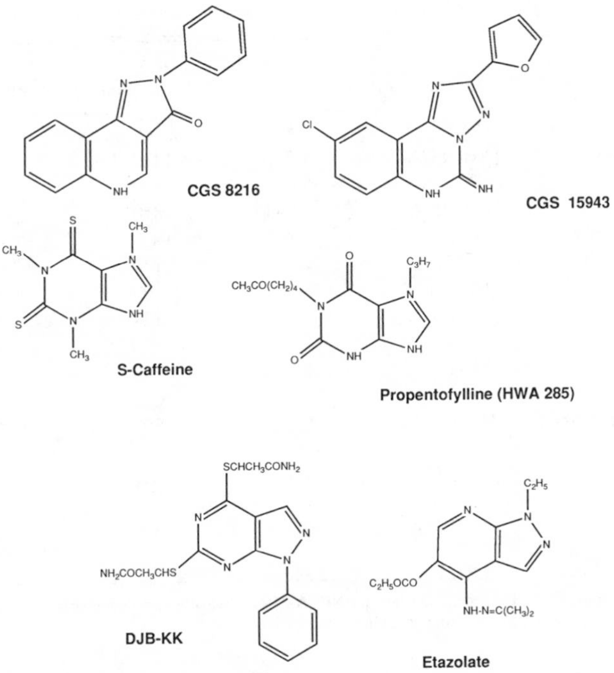

Figure 3   Atypical adenosine antagonists.

NECA may also label sites that are not adenosine receptors (40, 55). In the PC12 pheochromocytoma cell line, which is devoid of A_1 receptors, NECA binds only to A_2 receptors (56).

Use of antagonist radioligands for adenosine receptors has met with limited success. 1,3-Diethyl-8-phenylxanthine (DPX; Figure 2; 27), initially thought to label both A_1 and A_2 receptors (27), has unpredictable binding behavior. XAC and the related xanthine congeners XCC, PD 115,199, and PD 116,948 (Figure 2) have demonstrated useful binding characteristics (10, 57–59). Because of their high specific activity (100–150 Ci/mmole), these antagonists may aid assessing adenosine receptor pharmacology in peripheral tissues.

ATP RECEPTORS

Studies in peripheral tissues (51) provide the majority of evidence for the existence of ATP receptor–mediated processes. However, ATP-elicited responses not blocked by xanthines have been reported in the CNS (60). In many instances, the effects of ATP on cell function have been ascribed either to formation of adenosine from the nucleotide or to the possible chelation of calcium by the triphosphate side chain (47). The use of nonmetabolizable

Table 2 Characteristics of adenosine receptor binding in various mammalian tissue[a]

Tissue	Ligand	K_D (nM)	Bmax (fmole/mg protein)	Receptor	Reference
Rat brain	[³H]CPA	0.5	416	A_1	41
Rat striatum	[³H]NECA	3.5	1420	A_{2a}	40
	+ CPA	35.0	3600	A_{2b}	40
Rat brain	[¹²⁵I]HPIA	1.94	870	A_1	51
Guinea pig brain	[³H]CHA	2.4	1230	A_1	237
Guinea pig ileum	[³H]CHA	1.7	140	A_1	237
Rat mast cells	[³H]Ado	28	16,400[b]	A_2	237
Guinea pig atrium	[³H]NECA	4.3	127	A_1	238
Guinea pig ventricle	[³H]NECA	3.2	50	A_1	238
Rat kidney membranes	[³H]2-CADO	14900	2300	A_2	206
Bovine myocardium	[¹²⁵I]HPIA	1.1	31	A_1	51
Human neutrophils	[³H]NECA	230	9310	A_2	218

[a]Abbreviations: CPA, Cyclopentyladenosine; NECA, 5'N-ethylcarboxamidoadenosine; CHA, Cyclohexyladenosine; Ado, adenosine; and HPIA, Hydroxyphenylisopropyladenosine.
[b]Units in sites per cell.

analogs of ATP, including the α-β- and β-γ-methylene isosteres, provided definitive evidence of unique ATP recognition sites. These sites have recently (32) been subdivided into P_{2x} and P_{2y} subtypes on the basis of the actions of α-β-methylene ATP and 2-methylthio-ATP, respectively. Reliable antagonists for the P_2 receptor have proved difficult to identify. 3-O-3[N-(4-Azido-2-nitrophenyl)amino]proprionyl-ATP(ANAPP₃) has been a useful tool; it is a photolabile, irreversible blocker of P_2 receptors (61).

The stable ATP analog, [³H]AppNHp, bound irreversibly to rat brain membranes with affinities of 10^{-9} M (62). [³H]ATP has also been used to label ATP recognition sites in rabbit bladder membranes (63) that were distinct from ATPase sites. ANAPP₃ covalently labeled two recognition sites in guinea pig vas deferens smooth muscle (64). Because of the incubation conditions used to determine the covalent nature of [³H]-ANAPP₃ binding, kinetic parameters could not be established. ANAPP₃ may be metabolized to adenosine (65).

ADENOSINE AVAILABILITY

The physiological factors controlling the availability of adenosine in mammalian tissues remain unclear. As with other mediators of cellular communication, adenosine can be removed from the extracellular environment by uptake and degradation (deamination). The processes defining these events are well characterized (1, 66). The factors regulating the release of adenosine are, however, less clearly defined. In the heart, adenosine can be formed and released from hypoxic or ischemic myocardium (67, 68). The sources of cardiac adenosine are breakdown of either 5'-AMP or S-adenosyl-homocysteine (SAH; 69–71). The possible contribution of a novel phospho-glycerol adenosine tetraphosphate (71a) has yet to be evaluated.

In the CNS and nonmammalian models of the synapse (such as Torpedo; 72), electrical stimulation and K^+ depolarization can cause purine release (73–75). Adenosine release has been described as a "neuronal nonexocytotic release" process involving carrier mediation (75, 76). The form of adenosine released also contributes to the confusion surrounding its availability. Cyclic AMP, 5'-AMP, and ATP have all been identified as potential sources for extracellular adenosine (77–80). Antisera to a levulinic acid derivative of adenosine have enabled the tentative mapping of adenosine-containing neurones in rat brain (81). The distribution of immunoreactivity is comparable to that seen for A_1 receptors (82). In hippocampus, 5'-nucleotidase is co-localized with A_1 receptors (82), which may be a finding of potential functional relevance. Broken cell preparations from brain tissue have an apparently unlimited capacity to produce adenosine (29, 46, 83); thus, tissues must be pretreated with ADA to detect high-affinity binding sites. Removal of this enzyme reduces specific binding (83), indicating that the purine is being continuously produced. The source of this adenosine, and its relationship to the physiological availability of the nucleoside, has not yet been determined. Overall, therefore, other than those in distress states such as hypoxia or ischemia (5, 84), the factors regulating the physiological availability of adenosine are poorly understood.

Another facet of this issue is the "purinergic inhibitory tone." Because xanthine adenosine antagonists can increase neurotransmitter release (85), cell firing (86), and behavioral activity (87), it is generally agreed that adenosine is normally present extracellularly (5) and that it may fulfill a homeostatic role in target tissues. In the heart, for instance, the release of adenosine during hypoxia prevents an excessive mechanical load on cardiac tissue while at the same time it dilates the coronary vasculature to increase oxygen supply to the tissue (88). Similarly, during epileptic fits, adenosine can be released in brain tissue (89) and may act as an endogenous anti-convulsant. Although speculative, the relationship between hypothalamic ADA-containing neurons and jaw movement is suggested to be related to aggressive attack behavior and, consequently, to survival (90). In all these situations, adenosine acts as a protective agent, or, as termed by Newby (84), a "retaliatory metabolite." An endogenous adenosine tone has also been reported at the neuromuscular junction (91).

Uptake or deamination terminates the actions of adenosine as a neuromodulator (1, 66). High-affinity uptake mechanisms have been characterized (92). In rat brain a rapid-uptake system with a K_m value of 0.9 μM and a slower system with two components with K_m values of 1 and 5 μM have been described. Adenosine transport can be blocked in both directions such that many uptake inhibitors can prevent the purine from leaving the cell (92). Transport inhibitors such as dipyridamole (93) and, to a lesser extent, CV 1808 (Figure 1; 94) are effective vasodilators. Adenosine transport site can be labeled using either nitrobenzylthioinosine (NBI; 95), a ligand that is a selective adenosine uptake inhibitor, or dipyridamole (96). [^{3}H]NBI binds with high affinity (K_d = 50 pM) to mammalian brain tissue. Somewhat unexpectedly, [^{3}H]NBI does not require the removal of endogenous adenosine to facilitate its characterization. This difference may be due to the fact that NBI does not bind to the active site of the transporter mechanism but rather to a component protein. Also, dipyridamole is a relatively weak inhibitor of NBI binding (95), and higher concentrations of NBI than those used in binding are required for adenosine to depress cell firing (97). Inhibition of the catabolic enzyme, ADA, induces sleep (98, 99). Immunocytochemical studies of this enzyme (100) located a discrete plexus of ADA-containing neurons in the basal hypothalamus that innervate the striatum, amygdala, and cortex. A correlation between the regional distribution of ADA-immunoreactive neurons and NBI binding sites has been reported (101), suggesting that the systems are coinvolved in regulating the bioavailability of the purine.

SECOND MESSENGER SYSTEMS

Cyclic AMP

As indicated, cyclic AMP is the primary second messenger associated with adenosine receptor activation (6). The nucleoside is a ligand for the recognition site. In contrast to other cyclic nucleotide–modulated systems, cyclic AMP can also modulate the enzyme via direct interactions with the P site on the catalytic subunit (Table 1). In addition, it can contribute to the precursor pool of ATP used as a substrate by the enzyme. In intact slice preparations, the contribution of exogenous adenosine to this ATP pool is negligible (6) and cannot account for the increase in cyclic AMP associated with A_2 receptor activation. While cyclic AMP is a potent modulator of protein kinase activity (102), the physiological consequences of adenosine-related increases in cyclic AMP have yet to be demonstrated (29). The biphasic effects of R-PIA on glutamate release in cultured cerebellar neurons (103) in the absence and presence of pertussis toxin can be related to effects on both A_1 and A_2 receptors. In the absence of the toxin, R-PIA inhibits glutamate release. Pertussis toxin binds irreversibly to the N_i subunit (104) of adenylate cyclase.

This binding prevents A_1 receptor activation and reveals the involvement of an A_2 component in the adenosine agonist response and a concomitant increase in glutamate release. These toxin effects parallel similar effects on cyclic AMP formation.

Phosphatidylinositol Turnover

The recent surge of interest in the role of phospholipids as second messengers in the diacylglycerol–inositol triphosphate pathways (105) prompted evaluation of adenosine as an effector agent. While adenosine alone has no demonstrated effect, it can potentiate the effects of histamine (38).

Ion Fluxes

The effects of adenosine on ion movement in both central (30, 47, 73, 106) and peripheral (30, 107) tissues have been well documented. Adenosine has pre- and postsynaptic effects (30, 108–111), the former related to adenosine's indirect actions on the release of other neurotransmitters (see below) and the latter to its direct effects on cellular excitation. The ionic mechanisms involved reflect changes in calcium influx (30, 73, 112, 113), increases in potassium conductance (108, 109), and possibly regulation of sodium movement (113). Adenosine also has nonsynaptic effects in the hippocampal slice preparation (30, 114, 115) that probably result from an increase in K^+ conductance. Adenosine has an additional postsynaptic effect of long duration. It reduces neuronal excitability through calcium-dependent enhancement after hyperpolarizations (110). The effects of the purine on membrane conductance (106, 108, 113) are controversial (30). Synaptic transmission can be reduced by adenosine at concentrations that have no effect on membrane conductance potential (30). Presynaptic, rather than postsynaptic, actions, therefore, seem primarily responsible for the depressant actions of adenosine (114). The chronotropic and dromotropic actions of adenosine are also related to changes in K^+ conductance (107).

At the molecular level, direct interactions between adenosine and calcium have been reported (116, 117), although adenosine does not affect the positive inotropic actions of the dihydropyridine calcium agonist Bay K 8644 (118). Cyclic AMP does not appear to be an obligatory second messenger for the electrophysiological effects of adenosine (36). A third receptor subtype, termed A_3, may be involved in such effects (49).

Neurotransmitter Release

Adenosine is a potent and apparently ubiquitous modulator of neurotransmitter release. It has been reported to inhibit the release of aspartate, glutamate, norepinephrine, GABA, dopamine, serotonin, and acetylcholine (for reviews see 30, 47, 119). Adenosine has been reported to have biphasic effects on acetylcholine (120), and on norepinephrine and dopamine release (121), that may be related to the receptor subtype activated (103, 120). The role cyclic AMP plays in these effects on transmitter release is unclear (3, 29, 30).

From a physiological, as opposed to pharmacological, vantage point, the effects of adenosine on transmitter release are confusing. The concentrations of adenosine required to change in vitro release are higher than those necessary to change electrophysiological parameters. This discrepancy has been discussed (30) in relation to the effects of potassium on the various release systems. As mentioned, adenosine is generally thought to act presynaptically and to regulate calcium flux (37, 116), affecting stimulus–secretion coupling (73). Obtaining definitive evidence for the direct effects of adenosine on calcium fluxes has been difficult (30). Silinsky (73) has alternatively suggested that receptor activation may reduce the affinity of a strategic component of the secretory apparatus for calcium. Irrespective of the molecular events involved, the effects of adenosine on transmitter release need evaluation within the context of autoreceptor function (122).

Receptor activation involves a neurotransmitter released presynaptically that can modulate its own release, usually by feedback inhibition. Assigning a role in this process to the apparently nonspecific actions of adenosine has led to a good deal of confusion and has significantly contributed to the skepticism surrounding the therapeutic value of an agent affecting purinergic systems. At a behavioral level, adenosine has sedative activity (3) because it inhibits the release of glutamate and aspartate, the major excitatory transmitters in the brain. Adenosine can also inhibit the release of GABA, the major inhibitory neurotransmitter in the brain. Adenosine's sedative effect can be reconciled to its inhibition of GABA release because it disinhibits GABA-related tonic influences. The localization of A_1 receptor to axon terminals of excitatory neurons (76) is consistent with this reasoning.

However, many studies use a reductionist approach, that is, tissues are usually prelabeled with an excess of a chosen radioactive transmitter (or a precursor) that may not be stored (or released) in a manner analogous to that of the endogenous substance. Because of this bias, only the substance chosen to be studied actually is. In vivo, however, the effects of caffeine on dopamine metabolism are regionally selective (123). Other in vivo studies using more sophisticated assay techniques to measure endogenous release will provide further evidence for the selectivity of adenosine.

Adenosine can also affect monoamine synthesis. It affects the activity of tyrosine hydroxylase (124), increasing the enzyme's activity in the PC12 pheochromocytoma cell line while changing cyclic AMP levels.

STRUCTURE–ACTIVITY RELATIONSHIPS AT ADENOSINE RECOGNITION SITES

Defining receptor site function depends almost exclusively on identifying chemicals that selectively interact with the receptor in question. The major impetus in adenosine-related research was the observation that caffeine, the most widely used psychoactive agent in the world (3, 125), was an adenosine antagonist (22). Although almost twenty years have since passed, studies of purine nucleosides are directed more to their actions as antimetabolites (126) than as neuromodulatory agents. Thus, without exception, all known adenosine agonists are purine nucleosides (6), whereas antagonists, with few exceptions, are imidazol [3,4d]-pyrimidines (9, 10, 26, 57).

Studies of these agonists and antagonists have led to a considerable knowledge of the structure–activity relationship (SAR) for adenosine receptors (127, 128). Using avidin-biotin conjugates (129), investigators have examined the receptor topography for the brain A_1 receptor. As already discussed, substitutions in the N^6, 2, and 5' positions on the purine ring confer receptor site selectivity (39) and make the compound more resistant to degradation and uptake (6). Examination of many agonist analogs led to the postulation of models for the brain A_1 receptor (130) and for the coronary receptor. The coronary receptor has an SAR different from that for either A_1 or A_2 receptors (131). Adenosine analogs substituted in the N^6 position (CHA, CPA, R-PIA; Figure 1) are A_1 selective; 5'-substituted (NECA, MECA) and 2-substituted analogs (CV 1808) are active at A_2 receptor. Compounds substituted in both the N^6 and 5' positions tend to still be A_1 selective (130), but with reduced activity. The observed lower intrinsic activity and efficacy of adenosine itself have generally been assumed (3, 6, 16, 29, 30) to be the result of the endogenous compound's susceptibility to metabolic degradation and uptake. This susceptibility may still be a major factor and certainly is in receptor binding assays that include ADA. However, several adenosine agonists differ in their efficacy, as assessed by their ability to increase A_2 receptor–mediated cyclic AMP formation (46, 48, 132). The order of activity is: NECA > 2-CADO > CPA $\geq$ N^6-methyladenosine = adenosine N'-oxide > adenosine > R-PIA $\geq$ CHA > S-PIA. The position of the substitutions does not appear to be consistently related to the efficacy of the analogs, which have been suggested (132) to be partial agonists. However, P site (Table 1) activation may contribute to the efficacy of the analogs. The analogs probably do not interact with A_1 and A_2 receptor subtypes (103), as the binding profiles of these compounds show (40).

Substitutions in the 8-position of the xanthine molecule (Figure 2) increase adenosine antagonist activity considerably (9, 10, 26, 43, 57) in some instances and similarly decrease solubility (7). DPX, PACPX, and a series of 27 other xanthines exhibit receptor selectivity of the order: $A_1 > A_{2_b} > A_{2_a}$ (40). The activity of 8-cyclopentyltheophylline (CPT) when compared to that of CPA has led to the suggestion (40) that the cyclopentyl moiety of the xanthine and the purine both bind to the same region of the A_1 receptor. The xanthine therefore bound "backwards" compared to the nucleoside, with the pyrimidine ring of the xanthine corresponding to that of the purine (Figures 1 & 2). The functionalized congeners, XAC and XCC (Figure 2; 10), and PD 113,297 (Figure 2; 40; 133) are more soluble 8-substituted xanthines. PD 116,948 (Figure 2) is an A_1-selective antagonist, whereas PD 115,199, like NECA, is nonselective in its antagonist actions (59, 134). BW A1433U (Figure 2) is another potent xanthine antagonist (135).

Nonxanthine adenosine antagonists have also been described (Figure 3). CGS 8216, a pyrazoloquinoline that is a potent inverse agonist at the central benzodiazepine receptor (136), has weak adenosine antagonist activity (44). Subsequent chemical modification of this compound led to the identification of the triazoloquinazoline CGS 15943A (44), a potent A_2-selective adenosine antagonist with minimal benzodiazepine receptor interactions. The pyrazolopyridines etazolate and cartazolate also have adenosine antagonist activity (40, 129, 137), as does the pyrazolopyrimidine DJB-KK (138) (Figure 3). Two other xanthines, S-caffeine (139) and propentofylline (HWA 825; 140, 141), have somewhat unusual biological activity profiles. Their effects are opposite to those of the more classical xanthines. It has been speculated (140) that propentofylline may be the first xanthine adenosine agonist. It enhances the effects of adenosine (142).

PHYSIOLOGICAL IMPLICATIONS OF ADENOSINE RECEPTOR FUNCTION

Central Nervous System

Much of the receptor work on adenosine receptor function has been carried out using nervous tissue because this tissue has a higher density of these receptors than other tissues. Because of the ubiquitous distribution of the nucleoside and its receptors (82, 143) and the paucity of structurally dissimilar chemical entities to probe the adenosine receptor, adenosine's physiological role in CNS function has largely been defined by inference (29, 30).

ADENOSINE AND LOCOMOTOR ACTIVITY   Adenosine agonists decrease spontaneous motor activity (3) when administered either peripherally or directly into the brain. Sedative effects can also be observed (3, 21, 142). While A_2 receptor activation has been linked to the sedative and locomotor effects of adenosine (144), the relative bioavailability of the various agonists may also be a contributory factor (30). These effects of adenosine can be blocked by xanthines. However, adenosine at lower doses than those required to decrease locomotor performance can increase activity via mechanisms that cannot be blocked by caffeine (3).

ADENOSINE AND SLEEP   Adenosine is a potent sedative, eliciting a hypnotic state in various species including mammals (20, 21, 99, 145, 146). In rats, adenosine agonists increase deep sleep duration (146) and may increase REM sleep. Administration of the ADA-inhibitors EHNA (erythrohydroxynonyl-adenine; 98) or deoxycoformycin (99) can induce sleeplike states. The adenosine analog, 1-methylisoguanosine (doridosine), does not affect sleep (147), suggesting receptor selectivity for adenosine. The central stimulant activity of the xanthines (3, 125) is consistent with a sedative and hypnotic action for endogenous adenosine. The ethanol-sensitive "long-sleep" mouse is more sensitive to the sedative and hypothermic actions of R-PIA than the ethanol-insensitive "short-sleep" mouse (148). Such differences that have been related to increases in both the affinity and density of A_1 receptors in the long-sleep mouse (149).

ADENOSINE AND ANXIETY   Caffeine has well-documented anxiogenic activity (125, 150). Following the discovery of a central benzodiazepine receptor (151), considerable effort was expended in the search for an endogenous factor similar in function to the enkephalins at the opiate receptor (or receptors) that would be the endogenous anxiogenic and anxiolytic agent. Inosine, isolated from bovine brain, was found to be a weak inhibitor (IC_{50} = 10^{-3} M) of ligand binding to the benzodiazepine receptor. Isobutylmethyl-xanthine and 2-CADO were subsequently determined to be ligands for this receptor (151). The later identification of the β-carbolines (152) and various peptidic entities (153) that demonstrated activity similar to that of the ben-zodiazepines (IC_{50} values = 10^{-9} M) raised considerable debate about the physiological significance of the inosine interaction (151, 154, 155). Further-more, no correlation could be demonstrated for the effects of a series of anxiolytics on benzodiazepine and A_1 receptor binding (137).

Despite these negative data, a considerable amount of circumstantial evi-dence still links purines to the antianxiety and other properties of the ben-zodiazepines. Xanthines can antagonize the effects of benzodiazepines on cell firing (47) and behavior (155). Purines, like the benzodiazepines, are effec-tive muscle relaxants (156, 157). It has been suggested that the sedative effects of the benzodiazepines, but not their anxiolytic activity, involves some interaction with purine-related systems (155). The adenosine-uptake in-hibitor, dipyridamole, can inhibit benzodiazepine and A_1 receptor binding equally (137, 158) and has benzodiazepine agonist activity in vivo (159). The benzodiazepine antagonist, Ro 15-1788, can antagonize caffeine-induced seizures in mice (160). The effects of the prototypic anxiolytic, meprobamate, together with those of many other centrally active therapeutic agents (161), have been related to the ability of such compounds to weakly inhibit adenosine uptake (66). Benzodiazepine receptor antagonists cannot, however, inhibit the effects of diazepam on adenosine uptake (162). Given this series of relationships and the weak adenosine antagonist activity of the inverse agonist, CGS 8216 (136, 137), there may be similarities in the receptor topography and/or function of the central benzodiazepine receptor and the A_1 receptor.

ADENOSINE AND EPILEPSY   Caffeine and theophylline have convulsant activity at high doses (125), whereas adenosine can prevent audiogenic- (21), kainate-, picrotoxin-, and mercaptoproprionic acid– (145) induced seizures. Adenosine levels in brain increase markedly during seizure activity (163), and as already noted, the purine may function as an endogenous anticonvulsant (89). R-PIA prolongs postictal depression and decreases the frequency of spiking following amydaloid-kindled and metrazole-induced (164, 165) seizures. The effects of the anticonvulsant carbamazepine have been related to both diazepam and adenosine processes although an SAR was absent (166). Chronic treatment with carbamazepine can up-regulate A_1 receptors (166). The barbiturate anticonvulsants have micromolar affinity for the A_1 receptor (167).

ADENOSINE AND ANALGESIA   As with the other central processes in which adenosine may play a role, the association of adenosine with the mechanisms involved in analgesia is complex. Xanthines reduce morphine analgesia (168) and can elicit a "quasi-morphine withdrawal syndrome" (QMWS; 169), which involves an increase in norepinephrine turnover (170, 171). The α_2-adrenoceptor agonist clonidine can antagonize the QMWS phenomenon (172). Both adenosine and clonidine have been used to suppress responses to opiate withdrawal in humans (173) and animals (174). Xanthines reverse the respiratory depressant actions of morphine (175) and act as an analgesic adjuvant (176). This effect may be related to their ability to inhibit cyclooxygenase activity (177). Conflicting reports (168, 178) have suggested that xanthines have both analgesic and antinociceptive activity, as does adenosine (179). The analgesic actions of R-PIA can be blocked by theophylline but not by naloxone (180). Increases in adenosine receptor density have been found in morphine-dependent mice (181).

ADENOSINE AND DEPRESSION   It has been suggested, on the basis of the effects of antidepressants on cyclic AMP formation and their ability to potentiate the effects of adenosine, that certain of the effects of antidepressants involve adenosine-related processes (182, 183). Chronic electro-convulsive therapy (ECT), used in the treatment of depression, increases A_1 receptor density in rat brain (184). However, neither chronic antidepressant (185) nor lithium (184) treatment affects the affinity or density of A_1 receptors. Several antidepressants are weak inhibitors of adenosine uptake (183).

ADENOSINE AND SELF-MUTILATION BEHAVIORS   Large doses of caffeine can elicit a self-destructive behavior in rats (186) similar to that observed in Lesch–Nyhan syndrome (187), an X-linked disorder that results in a deficit in the purine-metabolizing enzyme hypoxanthine-guanine phosphoribosyltrans-ferase (HRGTPase). While chronic caffeine intake elicits a similar behavioral profile, rather than decreasing HRGPTase activity, the xanthine can actually increase it (186). This action suggests that the enzyme changes are co-incidental and that the primary lesion in this disorder is a hyperactivity of central dopaminergic systems, most notably at the level of the basal ganglia (188). A selective association between adenosine and dopamine occurs at the behavioral (189, 190) and anatomical (191) levels. This relationship is further emphasized by the demonstrated antipsychotic profile of adenosine agonists in animal models (192).

The relationship between α_2 adrenoceptor– and adenosine receptor– mediated events is further underlined by the fact that clonidine can induce self-mutilation (193). This effect is enhanced by caffeine and attenuated by adenosine (194).

Cardiovascular

Adenosine can regulate coronary blood flow (13, 18, 71) and has negative dromotropic, chronotropic, and inotropic effects on heart contractility (18, 107). These effects can be mediated directly through interactions with adeno-sine receptors. They can be indirectly mediated by either the inhibition of the release of other neurotransmitters affecting heart function or by the indirect antagonism of the myocardial actions of norepinephrine. The increase in coronary blood flow is mediated by A_2-receptor activation (195). The effects on cardiac rhythmicity that involve the suppression of impulse formation in the sinoatrial node and the blockade of impulse propagation in the atrioven-tricular node (107) involve an A_1 receptor (18, 107). Exogenously adminis-tered adenosine, due to its effects on cardiac conduction, has been suc-cessfully used in the treatment of supraventricular tachycardia (196). During hypoxia, ischemia, or reactive hyperemia, adenosine is freely available (13, 18). Thus, the observed effects of the purine on cardiac function are physi-ological rather than pharmacological. Purine effects on heart function have been directly compared with those of acetylcholine (197). Both compounds have negative ionotropic actions, shorten atrial transmembrane action potentials, activate K^+ channels, and elicit antiadrenergic effects in Purkinje cell fibers. The negative chronotropic effects of adenosine, unlike those seen with acetylcholine, are indirect, however (197, 198). This indirect action, like that related to the antagonism of catecholamine actions at the adenylate cyclase level (18), has not been demonstrated in the intact animal (193). Adenosine infusion can markedly decrease mean arterial pressure without affecting heart rate (199). In light of adenosine's lack of selectivity for either receptor subtype, this finding suggests (195) that A_2 receptors are more sensitive to adenosine than A_1 receptors. However, the A_1 receptor–mediated effects of adenosine may offset the reflex stimulation of the heart when arterial blood pressure decreases. A vagal component of the effects of the purine on heart function also exists (8, 13) that does not appear to be mediated through reflex mechanisms.

Xanthines have been used as cardiotonics (200) although their solubility and efficacy as adenosine antagonists result in the concomitant inhibition of phosphodiesterase activity and the generation of arrhythmias. The vasodilatory actions of a series of adenosine analogs have been ascribed to interactions with an atypical A_2 receptor (201).

The possibility that the centrally observed actions of adenosine may be indirect and mediated via alteration in blood pressure or changes in the cerebral blood flow has been an issue of some concern (202). While peripheral actions can contribute to the central effects of the purine, changes in CNS function have been reported to occur at purine doses well below those that cause observable changes in blood pressure (3).

Renal

Adenosine, in contrast to its effects in the coronary vasculature, is a vasoconstrictor in the kidney (19) and has biphasic effects on renin release (203). At low concentrations, activating A_1 receptors inhibits renin release and at higher concentrations, activating A_2 receptors stimulates renin release. While both receptor subtypes are present on afferent arterioles (mediating constriction and dilation, respectively), only A_2 receptors are present on efferent arterioles, and these mediate dilation. Adenosine can increase sodium excretion (204) and sympathetic nervous activity, and it reduces the glomerular filtration rate (205). Adenosine is released from macula densa cells in response to an increased sodium load, which may function as the signal transducer to modulate renin release. Binding sites for $[^3H]2$-CADO have been identified in kidney membranes (206).

Pulmonary

Theophylline is one of the most widely used antiasthmatic agents, acting as a bronchodilator (207). This effect has been traditionally ascribed to inhibition of phosphodiesterase activity, an effect that parallels the effects of β_2 adrenoceptor agonists and forskolin in increasing pulmonary cylic AMP levels (208). In rat mast cells and guinea pig lung tissue, adenosine potentiates the histamine release that results from an allergic challenge. In human basophils, however, adenosine inhibits mediator release (209, 210). This apparent dichotomy has been resolved by the work by Church & Holgate (211), who found that adenosine has biphasic effects on mediator release, which reflect the time of challenge after an allergic insult. Administration of adenosine to asthmatics causes bronchoconstriction but has no effect in normal subjects. Thus, the effects of theophylline as an antiasthmatic may be consistent with its actions as an adenosine antagonist. Examination of the agonist profile for the mediation of histamine release from rat mast cells (212) has provided evidence that a novel adenosine receptor, neither A_1 nor A_2, is involved in the mediation of autocoid release.

Adenosine and the Immune System

Adenosine can inhibit the mitogenic stimulation of lymphocytes by phytohemagglutinin and can inhibit the cytolytic actions of mouse lymphocytes (213). The purine modulates T-cell subset-specific antigen expression, facilitating T8 antigen expression and activating radioresistant suppressor activity (214). Defects in immune function have been linked to deficiencies in ADA activity. In Hodgkin's disease, both ADA and 5'-nucleotidase activity decrease (215). In acquired immune deficiency syndrome (AIDS), purine nucleoside phosphorylase and ADA activities are increased (216). Such an increase suggests that the cellular disorder in this disease probably results from abnormal lymphocyte differentiation. Adenosine can potently modulate neutrophil superoxide formation by interacting with A_2 receptors (217). It also prevents endothelial damage in cell cultures (218). The involvement of cyclic AMP in this effect is unclear (217). 2-CADO has immunosuppressant activity (219).

Gastrointestinal Function

Caffeine and theophylline can augment stress-related events (220). In rats restrained in the cold for 3 hr (221) or immobilized for 12 hr (222) a high incidence of gastric lesions occurs. CHA and R-PIA can also produce lesions in nonstressed animals. In studying the interaction of adenosine and clonidine in analgesia and self-mutilation and aggressive behavior, it was found that the α_2 adrenoceptor agonist, clonidine, could block the action of adenosine on gastric lesion formation. This stress-related phenomenon appears to be centrally mediated via A_1 receptors (221, 222). Adenosine receptors modulating gastric acid secretion are also present in the gastric fundus (223). The purine can also modulate pancreatic secretion (224).

Respiration

Adenosine can cause respiratory depression via a mechanism that can be blocked by aminophylline (225). When administered both centrally and peripherally, adenosine and related analogs can decrease inspiratory neural drive and prolong expiratory time. Aminophylline has been used to treat the paradoxical ventilatory response in infants, and i.v. adenosine can stimulate respiration (226) via a mechanism involving an increase in carotid-body chemoceptor discharge (227).

ADENOSINE RECEPTOR DYNAMICS

Treatment of animals with caffeine or theophylline can cause an up-regulation of A_1 receptors (228, 229), an effect associated with tolerance to the xanthines (230). Chronic carbamazepine (166) and opiate treatment (181) can increase receptor density. In contrast, in gerbils, transient ischemia can down-regulate A_1 receptors in the CA1 region of the hippocampus (231).

ADENOSINE UPTAKE

The physiological significance of the ability of various classes of psychotherapeutic agents to inhibit adenosine uptake has yet to be resolved, especially since the concentrations required to show significant effects are usually in the micromolar range. Nearly every class of centrally active therapeutic agents inhibits adenosine uptake (66). The side effects associated with the use of heterocyclic compounds (which can accumulate at high concentrations in brain bilayers) may be related to a relatively nonspecific effect on adenosine uptake.

ADENOSINE AND CELLULAR ENERGY CHARGES

The control of cerebral blood flow has been related to the redox state of NAD/NADH (232). However, cyclic AMP produced in response to A_2-receptor activation may be the primary mediator of the vasodilatory and vascular permeability changes (163, 233). In the context of the "retaliatory metabolite" hypothesis, and the production of adenosine under adverse conditions, some adenosine-related neuromodulatory events may involve an energy charge transfer (33). In hypoxia, purine release from brain slices is related to a decrease in energy charge (234).

THERAPEUTIC TARGETING OF ADENOSINE RECEPTOR MODULATORS

In considering the potential therapeutic applications of agents that either mimic or antagonize the actions of adenosine, it is clear that there are a variety of targets, many of which are attractive pharmacologically. Adenosine agonists may be effective as antihypertensive agents (8, 195), in the treatment of opiate withdrawal (174), as modulators of immune competence (215) and renin release (203), as antipsychotics (192), and as hypnotics (146). Conversely, antagonists may be useful as central stimulants (3), nootropics (141), cardiotonics (200), antistress agents (221), antiasthmatics (211), and in the treatment of respiratory disorders (225). As emphasized, this relative smorgasbord of therapeutic applications reflects the lack of tissue- and receptor-selective adenosine-receptor ligands. The demonstration of consistent species differences in adenosine-related systems (45, 235) further emphasizes the potential significance of adenosine in mammalian tissue function and the need for more selective agents (8).

Much research needs to be done to reach this goal. The consistent, but as yet undemonstrated, interactions between adenosine and opiate, α adrenoceptor, benzodiazepine receptor ligands, and, to a lesser extent, calcium channel–related processes further suggest that adenosine neuromodulation is not an epiphenomenon. In regard to the availability of endogenous adenosine under normal conditions, it has been suggested (29, 30, 236) that receptor density rather than purine availability is the primary factor determining responses to adenosine. This suggestion would be consistent with the selective activation of coronary A_2 receptors by nonselective agonists (195). Much of the work done in the past five years has, due to technical limitations, been confined to the A_1 receptor. The possibility that A_{2a}, A_{2b}, and P_2 receptors may play significant roles in tissue function cannot be discounted at this time.

Dunwiddie (30) has compared the role of adenosine as a neuromodulator with that of cyclic AMP in relation to protein kinase activation, where the location of the enzyme and its substrates regulates the final response to elevation of cyclic nucleotide levels. In any event, adenosine and related adenine nucleotides, like the peptides, represent unconventional neurotransmitters. They require new hypotheses to explain their role in tissue function (30). With the current rapid progress in the biological evaluation of adenosine as a neuromodulator, together with increased efforts in developing new chemical entities in this area, adenosine may be the first neuromodulator to aid significantly the understanding and treatment of human disease states where current therapy is either absent or limited.

ACKNOWLEDGMENTS

The author would like to thank Drs. Tom Dunwiddie, John Daly, John Carney, and Al Hutchison for helpful discussions, and Ruth Thompson, Natalie Johnson and Lenora Hall for excellent administrative support. Space limitations have necessitated literature citations being kept to a minimum.

Literature Cited

1. Arch, J. R. S., Newsholme, E. A. 1978. The control of the metabolism and the hormonal role of adenosine. *Essays Biochem.* 14:82–123
2. Alberts, B., Bray, D., Lewis, J., Raff, M., Roberts, K., Watson, J. D. 1983. *Molecular Biology of the Cell*, New York: Garland
3. Snyder, S. H. 1985. Adenosine as a neuromodulator. *Ann. Rev. Neurosci.* 8:103–24
4. Bradford, H. F. 1986. *Chemical Neurobiology*, pp. 158–59. New York: Freeman
5. Williams, M. 1984. Adenosine—a selective neuromodulator in the mammalian CNS? *Trends Neurosci.* 7:164–68
6. Daly, J. W. 1982. Adenosine receptors: target sites for drugs. *J. Med. Chem.* 25:197–207
7. Bruns, R. F., Daly, J. W., Snyder, S. H. 1983. Adenosine receptor binding: structure activity analysis generates extremely potent xanthine antagonists. *Proc. Natl. Acad. Sci. USA* 80:2077–80
8. Williams, M. 1985. Tissue and species differences in adenosine receptors and their possible relevance to drug development. In *Adenosine: Receptors and Modulation of Cell Function*, ed. V. Stefanovich, K. Rudolphi, P. Schubert, pp. 73–85. Oxford: IRL Press
9. Daly, J. W., Padgett, W., Shamin, M. T., Butts-Lamb P., Waters, J. 1985. 1,3-Dialkyl-8-(p-sulfophenyl)xanthines: potent water-soluble antagonists for A_1- and A_2 adenosine receptors. *J. Med. Chem.* 28:487–492
10. Jacobson, K. A., Kirk, K. L., Padgett, W. L., Daly, J. W. 1985. Functionalized congeners of 1,3-dialkylxanthines: preparation of analogs with high affinity for adenosine receptors. *J. Med. Chem.* 28:1334–40
11. Hanley, M. 1985. Peptide Binding Assays. In *Neurotransmitter Receptor Binding*, ed. H. I. Yamamura, S. J. Enna, M. J. Kuhar, pp. 91–102. New York: Raven. 2nd ed.

12. Schwartz, J. H. 1981. Chemical basis of synaptic transmission. In *Principles of Neural Science*, ed. E. R. Kandel, J. H. Schwartz, pp. 106–20. New York: Elsevier-North Holland
13. Drury, A. N., Szent-Gyorgi, A. 1929. The physiological activity of adenine compounds with especial reference to their actions upon the mammalian heart. *J. Physiol. London* 68:213–37
14. Williams, M. 1987. Purinergic receptors and central nervous system function. In *Psychopharmacology: A Third Generation of Progress*, ed. H. Meltzer. New York: Raven. In press
15. Honey, R. M., Ritchie, W. T., Thomson, W. A. R. 1930. The action of adenosine upon the human heart. *Quart. J. Med.* 23:485–89
16. Editorial. 1985. Adenosine revisited. *Lancet* 2:927–28
17. Berne, R. M., Knabb, R. M., Ely, S. W., Rubio, R. 1983. Adenosine in the local regulation of blood flow: a brief overview. *Fed. Proc.* 42:3136–42
18. Fredholm, B. B., Sollevi, A. 1986. Cardiovascular effects of adenosine. *Clin. Physiol.* 6:1–21
19. Osswald, H. 1983. Adenosine and renal function. In *Regulatory Function of Adenosine*, ed. R. M. Berne, T. W. Rall, R. Rubio, pp. 399–415. Boston: Nijhoff
20. Feldberg, W., Sherwood, S. L. 1954. Injections of drugs into the lateral ventricle of the cat. *J. Physiol. London* 123:148–67
21. Maitre, M., Ciesielski, L., Lehmann, A., Kempf, E., Mandel, P. 1974. Protective effect of adenosine and nicotinamide against audiogenic seizure. *Biochem. Pharmacol.* 23:2807–16
22. Sattin, A., Rall, T. W. 1970. The effect of adenosine and adenine nucleotides on the cyclic adenosine 3'5'-phosphate content of guinea pig cerebral cortex slices. *Mol. Pharmacol.* 6:13–23
23. Londos, C. Wolff, T. 1977. Two distinct adenosine-sensitive sites on adenyl-

ate cyclase. *Proc. Natl. Acad. Sci. USA* 74:5482–86

24. Londos, C., Wolff, J., Cooper, D. M. F. 1983. Adenosine receptors and adenylate cyclase interactions. See Ref. 19, pp. 17–32

25. Van Calker, D., Muller, M., Hamprecht, B. 1979. Adenosine regulates via two different types of receptors, the accumulation of cyclic AMP in cultured brain cells. *J. Neurochem.* 33:999–1005

26. Smellie, F. W., Davis, C. W., Daly, J. W., Wells, T. N. 1979. Alkylxanthines-inhibition of adenosine-elicited accumulation of cyclic AMP in brain slices and of brain phosphodiesterase activity. *Life Sci.* 24:2475–81

27. Bruns, R. F., Daly, J. W., Snyder, S. H. 1980. Adenosine receptors in brain membranes: binding of N^6-cyclohexyl[^{3}H]adenosine and 1,3-diethyl-8-[^{3}H]phenylxanthine. *Proc. Natl. Acad. Sci. USA* 77:5547–51

28. Stone, T. W. 1981. Physiological roles for adenosine and adenosine 5'-triphosphate in the nervous system. *Neuroscience* 6:523–45

29. Williams, M. 1984. Mammalian adenosine receptors. *Handb. Neurochem.* 6:1–28

30. Dunwiddie, T. V. 1985. The physiological roles of adenosine in the central nervous system. *Int. Rev. Neurobiol.* 27:63–139

31. Burnstock, G. 1983. A comparison of receptors for adenosine and adenine nucleotides. See Ref. 19, pp. 49–62

32. Burnstock, G., Kennedy, C. 1985. Is there a basis for distinguishing two types of P_2-purinoceptor? *Gen. Pharmac.* 16:433–40

33. Atkinson, D. E. 1968. Energy charge of the adenylate pool as a regulatory parameter. *Biochemistry* 7:4030–34

34. Haslam, R. J., Davidson, M. M. L., Desjardins, T. V. 1978. Inhibition of adenylate cyclase by adenosine analogues in preparations of broken and intact human platelets. Evidence for the unidirectional control of platelet function by cyclic AMP. *Biochem. J.* 176:83–95

35. Dolphin, A. C., Archer, E. A. 1983. An adenosine agonist inhibits and a cyclic AMP analogue enhances the release of glutamate but not GABA from slices of rat dentate gyrus. *Neurosci. Lett.* 43:49–54

36. Dunwiddie, T. W., Fredholm, B. B. 1984. Adenosine receptors mediating inhibitory electrophysiological responses in rat hippocampus are different from receptors mediating cAMP formation. *Naunyn Schmiedebergs Arch. Pharmacol.* 326:294–301

37. Riberio, J. A., Sa-Almedia, A. M., Namordo, J. M. 1979. Adenosine and adenosine triphosphates decrease $^{45}Ca^{2+}$ uptake by synaptosomes stimulated by potassium. *Biochem. Pharmacol.* 28:1297–300

38. Hollingsworth, E. B., De La Cruz, R. A., Daly, J. W. 1986. Accumulations of inositol phosphates and cyclic AMP in brain slices: synergistic interactions of histamine and 2-chloroadenosine. *Eur. J. Pharmacol.* 122:45–50

39. Hamprecht, B., Van Calker, D. 1985. Nomenclature of adenosine receptors. *Trends Pharmacol. Sci.* 6:153–54

40. Bruns, R. F., Lu, G. H., Pugsley, T. A. 1986. Characterization of the A_2 adenosine receptor labeled by [^{3}H]NECA in rat striatal membranes. *Mol. Pharmacol.* 29:331–46

41. Williams, M., Braunwalder, A., Erickson, T. E. 1986. Evaluation of the binding of the A-1 selective adenosine radioligand, cyclopentyladenosine (CPA), to rat brain tissue. *Naunyn Schmiedebergs Arch. Pharmacol.* 332:179–83

42. Deleted in proof

43. Schwabe, U., Ukena, D., Lohse, M. J. 1985. Xanthine derivatives as antagonists at A_1 and A_2 adenosine receptors. *Naunyn Schmiedebergs Arch. Pharmacol.* 330:212–21

44. Williams, M., Francis, J., Ghai, G., Psychoyos, S., Braunwalder, A., et al. 1987. Biochemical characterization of CGS 15943A, a novel, non-xanthine adenosine antagonist. *J. Pharmacol. Exp. Ther.* In press

45. Stone, G. A., Snowhill, E. W., Weeks, B., Williams, M. 1986. Species differences in adenosine A-2 receptor binding in mammalian striatal membranes. *Abstr. Soc. Neurosci.* 12:799

46. Premont, J., Perez, M., Blanc, G., Tarsin, J. P., Thierry, A. M., et al. 1979. Adenosine-sensitive adenylate cyclase in rat brain homogenates: kinetic characteristics, specificity, topographical, subcellular and cellular distribution. *Mol. Pharmacol.* 16:790–804

47. Phillis, J. W., Wu, P. H. 1981. The role of adenosine and its nucleotides in central synaptic transmission. *Prog. Neurobiol.* 16:187–93

48. Daly, T. W., Butts-Lamb, P., Padgett, W. 1983. Subclasses of adenosine re-

ceptors in the central nervous system: interaction with caffeine and related methylxanthines. *Cell. Mol. Neurobiol.* 3:69–80

49. Ribeiro, J. A., Sebastiao, A. M. 1986. Adenosine receptors and calcium: basis for proposing a third (A$_3$) adenosine receptor. *Prog. Neurobiol.* 26:179–209

50. Schwabe, U., Trost, T. 1980. Characterization of adenosine receptors in rat brain by (−)(^{3}H)N^6-phenylisopropyladenosine. *Naunyn Schmiedebergs Arch. Pharmacol.* 313:179–88

51. Linden, J., Hollen, C. E., Patel, A. 1985. The mechanism by which adenosine and cholinergic agents reduce contractility in rat myocardium. Correlation with cyclic adenosine monophosphate and receptor densities. *Circ. Res.* 56:728–35

52. Yeung, S.-M. H., Green, R. D. 1984. [^{3}H]-5'N-ethylcarboxamide adenosine binds to both Ra and Ri receptors in rat striatum. *Naunyn Schmiedebergs Arch. Pharmacol.* 325:218–25

53. Ukena, D., Poeschla, E., Hutteman, E., Schwabe, U. 1984. Effects of N-ethylmaleimide on adenosine receptors of rat fat cells and human platelets. *Naunyn Schmiedebergs Arch. Pharmacol.* 327:247–53

54. Fredholm, B. B., Lindren, E., Lindstrom, K. 1985. Treatment with N-ethylmaleimide selectively reduces adenosine receptor-mediated decreases in cyclic AMP accumulation in rat hippocampal slices. *Br. J. Pharmacol.* 86:509–13

55. Barnes, E. M. Jr., Thampy, K. G. 1982. Subclasses of adenosine receptors in brain membranes from adult tissue and from primary cultures of chick embryo. *J. Neurochem.* 39:647–52

56. Williams, M., Abreu, M., Jarvis, M. F., Noronha-Blob, L. 1987. Characterization of adenosine receptors in the PC12 pheochromocytoma cell line using radioligand binding-evidence for A-2 selectivity. *J. Neurochem.* In press

57. Jacobson, K. A., Kirk, K. L., Padgett, W. L., Daly, J. W. 1986. A functionalized congener approach to adenosine receptor antagonists: amino acid conjugates of 1,3-dipropylxanthine. *Mol. Pharmacol.* 29:126–33

58. Ukena, D., Jacobson, K. A., Kirk, K. L., Daly, J. W. 1986. A [^{3}H]amine congener of 1,3-dipropyl-8-phenylxanthine: a new radioligand for A$_2$ adenosine re-

ceptors of human platelets. *FEBS Lett.* 199:269–74

59. Bruns, R. F., Lu, G. H., Pugsley, T. A. 1986. Adenosine receptor subtypes: binding studies. *Pfluegers Arch.* 407:54 (Suppl.)

60. Salter, M. W., Henry, T. L. 1985. Effects of adenosine 5'-monophosphate and adenosine 5'-triphosphate on functionally identified neurons in the cat spinal horn. *Neuroscience* 15:815–25

61. Fedan, J. S., Hogaboom, G. K., O'Donnell, J. P., Westfall, D. P. 1985. Use of photoaffinity labels as P$_2$-purinoceptor antagonists. In *Methods Used in Pharmacology. Methods Used in Adenosine Research*, ed. D. M. Paton, 6:279–92. New York: Plenum

62. Williams, M., Risley, E. A. 1980. Binding of ^{3}H-adenyl-5-imidodiphosphate (AppNHp) to rat brain synaptic membranes. *Fed. Proc.* 39:1009

63. Levin, R. M., Jacoby, R., Wein, A. J. 1983. High affinity, divalent ion-specific binding of ^{3}H-ATP to homogenate derived from rabbit urinary bladder. *Mol. Pharmacol.* 23:1–7

64. Fedan, J. S., Hogaboom, G. K., O'Donnell, J. P., Jeng, C. J., Guillory, G. 1985. Interaction of [^{3}H]arylazido aminopropronyl ATP ([^{3}H]ANAPP$_3$) with P$_2$-purinergic receptors in the smooth muscle of the isolated guinea pig vas deferens. *Eur. J. Pharmacol.* 108:49–61

65. Frew, R., Lundy, R. M. 1986. Arylazido aminopropionyl ATP (ANAPP$_3$): interaction with adenosine receptors in longitudinal smooth muscle of the guinea-pig ileum. *Eur. J. Pharmacol.* 123:395–400

66. Wu, P. H., Phillis, J. W. 1984. Uptake by central nervous tissues as a mechanism for the regulation of extracellular adenosine concentrations. *Neurochem. Int.* 6:613–32

67. Olsson, R. A., Snow, J. A., Gentry, M. K. 1978. Adenosine metabolism in canine myocardial reactive hyperemia. *Circ. Res.* 42:358–62

68. Rubio, R., Wiedmeier, V. T., Berne, R. M. 1974. Relationship between coronary flow and adenosine production and release. *J. Mol. Cell. Cardiol.* 6:561–66

69. Rubio, R., Berne, R. M., Dobson, J. G. Jr. 1973. Sites of adenosine production in cardiac and skeletal muscle. *Am. J. Physiol.* 225:938–53

70. Schraeder, J., Schutz, W., Bardenheuer, H. 1981. Role of S-adenosylhomocysteine hydrolase in aden-

osine metabolism in mammalian heart. *Biochem. J.* 196:65–70

71. Sparks, H. V., Bardenheuer, H. 1986. Regulation of adenosine formation by the heart. *Circ. Res.* 58:193–201

71a. Lawson, R., Mowbray, J. 1986. Purine nucleotide metabolism: The discovery of a major new oligomeric adenosine tetraphosphate derivative in rat heart. *Int. J. Biochem.* 18:407–13

72. Israel, M., Lesbats, B., Manaranche, R., Muenier, F. M., Franchon, P. 1980. Retrograde inhibition of transmitter release by ATP. *J. Neurochem.* 34:923–32

73. Silinsky, E. 1985. Processes by which purines inhibit transmitter release. In *Purines: Pharmacology and Physiological Roles*, ed. T. W. Stone, pp. 67–73. Deerfield Beach, Fla: VCH Publications

74. Fredholm, B. B., Hedqvist, P. 1980. Modulation of neurotransmission by purine nucleotides and nucleosides. *Biochem. Pharmacol.* 29:1633–43

75. Jonzon, B., Fredholm, B. B. 1985. Release of purines, noradrenaline and GABA from rat hippocampal slices by field stimulation. *J. Neurochem.* 44:217–24

76. Goodman, R. R., Kuhar, M. J., Hester, L., Snyder, S. H. 1983. Adenosine receptors: autoradiographic evidence for their location on axon terminals of excitatory neurons. *Science* 220:967–68

77. Pons, F., Bruns, R. F., Daly, J. W. 1980. Depolarization-evoked accumulation of cyclic AMP in brain slices: the requisite intermediate adenosine is not derived from hydrolysis of released ATP. *J. Neurochem.* 34:1319–23

78. Newman, M. E., McIwain, H. 1977. Adenosine as a constituent of the brain and of isolated cerebral tissues, and its relationship to the generation of adenosine 3'5'-cyclic monophosphate. *Biochem. J.* 164:131–17

79. McDonald, W. F., White, T. D. 1984. Adenosine released from synaptosomes is derived from the extracellular dephosphorylation of released ATP. *Prog. Neuropsychopharmacol. Biol. Psychiatr.* 8:487–94

80. Marangos, P. J., Boulenger, T. P. 1985. Basic and clinical aspects of adenosinergic neuromodulation. *Neurosci. Biobehav. Rev.* 9:421–30

81. Braas, K. M., Newby, A. C., Wilson, V. S., Snyder, S. H. 1986. Adenosine containing neurons in the brain localized by immunocytochemistry. *J. Neurosci.* 6:1952–61

82. Goodman, R. R., Snyder, S. H. 1982. Autoradiographic localization of adeno-

sine receptors in rat brain using [³H]cyclohexyladenosine. *J. Neurosci.* 2:1230–41

83. Patel, J., Marangos, P. J., Stivers, J., Goodwin, F. K. 1982. Characterization of adenosine receptors in brain using N⁶ cyclohexyl[³H]adenosine. *Brain Res.* 237:203–14

84. Newby, A. C. 1984. Adenosine and the concept of "retaliatory metabolites." *Trends Biochem. Sci.* 9:42–44

85. Harms, H. H., Wardeh, G., Mulder, A. H. 1978. Adenosine modulates depolarization-induced release of ³H-noradrenaline from slices of rat brain neocortex. *Eur. J. Pharmacol.* 49:305–8

86. Fredholm, B. B., Dunwiddie, T. V., Bergman, B., Lindstrom, K. 1984. Levels of adenosine and adenine nucleotides in slices of rat hippocampus. *Brain Res.* 295:127–36

87. Carney, J. M., Logan, L., McMaster, S. B., Seale, T. W. 1985. Can we understand the CNS pharmacology of xanthines when we understand CNS adenosine systems? See Ref. 8, pp. 199–208

88. Berne, R. M. 1963. Cardiac nucleotides in hypoxia: possible role in regulation of coronary blood flow. *J. Physiol. London* 204:317–22

89. Dragunow, M., Goddard, G. V., Laverty, R. 1985. Is adenosine an endogenous anticonvulsant? *Epilepsia* 26:480–87

90. Nagy, J. I., Buss, M., Daddona, P. E. 1986. On the innervation of trigeminal mesencephalic primary afferent neurons by adenosine deaminase containing projections from the hypothalamus in the rat. *Neuroscience* 17:141–56

91. Sebastiao, A. M., Riberio, J. A. 1986. Enhancement of transmission at the frog neuromuscular junction by adenosine deaminase: evidence for an inhibitory role of endogenous adenosine on neuromuscular transmission. *Neurosci. Lett.* 62:267–70

92. Bender, A. S., Wu, P. H., Phillis, J. W. 1981. The rapid uptake and release of [³H]-adenosine by rat cerebral cortical synaptosomes. *J. Neurochem.* 36:651–60

93. Moritaki, H. 1983. Possible mechanism of potentiation of the action of adenosine by some vasodilators. In *Physiology and Pharmacology of Adenosine Derivatives*, ed. J. W. Daly, Y. Kuroda, J. W. Phillis, H. Shimizu, M. Ui, pp. 197–207. New York: Raven

94. Taylor, D. A., Williams, M. 1982. Interaction of 2-phenylaminoadenosine

(CV 1808) with adenosine systems in rat tissues. *Eur. J. Pharmacol.* 86:35–42

95. Hammond, J. R., Clanachan, A. S. 1985. Species differences in the binding of [^{3}H]nitrobenylthioinosine to the nucleoside transport system in mammalian central nervous system membranes. Evidence for interconvertible forms of the binding site/transporter complex. *J. Neurochem.* 45:527–35

96. Marangos, P. J., Houston, M., Montgomery, P. 1985. [^{3}H]Dipyridamole: a new ligand probe for brain adenosine uptake sites. *Eur. J. Pharmacol.* 117:393–94

97. Sanderson, G. Schofield, C. N. 1986. Effects of adenosine uptake blockers and adenosine on evoked potentials of guinea-pig olfactory cortex. *Pfluegers Arch.* 406:25–30

98. Mendelson, W. B., Kuruvilla, A., Watlington, T., Goehl, K., Paul, S. M., Skolnick, P. 1983. Sedative and electroencephalographic actions of erythro-9-(2-hydroxy-3-nonyl)adenine (EHNA): Relationship to inhibition of brain adenosine deaminase. *Psychopharmacology* 79:126–29

99. Radulovacki, M., Virus, R. M., Djuricic-Nedelson, M., Green, R. D. 1983. Hypnotic effects of deoxycorformycin in rats. *Brain Res.* 271:392–95

100. Nagy, J. I., Labella, F., Buss, M., Dadonna, P. E. 1984. Immunohistochemistry of adenosine deaminase: implications for adenosine neurotransmission. *Science* 224:166–68

101. Nagy, J. I., Geiger, J. D., Daddona, P. E. 1985. Adenosine uptake sites in rat brain: identification using [^{3}H]nitrobenzylthioinosine and co-localization with adenosine deaminase. *Neurosci. Lett.* 55:47–53

102. Browning, M. D., Huganir, R., Greengard, P. 1985. Protein phosphorylation and neuronal function. *J. Neurochem.* 45:11–23

103. Dolphin, A. C., Prestwich, S. A. 1985. Pertussis toxin reverses adenosine inhibition of neuronal glutamate release. *Nature* 316:148–51

104. Ui, M., Katada, T., Murayama, T., Kurose, T., Yajima, M., et al. 1984. Islet activating protein, pertussis toxin: a specific uncoupler of receptor-mediated inhibition of adenylate cyclase. *Adv. Cyclic Nucleotide Res.* 17:145–51

105. Berridge, M. J., Irvine, R. F. 1984. Inositol triphosphate, a novel second messenger in cellular signal transduction. *Nature* 312:315–21

106. Siggins, G. R., Schubert, P. 1981. Adenosine depression of hippocampal neurons in vitro: an intracellular study of dose-dependent actions on synaptic and membrane potential. *Neurosci. Lett.* 23:55–60

107. Bellardinelli, L., West, A., Crampton, R., Berne, R. M. 1983. Chronotropic and dromomotropic effects of adenosine. See Ref. 19, pp. 377–98

108. Segal, M. 1982. Intracellular analysis of a postsynaptic action of adenosine in the rat hippocampus. *Eur. J. Pharmacol.* 79:193–99

109. Trussell, L. O., Jackson, M. B. 1985. Adenosine-activated potassium conductance in cultured striatal neurons. *Proc. Natl. Acad. Sci. USA* 82:4857–61

110. Greene, R. A. W., Haas, H. L. 1985. Adenosine actions on CA$_1$ pyramidal neurones in rat hippocampal slices. *J. Physiol. London* 366:119–27

111. Schofield, C. N. 1978. Depression of evoked potentials in brain slices by adenosine compounds. *Br. J. Pharmacol.* 63:239–44

112. Kuroda, Y. 1985. Modulation of calcium channels through different adenosine receptors; ADO-1 and ADO-2. See Ref. 8, pp. 233–40

113. Proctor, W. R., Dunwiddie, T. V. 1983. Adenosine inhibits calcium spikes in hippocampal pyramidal neurons in vitro. *Neurosci. Lett.* 35:197–201

114. Dunwiddie, T. V., Haas, H. L. 1985. Adenosine increases synaptic facilitation in the in vitro rat hippocampus: evidence for a presynaptic site of action. *J. Physiol. London* 369:365–77

115. Schubert, P. 1985. Synaptic and nonsynaptic modulation by adenosine: a differential action on K- and Ca-fluxes. See Ref. 8, pp. 117–27

116. Phillis, J. W., Swanson, T. H., Barraco, R. A. 1984. Interactions between adenosine and nifedipine in the rat cerebral cortex. *Neurochem. Int.* 6:693–99

117. Murphy, K. M. M., Snyder, S. H. 1982. Adenosine receptor binding and specify receptors for calcium channel drugs. In *Calcium Entry Blockers Adenosine and Neurohumors: Advances In Coronary Vascular and Cardiac Control*, ed. G. F. Merrill, H. R. Weiss, pp. 295–306. Baltimore: Urban & Schwarzenberg

118. Bohm, M., Burmann, H., Meyer, W., Nose, M., Schmitz, W., Scholz, H. 1985. Positive inotropic effect of Bay K 8644: cAMP-independence and lack of inhibitory effect of adenosine. *Naunyn Schmiedebergs Arch. Pharmacol.* 329: 447–50

119. Stone, T. W. 1981. Physiological roles for adenosine and adenosine 5'-triphosphate in the nervous system. *Neuroscience* 6:523–45

120. Spignoli, G., Pedata, F., Pepeu, G. 1984. A_1 and A_2 adenosine receptors modulate acetylcholine release from brain slices. *Eur. J. Pharmacol.* 97:341–43

121. Ebstein, R. P., Daly, T. W. 1982. Release of norepinephrine and dopamine from brain vesicular preparations: effects of calcium antagonists. *Cell. Mol. Neurobiol.* 2:205–13

122. Carlsson, A. 1975. Receptor-mediated control of dopamine metabolism. In *Pre- and Postsynaptic Receptors*, ed. E. Usdin, W. E. Bunney, Jr., pp. 49–67. New York: Dekker

123. Govoni, S., Perkov, V., Montefusco, O., Missale, C., Battaini, F., et al. 1984. Differential effects of caffeine on dihydroxyphenylacetic acid concentration in various rat brain dopaminergic structures. *J. Pharm. Pharmacol.* 36:458–60

124. Koboyashi, K., Kuroda, Y., Yoshioka, M. 1981. Change of cyclic AMP level in synaptosomes from cerebral cortex: increase by adenosine derivatives. *J. Neurochem.* 36:86–91

125. Snyder, S. H., Sklar, P. 1984. Behavioral and molecular actions of caffeine: focus on adenosine. *J. Psychiatr. Res.* 18:91–106

126. Robins, R. K., Revankar, G. R. 1985. Purine analogs and related nucleosides and nucleotides as antitumor agents. *Med. Res. Rev.* 5:273–96

127. Bruns, R. F. 1979. Adenosine receptor activation in human fibroblast: nucleoside agonists and antagonists. *Can. J. Physiol. Pharmacol.* 58:673–91

128. Bruns, R. F. 1981. Adenosine antagonism by purines, pteridines and benzopteridines in human fibroblasts. *Biochem. Pharmacol.* 30:325–33

129. Jacobson, K. A., Kirk, K. L., Padgett, W., Daly, J. W. 1985. Probing the adenosine receptor with adenosine and xanthine biotin conjugates. *FEBS Lett.* 184:30–35

130. Daly, J. W. 1985. Adenosine receptors in the central nervous system: structure activity relationships for agonists and antagonists. See Ref. 73, pp. 5–15

131. Kusachi, S., Thompson, R. D., Yamada, N., Daly, D. T., Olsson, R. A. 1985. Coronary Adenosine receptor: Structure of the N^6 aryl subregion. *J. Med. Chem.* 28:1636–43

132. Bazil, C. W., Minneman, K. P. 1986. An investigation of the low intrinsic activity of adenosine and its analogs at low affinity (A2) adenosine receptors in rat cerebral cortex. *J. Neurochem.* 47:547–53

133. Bruns, R. F., Lu, G. H., Pugsley, T. A. 1985. Towards selective adenosine antagonists. See Ref. 8, pp. 51–58

134. Bruns, R. F., Fergus, J. H., Badger, E. W., Bristol, J. A., Santay, L. A., Hays, S. J. 1986. PD 115,199: Antagonist ligand for adenosine A_2 receptors. *Fed. Proc.* 45:801

135. Leighton, H. J., Daluge, S., Craig, R., Parmeter, L. L. 1986. Classification of purine receptors in electrically stimulated guinea pig ileum and guinea pig left atria using the potent purine receptor antagonist BW A1433U. *Pfluegers Arch.* 407:531 (Suppl.)

136. Czernik, A. J., Petrack, B., Kalinsky, H. J., Psychoyos, S., Cash, W. D., et al. 1982. CGS 8216: Receptor binding characteristics of a potent benzodiazepine antagonist. *Life Sci.* 30:363–72

137. Williams, M., Risley, E. A., Huff, J. R. 1981. Interaction of putative anxiolytic agents with central adenosine receptors. *Can. J. Physiol. Pharmacol.* 59:897–900

138. Davies, L. P., Chen Chow, S., Skerritt, J. H., Brown, D. J., Johnston, G. A. R. 1984. Pyrazolo[3,4-d]Pyrimidines as adenosine antagonists. *Life Sci.* 34:2117–28

139. Fassina, G., Gaion, L. M., Caparrotta, L., Carponedo, F. 1985. A caffeine analogue (1,3,7-trimethyl-6-thioxo-2-oxopurine) with a negative inotropic and chronotropic effect. *Naunyn Schmiedebergs Arch. Pharmacol.* 330:222–26

140. Grome, J. J., Stefanovich, V. 1985. Differential effects of xanthine derivatives on local cerebral blood flow and glucose utilization in the conscious rat. See Ref. 8, pp. 453–57

141. Hindmarch, I., Subhan, Z. 1985. A preliminary investigation of "Albert 285" HWA 285 on psychomotor performance, mood and memory. *Drug Dev. Res.* 5:379–86

142. Fredholm, B. B., Lindstrom, K. 1986. The xanthine derivative 1-(5'-oxohexyl)-3-methyl-7-propyl xanthine (HWA 285) enhances the actions of adenosine. *Acta Pharmacol. Toxicol.* 58:187–92

143. Snowhill, E. A., Williams, M. 1986. Autoradiographic evaluation of the binding of [^{3}H]cyclohexyladenosine to aden-

osine A-1 receptor in rat tissues. *Neurosci. Lett.* 68:41–46

144. Barraco, R. A., Coffin, V. L., Altman, H. J., Phillis, J. W. 1983. Central effects of adenosine analogues on locomotor activity in mice and antagonism of caffeine. *Brain Res.* 272:392–95

145. Dunwiddie, T. V., Worth, T. 1982. Sedative and anticonvulsant effects of adenosine analogs in mouse and rat. *J. Pharmacol. Exp. Ther.* 220:70–76

146. Radulovacki, M., Virus, R. M., Djuricic-Nedelson, M., Green, R. D. 1984. Adenosine analogs and sleep in rats. *J. Pharmacol. Exp. Ther.* 228:268–74

147. Virus, R. M., Rapoza, D., Crane, R. C. 1985. Lack of effect of 1-methylisoguanosine on sleep in rats. *Neuropharmacology* 24:547–49

148. Proctor, W. R., Dunwiddle, T. V. 1984. Behavioral sensitivity to purinergic drugs parallel ethanol sensitivity in selectively bred mice. *Science* 224:519–21

149. Fredholm, B. B., Zahniser, N. R., Weiner, G. R., Proctor, W. R., Dunwiddle, T. V. 1985. Behavioral sensitivity to PIA in selectively bred mice is related to a number of A_1 adenosine receptors but not to cyclic AMP accumulation in brain slices. *Eur. J. Pharmacol.* 111:133–36

150. Charney, D. S., Galloway, M. P., Heninger, G. R. 1984. The effects of caffeine on plasma MPHG, subjective anxiety, autonomic symptoms and blood pressure in healthy humans. *Life Sci.* 35:135–44

151. Williams, M. 1983. Anxioselective anxiolytics. *J. Med. Chem.* 26:619–28

152. Braestrup, C., Nielsen, M., Olsen, C. E. 1980. Urinary and brain β-carboline-3-carboxylates as potent inhibitors of brain benzodiazepine receptors. *Proc. Natl. Acad. Sci. USA* 77:2288–92

153. Costa, E., Guidotti, A. 1985. Endogenous ligands for benzodiazepine recognition sites. *Biochem. Pharmacol.* 34:3399–403

154. Haefely, W., Kyburz, E., Gerecke, M., Mohler, H. 1985. Recent advances in the molecular pharmacology of benzodiazepine receptors and in the structure activity relationships of their agonists and antagonists. *Adv. Drug Res.* 14:165–322

155. Williams, M., Yokoyama, N. 1986. Anxiolytics, anticonvulsants and sedative-hypnotics. *Ann. Rep. Med. Chem.* 21:11–20

156. Turski, L., Schwarz, M., Turski, W. A., Ikonomidou, C., Sontag, K.-H.

1984. Effect of aminophylline on muscle relaxant action of diazepam and phenobarbitone in genetically spastic rats: further evidence for a purinergic mechanism in the action of diazepam. *Eur. J. Pharmacol.* 103:99–105

157. Bruns, R. F., Katims, J. J., Annau, Z., Snyder, S. H., Daly, T. W. 1983. Adenosine receptor interactions and anxiolytics. *Neuropharmacology* 22:1523–29

158. Davies, L. P., Cook, A. F., Poonian, A. M., Taylor, K. M. 1980. Displacement of [^{3}H]diazepam binding in rat brain by dipyridamole and by 1-methylisoguanosine, a natural marine product with muscle relaxant activity. *Life Sci.* 26:1089–97

159. Davies, L. P., Chow, S. C., Johnston, G. A. R. 1984. Interaction of purines and related compounds with photoaffinity-labeled benzodiazepine receptors in rat brain membranes. *Eur. J. Pharmacol.* 97:325–29

160. Albertson, T. E., Bowyer, J. F., Paule, M. G. 1982. Modification of the anticonvulsant efficacy of diazepam by Ro-15-1788 in the kindled amygdaloid seizure model. *Life Sci.* 31:1597–601

161. Phillis, J. W., Delong, R. E. 1984. A purinergic component in the central actions of meprobamate. *Eur. J. Pharmacol.* 101:295–97

162. Morgan, P. F., Lloyd, H. G., Stone, T. W. 1983. Inhibition of adenosine accumulation by a CNS benzodiazepine antagonist (Ro 15-1788) and a peripheral benzodiazepine receptor ligand (Ro 5-4864). *Neurosci. Lett.* 41:183–88

163. Winn, H. R., Morii, S., Berne, R. M. 1985. The role of adenosine in the autoregulation of cerebral blood flow. *Ann. Biomed. Eng.* 13:321–28

164. Rosen, J. B., Berman, R. F. 1985. Prolonged postictal depression in amygdaloid kindled rats by the adenosine analog, L-PIA. *Exp. Neurol.* 90:549–57

165. Burley, E. S., Ferrendelli, J. A. 1984. Regulatory effects of neurotransmitter on electroshock and pentylenetetrazol seizures. *Fed. Proc.* 43:2521–24

166. Marangos, P. J., Weiss, S. B. B., Montgomery, P., Patel, J., Narang, P. K., et al. 1985. Chronic carbamazepine treatment increases brain adenosine receptors. *Epilepsia* 26:493–98

167. Lohse, M. J., Klotz, K.-N., Jakobs, K. H., Schwabe, U. 1985. Barbiturates are selective antagonists at A_1 adenosine receptors. *J. Neurochem.* 45:1761–70

168. Ho, I. K., Lo, H. H., Way, E. L. 1973.

Cyclic adenosine monophosphate antagonism of morphine analgesia. *J. Pharmacol. Exp. Ther.* 185:336–46

169. Collier, H. O. J., Cuthbert, N. J., Francis, D. L. 1981. Character and meaning of quasi-morphine withdrawal phenomena elicted by methyl-xanthines. *Fed. Proc.* 40:1513–18

170. Reinhard, R. J. F. Jr., Galloway, M. P., Roth, R. H. 1983. Noradrenergic stimulation of serotonin synthesis and metabolism. II. Stimulation by 3-isobutyl-1-methylxanthine. *J. Pharmacol. Exp. Ther.* 226:764–69

171. Galloway, M., Roth, R. 1983. Clonidine prevents methylxanthine stimulation of norepinephrine metabolism in rat brain. *J. Neurochem.* 40:246–51

172. Grant, S. J., Redmond, D. E. 1982. Methylxanthine activation of noradrenergic unit activity and reversal by clonidine. *Eur. J. Pharmacol.* 85:1094–109

173. Gold, M. S., Pottash, A. C., Sweeney, D. R., Kleber, H. D. 1980. Opiate withdrawal using clonidine. A safe, effective and rapid nonopiate treatment. *J. Am. Med. Assoc.* 243:343–46

174. Collier, H. O. J., Plant, N. T., Tucker, J. F., Von Uexkull, A. 1984. Inhibition with adenosine derivatives of opiate withdrawal effects. *Br. J. Pharmacol,* 81:1–131

175. Arnanda, J. V., Thurman, T. 1970. Methylxanthines in apnea of prematurity. *Clin. Perinatol.* 6:87–108

176. Laska, E. M., Sunshine, A., Mueller, F., Elvers, W. B., Siegel, C., Rubin, A. 1984. Caffeine as an analgesic adjuvant. *J. Am. Med. Assoc.* 251:1711–18

177. Whorton, A. R., Collawn, J. B., Montgomery, M. E., Young, S. L., Kent, R. S. 1985. Arachidonic acid metabolism in cultured aortic endothelial cells. Effect of cAMP and 3-isobutyl-1-methylxanthines. *Biochem. Pharmacol.* 34:119–23

178. Gourley, D. R. H., Beckner, S. K. 1973. Antagonism of morphine analgesia by adenine, adenosine and adenine nucleotides. *Proc. Soc. Exp. Biol. Med.* 144:774–80

179. Yarbrough, B. V., McGuffin-Clineschmidt, J. 1981. In vivo behavioral assessment of central nervous system purinergic receptor. *Eur. J. Pharmacol.* 76:137–44

180. Ahlijanian, M. K., Takemori, A. E. 1985. Effects of $(-)N^6(R$-phenylisopropyl)-adenosine (PIA) and caffeine on nociception and morphine-induced analgesia, tolerance and dependence in mice. *Eur. J. Pharmacol.* 112:171–79

181. Ahlijanian, M. K., Takemori, A. E. 1986. Changes in adenosine receptor sensitivity in morphine-tolerant and -dependent mice. *J. Pharmacol. Exp. Ther.* 236:615–620

182. Sattin, A., Stone, T. W., Taylor, D. A. 1978. Biochemical and electropharmaceutical studies with tricyclic antidepressants in rat and guinea pig cerebral cortex. *Life Sci.* 23:2621–26

183. Phillis, J. W. 1984. Potentiation of the action of adenosine on cerebral cortical neurones by the tricyclic antidepressants. *Br. J. Pharmacol.* 83:567–75

184. Newman, M., Zohar, J., Kalian, M., Belmaker, R. H. 1984. The effects of chronic lithium and ECT on A_1 and A_2 adenosine receptor systems in rat brain. *Brain Res.* 291:188–92

185. Williams, M., Risley, E. A., Robinson, J. L. 1983. Chronic in vivo treatment with desmethylimipramine and mianserin does not alter adenosine A_1 radioligand being in rat cortex. *Neurosci. Lett.* 35:47–51

186. Minana, M. D., Portoles, M., Jorda, G., Grisolia, S. 1984. Lesch–Nyhan syndrome, caffeine model: increase of purine and pyrimidine enzymes in rat brain. *J. Neurochem.* 43:1556–60

187. Nyhan, W. L., Oliver, W. J., Lesch, M. 1965. A familial disorder of uric acid metabolism and central nervous system function. *J. Pediatr.* 67:257–63

188. Lloyd, K. G., Hornykiewicz, O., Davidson, L., Shannak, K., Farley, I., et al. 1981. Biochemical evidence of dysfunction of brain neurotransmitters in the Lesch–Nyhan Syndrome. *N. Engl. J. Med.* 305:1106–11

189. Fredholm, B. B., Herrara-Marschitz, M., Jonzon, B., Lindstrom, K., Ungerstedt, U. 1983. On the mechanism by which methylxanthines enhance apomorphine induced rotation behavior in the rat. *Pharmacol. Biochem. Behav.* 19:535–41

190. Green, R. D., Proudfit, H. K., Yeung, S.-M. H. 1982. Modulation of striatal dopaminergic function by local injection of 5'-N-ethylcarboxamide adenosine. *Science* 218:58–61

191. Williams, M., Jarvis, M. J. 1987. Adenosine antagonists as potential therapeutic agents. *Pharmacol. Biochem. Behav.* In press

192. Heffner, T. G., Downs, D. A., Bristol, J. A., Bruns, R. F., et al. 1985. Antipsychotic-like effects of adenosine re-

ceptor agonists. *Pharmacologist* 27: 293

193. Ushijima, I., Katsuragi, T., Furukawa, T. 1984. Involvement of adenosine receptor activities in aggressive responses produced by clonidine in mice. *Psychopharmacology,* 83:335–39

194. Holloway, W. R. Jr., Thor, D. H. 1985. Interactive effects of caffeine, 2-chloroadenosine and haloperidol on activity, social investigation and play fighting in juvenile rats. *Pharmacol. Biochem. Behav.* 22:421–26

195. Evans, D. B., Schenden, J. A., Bristol, J. A. 1982. Adenosine receptors mediating cardiac depression. *Life Sci.* 30:2425–32

196. Dimarco, J. P., Sellers, T. D., Lerman, B. D., Greenberg, M. L., Berne, R. M., Belardinelli, L. 1985. Diagnostic and therapeutic use of adenosine in patients with supraventricular tachyarrhythmias. *J. Am. Coll. Cardiol.* 6:417–25

197. Rardon, D. P., Bailey, J. C. 1984. Adenosine attenuation of the electrophysiological effects of isoproterenol on canine cardiac purkinje fibers. *J. Pharmacol. Exp. Ther.* 228:792–98

198. Schutz, W., Freissmuth, M. 1985. Adenosine receptors in the heart: controversy about signal transmission. *Trends Pharmacol. Sci.* 6:310–11

199. Collis, M. G., Keddie, J. R., Pettinger, S. J. 1983. 2-Chloroadenosine lowers blood pressure in the conscious dog without reflex tachycardia. *Br. J. Pharmacol.* 80: 385 pp.

200. Lucchesi, B. R., Patterson, E. S. 1984. Antiarrhythmic drugs. In *Cardiovascular Pharmacology,* ed. M. Antonaccio, pp. 329–414, New York: Raven. 2nd ed.

201. Leung, E., Johnston, C. I., Woodcock, E. A. 1985. An investigation of the receptors involved in the coronary vasodilatory effect of adenosine analogues. *Clin. Exp. Pharmacol. Physiol.* 12:515–19

202. Barraco, R. A., Aggarawal, A. K., Phillis, J. W., Moron, M. A., Wu, P. H. 1986. Dissociation of the locomotor and hypotensive effects of adenosine analogues in the rat. *Neurosci. Lett.* 48:139–44

203. Itoh, S., Carretero, O. A., Murray, R. D. 1985. Possible role of adenosine in the macula densa mechanism of renin release in rabbits. *J. Clin. Invest.* 76:1412–17

204. Lang, M. A., Preston, A. S., Handler, J. S., Forrest, J. N. 1985. Adenosine stimulates sodium transport in kidney

A6 epithelia in culture. *Am. J. Physiol.* 249:C330–36

205. Hall, J. E., Granger, J. P. 1986. Renal hemodynamics and arterial pressure during chronic intrarenal adenosine infusion in conscious dogs. *Am. J. Physiol.* 250:F32–39

206. Wu, P. H., Churchill, P. C. 1985. 2-chloro[^{3}H]-adenosine binding in isolated rat kidney membranes. *Arch. Int. Pharmacodyn.* 273:83–87

207. Cushley, M. J., Tattersfield, A. E., Holgate, S. T. 1983. Inhaled adenosine and guanosine on airway resistance in normal and asthmatic subjects. *Br. J. Clin. Pharmacol.* 15:161–65

208. Holgate, S. T., Lewis, R. A., Austen, K. F. 1980. Role of adenylate cyclase in immunologic release of mediators from rat mast cells and agonist and antagonist effects of purine- and ribose-modified adenosine analogs. *Proc. Natl. Acad. Sci. USA* 77:6800–4

209. Holgate, S. T., Mann, J. S., Cushley, M. J. 1984. Adenosine as a bronchoconstrictor mediator in asthma and its antagonism by methylxanthines. *J. Allergy Clin. Immunol.* 74:302–6

210. Marone, G., Findlay, S. R., Lichtenstein, L. M. 1979. Adenosine receptors on human basophils. Modulation of histamine release. *J. Immunol.* 123:1473–77

211. Church, M. K., Holgate, S. T. 1986. Adenosine and asthma. *Trends Pharmacol. Sci.* 7:49–50

212. Church, M. K., Hughes, P. J. 1985. Adenosine potentiates immunological histamine release from rat mast cells by a novel cyclic AMP-independent cell-surface action. *Br. J. Pharmacol.* 85:3–5

213. Marone, G., Ambrosio, G., Bonaduce, D., Genovese, A., Triggiani, M., Condorelli, M. 1984. Adenosine receptors on human inflammatory cells. *Int. Arch. Allergy Appl. Immunol.* 74:356–61

214. Moroz, C., Twig, S. 1985. The regulatory role of adenosine activated T-lymphocyte subset on the immune response in humans. II. Adenosine induced expression of T-8 antigen. *Biomed. Pharmacother.* 39:145–49

215. Giblett, E. R. 1985. ADA and PNP deficiencies: how it all began. *Ann. N. Y. Acad. Sci.* 451:1–8

216. Murray, J. L., Loftin, K. C., Munn, C. G., Reuben, J. M., Mansell, P. W. A., Hersh, E. M. 1985. Elevated adenosine deaminase and purine nucleoside phosphorylase activity in peripheral blood null lymphocytes from patients with ac-

quired immune deficiency syndrome. *Blood* 65:1318–23

217. Cronstein, B. N., Kramer, S. B., Weissman, G., Hirshhorn, R. 1983. Adenosine: a physiologic modulator of superoxide anion generation by human neutrophils. *J. Exp. Med.* 158:1160–77

218. Cronstein, B. N., Rosenstein, E. D., Kramer, S. b., Weissmann, G., Hirshhorn, R. 1985. Adenosine: a physiologic modulator of superoxide anion generation by human neutrophils. Adenosine acts via an A_2 receptor on human neutrophils. *J. Immunol.* 135:1366–71

219. Samet, M. K. 1985. Inhibition of antibody production by 2-chloroadenosine. *Life Sci.* 37:225–33

220. Henry, J., Stephens, P. 1980. Caffeine as an intensifier of stress-indirect hormonal and pathophysiologic changes in mice. *Pharmacol. Biochem. Behav.* 13:719–24

221. Geiger, J. D., Glavin, G. B. 1985. Adenosine receptor activation in brain reduces stress-induced ulcer formation. *Eur. J. Pharmacol.* 115:185–90

222. Ushijima, I., Mizuki, Y., Yamada, M. 1985. Development of stress-induced gastric lesions involves central adenosine A_1-receptor stimulation. *Brain Res.* 339:351–55

223. Gerber, J. G., Nies, A. S., Payne, N. A. 1985. Adenosine receptors on canine parietal cells modulate gastric acid secretion to histamine. *J. Pharmacol. Exp. Ther.* 233:623–27

224. Yamagishi, F., Homma, N., Haruta, K., Iwatsuki, K., Chiba, S. 1985. Adenosine potentials secretion-stimulated pancreatic exocrine secretion in the dog. *Eur. J. Pharmacol.* 118:203–9

225. Wessburg, P., Hedner, J., Hedner, T., Persson, B., Jonason, J. 1985. Adenosine mechanisms in the regulation of breathing in the rat. *Eur. J. Pharmacol.* 106:59–67

226. Lagercrantz, H., Yamamoto, Y., Fredholm, B. B., Prabhakar, N., Euler, C. 1984. Adenosine analogues depress ventillation in rabbit neonates. Theophylline stimulation of respiration via adenosine receptors? *Pediatr. Res.* 18:387–90

227. McQueen, D. S., Ribeno, T. A. 1981. Effect of adenosine on carotid chemoreceptor activity in the rat. *Br. J.*

228. Fredholm, B. B. 1982. Adenosine actions and adenosine receptor after one week treatment with caffeine. *Acta Physiol. Scand.* 115:283–86

229. Murray, T. F. 1982. Up-regulation of rat cortical adenosine receptors following chronic administration of theophylline. *Eur. J. Pharmacol.* 82:113–14

230. Chou, D. T., Khan, S., Forde, J., Hirsh, K. R. 1985. Caffeine tolerance: behavioral, electrophysiological and neurochemical evidence. *Life Sci.* 36:2347–58

231. Onodera, H., Kogure, K. 1985. Autoradiographic visualization of adenosine A_1 receptors in the gerbil hippocampus: changes in the receptor density after transient ischemia. *Brain Res.* 345:406–8

232. Dora, E. 1985. Effect of adenosine and its stabile analogue 2-chloroadenosine on cerebrocortical microcirculation and NAD/NADH redox state. *Pfluegers Arch.* 404:208–13

233. Li, Y.-O., Fredholm, B. B. 1985. Adenosine analogues stimulate cyclic AMP formation in rabbit cerebral microvessels via adenosine A_2-receptors. *Acta Physiol. Scand.* 124:253–59

234. Fredholm, B. B., Duner-Engstrom, M., Fastbom, J., Jonzon, B., Lindgren, E., et al. 1987. Interactions between the neuromodulator adenosine and classical transmitters. *Proc. 3rd Int. Symp. Adenosine. Munich, Fed. Republ. Germany:* Springer-Verlag. In press

235. Murphy, K. M. M., Snyder, S. H. 1982. Heterogeneity of adenosine A_1 receptor binding in brain tissue. *Mol. Pharmacol.* 21:250–57

236. Lee, K. S., Reddington, M., Schubert, P., Kreutzberg, G. 1983. Regulation of the strength of adenosine modulation in the hippocampus by a differential distribution of the density of A_1 receptors. *Brain Res.* 260:156–59

237. Marquardt, D. L., Wasserman, S. I. 1985. [^{3}H]Adenosine binding to rat mast cells—pharmacologic and functional characterization. *Agents Actions* 16:453–61

238. Abreu, M. E., Valentine, H. L. 1986. Pharmacologic profile of adenosine receptor binding sites in guinea pig atrium and ventricle. *Pfluegers Arch.* 407:547 (Suppl.)

Ann. Rev. Pharmacol. Toxicol. 1987. 27:347–69

CALCIUM CHANNEL LIGANDS

D. J. Triggle

Department of Biochemical Pharmacology, School of Pharmacy, State University of New York at Buffalo, Buffalo, New York 14260

R. A. Janis

Miles Institute for Preclinical Pharmacology, P. O. Box 1956, New Haven, Connecticut 06509

INTRODUCTION

The Ca^{2+} channel blockers, diltiazem, nifedipine, and verapamil, are now well-established members of the therapeutic armamentarium employed in cardiovascular disease including, but not limited to, angina in its several forms, hypertension, some cardiac arrhythmias including supraventricular tachycardia, congestive heart failure, and hypertrophic cardiomyopathy. Several reviews detail these and related clinical uses (1–8). The introduction of these agents into cardiovascular medicine has had several major and related consequences.

Investigators are examining the efficacy of Ca^{2+} blockers in a number of additional disorders both within and without the cardiovascular system, including achalasia, asthma, atherosclerosis, dysmenorrhea, intestinal spasm, labyrinthine disorders, migraine, peripheral vascular disorders, premature labor, and urinary incontinence.

In addition to diltiazem, nifedipine, and verapamil, a large number of related agents are coming into use or are under clinical investigation. In the 1,4-dihydropyridine (nifedipine) category these related agents include felodipine, nicardipine, nitrendipine, nisoldipine, nimodipine, and PN 200-110. Among the phenylalkylamine (verapamil) class they include gallopamil and tiapamil (Figure 1). As a consequence of this high level of clinical activity, discrete sections or chapters on Ca^{2+} channel antagonists are appearing in standard texts of pharmacology (9, 10).

347

0362-1642/87/0415-0347$02.00

The Ca^{2+} channel blockers are drugs acting specifically at defined pathways of Ca^{2+} mobilization. This realization spurred considerable interest in their use as probes with which to characterize, isolate, and reconstitute Ca^{2+} channels (see 2, 4, 11–18 for reviews). The introduction of Ca^{2+} channel activators of the 1,4-dihydropyridine class, including Bay K 8644, provided a further stimulus (19–22, Figure 1). This latter development suggests *Ca^{2+} channel ligand* as a global term for drugs acting at Ca^{2+} channels.

Investigators recognized early that the Ca^{2+} channel antagonists were not uniformly effective in all tissues. They also realized that 1,4-dihydropyridines are smooth muscle selective (compared to the verapamil and diltiazem structures) and that neuronal tissues are, despite the presence of ligand-binding sites, frequently insensitive to these drugs. Such phenomena are now explained according to the concepts of state-dependent binding of Ca^{2+} channel ligands (23, 24) and of multiple classes of voltage-dependent Ca^{2+} channels that differ in their kinetic and permeation characteristics and in their pharmacological sensitivity (25). Additionally, introduction of the Ca^{2+} channel antagonists into both clinical and basic sciences focuses additional attention on the general regulatory role of Ca^{2+} in cell function (26).

The literature of the Ca^{2+} channel ligands has expanded dramatically in the

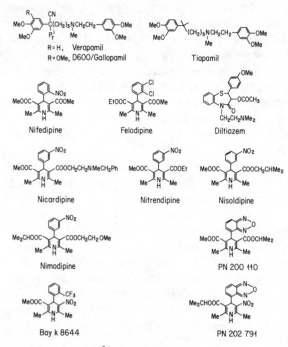

Figure 1 Structural formulas of Ca^{2+} channel ligands.

past several years. This review concentrates primarily on developments during 1985 and 1986 and refers only selectively to the earlier literature (27–30). It covers only the Ca^{2+} channels of the plasmalemma and associated structures and does not discuss the intracellular channels of the endoplasmic and sarcoplasmic structures. We organize this review around five main areas: (a) structure-function relationships; (b) properties and function of binding sites; (c) the basis of tissue selectivity; (d) regulation of Ca^{2+} channels; and (e) prospects for the future.

STRUCTURE–FUNCTION RELATIONSHIPS

Evidence for Specific Sites

The chemical and pharmacological heterogeneity of the major classes of Ca^{2+} channel ligands suggested that they interact at different sites and by different mechanisms to modulate Ca^{2+} currents. Consequently, no single all-embracing structure–function relationship could describe Ca^{2+} channel ligands (17). Radioligand-binding data validate this conclusion and generate a model for channel ligand binding of three discrete, allosterically linked binding sites for the major 1,4-dihydropyridine, phenylalkylamine, and benzothiazepine categories (See "Properties and Function of Binding Sites"; 11–14, 16). These linked interactions have been demonstrated in several pharmacological preparations (31–33). Structure–function relationships must therefore be interpreted in terms of interaction at these separate receptor sites.

Few significant advances in data accumulation for structure-activity relationships have occurred since the last comprehensive review (34), but developments in the 1,4-dihydropyridine field continue. Additional solid-state (35–37) and solution conformation (38) determinations are consistent with previous reports (39) that active 1,4-dihydropyridine molecules contain the substituted 4-phenyl ring positioned above and in the vertical plane of the 1,4-dihydropyridine ring, which itself is in a flattened boat conformation. Synthesis of rigid analogs in which the dihedral angle between the two rings is restricted confirms this proposal (40). Extensive comparisons of the pharmacological activities of a series of 1,4-dihydropyridines in smooth muscle, vascular and nonvascular (41, 42), confirm the previous observations (17, 43, 44) that despite quantitative tissue-dependent differences in activity the rank order is constant. This finding is consistent with the variable expression of a single structure–function relationship (See "The Basis of Tissue Selectivity"). Antibodies directed against 1,4-dihydropyridines show binding properties very similar to those exhibited by the membrane receptor, save for the absence of allosteric interactions with other structural categories of ligands and the independence of binding from divalent cations (45).

Orientational aspects of drug-receptor interactions are receiving increasing attention. In principle, ligand approaches to ion channel extra- or intracellular binding sites may involve aqueous or membrane pathways. Such considerations are important with respect to both the rate (two- and three-dimensional diffusion; 46) and the extent (binding site availability) of the ligand-channel interaction. A model has been advanced for the 1,4-dihydropyridine interaction in which these hydrophobic molecules partition into the lipid bilayer and then diffuse laterally to a specific binding site (47, 48). If this model is correct, the implications for drug design may be quite important, since the partitioning and diffusion pathways may determine both ligand affinity and access to different channel states.

Antagonist and Activator Ligands

1,4-Dihydropyridine activators and antagonists differ only in minor structural aspects (Figure 1). Very limited structure-activity data are available for activators. The presence of a 3-nitro or 2,3-lactone substitution in the 1,4-dihydropyridine ring is important, but not sufficient, for significant activity. The solid-state structures of Bay K 8644 and CGP 28 392 are very similar to those for antagonist 1,4-dihydropyridines (49). The common conformational features of activators and antagonists are consistent with the suggestion that they interact at a common site (50–53). However, the enhanced 1,4-dihydropyridine ring planarity and acidity of the $-NH$ proton, together with subtle differences in ester orientation in activator molecules, could contribute to the relative ability of 1,4-dihydropyridines to stabilize open and closed channel states (49). Of these electronic and structural differences, the most important may be the asymmetric disposition and function of binding sites for C_3 and C_5 substituents (49); this speculation is supported by the remarkable enantiomeric selectivity of Bay K 8644 and PN 202 791, where the S- and R-enantiomers are activator and antagonist, respectively (53–58). Binding of 1,4-dihydropyridines is dominated by hydrophobic interactions. In contrast to other receptor systems, including β-adrenoceptors (59), thermodynamic discrimination between activator and antagonist species was not observed (60).

Structure-Function Correlations

Radioligand-binding data from neuronal and skeletal muscle preparations yield structure-activity correlations very similar to those from cardiac and smooth muscle, despite the former studies' frequent absence of easily demonstrable pharmacologic effects (2, 16, 17). This absence is particularly obvious for neuronal tissue, where the binding data are virtually identical to those derived from functional preparations. Some binding sites may be nonfunctional or uncoupled (61, 62). However, resolution of this anomaly is probable, in part, through state dependence of ligand interaction, in which radioligand binding gains access to a state that is pharmacologically inaccess-

Table 1   Properties of major Ca^{2+} channel types[a]

	Persistent	Transient
Activation	-10 mV	-50 mV
Peak	$+20$ mV	-10 mV
Tails	fast	slow
Inactivation	slow, incomplete	fast, complete
Permeation	$Ba^{2+} > Sr^{2+} > Ca^{2+}$	$Ca^{2+} \sim Sr^{2+} \sim Ba^{2+}$
Stability	labile	stable
Metal^{2+}	sensitive	less sensitive
Organic antagonists	sensitive[b]	insensitive or much less sensitive

[a]This table was compiled using data from various publications encompassing several tissue types. We do not intended to indicate that there are only two channel classes with precisely the characteristics defined above.
[b]Sensitivity of this channel type to 1,4-dihydropyridines is $\leq 10^{-9}$ M in smooth and cardiac muscle, but $\geq 10^{-6}$ M in many neuronal systems.

ible (See "The Basis of Tissue Selectivity"). The existence of different Ca^{2+}-channel classes with different pharmacological specificity may also aid this understanding. Accordingly, quantitatively and qualitatively different structure–activity relationships should exist. Examples of both are known. Quantitative variations in the expression of a structure–activity relationship are consistent with state-dependent interactions (See "The Basis of Tissue Selectivity"; 41–44), and considerable electrophysiological data document the existence of at least two kinetically and pharmacologically distinct voltage-dependent Ca^{2+} channels (Table 1) in neurons (63–67), cardiac, skeletal and smooth muscle (68–71), and secretory cells (72).

The recognition of distinct Ca^{2+}-channel types and processes underlies the search for new structures and the possible reevaluation of existing activities. Comparatively little information is available currently, but the area is ripe for rapid development.

New Channel Ligands

Some of the actions of benzodiazepines have been interpreted in terms of Ca^{2+} channel modulation, but whether these effects are primary or secondary remains to be determined (73). Peripheral, rather than central, benzodiazepine ligands appear to be the more active, although the function of the peripheral site is unknown and appears physically distinct from the 1,4-dihydropyridine-sensitive Ca^{2+} channel (74, 75). Insufficient data are available to establish whether benzodiazepines are selective for a particular channel class. The peripheral ligand PK 11195 has been suggested to function by stabilizing the resting state of the 1,4-dihydropyridine-sensitive channel and thus may serve to antagonize both Ca^{2+}-channel antagonists and activators (76, 77).

Organization of pharmacological and structural knowledge of the Na^+ channel was greatly assisted by the existence of specific toxins. Such toxins and related materials for the Ca^{2+} channel are becoming available (78). They include the dinoflagellate toxin, maitotoxin (79, 80); atrotoxin from *Crotalus atrox* venom (81); β-leptinotarsin-h from the hemolymph of the beetle *Leptinotarsa haldemani* (82); and w-conotoxin GVIA, a toxin from fish-eating molluscs of the *Conus* genus (83, 84). The conotoxins affect several ion channels and receptors. GVIA, with 27 amino acids, is of particular interest. It blocks presynaptic Ca^{2+} channels with a pharmacological and radioligand-binding profile that distinguishes it from the sites controlled by the dihydropyridine, verapamil, and diltiazem class of ligands (85, 86). This toxin probably defines the *L*- and N-channels of neurons, rather than the long-lasting 1,4-dihydropyridine-sensitive *L*-channels that appear currently to dominate the cardiovascular system.

Voltage-dependent Ca^{2+} channels are modulated by a number of neurotransmitters and neuropeptides including catecholamines, acetylcholine, histamine, serotonin, adenosine, somatostatin, and opiates (28, 87). The existence of both antagonist and activator 1,4-dihydropyridine ligands (88) raises questions concerning the existence of endogenous regulators and the physiological basis of excitatory and inhibitory ligand control of Ca^{2+} channels. Thus, the central issue becomes communication between receptor and channel: how are these macromolecules linked? Phosphorylation through the cAMP-dependent protein kinase plays an indirect role in control (89). However, recent evidence indicates that guanine nucleotide–binding (G) proteins are involved in both turning on and turning off Ca^{2+} channels (90–92). One possible explanation is that the G proteins couple directly channels and receptors. Such membrane organization would have important implications to both Ca^{2+} channel organization and the definition of structure–activity relationships for ligand modulation of Ca^{2+} channels.

PROPERTIES AND FUNCTION OF BINDING SITES

General Properties

The characteristics of the sites for nonpeptide Ca^{2+} channel ligands, as revealed by radioligand-binding studies, have been reviewed several times (11–14, 16–18, 29, 93). Quite generally, membranes from different tissues have very similar affinities for 1,4-dihydropyridine ligands ($\sim 10^{-10}$M for nitrendipine), except for skeletal muscle, which has an approximately 10-fold lower affinity. These affinities are all similarly temperature dependent over the temperature range 0–37°C, consistent with an identity or near identity of the 1,4-dihydropyridine binding site in several preparations (60). The relationship of this site to the permeation machinery of the channel remains unknown (94). The thermodynamic data are consistent with a dominantly hydrophobic interaction of the ligands; activators and antagonists were not distinguished, perhaps reflecting ligand binding to a depolarized, inactivated channel state. Recent size and immunoreactivity studies (95) support the finding that the recognition site of the 1,4-dihydropyridine receptor is very similar in different tissues. The densities of binding sites for 1,4-dihydropyridines in purified or partially purified membranes are: skeletal muscle t-tubules (> 65 pmol/mg), cardiac sarcolemma (1–2 pmol/mg), synaptosomal membranes (0.6 pmol/mg), nonvascular and vascular smooth muscle sarcolemma (0.8 and 0.2 pmol/mg, respectively). Vascular smooth muscle, the major target tissue for nifedipine and related drugs, appears to have the lowest density of sites for these drugs (11, 12, 16). Studies of single channel conductances (96) confirm that differences exist between Ca^{2+} channels of similar pharmacological sensitivity.

1,4-Dihydropyridine receptors are susceptible to proteases, phospholipases, -SH reagents, heat, and divalent cations (11–14, 93). Despite the previously mentioned similarities between receptors in different tissues, skeletal muscle binding sites do appear to be biochemically distinguishable by several criteria, including susceptibility to EDTA, -SH reagents, and 1,4-dihydropyridines (93). The receptors in neuronal membranes may differ from those in heart in their sensitivity to monovalent and divalent cations (97). These results indicate that receptors in different tissues may exhibit differences in their associated regulatory sites for cations and other substances.

Purification on lectin columns shows these receptors to be glycoproteins. The high-affinity binding site of the 1,4-dihydropyridine receptor is also susceptible to voltage, as both electrophysiological and ligand-binding studies show (98; See "The Basis of Tissue Selectivity"). The voltage-dependent interactions, together with the correlations between pharmacology and binding and the reconstitution experiments, provide strong evidence for the association between high-affinity sites for 1,4-dihydropyridines and Ca^{2+} channels.

The binding of each of the main classes of Ca^{2+} channel ligands to membranes from excitable cells, except for those in skeletal muscle, is dependent on micromolar concentrations of divalent cations (11–14, 16, 93). In addition, millimolar concentrations of extracellular Ca^{2+} inhibit the binding of verapamil- and diltiazem-like ligands (99). Whether the high-affinity divalent cation–binding sites within the Ca^{2+} channel (44) are the same sites required for the binding of these drugs remains to be determined. Ca^{2+} produces Ca^{2+}-dependent inactivation at a site that is unlikely to promote the binding of these drugs, since Mg^{2+} also promotes drug binding but does not cause channel inactivation.

Localization

Studies with [³H]nitrendipine suggest very strongly that the high-affinity binding sites for this drug are associated with Ca^{2+} channels in the plasma membrane and its invaginations in excitable cells (11–14, 16, 93). Electrophysiological studies using dialyzed cells confirm this localization (100). Reconstitution of purified skeletal muscle t-tubular membranes (96, 101), solubilized Ca^{2+} channel protein (102), and cardiac sarcolemma (96, 103) further establish the sarcolemmal localization of these binding sites.

Both ligand-binding and autoradiographic studies (104, 105) show that high-affinity binding sites for 1,4-dihydropyridines exist in synaptic areas of the brain. Behavioral (106, 107) and biochemical (66, 108) studies indicate that the binding sites for Bay K 8644, and therefore other 1,4-dihydropyridines, represent functional sites on neurons. Central effects of Ca^{2+} channel antagonists are also seen, but usually only under special conditions, presumably those needed to produce a channel state that permits antagonist interaction. Collectively these results indicate that at least some of these high-affinity binding sites in the brain are on Ca^{2+} channels (16, 17, 66, 107, 108).

Electrophysiological studies reveal large numbers of Ca^{2+} channels in skeletal muscle, which is consistent with the high binding-site density of t-tubules (11–14, 16). However, electrophysiological estimates of functional Ca^{2+} channel density suggest that if these sites are on Ca^{2+} channels, then most may not represent functional channels (62). The finding that only 2–3% of purified 1,4-dihydropyridine-binding site–channel complex was reconstituted into functional channels is consistent with this hypothesis (102). Most of the 1,4-dihydropyridine-binding sites in skeletal muscle may be located on the abundant voltage-sensing sites involved in coupling t-tubule excitation to Ca^{2+} release from the sarcoplasmic reticulum (109).

Correlation Between Ligand Binding and Function

Many studies with smooth and cardiac muscle indicate that high-affinity binding of 1,4-dihydropyridines is that to Ca^{2+} channels. The correlation of the potencies of these drugs for inhibition of 1,4-dihydropyridine binding and for pharmacological response provided the first direct evidence for this view (10–12, 16–18). Recent reports extend these observations to a variety of smooth muscles (41, 42). The correlations obtained suggested that the same Ca^{2+} channels were activated in the different smooth muscles studied, regardless of the nature of stimulant (K^+ depolarization or specific agonist). These correlations also extend to the allosteric interactions between ligands of different structural categories that are seen in both binding and pharmacological experiments (31–33). Similarly, ligand-binding studies suggesting that no direct competition occurs between Ca^{2+} and 1,4-dihydropyridines were confirmed electrophysiologically (110).

The various reconstitution experiments mentioned above also support the view that the ligand-binding sites are associated with Ca^{2+} channels. Unfortunately, in the only case in which purified proteins were reconstituted into vesicles, the degree of incorporation was poor (102). Also, as already noted, evidence shows that for cells in skeletal muscle, most of the binding may be to a protein, the voltage sensor. The voltage sensor may be closely related to, but is not itself, the Ca^{2+} channel (109).

Studies on neuroleptics and antidiarrheal agents (104) show that ligand binding can be used to predict effects on Ca^{2+} channels. To date no drugs inhibit 1,4-dihydropyridine binding without affecting Ca^{2+} channels (17).

There are at least three distinguishable sites for Ca^{2+} channel ligands, one each for 1,4-dihydropyridine, verapamil, and diltiazem analogs. Several studies on purified membranes from skeletal and cardiac muscle (99, 103, 111) indicate that the ratio of these binding sites is $1:1:1$. Less-pure membranes yield different stoichiometries (13, 112). Other workers suggest that diltiazem and verapamil share common, or have overlapping, binding sites (104, 112). The differences to pH, temperature, -SH reagents, and 1,4-dihydropyridines (99) in the sensitivity of binding of these two ligand classes make this suggestion unlikely.

The binding sites are allosterically coupled such that at 37°C 1,4-dihydropyridine antagonists and diltiazem reciprocally stimulate binding (11–14, 16, 99, 111). Verapamil (and phenylalkylamines) and 1,4-dihydropyridines are mutually inhibitory independent of temperature (99, 111). Solubilized membranes from cardiac (113) and skeletal muscle (13, 14) also display these allosteric interactions. Diltiazem and verapamil also show mutual inhibition of binding. In contrast to the effects of 1,4-dihydropyridine antagonists, activators such as Bay K 8644 inhibit diltiazem binding in heart membranes (99) and stimulate it in brain membranes, but only at high concentrations (114).

At present these studies of ligand interactions present a complex picture. Transitions probably occur between different states of each receptor during ligand binding and a preexisting equilibrium likely exists between different affinity states of each binding site (115). Interpretations of radioligand-binding data are complicated by three realizations: that the membrane studies may reflect a dominantly inactivated channel state, that chiral 1,4-dihydropyridines may generate enantiomeric-specific activation and antagonism, and that one identified low-affinity 1,4-dihydropyridine binding site represents the adenosine transporter (116, 117). Similarly, the low-affinity phenylalkylamine binding site present in sarcoplasmic reticulum may not be related to the high-affinity Ca^{2+} channel component (118).

Isolation

Several laboratories have reported the isolation of the skeletal muscle 1,4-dihydropyridine t-tubule channel complex, and its reconstitution from the solubilized protein has been reported (102). In this latter preparation, subunits of 135, 50, and 33 kd were reported, but others have not detected the 50-kd component (95). The large 140-kd glycoprotein is bound to the smaller subunit (33 kd) by disulfide bridges (170 kd; 95). 1,4-Dihydropyridine receptors from cardiac and smooth muscle appear composed of 135- and 33-kd subunits. Antisera to the small subunit from skeletal muscle reacted with the small or large components from smooth and cardiac muscle under reducing or nonreducing conditions, respectively. Thus, the size and immunohistochemical characteristics in the three types of muscle appear very similar. Other immunological (45) and genetic (119) approaches are likely to be extremely useful for further channel purification and characterization.

THE BASIS OF TISSUE SELECTIVITY

Ca^{2+} channel antagonists show significant tissue selectivity both pharmacologically and therapeutically. In principle such selectivity may have its origin in the following factors, either alone or in combination:

1. Pharmacokinetic factors: tissue distribution and time course;
2. Ca^{2+} source mobilized: relative use of intra- and extracellular pools;
3. Ca^{2+} channel class: different pharmacological profile of channel classes;
4. State-dependent interactions: affinity of drug depends on channel state;
5. Nonspecific effects: ability to interact at other sites (receptors, etc); and
6. Pathologic state: organ or tissue state may influence above factors.

All of the preceding factors may be important, depending upon circumstance, but recent investigations focus on the existence of discrete channel categories with differing pharmacological sensitivities (See "Structure-Activity Relationships") and on the role of state-dependent phenomena in defining Ca^{2+} channel–ligand interactions.

Ligand affinity for channels may vary dramatically between resting, open, and inactivated states, according to stimulus frequency and membrane potential (23, 24, 28, 30). Use-dependent blockade, in which the inhibitory activity of a drug increases with increasing frequency of stimulation, reflects a preferential ligand interaction with, or access to, an activated or inactivated channel state. This occurrence has been described for verapamil, diltiazem, and their analogs (for reviews see 30, 120). These use-dependent actions are also influenced by the level of the membrane potential between stimuli -hyperpolarization and depolarization reducing and increasing, respectively, the extent of use-dependent blockade.

Until recently the 1,4-dihydropyridines were assumed to behave very differently and to exhibit little, if any, state-dependent interaction (see, for example, 121, 122). However, both activator and antagonist 1,4-dihydropyridines show significant voltage-dependent and, under the appropriate circumstances, frequency-dependent interactions (57, 71, 98, 110, 123–129). Original studies by Sanguinetti & Kass (124, 125) and by Bean (126) indicated that 1,4-dihydropyridine block of cardiac Ca^{2+} channels was strongly enhanced by membrane depolarization, was frequency dependent at pulse frequencies greater than 1 Hz, and occurred preferentially at inactivated Ca^{2+} channel states. Indeed, the high-affinity interactions occurring in depolarized preparations, $K_D \sim 10^{-9}$–10^{-10} M, are very similar to those derived from radioligand-binding experiments in membrane preparations. The significantly lower affinities observed in polarized preparations, $K_D \sim 10^{-7}$–10^{-6} M, contribute in large part to the observed discrepancies between 1,4-dihydropyridine binding and pharmacological actions in cardiac cells (11, 12, 16, 17, 29). The 1,4-dihydropyridine block of Ca^{2+} currents is enhanced by depolarizing prepulses and relieved by hyperpolarization, as subsequent investigations show (57, 71, 98, 127–129). Thus, 1,4-dihydropyridines interact with differing affinities at the resting, open, and inactivated states of the Ca^{2+} channel in a structure-dependent fashion. Nicardipine, which differs from other 1,4-dihydropyridines by the presence of a basic amine function, shows both the frequency-dependence characteristics of verapamil and diltiazem and the potential-dependence characteristics of 1,4-dihydropyridines (125).

The extent to which 1,4-dihydropyridines stabilize different channel states determines the activator-antagonist properties of this ligand series. Thus, Hess et al (77) indicate that Ca^{2+} channels possess three basic gating modes, 0, 1, and 2, which are characterized by no openings because of channel unavailability, brief openings, and long-lasting openings that appear rarely, respectively. 1,4-Dihydropyridine antagonists favor state 0; activators favor state 2. 1,4-Dihydropyridine ligand interaction with, and discrimination between, Ca^{2+} channel states exhibits many interesting subtleties and complexities. The previously noted enantiomeric selectivity of chiral 1,4-dihydropyridines (54–58) presumably reflects a configurational change in the several channel states. However, whether a single 1,4-dihydropyridine enantiomer can exhibit both activation and antagonism is not yet resolved. Tension studies in smooth and cardiac muscle (55, 58) and current studies in myocytes (130) show that the (−)-activator isomer of Bay K 8644 is both an activator and antagonist, according to membrane potential, whereas the (+)-enantiomer is solely antagonistic. However, in pituitary cells, where the Ca^{2+} channels are very slowly inactivated, (−)Bay K 8644 exhibited activator properties only (131). These state-dependent ligand interactions depend both on the relative availability of the different channel states and on the relative

REGULATION

The cardiovascular crises that may follow abrupt clonidine or propranolol

ligand affinities for these states (77, 110, 129). Accordingly, the expression of activator and/or antagonist properties of a 1,4-dihydropyridine depends on the one hand on the chemical and configurational properties of the ligand and, on the other hand, on channel characteristics and channel-state dominance.

The preceding considerations suggest that discrete affinity states should therefore be accessible to radioligand-binding experiments. Although both high- and low-affinity sites have been detected for 1,4-dihydropyridine and verapamil ligands (11–14, 16, 17, 98, 112, 132–135), many studies attempting to demonstrate state (voltage)-dependent binding have serious limitations. Nonspecific binding levels may be unacceptably high at the concentrations necessary to detect low-affinity binding. Many studies have been carried out in depolarized (inactivated) membrane fragments, and the low-affinity sites described have not been pharmacologically characterized. These sites could represent other sites such as the adenosine transporter (116, 117), or they could represent intracellular sites of unknown significance (99, 112, 135). However, a component of voltage-dependent [^{3}H]nitrendipine binding that is lost upon hyperpolarization has been detected in cardiac sarcolemmal vesicles (134). In cultured cardiac cells PN 200–110 binding is voltage dependent, with K_D values of 0.73×10^{-9} M and 0.06×10^{-9} M at -40 and 0 mV, respectively (98). These and similar data obtained in competition studies (98), although not revealing K_D differences of the magnitude expected from electrophysiological observations, are nonetheless encouraging. They suggest a radioligand-binding correlate to state-dependent ligand interactions at the Ca^{2+} channel. Importantly, differential access, rather than differential binding, may also underlie state-dependent interactions (136). Other factors besides these several listed factors may contribute to tissue selectivity of the Ca^{2+} channel ligands. One such factor is the distribution of different channel types at both the organ and cellular levels. It will be important to determine how channel types are distributed between nodal and nonnodal regions in cardiac tissue and between cell bodies, dendrites, and terminals in neurons.

REGULATION

The availability of ligands for at least two categories of voltage-dependent Ca^{2+} channels makes it possible to determine the conditions, mechanisms, and consequences of the regulation of Ca^{2+} channels and the associated drug binding sites under physiological and pathological conditions. How closely such regulation follows the patterns established for other membrane effectors remains to be determined (137). Most studies to date focus only on radioligand-binding changes; correlates to functional channel changes are needed.

The cardiovascular crises that may follow abrupt clonidine or propranolol withdrawal are well documented (138, 139). Several clinical reports are now available concerning Ca^{2+} channel antagonist withdrawal (140–147). Possible withdrawal symptoms were reported in some (140–143, 146), but not other (144, 145, 148), studies, following abrupt termination of diltiazem, verapamil, or nifedipine therapy. Tachyphylaxis to verapamil was reported in one case (148). Reactivity studies in rats chemically treated with D600 (gallopamil, methoxyverapamil) or in humans following nifedipine or verapamil treatment (149, 150) indicate a hyperresponsiveness that may reflect a compensatory effect. With the exception of a report on verapamil (143), an objective withdrawal phenomenon occurs in very few patients (144). Binding studies are inconclusive. 1,4-Dihydropyridine binding site density is unaffected or reduced in heart (151, 152) and reduced in brain (151, 153) following chronic treatment with nifedipine or verapamil. Exposure to Bay K 8644 produces both down-regulation (high dose) and up-regulation (low dose) of cardiac 1,4-dihydropyridine binding sites (P. Gengo & D. J. Triggle, unpublished data).

These reports represent initial attempts to define the channel regulation mediated by Ca^{2+} channel ligands. Such channel regulation may differ from that of membrane receptors for hormones and neurotransmitters because such receptors are tonically regulated by endogenous receptor-directed signals. Endogenous signals for the Ca^{2+} channel may be Ca^{2+} itself, endogenous factors presently unknown, or the input from associated activating or inhibitory receptors. Channel traffic and intracellular Ca^{2+} accumulation is one component of Ca^{2+} channel inactivation (154). Epidemiological and other studies (155, 156) suggest that reduced serum Ca^{2+} levels may be associated with hypertension. Whether chronic changes in Ca^{2+} levels are reflected in changes in Ca^{2+} channels or in other specific components of the Ca^{2+} regulatory machinery of the cell is not known.

It is not clear whether, and under what conditions, Ca^{2+} channels and membrane receptors may coregulate. In rats, chronic antagonist and agonist treatment, which up- and down-regulates β-adrenoceptors and muscarinic receptors, respectively, did not affect 1,4-dihydropyridine-binding-site density (157). However, denervation by reserpine or 6-hydroxydopamine increases both cardiac β-adrenoceptors and Ca^{2+} channels (158, 159). This finding suggests a role for neuronal influences on channel ligand–binding sites other than, or additional to, the tonic sympathetic activity. Consistent with this suggestion, nitrendipine-binding-site density is higher in cultured chick heart cells than in similarly aged cells from functioning hearts (160). Cardiac tissue from patients chronically treated with β-blockers or Ca^{2+} channel antagonists contains elevated β-adrenoceptor density (161), suggesting coregulation. Coregulation of Ca^{2+} channels and receptors, if it indeed occurs, may be uni- or bidirectional and may involve indirect or direct linkages between the two membrane components. Thus, in skeletal muscle (162) and neuronal cell lines (163), elevation of cellular c-AMP levels by various agents is associated with increases in or the appearance of 1,4-dihydropyridine binding sites. c-AMP-dependent protein kinase–mediated phosphorylation is associated with Ca^{2+} channel activation in excitable tissues (164, 165); it may also be associated with Ca^{2+} channel expression. Channels and receptors may also have shared components through which communication occurs. A guanine nucleotide–binding (G) protein is (as measured by the effect of nucleotides and pertussis toxin) involved in the coupling of inhibitory norepinephrine and GABA signals to Ca^{2+} channels in dorsal root ganglia (90, 91). G proteins may couple directly receptors and channels.

Ca^{2+} channels are also regulated under pathological conditions. At least two diseases described are associated with alterations in Ca^{2+} channel ligand binding. Embryonic muscular dysgenesis in mice is characterized by disorganized triadic structure and decreased 1,4-dihydropyridine-binding sites in skeletal muscle; cardiac muscle was not affected. These changes could be directly linked to the observed defect in excitation-contraction coupling (166). The Syrian cardiomyopathic hamster has been reported to have higher densities of 1,4-dihydropyridine-binding sites in muscle and brain (167). This change may underline both the pathology, calcium-induced necrosis, and the therapeutic efficacy of Ca^{2+}-channel antagonists in this condition and in human hypertrophic obstructive cardiomyopathy. However, others have not found evidence for alterations in cardiac 1,4-dihydropyridine binding sites in this animal model (167a). Both elevated and reduced [^{3}H]nitrendipine binding have been reported in brains of DOCA- and spontaneously hypertensive rats (168, 169); how significant, if at all, these changes are to hypertension remains to be defined. A reduced dietary Na^+ intake increases nitrendipine-binding-site density in adrenal glomerulosa cell membranes, but is without effect in vascular and nonvascular smooth muscle (170). Thus, enhanced glomerulosa cell sensitivity to angiotensin during Na^+ reduction may in part reflect the increased number of Ca^{2+} channels as well as the increased number of angiotensin receptors.

Further studies demonstrating channel changes with physiological and pathological events will undoubtedly be forthcoming. Currently, many studies are based on equating changes in ligand-binding properties with changes in channel function. This assumption may not be unreasonable. However, correlative studies are needed, since binding and function are not necessarily coregulated (171). Ontogenic (171) and aging (172, 173) studies have described binding site changes, but have not measured function. This limitation is very important, since studies of the development of 1,4-dihydropyridine binding sites and of functional Ca^{2+} channels in chick heart show clearly that the two events are temporally distinct (160) and that nonfunctional or uncoupled binding sites exist early in development.

PROSPECTS FOR THE FUTURE

In the past few years particularly dramatic progress has been made in the area of Ca^{2+} channel drugs. The introduction of these drugs into clinical medicine, the subsequent development of the radioligand-binding assay, and the electrophysiological assault on the Ca^{2+} channel have greatly contributed to this progress. The recent introduction of Ca^{2+} channel activators spurred more research in an already active field.

Currently, most research is centered on classifying Ca^{2+} channel categories by biochemical and electrophysiological techniques. Undoubtedly in the next few years major developments will occur in the areas of new channel ligands, genetic analyses of channel structure and function, development of new therapeutic areas (including particularly neuronal sites), and identification of Ca^{2+} channel defects with human disease states. The recent identification of Ca^{2+} channel ligand-binding sites in plants raises important questions about the functions and possible exploitation of these sites (174, 175).

Increasing pharmacological awareness of the spectrum of events, both specific and nonspecific, modulated by the Ca^{2+} channel ligands will also serve to focus attention on areas other than Ca^{2+} channel modulation. Some categories of Ca^{2+} channel blockers, notably verapamil, lower the resistance of malignant cells to a number of antitumor agents. This action is receiving considerable attention, although it is probably unrelated to channel blockade (176). Similarly, we may expect continued elucidation of the roles of Ca^{2+} channel ligands in cell protection and of the relationship of the observed protection to channel blockade (177–179). Finally, the significance of Ca^{2+} channel blockade to the development of atherosclerotic lesions and tissue calcification (2, 180–182) requires further investigation to determine the cellular and molecular basis of the observed protection.

The exploration of these future directions makes it very probable that Ca^{2+} channel ligands will enjoy prominent pharmacological and therapeutic roles for many years to come. Patient and scientist alike will benefit from this progress.

ACKNOWLEDGMENTS

Preparation of this review was assisted by grants from the National Institutes of Health (HL 16003, HL 31178).

Literature Cited

1. Urthaler, F. 1986. Review: Role of calcium channel blockers in clinical medicine. *Am. J. Med. Sci.* 292:217–30
2. Fleckenstein, A. 1983. *Calcium Antagonism in Heart and Smooth Muscle. Experimental Facts and Therapeutic Prospects.* New York: Wiley. 399 pp.
3. Opie, L. H., ed. 1984. *Calcium Antagonists and Cardiovascular Disease.* New York: Raven
4. Fleckenstein, A., van Breemen, C., Gross, R., Hoffmeister, F., eds. 1985. *Cardiovascular Effects of Dihydropyridine-Type Calcium Antagonists and Agonists.* Berlin/Heidelberg: Springer-Verlag. 511 pp.
5. Baky, S. 1984. Verapamil. In *New Drugs Annual,* ed. A. Scriabine, 2:71–102. New York: Raven
6. Flaim, S. 1984. Diltiazem. See Ref. 4, pp. 123–56
7. Chaffman, M., Brogden, R. N. 1985. Diltiazem. A review of its pharmacological properties and therapeutic efficacy. *Drugs* 29:387–454
8. Sorkin, E. M., Clissold, S. P., Brogden, R. N. 1985. Nifedipine. A review of its pharmacodynamic and pharmacokinetic properties, and therapeutic efficacy, in ischaemic heart disease, hypertension and related cardiovascular disorders. *Drugs* 30:182–274
9. Needleman, P., Corr, P. B., Johnson, E. M. Jr. 1985. Drugs used for the treatment of angina: organic nitrates, calcium channel blockers, and β-adrenergic antagonists. In The *Pharmacological Basis of Therapeutics,* ed. A. G. Gilman, L. S. Goodman, T. W. Ralland, F. Murad. pp. 806–26. New York: Macmillan. 7th ed.
10. Swamy, V. C., Triggle, D. J. 1986. The calcium channel blockers. In *Modern Pharmacology,* ed. C. R. Craig, R. E. Stitzel. pp. 373–80. Boston: Little, Brown. 2nd ed.
11. Triggle D. J., Janis, R. A. 1984. Calcium channel antagonists: new perspectives from the radioligand binding assay. In *Modern Methods in Pharmacology,* ed. N. Back, S. Spector, 2:1–28. New York: Liss
12. Janis, R. A., Triggle, D. J. 1984. 1,4-Dihydropyridine Ca^{2+} channel activators: a comparison of binding characteristics with pharmacology. *Drug Dev. Res.* 4:257–74
13. Glossmann, H., Ferry, D. R. 1985. Assay for calcium channels. *Methods Enzymol.* 109:513–51

14. Glossmann, H., Ferry, D. R., Goll, A., Striessnig, J., Zernig, G. 1985. Calcium channels and calcium channel drugs: recent biochemical and biophysical findings. *Arzneim. Forsch.* 35:1917–35
15. Spedding, M. M. 1985. Activators and inactivators of Ca^{++} channels: new perspectives. *J. Pharmacol.* 16:319–43
16. Triggle, D. J., Janis, R. A. 1987. Calcium channels and calcium channel ligands. In *Receptor Pharmacology and Function,* ed. M. Williams, R. A. Glennon, P. B. M. W. M. Timmermans. New York: Dekker. In press
17. Janis, R. A., Silver, P., Triggle, D. J. 1987. Drug action and cellular calcium regulation. *Adv. Drug Res.* In press
18. Triggle, D. J., Venter, J. C., eds. 1987. *Structure and Physiology of the Slow Inward Calcium Channel.* New York: Liss. In press
19. Takenaka, T., Maeno, H. 1982. A vasoconstrictive compound 1,4-dihydropyridine derivative. *Jpn. J. Pharmacol.* 32:139
20. Troug, A. G., Brunner, H., Criscione, L., Fallert, M., Kuhnis, H., et al. 1985. Cg28392, a dihydropyridine Ca^{2+} entry stimulator. See Ref. 25, pp. 441–52
21. Schramm, M., Thomas, G., Towart, R., Franckowiak, G. 1983. Novel dihydropyridines with positive inotropic action through activation of Ca^{2+} channels. *Nature* 303:535–37
22. Preuss, K. C., Gross, G. J., Brooks, H. L., Warltiet, D. C. 1985. Slow channel calcium activators, a new group of pharmacological agents. *Life Sci.* 37:1271–78
23. Hill, B. 1977. Local anesthetics: hydrophilic and hydrophobic pathways for the drug-receptor reaction. *J. Gen. Physiol.* 69:497–515
24. Hondeghem, L. M., Katzung, B. G. 1977. Time- and voltage-dependent interactions of antiarrhythmic drugs with cardiac sodium channels. *Biochim. Biophys. Acta* 472:373–98
25. Rubin, R. P., Weiss, G. B., Putney, J. W., eds. 1985. *Calcium in Biological Systems.* New York: Plenum. 737 pp.
26. Rasmussen, H. 1986. The calcium messenger system. *N. Engl. J. Med.* 314:1094–101; 1164–70
27. Fleckenstein, A. 1977. Specific pharmacology of calcium in myocardium, cardiac pacemakers, and vascular smooth muscle. *Ann. Rev. Pharmacol. Toxicol.* 17:149–66
28. Tsien, R. W. 1983. Calcium channels in

excitable cell membranes. *Ann. Rev. Physiol.* 45:341–58
29. Schwartz, A., Triggle, D. J. 1984. Cellular action of calcium channel–blocking drugs. *Ann. Rev. Med.* 35:325–40
30. Hondeghem, L. M., Katzung, B. G. 1984. Antiarrhythmic agents: the modulated receptor mechanism of action of sodium and calcium channel–blocking drugs. *Ann. Rev. Pharmacol. Toxicol.* 24:387–23
31. Spedding, M. 1983. Functional interactions of calcium-antagonists in K^+-depolarized smooth muscle. *Br. J. Pharmacol.* 80:485–88
32. Yousif, F., Triggle, D. J. 1985. Functional interactions between organic calcium channel antagonists in smooth muscle. *Can. J. Physiol. Pharmacol.* 63:193–95
33. DePover, A., Grupp, I. L., Grupp, G., Schwartz, A. 1983. Diltiazem potentiates the negative inotropic action of nimodipine in heart. *Biochem. Biophys. Res. Commun.* 114:922–29
34. Mannhold, R., Rodenkirchen, R., Bayer, R. 1982. Quantitative and qualitative structure-activity relationships of specific Ca antagonists. *Prog. Pharmacol.* 5:25–52
35. Fossheim, R. 1985. Crystal structure of the calcium channel antagonist: 3,5-bis(methoxycarbonyl) - 2,6 - dimethyl - 4 - (2 - trifluoromethylphenyl) - 1,4 - dihydropyridine. *Acta Chem. Scand. Ser. B* 39:785–90
36. Fossheim, R. 1986. Crystal structure of the dihydropyridine Ca^{2+} antagonist felodipine. Dihydropyridine binding prerequisites assessed from crystallographic data. *J. Med. Chem.* 29:305–7
37. Langs, D. A., Triggle, D. J. 1985. Conformational features of calcium channel agonist and antagonist analogs of nifedipine. *Mol. Pharmacol.* 27:544–48
38. Goldmann, S., Geiger, W. 1984. Rotational barriers of 4-aryl-1,4-dihydropyridines. *Ang. Chem. (Int. Ed.)* 23:301–2
39. Fossheim, R., Svarteng, K., Mostad, A., Rømming, C., Shefter, E., Triggle, D. J. 1982. Crystal structures and pharmacological activity of calcium channel antagonists. *J. Med. Chem.* 25:126–31
40. Seidel, W., Meyer, H., Born, L., Kazda, S., Dompert, W. 1984. Rigid calcium antagonists of the nifedipine-type: geometric requirements for the dihydropyridine receptor. In *QSAR and Strategies in the Design of Bioactive Compounds. Proc. 5th Eur. Symp. Quant. Struct. Act. Relat. Bad Segeberg. 1984,* ed. J. K. Seydel, pp. 366–69. Weinheim, Fed. Rep. Germany: VCH Verlag
41. Yousif, F. B., Bolger, G. T., Ruzycky, A., Triggle, D. J. 1985. Ca^{2+} channel antagonist actions in bladder smooth muscle: comparative pharmacologic and [^{3}H]nitrendipine binding studies. *Can. J. Physiol. Pharmacol.* 63:453–62
42. Yousif, F. B., Triggle, D. J. 1986. Inhibitory actions of a series of Ca^{2+} channel antagonists against agonist and K^+ depolarization–induced responses in smooth muscle: an assessment of selectivity of action. *Can. J. Physiol. Pharmacol.* 64:273–83
43. Triggle, D. J. 1981. Calcium antagonists: basic chemical and pharmacological aspects. In *New Perspectives on Calcium Antagonists,* ed. G. B. Weiss, pp. 1–18. Bethesda, MD: Am. Physiol. Soc.
44. Triggle, D. J., Janis, R. A. 1984. Nitrendipine: binding sites and mechanisms of action. In *Nitrendipine,* eds. A. Scriabine, S. Vanov, K. Deck, pp. 33–52. Baltimore: Urban & Schwarzenberg
45. Campbell, K. P., Sharp, A., Strom, M., Kahl, S. D. 1986. High-affinity antibodies to the 1,4-dihydropyridine Ca^{2+} channel blockers. *Proc. Natl. Acad. Sci. USA* 83:2792–96
46. Berg, H. C., Purcell, E. M. 1977. Physics of chemoreception. *Biophys. J.* 20:193–19
47. Rhodes, D. G., Sarmiento, J. G., Herbette, L. G. 1985. Kinetics of binding of membrane-active drugs to receptor sites. Diffusion-limited rates for a membrane bilayer approach of 1,4-dihydropyridine calcium channel antagonists to their active site. *Mol. Pharmacol.* 27:612–23
48. Chester, D. W., Herbette. L. G., Mason, R. P., Joslyn, A. F., Triggle, D. J., Koppel, D. E. 1986. Diffusion of dihydropyridine calcium channel antagonists in cardiac sarcolemmal lipid multibilayers. *Biophys. J.* In press
49. Langs, D. A., Triggle, D. J. 1985. Conformational features of calcium channel agonist and antagonist analogs of nifedipine. *Mol. Pharmacol.* 27:544–48
50. Rampe, D., Janis, R. A., Triggle, D. J. 1984. Bay K 8644, a 1,4-dihydropyridine Ca^{2+} channel activator: dissociation of binding and functional effects in brain synaptosomes. *J. Neurochem.* 43:1688–92
51. Janis, R. A., Sarmiento, J. G., Maurer, S. C., Bolger, G. T., Triggle, D. J.

1984. Characteristics of the binding of [^{3}H]nitrendipine to rabbit ventricular membranes: modifications by other Ca^{2+} channel antagonists and by the Ca^{++} channel agonist Bay K 8644. *J. Pharmacol. Exp. Ther.* 231:8–15

52. Su, C. M., Swamy, V. C., Triggle, D. J. 1984. Calcium channel activation in vascular smooth muscle by Bay K 8644. *Can. J. Physiol. Pharmacol.* 62:1401–10

53. Wei, X. Y., Luchowski, E. M., Rutledge, A., Su, C. M., Triggle, D. J. 1986. A pharmacologic and radioligand binding analysis of the action of 1,4-dihydropyridine activator-antagonist pairs in smooth muscle. *J. Pharmacol. Exp. Ther.* 239:144–53

54. Hof, P. R., Rugg, V. T., Hof, A., Vogel, A. 1985. Stereoselectivity at the calcium channel: opposite action of the enantiomers of a 1,4-dihydropyridine. *J. Cardiovasc. Pharmacol.* 7:689–93

55. Franckowiak, G., Bechem, M., Schramm, M., Thomas, G. 1985. The optical isomers of the 1,4-dihydropyridine Bay K 8644 show opposite effects on Ca^{2+} channels. *Eur. J. Pharmacol.* 114:223–26

56. Kongsamut, S., Kamp, T. J., Miller, R. J. 1985. Calcium channel agonist and antagonist effects of the stereoisomers of the dihydropyridine 202–791. *Biochem. Biophys. Res. Commun.* 130:141–48

57. Williams, J. S., Grupp, I. L., Grupp, G., Vaghy, P. L., Dumont, L., Schwartz, A. 1985. Profile of the oppositely acting enantiomers of the dihydropyridine 202–791 in cardiac preparations: receptor binding, electrophysiological, and pharmacological studies. *Biochem. Biophys. Res. Commun.* 131:13–21

58. Wei, X. Y., Triggle, D. J. 1987. Comparative radioligand binding and pharmacological activities of the enantiomers of Bay K 8644 and other 1,4-dihydropyridines. *Symp. Calcium Antagonists. Pharmacol. Clin. Res. N. Y. Acad. Sci.* Feb. 10–13 (Abstr.)

59. Weiland, G. A., Minneman, K. P., Molinoff, P. B. 1979. Fundamental differences between the molecular interactions of agonists and antagonists with the β-adrenergic receptor. *Nature* 281:114–17

60. Rampe, D., Luchowski, E., Rutledge, A., Janis, R. A., Triggle, D. J. 1986. Comparative aspects of [^{3}H]1,4-dihydropyridine Ca^{2+} channel antagonist and activator binding to neuro-

nal and muscle membranes. *Can. J. Physiol. Pharmacol.* In press

61. Triggle, D. J., Janis, R. A. 1984. The 1,4-dihydropyridine receptor: a regulatory component of the Ca^{2+} channel. *J. Cardiovasc. Pharmacol.* 6:S949–55

62. Schwartz, L. M., McCleskey, E. W., Almers, W. 1985. Dihydropyridine receptors in muscle are voltage-dependent but most are not functional calcium channels. *Nature* 314:747–51

63. Nowycky, M., Fox, A. P., Tsien, R. W. 1985. Three types of neuronal calcium channel with different calcium agonist sensitivity. *Nature* 316:440–43

64. Bossu, J. L., Feltz, A., Thomann, J. M. 1985. Depolarization elicits two distinct calcium currents in vertebrate sensory neurones. *Pfluegers Arch.* 403:360–68

65. Fedulova, S. A., Kostyuk, P. G., Veselovsky, N. S. 1985. Two types of calcium channels in the somatic membrane of new-born rat dorsal root ganglion neurones. *J. Physiol. London* 359:431–46

66. Miller, R. J. 1987. Calcium channels in neurones. See Ref. 18. In press

67. Penner, R., Dreyer, F. 1986. Two different presynaptic calcium currents in mouse motor nerve terminals. *Pfluegers Arch.* 406:190–97

68. Nilius, B., Hess, P., Lansman, J. B., Tsien, R. W. 1985. A novel type of cardiac calcium channel in ventricular cells. *Nature* 316:443–46

69. Bean, B. P. 1985. Two kinds of calcium channels in canine atrial cells. Differences in kinetics, selectivity and pharmacology. *J. Gen. Physiol.* 86:1–30

70. Friedman, M. E., Suarez-Kurtz, G., Kaczorowski, G. J., Katz, G. M., Reuben, J. P. 1986. Two calcium currents in a smooth muscle cell line. *Am. J. Physiol.* 250:H699–703

71. Cognard, C., Lazdunski, M., Romey, G. 1986. Different types of Ca^{2+} channels in mammalian skeletal muscle cells in culture. *Proc. Natl. Acad. Sci. USA* 83:517–21

72. Matteson, D. R., Armstrong, C. M. 1986. Properties of two types of calcium channels in clonal pituitary cells. *J. Gen. Physiol.* 87:161–82

73. Rampe, D., Triggle, D. J. 1986. Benzodiazepines and calcium channel function. *Trends Pharmacol. Sci.* In press

74. Doble, A., Benavides, J., Ferris, O., Bertrand, P., Menager, J., et al. 1985. Dihydropyridine and peripheral type benzodiazepine binding sites: subcellular distribution and molecular size

determination. *Eur. J. Pharmacol.* 119:153–67

75. Bolger, G. T., Weissman, B. A., Luedens, H., Barrett, J. E., Witkin, J., et al. 1986. Dihydropyridine calcium channel antagonist binding in non-mammalian vertebrates: characterization and relationship to "peripheral-type" binding sites for benzodiazepines. *Brain Res.* 368:351–56

76. Mestre, M., Carriot, T., Belin, C., Uzan, A., Renault, C., et al. 1985. Electrophysiological and pharmacological evidence that peripheral type benzodiazepine receptors are coupled to calcium channels in the heart. *Life Sci.* 36:391–400

77. Hess, P., Lansman, J. B., Tsien, R. W. 1984. Different modes of Ca^{2+} channel gating favoured by dihydropyridine Ca^{2+} agonists and antagonists. *Nature* 311:538–44

78. Miller, R. J. 1984. Toxin probes for voltage sensitive calcium channels. *Trends Neurosci.* 7:309–12

79. Freedman, S. B., Miller R. J., Miller, D. B., Tindall, D. R. 1984. Interactions of maitotoxin with voltage-sensitive calcium channels in cultured neuronal cells. *Proc. Natl. Acad. Sci. USA* 8:4582–85

80. Login, I. S., Judd, A. M., Cronin, M. J., Koike, K., Schettini, G., et al. 1985. The effects of maitotoxin on $^{45}Ca^{2+}$ flux and hormone release in GH_3 rat pituitary cells. *Endocrinology* 116:622–27

81. Hamilton, S. L., Yatani, A., Hawkes, M. J., Redding, K., Brown, A. M. 1985. Atrotoxin: a specific agonist for calcium currents in heart. *Science* 229:182–84

82. Crosland, R. D., Hsiao, T. H., McClure, W. O. 1984. Purification and characterization of β-leptinotursin-h, an activator of presynaptic calcium channels. *Biochemistry* 23:734–41

83. Olivera, B. M., Gray, W. R., Zeikus, R., McIntosh, J. M., Varga, J., et al. 1985. Peptide neurotoxins from fish-hunting cone snails. *Science* 230:1338–43

84. Cruz, L. J., Gray, W. R., Yoshikami, D., Olivera, B. M. 1985. *Conus* venoms: a rich source of neuroactive peptides. *J. Toxicol. Toxin Rev.* 4:107–32

85. Kerr, L. M., Yoshikami, D. 1984. A venom peptide with a novel presynaptic blocking action. *Nature* 308:282–84

86. Cruz, L. J., Olivera, B. M. 1986. Calcium channel antagonists. w-Conotoxin defines a new high affinity site. *J. Biol. Chem.* 261:6230–33

87. Reuter, H. 1983. Calcium channel modulation by neurotransmitters, enzymes and drugs. *Nature* 301:509–74

88. Gross, R., Bechem, M., Kayser, M., Schramm, M., Tariel, R., Thomas, G. 1985. Effects of calcium agonistic 1,4-dihydropyridine Bay k 8644 on the heart. See Ref. 4, pp. 218–32

89. Levitan, I. B. 1985. Phosphorylation of ion channels. *J. Membr. Biol.* 87:177–90

90. Stevens, C. F. 1986. Modifying channel function. *Nature* 319:622

91. Holz, G. G., Rane, S. G., Dunlap, K. 1986. GTP-binding proteins mediate transmitter inhibition of voltage-dependent calcium channels. *Nature* 319:670–72

92. Breitwieser, G. E., Szabo, G. 1986. Uncoupling of cardiac muscarinic and β-adrenergic receptors from ion channels by a guanine nucleotide analogue. *Nature* 317:538–40

93. Janis, R. A., Bellemann, P., Sarmiento, J. G., Triggle, D. J. 1985. The dihydropyridine receptors. See Ref. 4, pp. 140–55

94. Hess, P., Tsien, R. W. 1984. Mechanism of ion permeation through the Ca^{2+} channel. *Nature* 309:453–56

95. Schmid, A., Barhanin, J., Coppola, J., Borsotto, M., Lazdunski, M. 1986. Immunochemical analysis of subunit structures of 1,4-dihydropyridine receptors associated with voltage-dependent Ca^{2+} channels in skeletal, cardiac and smooth muscles. *Biochemistry* 25:3492–95

96. Rosenberg, P. L., Hess, P., Tsien, R. W., Smilowitz, H., Reeves, J. P. 1986. Calcium channels in planar lipid bilayers: insights into mechanisms of ion permeation and gating. *Science* 231:1504–66

97. Bolger, G. T., Skolnick, P. 1986. Novel interactions of cations with dihydropyridine calcium antagonist binding sites in brain. *Br. J. Pharmacol.* 88:857–66

98. Reuter, H., Porzig, H., Kokubun, S., Prodhum, B. 1986. Voltage-dependent binding and action of 1,4-dihydropyridine enantiomers in intact cardiac cells. In *Proteins in Excitable Membranes*, ed. B. Hille, P. M. Fambrough. New York: Wiley. In press

99. Garcia, M. L., King, V. J., Siegl, P. K. S., Reuben, J. P., Kaczorowski, G. J. 1986. Binding of Ca^{2+} entry blockers to cardiac sarcolemmal membrane vesicles. *J. Biol. Chem.* 261:8146–51

100. Tsien, R. W., Bean, B. P., Hess, P., Lansman, J. B., Nilius, B., Nowycky,

M. C. 1986. Mechanisms of calcium channel modulation by β-adrenergic agents and dihydropyridine calcium agents. *J. Mol. Cell. Cardiol.* 18:691–710

101. Affolter, H., Coronado, R. 1985. Agonists Bay k 8644 and CGP 28 392 open calcium channels reconstituted from skeletal muscle transverse tubules. *Biophys. J.* 48:341–47

102. Curtis, B. M., Catterall, W. A. 1986. Reconstitution of the voltage-sensitive calcium channel purified from skeletal muscle transverse tubules. *Biochemistry* 25:3077–83

103. Ehrlich, B. E., Schen, C. R., Garcia, M. L., Kaczorowski, G. J. 1985. Incorporation of calcium channels from cardiac sarcolemmal membrane vesicles into planar lipid bilayers. *Proc. Natl. Acad. Sci. USA* 83:193–97

104. Snyder, S. H., Reynolds, I. 1985. Calcium antagonist drugs: receptor interactions that clarify therapeutic effects. *N. Engl. J. Med.* 313:995–1001

105. Gould, R. J., Murphy, K. M. M., Snyder, S. H. 1985. In vitro autoradiography of [3H]nitrendipine localizes calcium channels to synaptic rich zones. *Brain Res.* 330:217–23

106. Bolger, G. T., Weissman, B. A., Skolnick, P. 1985. The behavioral effects of the calcium agonist Bay k 8644 in the mouse: antagonism by the calcium antagonist nifedipine. *Naunyn-Schmiedebergs Arch. Pharmacol.* 328:373–77

107. Ramkumar, V., El-Fakahay, E. S. 1986. The current status of the dihydropyridine calcium channel antagonist binding sites in the brain. *Trends Pharmacol. Sci.* 7:171–72

108. Kendall, D. A., Nahorski, S. R. 1985. Dihydropyridine calcium channel activators and antagonists influence depolarization-evoked inositol phospholipid hydrolysis. *Eur. J. Pharmacol.* 115:31–36

109. Rious, E., Brum, G., Stefani, E. 1986. E-C coupling effects of interventions that reduce slow Ca^{2+} currents suggest a role of t-tubule Ca^{2+} channels in skeletal muscle function. *Biophys. J.* 49:13a

110. Kass, R. S., Sanguinetti, M. C., Bennett, P. E., Coplin, B. E., Krafte, D. S. 1985. Voltage-dependent modulation of cardiac Ca^{2+} channels by dihydropyridines. See Ref. 4, pp. 198–215

111. Galazzi, J.-P., Borsotto, M., Barhanin, J., Fosset, M., Lazdunski, M. 1986. Characterization and photoaffinity labeling of receptor sites for the Ca^{2+} channel inhibitors, d-*cis*-diltiazen,(±)-bepridil, desmethoxyverapamil and (+)-PN 200 110 in skeletal muscle transverse tubule membranes. *J. Biol. Chem.* 261:1393–97

112. Reynolds, I. J., Snowman, A. M., Snyder, S. H. 1986. (–)-[3H]-Desmethoxyverapamil labels multiple Ca^{2+} channel modulator receptors in brain and skeletal muscle membranes: differentiation by temperature and dihydropyridines. *J. Pharmacol. Exp. Ther.* 237:731–38

113. Ruth, P., Flockerzi, U., Oeken, H. J., Hofmann, F. 1986. Solubilization of the bovine cardiac sarcolemmal binding sites for calcium blockers. *Eur. J. Biochem.* 155:613–20

114. Schoemaker, H., Langer, S. Z. 1985. [3H]Diltiazem binding to calcium channel antagonist recognition sites in rat cerebral cortex. *Eur. J. Pharmacol.* 111:273–77

115. Weiland, G. A., Oswald, R. E. 1985. The mechanism of binding of dihydropyridine calcium channel blockers to rat brain membranes. *J. Biol. Chem.* 260:8456–64

116. Marangos, P. J., Finkel, M. S., Verma, A., Maturi, M. F., Patel, J., Patterson, R. E. 1984. Adenosine uptake sites in dog heart and brain; interaction with calcium antagonists. *Life Sci.* 35:1109–16

117. Striessnig, J., Zernig, G., Glossmann, H. 1985. Human red-blood-cell Ca^{2+} antagonist binding sites: Evidence for an unusual receptor coupled to the nucleoside transporter. *Eur. J. Biochem.* 150:67–77

118. Oeken, H.-J., von Nettelbladt, E., Zimmer, M., Flockerzi, V., Ruth, P., Hofmann, F. 1986. Cardiac sarcoplasmic reticulum contains a low-affinity site for phenylalkylamines. *Eur. J. Biochem.* 156:661–67

119. Dascal, N., Snutch, J. P., Lubbert, H., Davidson, N., Lester, H. A. 1986. Expression and modulation of voltage-gated calcium channels after RNA injection in *Xenopus* oocytes. *Science* 231:1147–50

120. Hurwitz, L. 1986. Pharmacology of calcium channels and smooth muscle. *Ann. Rev. Pharmacol. Toxicol.* 26:225–58

121. Bayer, R., Kaufmann, R., Mannhold, R., Rodenkirchen, R. 1982. The actions of specific Ca antagonists on cardiac electrical activity. *Prog. Pharmacol.* 5:53–85

122. Kass, R. S. 1982. Nisoldipine: a new, more selective, calcium current blocker

123. Lee, K. S., Tsien, R. W. 1983. Mechanism of calcium channel blockade by verapamil, D600, diltiazem and nitrendipine in single dialysed heart cells. *Nature* 302:790–94

in cardiac Purkinje fibers. *J. Pharmacol. Exp. Ther.* 223:446–56

124. Sanguinetti, M. C., Kass, R. S. 1984. Regulation of cardiac calcium current and contractile activity by the dihydropyridine Bay k 8644 is voltage-dependent. *J. Mol. Cell. Cardiol.* 16:667–70

125. Sanguinetti, M. C., Kass, R. S. 1984. Voltage-dependent block of calcium channel current in the calf cardiac Purkinje fiber by dihydropyridine calcium channel antagonists. *Circ. Res.* 55:336–48

126. Bean, B. P. 1984. Nitrendipine block of cardiac calcium channels: high affinity binding to the inactivated state. *Proc. Natl. Acad. Sci. USA* 81:6388–92

127. Uehara, V., Hurre, J. R. 1985. Interactions of organic calcium channel antagonists with calcium channels in single frog atrial cells. *J. Gen. Physiol.* 85:621–47

128. Gurney, A. M., Nerbonne, J. M., Lester, H. A. 1985. Photo-induced removal of nifedipine reveals mechanisms of calcium antagonist action on single heart cells. *J. Gen. Physiol.* 86:353–79

129. Sanguinetti, M. C., Krafte, D. S., Kass, R. S. 1986. Voltage-dependent modulation of Ca channel current in heart cells by Bay k 8644. *J. Gen. Physiol.* 88:369–92

130. Kass, R. S. 1986. Voltage-dependent modulation of cardiac Ca channel current by the optical isomers of Bay k 8644: implications for channel gating. *Circ. Res.* In press

131. McCarthy, R. T., Cohen, C. J. 1986. The enantiomers of Bay k 8644 have different effects on Ca channel gating in rat anterior pituitary cells. *Biophys. J.* 49:432 (Abstr.)

132. Green, F. J., Farmer, B. B., Wiseman, G. L., Jose, M. J. L., Watanabe, A. M. 1985. Effect of membrane depolarization on binding of [^{3}H]nitrendipine to rat cardiac myocytes. *Circ. Res.* 56:576–85

133. Ptasienski, J., McMahon, K. K., Hosey, M. M. 1985. High and low affinity states of the dihydropyridine and phenylalkylamine receptors on the cardiac calcium channel and their interconversion by divalent cations. *Biochem. Biophys. Res. Commun.* 129:910–17

134. Schilling, W. P., Drews, J. A. 1986.

135. Sarmiento, J. G., Shrinkhande, A. V., Janis, R. A., Triggle, D. J. 1987. [^{3}H]Bay K 8644, a 1,4-dihydropyridine Ca^{++} channel activator: Characteristics of binding to high and low affinity sites in cardiac membranes. *J. Pharmacol. Exp. Ther.* In press

Voltage-sensitive nitrendipine binding in an isolated cardiac sarcolemma preparation. *J. Biol. Chem.* 261:2750–58

136. Starmer, C. F. 1986. Theoretical characterization of ion channel blockade: ligand binding to periodically accessible receptors. *J. Theor. Biol.* 119:235–49

137. Poste, G., Crooke, S. T., eds. 1985. *Mechanisms of Receptor Regulation.* New York: Plenum

138. Frishman, W. H., Klein, N., Strom, J., Cohen, M. N., Shamoon, H., et al. 1982. Comparative effects of abrupt withdrawal of propranolol and verapamil in angina pectoris. *Am. J. Cardiol.* 50:1191–95

139. Reid, J. L. 1981. The clinical pharmacology of clonidine and related central antihypertensive agents. *Br. J. Clin. Pharmacol.* 12:295–302

140. Moses, J. W., Wertheimer, J. H., Bodenheimer, M. M., Banka, V. S., Feldman, M., Helfant, R. H. 1981. Efficacy of nifedipine in rest angina refractory to propranolol and nitrates in patients with obstructive coronary artery disease. *Ann. Intern. Med.* 94:425–29

141. Kay, R., Blake, J., Rubin, D. 1982. Possible coronary spasm rebound to abrupt nifedipine withdrawal. *Am. Heart J.* 103:308

142. Schick, E. C., Liang, C.-S., Heupler, F. A., Kahl, F. R., Kent, K. M., et al. 1982. Randomized withdrawal from nifedipine: placebo-controlled study in patients with coronary artery spasms. *Am. Heart J.* 104:690–97

143. Subramanian, V. B. 1983. Calcium antagonist withdrawal syndrome: objective demonstration with frequency-modulated ambulatory ST-segment monitoring. *Br. Med. J.* 286:520–21

144. Raftery, E. B. 1984. Cardiovascular drug withdrawal syndromes. A potential problem with calcium antagonists. *Drugs* 28:371–74

145. Schroeder, J. S., Walker, S. D., Skalland, M. L., Hemberger, J. A. 1985. Absence of rebound from diltiazem therapy in Prinzmental's variant angina. *J. Am. Coll. Cardiol.* 6:174–78

146. Mehta, J., Lopez, L. 1985. Calcium blocker withdrawal phenomenon: increase in affinity of alpha$_2$-adrenoceptor

for agonist as a potential mechanism. *Circ. Suppl.* 3:1105 (Abstr.)

147. Gottlieb, S. O., Gerstenblith, G. 1985. Safety of acute calcium antagonist withdrawal studies in patients with unstable angina withdrawn from nifedipine. *Am. J. Cardiol.* 55:27E–30E

148. Aderka, D., Levy, A., Pinkhas, J., Tiqva, P. 1986. Tachyphylaxis to verapamil. *Arch. Intern. Med.* 146:207

149. Pang, C. C. Y., Sutter, M. C. 1985. Chronic treatment of rats with D-600 causes a compensatory decrease in the calcium requirement for contractility of vascular smooth and cardiac muscles. *Can. J. Physiol. Pharmacol.* 63:495–99

150. Nelson, D. O., Mangel, A. W., Graham, C. A., Frederiksen, J. W., Green, E. J., et al. 1984. Altered human vascular activity following withdrawal from calcium channel blockers. *J. Cardiovasc. Pharmacol.* 6:1249–50

151. Gengo, P. J. 1985. *Characterization of the persistent actions of the novel calcium channel blocker O-NCS and the metabolism and regulation of the 1,4-dihydropyridine binding site in rat brain, smooth and cardiac muscle.* PhD dissertation. State Univ. of New York at Buffalo

152. Nishiyama, T., Kobayashi, A., Haga, T., Yamazaki, N. 1986. Chronic treatment with nifedipine does not change the number of [^{3}H]nitrendipine and [^{3}H]dihydroalprenolol binding sites. *Eur. J. Pharmacol.* 121:167–72

153. Panza, G., Grebb, J. A., Sanna, E., Wright, A. G., Hanbauer, I. 1985. Evidence for down-regulation of [^{3}H]nitrendipine recognition sites in mouse brain after long-term treatment with nifedipine or verapamil. *Neuropharmacology* 24:1113–17

154. Eckert, R., Chad, J. E. 1984. Inactivation of Ca channels. *Prog. Biophys. Mol. Biol.* 44:218–67

155. Lau, K., Eby, B. 1985. The role of calcium in genetic hypertension. *Hypertension* 7:657–67

156. McCarron, D. A. 1985. Is calcium more important than sodium in the pathogenesis of essential hypertension? *Hypertension* 7:607–27

157. Skattebøl, A. 1986. *Regulation of putative Ca^{2+} channels in the brain.* PhD dissertation. State Univ. of New York at Buffalo

158. Powers, R. E., Colucci, W. S. 1985. An increase in putative voltage-dependent calcium channel number following reserpine treatment. *Biochem. Biophys. Res. Commun.* 132:844–49

159. Skattebøl, A., Triggle, D. J. 1986. 6-Hydroxydopamine treatment increases β-adrenoceptors and Ca^{2+} channels in rat heart. *Eur. J. Pharmacol.* 127:287–89

160. Renaud, J.-F., Kazazoglou, T., Schmid, A., Romey, G., Lazdunski, M. 1984. Differentiation of receptor sites for [^{3}H]nitrendipine in chick hearts and physiological relation to the slow Ca^{2+} channel and to excitation-contraction coupling. *Eur. J. Biochem.* 139:673–81

161. Hedberg, A., Kempf, F., Josephson, M. E., Molinoff, P. B. 1985. Co-existence of beta-1 and beta-2 adrenergic receptors in the human heart: effects of treatment with receptor antagonists or calcium entry blockers. *J. Pharmacol. Exp. Ther.* 234:561–68

162. Schmid, A., Renaud, J.-P., Lazdunski, M. 1985. Short-term and long-term effects of β-adrenergic effectors and cyclic AMP on nitrendipine-sensitive voltage-dependent Ca^{2+} channels of skeletal muscle. *J. Biol. Chem.* 260:13041–46

163. Freedman, S. B., Dawson, G., Villereal, M. L., Miller, R. J. 1984. Identification and characterization of voltage-sensitive calcium channels in neuronal clonal cell lines. *J. Neurosci.* 4:1453–67

164. Brum, G., Fluckerzi, V., Hofmann, F., Osterrieder, W., Trautwein, W. 1983. Injection of catalytic subunit of cAMP-dependent protein kinase into isolated cardiac myocytes. *Pfluegers Arch.* 398:147–54

165. Doroshenko, P. A., Kostyuk, P. G., Martynyuk, A. E., Kursky, M. D., Vorobetz, Z. D. 1984. Intracellular protein kinase and calcium inward currents in perfused neurones of the snail *Helix pomatia. Neuroscience* 11:263–67

166. Pinçon-Raymond, M., Rieger, F., Fosset, M., Lazdunski, M. 1985. Abnormal transverse tubule system and abnormal amount of receptors for Ca^{2+} channel inhibitors of the 1,4-dihydropyridine family in skeletal muscle from mice with embryonic muscular dysgenesis. *Dev. Biol.* 112:458–66

167. Wagner, J. A., Reynolds, I. J., Weisman, H. F., Dudeck, P., Weisfeldt, M. L., Snyder, S. H. 1986. Calcium antagonist receptors in cardiomyopathic hamster: selective increases in heart, muscle and brain. *Science* 232:515–18

167a. Howlett, S. E., Gordon, T. 1986. [^{3}H]Nitrendipine binding to the cardiac muscle of normal and dystrophic hamsters. *Proc. Int. Union Physiol. Sci.*

XVI. *XXXth Congr.* p. 231. *Vancouver, Canada:* Int. Union Physiol.
168. Ishii, K., Kano, T., Kurobe, Y., Ando, J. 1983. Binding of [³H]nitrendipine to heart and brain membranes from normotensive and spontaneously hypertensive rats. *Eur. J. Pharmacol.* 88:277–78
169. Lee, H. R., Watson, M., Yamamura, H. I., Roeske, W. R. 1985. Decreased [³H]nitrendipine binding in the brainstem of deoxycorticosterone NaCl hypertensive rats. *Life Sci.* 37:971–77
170. Schiebinger, R. J., Kontrimus, K. 1985. Dietary intake of sodium chloride in the rat influences [³H]nitrendipine binding to adrenal glomerulosa cell membranes but does not alter binding to vascular smooth muscle membranes. *J. Clin. Invest.* 76:2165–70
171. Rampe, D., Ferrante, J., Triggle, D. J. 1986. The ontogeny of [³H]nitrendipine binding sites and ⁴⁵Ca²⁺ uptake processes in brain synaptosomes from spontaneously hypertensive rats. *Dev. Brain Res.* 29:189–92
172. Battaini, F., Govoni, S., Rius, R. A., Trabucchi, M. 1985. Age-dependent increase in [³H]verapamil binding to rat cortical membranes. *Neurosci. Lett.* 61:67–71
173. Govoni, S., Rius, R. A., Battaini, F., Bianchi, A., Trabucchi, M. 1985. Age-related reduced affinity in [³H]nitrendipine labeling of brain voltage-dependent calcium channels. *Brain Res.* 333:374–77
174. Andrejauskas, E., Hertel, R., Marmé, D. 1985. Specific binding of the calcium antagonist [³H]verapamil to membrane fractions from plants. *J. Biol. Chem.* 260:5411–14

175. Hetherington, A. M., Trewavas, A.-J. 1984. Binding of nitrendipine, a calcium channel blocker, to pea shoot membranes. *Plant Sci. Lett.* 35:109–13
176. Simpson, W. G. 1985. The calcium channel blocker verapamil and cancer chemotherapy. *Cell Calcium* 6:449–67
177. Poole-Wilson, P. A., Harding, D. P., Bourdillan, P. D. V., Tones, M. A. 1984. Calcium out of control. *J. Mol. Cell. Cardiol.* 16:175–87
178. Dubinsky, B., Sierchio, J. N., Temple, D. E., Ritchie, D. M. 1984. Flunarazine and verapamil: effecs on central nervous system and peripheral consequences of cytotoxic hypoxia in rats. *Life Sci.* 34:1298–306
179. Landon, E. J., Naukam, R. J., Rama Sastry, B. V. 1986. Effects of calcium channel blocking agents on calcium and centrilobular necrosis in the liver of rats treated with hepatotoxic agents. *Biochem. Pharmacol.* 35:697–705
180. Nilsson, J., Sjölund, M., Palmberg, L., Von Euler, A. M., Jonzon, B., Thyberg, J. 1985. The calcium antagonist nifedipine inhibits arterial smooth muscle cell proliferation. *Atherosclerosis* 58:109–22
181. Henry, P. D. 1985. Atherosclerosis, calcium and calcium antagonists. *Circulation* 72:456–59
182. Habib, J. B., Bossalar, C., Wells, S., Williams, C., Morrisett, J. D., Henry, P. D. 1986. Preservation of endothelium-dependent vascular relaxation in cholesterol-fed rabbit by treatment with the calcium blocker PN 200 110. *Circ. Res.* 58:305–9

Ann. Rev. Pharmacol. Toxicol. 1987. 27:371–84

BIOCHEMICAL AND MOLECULAR GENETIC ANALYSIS OF HORMONE-SENSITIVE ADENYLYL CYCLASE

Gerald F. Casperson and Henry R. Bourne

Departments of Pharmacology and Medicine and the Cardiovascular Research Institute, University of California, San Francisco, California 94143-0450

INTRODUCTION AND SCOPE

The hormone-sensitive adenylyl cyclase of vertebrate cells detects external hormonal signals and transduces them across the plasma membrane into changes in the rate of cAMP synthesis. Each of these events—detection, transduction, and cAMP synthesis—involves a distinct class of membrane proteins. Receptors, integral membrane proteins with specific binding sites for endogenous ligands and drugs, detect the signal. Depending upon the type of receptor, the ligand–receptor interaction results in inhibition or stimulation of cAMP synthesis by the catalytic adenylyl cyclase (C)[1], an integral membrane protein whose enzymatic site faces the cytoplasm. A family of GTP-binding regulatory (G) proteins conveys information between the liganded receptor and the catalyst.

The G-proteins comprise the central element of this signal transduction system. These proteins interact with the receptor–ligand complex, bind GTP, and become activated. They then interact with the catalyst to alter the rate of cAMP synthesis; finally, they terminate their effect on adenylyl cyclase and return to the basal state by hydrolyzing GTP to GDP. Our understanding of

---

[1]Abbreviations: β-AR, β-adrenergic receptor; GTPγS, Guanosine-5'-O-(3-thiodiphosphate); Gpp[NH]p, guanylyl imidodiphosphate; G_s, G_i, G_o, holo-G-proteins consisting of α, β, and γ subunits; α_s, α_i, α_o, alpha subunits of the respective G-proteins; $\beta\gamma$, beta and gamma subunits of the G-proteins; R*, photoexcited rhodopsin; PDE, cGMP phosphodiesterase; SDS, sodium dodecyl sulfate.

0362-1642/87/0415-0371$02.00

the functioning of this complex system derives from biochemistry, genetics, and, more recently, from molecular biology. We discuss the biochemistry of the G-proteins in light of information gained from study of the nucleic acid sequences that encode their components. We discuss only briefly earlier work, such as the discovery of GTP effects on adenylyl cyclase and of the G-proteins themselves. The pharmacology and regulation of the receptors themselves similarly fall outside the scope of this review.

THE G-PROTEINS

Both stimulation and inhibition of adenylyl cyclase by hormones require GTP. Indeed, hydrolysis-resistant analogs of GTP (GTPγS and Gpp[NH]p) in many cases exert these effects without hormone. The sites of action of guanine nucleotides (and of aluminofluoride ion, which mimics the effects of GTP analogs) are G_i and G_s. These proteins couple inhibitory and stimulatory receptors, respectively, to the catalytic adenylyl cyclase. The function of a third G-protein, G_o, discussed below, is not known.

Recent purification of G_s, G_i, and G_o (1–4) and subsequent study of the purified proteins (for review see 5) showed that each is an $\alpha\beta\gamma$ heterotrimer. The α subunits contain a single GTP binding site, GTPase activity, and sites for modification by either of two bacterial exotoxins: cholera toxin for the α subunit of G_s (α_s) and pertussis toxin for α_i and α_o. The α subunits differ among the various G-proteins, whereas β (35 or 36 kd) and γ (6–10 kd) appear the same.

Figure 1 shows a generalized scheme for the G-protein regulatory cycle, first proposed by Cassel & Selinger (6, 7) and later elaborated by Gilman and coworkers (5, 8). The hormone-receptor complex promotes GTP binding and activation of the G-proteins. Activated α-GTP dissociates from $\beta\gamma$, and the dissociated form of the G-protein affects the catalyst. Hydrolysis of GTP to GDP by α, and reassociation of α with $\beta\gamma$, deactivates the G-protein and returns the system to the basal state.

G_s, The Stimulatory Guanine Nucleotide–Binding Regulatory Protein

Somatic-cell genetics laid the groundwork for the discovery and subsequent purification of G_s. Bourne and coworkers (9) isolated cyc^-, a hormone-resistant mutant of the S49 mouse lymphoma cell line. Cyc$^-$ membranes lack G_s activity (10) and the 52- and 45-kd cholera toxin substrates (11). Gilman and coworkers subsequently exploited this system by utilizing cyc^- membranes as a bioassay to purify G_s (see 8). G_s, purified from rabbit liver, contains either the 52-kd or the 45-kd cholera toxin substrate as its α subunit, associated in 1:1:1 stoichiometry with β and γ (3, 12). The 52-kd α_s is not

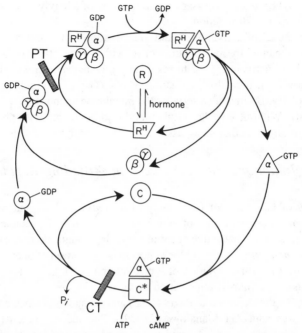

Figure 1   The G-protein regulatory cycle. Abbreviations: R, unliganded receptor; R^H, liganded receptor; C, inactive catalyst; C*, activated catalyst; α, β, γ, G-protein subunits. Stippled bars indicate the points at which cholera toxin (CT) and pertussis toxin (PT) block the cycle by ADP-ribosylation of α.

found in all tissues (3, 13, 14); we discuss its relationship to the 45-kd α_s in a later section.

G$_s$ binds hydrolysis-resistant GTP analogs in a magnesium-dependent manner (3). Binding of GTP analogs, in vitro, results in activation of G$_s$, as assessed by its ability to stimulate cAMP synthesis in *cyc$^-$* membranes. Activation of G$_s$ closely parallels GTP analog binding. Both require guanine nucleotide, Mg^{2+}, and have a similar time course (15, 16). Ligands that do not activate purified G$_s$ (GTP, GDP, GMP, and ITP) compete for GTPγS binding and activation with similar affinities (16). Thus, binding of GTP analogs and activation of G$_s$ occur more or less simultaneously. Several other events occur concomitantly with GTP binding and activation. G$_s$ releases bound GDP (7, 17), and α_s dissociates from $\beta\gamma$ (3, 12, 18) and undergoes conformational change (19). The precise mechanism and timing of these events are not yet known.

Whatever the mechanism of G$_s$ activation, stimulation of the catalyst requires only α_s. Activated α_s, separated from $\beta\gamma$, stimulates cAMP production in *cyc$^-$* membranes (13) and stimulates purified C in phospholipid vesicles (20). $\beta\gamma$ is not necessary for stimulation of adenylyl cyclase; indeed, it antagonizes the stimulation (21).

Upon removal of activating ligand, deactivation of G_s occurs very slowly and is accompanied by reassociation of α_s with $\beta\gamma$ (13, 16, 21). Addition of purified $\beta\gamma$ to activated G_s or to resolved, activated α_s increases the rate of deactivation (21); indeed, deactivation of α_s-GTPγS absolutely requires the presence of $\beta\gamma$. $\beta\gamma$ may also serve as the membrane anchor for α_s (and α_i and α_o as well). Without $\beta\gamma$, the α subunits do not associate with phospholipid vesicles; $\beta\gamma$, on the other hand, associates readily with vesicles in the absence of α (22).

G_i, The Inhibitory Guanine Nucleotide–Binding Regulatory Protein

Discovery of G_i came not from study of adenylyl cyclase, but rather from research into the mechanism of action of a bacterial toxin secreted by *Bordetella pertussis,* the causative agent in whooping cough. Pertussis toxin (also called *islet-activating protein*) blocks hormonal inhibition of adenylyl cyclase by catalyzing ADP-ribosylation of the α subunit of G_i (23, 24). This toxin-labeling assay facilitated purification of G_i (25, 26).

Like G_s, G_i dissociates into its α (41-kd) and $\beta\gamma$ subunits when activated by hydrolysis-resistant GTP analogs (27–29). Purified G_i reconstitutes α_2-adrenergic inhibition of adenylyl cyclase in platelet membranes whose endogenous G_i has been inactivated by pertussis toxin (27). Experiments in which purified α and $\beta\gamma$ subunits of G_i were added to platelet membranes suggested that G_i inhibited adenylyl cyclase by releasing $\beta\gamma$, which then deactivated α_s (27, 29). This model fails to account for the findings that α_i inhibits adenylyl cyclase when added to *cyc⁻* membranes (28) and that somatostatin inhibits adenylyl cyclase in *cyc⁻* membranes via G_i (28) even though *cyc⁻* lacks detectable α_s or indeed any α_s mRNA (30). Further study indicates that $\beta\gamma$ may directly inhibit the purified catalyst and that α_i competes with α_s for binding to C (T. Katada, personal communication). Thus G_i may inhibit adenylyl cyclase through both its α and $\beta\gamma$ subunits.

G_o, The "Other" G-Protein

G_o was also discovered and purified because pertussis toxin ADP-ribosylates its α subunit (39 kd) (4, 31). Like G_s and G_i, G_o dissociates into α and $\beta\gamma$ subunits on binding of GTP analogs. G_o couples in vitro to muscarinic receptors (32), but thus far has no demonstrated role in hormonal control of adenylyl cyclase.

THE β-ADRENERGIC RECEPTOR AND THE CATALYST

The β-adrenergic receptor (β-AR) and C have now been purified and reconstituted with G-proteins into phospholipid vesicles. β-ARs are single, glycosylated polypeptides with protein molecular weights of about 49,000 (33). The catalyst is a single polypeptide with a molecular weight of 120,000 (34).

β-ARs in intact membranes show biphasic agonist binding curves, which indicate two classes of binding sites with differing affinities. Activation of G_s with GTP analogs converts nearly all receptors to the low-affinity form. Two purified proteins, G_s and β-AR, are sufficient to reconstitute this effect in phospholipid vesicles. Receptors reconstituted alone into phospholipid vesicles exhibit low affinity for agonist. β-ARs reconstituted with G_s show biphasic agonist binding curves characteristic of intact membranes; activation of G_s with GTP analogs restores the receptors to their low-affinity form (35, 36).

This shift in receptor affinity results from dissociation of the β-AR:G_s complex. In the absence of guanine nucleotide, agonist-bound (high-affinity) β-AR and G_s exist as a stable complex. Activation of G_s by guanine nucleotide causes dissociation of the complex and a decrease in receptor affinity for agonist (37).

GTP analogs activate purified G_s slowly (3). In phospholipid vesicles containing β-AR and G_s, agonist occupancy of the receptor greatly increases the rate of GTP analog binding and of activation of G_s (38–40), and stimulates GTP hydrolysis (35, 36, 40–42). The presence or absence of the catalyst has little effect on G_s activation or stimulation of GTPase activity by liganded receptors (42). Addition of C to vesicles containing β-AR and G_s forms a complete system for positive regulation of cAMP synthesis. In the reconstituted system, β-adrenergic agonists stimulate cAMP synthesis in a GTP-dependent fashion (20).

Thus three proteins, β-AR, C, and G_s, form a functional adenylyl cyclase system. When reconstituted into phospholipid vesicles, these proteins display all the properties of the β-adrenergic hormone-sensitive adenylyl cyclase in intact membranes. They demonstrate hormonal stimulation of GTPase activity and cAMP synthesis, hormone- and GTP-dependent G-protein activation, and the effects of GTP analogs on affinity of the β-AR for ligands. The relatively modest hormonal stimulation of cAMP synthesis in the reconstituted system, however, may indicate that optimal performance of the system requires other proteins (20).

THE G-PROTEINS: FUNCTION VERSUS STRUCTURE

Any discussion of the G-proteins must include transducin, the protein that couples photoexcited rhodopsin (R*) to stimulation of a cGMP-phosphodiesterase (PDE) in vertebrate rod outer segments. Like G_s, G_i, and G_o, transducin is an $\alpha\beta\gamma$ heterotrimer. The α and γ subunits of transducin have molecular weights of 39,000 and 8,000, respectively; the β-chain behaves as a single 36-kd polypeptide on SDS-polyacrylamide gels (43, 44). Like hormones and β-AR, light and rhodopsin stimulate GTP binding and activation of transducin. The α subunit of transducin (α_t) dissociates from $\beta\gamma_t$ when activated by guanine nucleotide and, like α_s, stimulates its target enzyme, PDE (see 45 for review).

The G-proteins share more than their GTP regulatory cycle. Cholera toxin ADP-ribosylates the α subunits of transducin (46, 47) and of G_s (11, 48). In each case, the preferred toxin substrate is the activated, GTP form of the G-protein; light and GTP analogs enhance modification of transducin, just as hormone and GTP analogs increase labeling of G_s. Modification of both proteins by cholera toxin inhibits GTPase activity and results in persistent activation. Pertussis toxin catalyzes ADP-ribosylation of the α subunits of transducin (49, 50), G_i (23, 24, 26), and G_o (2, 4). In contrast to cholera toxin, pertussis toxin preferentially modifies the deactivated form of these proteins. Light or hormone and GTP analogs inhibit the toxin-catalyzed modification. Pertussis toxin–modified G-proteins remain persistently deactivated because they cannot interact with activated receptor (see Figure 1).

Several observations indicate that the α subunits of transducin, G_i, and G_o comprise a structurally related subgroup. Transducin and G_i interact much more effectively with R* than does G_s, whereas the reverse is true of the β-AR (40, 51). Antibodies against α_t cross-react with α_i and α_o but not with α_s (52). Similarly, antibodies to α_o cross-react with α_i but not α_s (31).

The 36-kd β subunits of all four G-proteins are very similar and may be identical. These β-chains are immunologically indistinguishable (31, 52, 53) and have similar peptide maps (54). The 35-kd β subunits differ immunologically from the 36-kd proteins (52). Transducin contains only the 36-kd β-chain.

PRIMARY STRUCTURE OF THE G-PROTEINS AND THE β-ADRENERGIC RECEPTOR

With the isolation and sequencing of cDNAs (55–61), the primary structures of the G-proteins can now be directly compared. Figure 2 shows pairwise comparisons of amino acid homologies among the G-proteins. The degree of homology between transducin, G_i, and G_o (about 65% allowing for conservative substitutions) confirms the conclusion, based on immunological and functional evidence, that these proteins form a closely related subgroup. G_s, the most divergent of the G proteins, shares about 45% homology with each of the others and contains extra sequences.

Examination of cDNAs encoding the 45- and 52-kd α_s chains resolves the question of their origin (58; A. G. Gilman, personal communication). The two cDNAs are identical except for one stretch of bases within the coding region; this stretch in the 52-kd α_s cDNA encodes 15 amino acids not encoded by the cDNA that specifies the 45-kd polypeptide. The mRNAs that correspond to these two cDNAs are probably derived by alternative splicing of exons from a single α_s gene.

Two other families of GTP-binding proteins, the bacterial elongation factors and the ras proteins, contain four regions of homology implicated in GTP binding and hydrolysis (62). The G-proteins contain sequences homologous to these regions (Figure 2), indicating a common origin for the three groups of proteins. Especially striking is the finding that the predicted secondary structures of these regions in the G-protein α chains closely resemble the solved crystal structure (63) of elongation factor-Tu (EF-Tu; S. Masters, R. Stroud & H. Bourne, unpublished).

The function of other portions of the G-proteins can also be predicted. Part

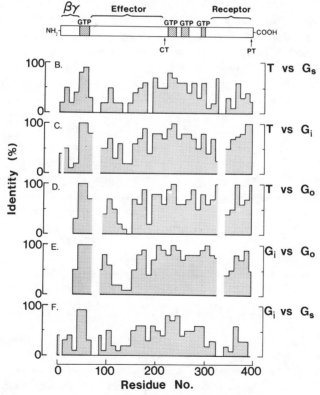

Figure 2 Comparison of amino acid sequences of the G-protein α subunits. The percentage of identical amino acid residues, averaged over blocks of 10 residues, is plotted versus position for pairs of α chains. The X-axis coordinates refer to residue numbers in α_s. Because α_s is longer than the other G-protein α chains, the plots have gaps. Regions implicated in GTP binding (62) and in interactions with $\beta\gamma$, effectors, and detectors are indicated in the diagram at the top.

of the area between the first and second GTP-binding regions (α_s residues 61–132) is poorly conserved among the G-proteins and may contain the effector binding domain. The highly conserved area preceding the second GTP contact site (α_s residues 133–204) is a good candidate for interaction with $\beta\gamma$. The analogous region of EF-Tu participates in aminoacyl tRNA binding (63). Just as GTP regulates the affinity of EF-Tu for aminoacyl tRNA (64), this region of the G-proteins may participate in GTP-dependent interaction with both the effector and $\beta\gamma$. The amino terminus of α_t is clearly required for interaction with $\beta\gamma$ because no interaction occurs when the N-terminal 18 amino acids are proteolytically removed (65). Poor conservation of amino acid sequence among the G-proteins in this region suggests, however, that it may not contain the actual $\beta\gamma$ contact site (Figure 2).

The 25 carboxy-terminal amino acid residues of the α chains may participate in receptor binding. The degree of homology in this region between pairs of G-proteins (Figure 2) correlates very well with their preference for interaction with R* or β-AR. Both α_t and α_i interact well with R* and are highly homologous in this region, whereas α_s interacts poorly with R* and is quite divergent. Pertussis toxin–catalyzed modification of a cysteine near the C-terminus blocks functional interaction of α_t with R* (49). Furthermore, this region of transducin is highly homologous to that of an internal sequence of another retinal protein, arrestin (66), which competes with transducin for binding to R*.

Recently, Dixon et al (67) isolated the gene and cDNA encoding the hampster β-AR. The predicted amino acid sequence of the hampster β-AR shows striking similarities to that of the rhodopsins. Like the rhodopsins, the β-AR contains 7 hydrophobic amino acid sequences of 20–25 residues. These regions are thought to span the membrane. Similarities in amino acid sequence in these regions between the β-AR and opsin suggests a common mode of action (67). Thus, similarities between GTP-dependent signal-transduction systems extend beyond the G-proteins themselves to receptors for such disparate signals as photons and catecholamines.

THE YEAST ADENYLYL CYCLASE SYSTEM

The adenylyl cyclase system of the yeast *Saccharomyces cerevisiae* deserves brief mention because of its similarity to vertebrate adenylyl cyclase and because of the enormous potential for genetic exploitation of the yeast system.

Matsumoto and his coworkers isolated yeast mutants with alterations in cAMP metabolism (see 68 for review). Their approach illustrates the power of the yeast system. Because wild-type yeast take up cAMP poorly, these investigators began by isolating mutants from an adenine-requiring strain that could use exogenous cAMP as an adenine source. From these mutants (designated *cam*), Matsumoto et al then isolated cells with mutations causing them to require cAMP for growth. Mutations in three genes resulted (69). One of these, *CYR1*, encodes the catalytic adenylyl cyclase (70, 71).

Biochemically, yeast adenylyl cyclase strikingly resembles that of vertebrate cells. Initial biochemical characterization of the yeast system showed that at the minimum it contains distinct stimulatory guanine nucleotide–binding regulatory and catalytic proteins (72). The genes encoding the yeast catalyst and regulatory proteins have now been isolated: the catalyst *(CYR1)* by complementation of *cyr1⁻* mutants (70, 73, 74) and the regulatory proteins *(RAS1* and *RAS2)* by virtue of their homology to the viral *Ha-ras* oncogene (75, 76). *CYR1* encodes a potential polypeptide of 2026 amino acid residues with a molecular weight of 225,000. The catalytic activity resides in a C-terminal domain of about 60 kd (74).

RAS1 and *RAS2* encode proteins of 308 and 322 amino acids, respectively. The amino acid sequences of the amino-terminal half of the yeast RAS proteins exhibit considerable homology (80% over the N-terminal 80 residues and 60% over the next 80) to the mammalian ras proteins (76), including the four GTP-binding regions (62). Interestingly, the yeast RAS proteins show no more homology to vertebrate G-proteins than do the mammalian ras proteins. Also, $p21^{ras}$ substitutes for yeast RAS proteins in supporting GTP-dependent cAMP synthesis (77), but clearly does not regulate adenylyl cyclase in vertebrates (see 78).

The yeast adenylyl cyclase system thus resembles two different signal-transduction systems in higher organisms: the hormone-sensitive adenylyl cyclase system and the $p21^{ras}$ system, whose effector and detector elements have not yet been identified.

FURTHER GENETIC STUDY OF HORMONE-SENSITIVE ADENYLYL CYCLASE

Biochemical studies reviewed here describe an overall scheme for hormonal control of adenylyl cyclase. Isolation of the genes encoding components of the system allows investigators to address more specific questions concerning the molecular mechanisms of signal transduction. In vitro mutagenesis of these genes will provide information on the structure and function of the proteins and provide answers to such questions as: How does the liganded receptor facilitate activation of the G-proteins? What is the nature of the activation event? How does the activated G-protein effect a change in the rate of cAMP synthesis?

The yeast system will be particularly useful for such studies. Techniques available in yeast allow replacement of a gene in the chromosome with a modified version produced by selective in vitro mutagenesis. The function of the mutant protein may then be studied in vivo and in native membranes. For example, substitution of valine for glycine at position 19 in *RAS2* results in constitutive activation of adenylyl cyclase (77). Substitution of valine for glycine at the analogous position in the mammalian ras gene products activates their oncogenic potential (79). The question of additional, undiscovered components of the adenylyl cyclase system may also be addressed in yeast. Our knowledge of the physiological role of cAMP in this organism should allow isolation of mutations in any component of the system.

G-proteins function as signal transducers in systems other than adenylyl cyclase (see 80 for review). How many G-proteins are there? Which of these regulate newly discovered effectors such as phospholipase C and potassium channels? Which are involved in tyrosine kinase–mediated processes? What, if any, is the role of developmental regulation of G-protein expression? With the tools at hand we may now address such questions.

A final set of questions concerns the evolutionary origin of signal transduction. The remarkable conservation of structure and function in receptors such as rhodopsin and the β-AR, and in the GTP-binding proteins, including bacterial elongation factors, transducin, and the yeast and vertebrate G-proteins, through eons of evolutionary time demonstrates their utility as signal detectors and transducers. Understanding the evolution of these systems will provide us with a more precise knowledge of their design and function.

ACKNOWLEDGMENTS

Work from the authors' laboratory was funded by grants from the National Institutes of Health. G. F. Casperson is the recipient of a fellowship from the Bank of America–Giannini Foundation.

Literature Cited

1. Codina, J., Hildebrandt, J. D., Sekura, R. D., Birnbaumer, M., Bryan, J., et al. 1984. N_s and N_i, the stimulatory and inhibitory regulatory components of adenylate cyclases: Purification of the human erythrocyte proteins without the use of activating regulatory ligands. *J. Biol. Chem.* 259:5871–86
2. Neer, E. J., Lok, J. M., Wolf, L. G. 1984. Purification and properties of the inhibitory guanine nucleotide regulatory unit of brain adenylate cyclase. *J. Biol. Chem.* 259:14222–29
3. Sternweis, P. C., Northup, J. K., Smigel, M. D., Gilman, A. G. 1981. The regulatory component of adenylate cyclase: Purification and properties. *J. Biol. Chem.* 256:11517–26
4. Sternweis, P. C., Robishaw, J. D. 1984. Isolation of two proteins with high affinity for guanine nucleotides from membranes of bovine brain. *J. Biol. Chem.* 259:13806–13
5. Smigel, M. D., Ross, E. M., Gilman, A. G. 1984. Role of the β-adrenergic receptor in the regulation of adenylate cyclase. In *Cell Membranes, Methods, and Reviews*, ed. W. Frazier, E. Elson, L. Glaser, pp. 247–95. New York: Plenum
6. Cassel, D., Selinger, Z. 1977. Mechanism of adenylate cyclase activation by cholera toxin: Inhibition of GTP hydrolysis at the regulatory site. *Proc. Natl. Acad. Sci. USA* 74:3307–11
7. Cassel, D., Selinger, Z. 1978. Mechanism of adenylate cyclase activation through the β-adrenergic receptor: Catecholamine-induced displacement of

bound GDP by GTP. *Proc. Natl. Acad. Sci. USA* 75:4155–59

8. Ross, E. M., Gilman, A. G. 1980. Biochemical properties of hormone-sensitive adenylate cyclase. *Ann. Rev. Biochem.* 49:533–64

9. Bourne, H. R., Coffino, P., Tomkins, G. M. 1975. Selection of a variant lymphoma cell deficient in adenylate cyclase. *Science* 187:750–52

10. Ross, E. M., Gilman, A. G. 1977. Resolution of some components of adenylate cyclase necessary for catalytic activity. *J. Biol. Chem.* 252:6966–69

11. Johnson, G. L., Kaslow, H. R., Bourne, H. R. 1978. Genetic evidence that cholera toxin substrates are regulatory components of adenylate cyclase. *J. Biol. Chem.* 253:7120–23

12. Hildebrandt, J. D., Codina, J., Risinger, R., Birnbaumer, L. 1984. Identification of a γ subunit associated with the adenylate cyclase regulatory proteins N_s and N_i. *J. Biol. Chem.* 259:2039–42

13. Northup, J. K., Smigel, M. D., Sternweis, P. C., Gilman, A. G. 1983. The subunits of the stimulatory regulatory component of adenylate cyclase: Resolution of the activated 45,000-dalton (α) subunit. *J. Biol. Chem.* 258:11369–76

14. Northup, J. K., Sternweis, P. C., Smigel, M. D., Schleifer, L. S., Ross, E. M., Gilman, A. G. 1980. Purification of the regulatory component of adenylate cyclase. *Proc. Natl. Acad. Sci. USA* 77:6516–20

15. Hanski, E., Gilman, A. 1982. The guanine nucleotide-binding regulatory component of adenylate cyclase in human erythrocytes. *J. Cyclic Nucleotide Res.* 8:323–36

16. Northup, J. K., Smigel, M. D., Gilman, A. G. 1982. The guanine nucleotide activating site of the regulatory component of adenylate cyclase: Identification by ligand binding. *J. Biol. Chem.* 257:11416–23

17. Murayama, T., Ui, M. 1984. [³H]GDP release from rat and hamster adipocyte membranes independently linked to receptors involved in activation or inhibition of adenylate cyclase. Differential susceptibility to two bacterial toxins. *J. Biol. Chem.* 259:761–69

18. Hanski, E., Sternweis, P. C., Northup, J. K., Dromerick, A. W., Gilman, A. G. 1981. The regulatory component of adenylate cyclase: Purification and properties of the turkey erythrocyte protein. *J. Biol. Chem.* 256:12911–19

19. Hudson, T. H., Roeber, J. F., Johnson, G. L. 1981. Conformational changes of

20. May, D. C., Ross, E. M., Gilman, A. G., Smigel, M. D. 1985. Reconstitution of catecholamine-stimulated adenylate cyclase activity using three purified proteins. *J. Biol. Chem.* 260:15829–33

21. Northup, J. K., Sternweis, P. C., Gilman, A. G. 1983. The subunits of the stimulatory regulatory component of adenylate cyclase. Resolution, activity, and properties of the 35,000-dalton (β) subunit. *J. Biol. Chem.* 258:11361–68

22. Sternweis, P. C. 1986. The purified α subunits of G_o and G_i from bovine brain require βγ for association with phospholipid vesicles. *J. Biol. Chem.* 261:631–37

23. Bokoch, G. M., Katada, T., Northup, J. K., Hewlett, E. L., Gilman, A. G. 1983. Identification of the predominant substrate for ADP-ribosylation by islet-activating protein. *J. Biol. Chem.* 258:2072–75

24. Katada, T., Ui, M. 1982. ADP ribosylation of the specific membrane protein of C6 cells by islet-activating protein associated with modification of adenylate cyclase activity. *J. Biol. Chem.* 257:7210–16

25. Bokoch, G. M., Katada, T., Northup, J. K., Ui, M., Gilman, A. G. 1984. Purification and properties of the inhibitory guanine nucleotide-binding regulatory component of adenylate cyclase. *J. Biol. Chem.* 259:3560–67

26. Codina, J., Hildebrandt, J., Iyengar, R., Birnbaumer, L., Sekura, R. D., Manclark, C. R. 1983. Pertussis toxin substrate, the putative N_i component of adenylate cyclases, is an αβ heterodimer regulated by guanine nucleotide and magnesium. *Proc. Nat. Acad. Sci. USA* 80:4276–80

27. Katada, T., Bokoch, G. M., Northup, J. K., Ui, M., Gilman, A. G. 1984. The inhibitory guanine nucleotide-binding regulatory component of adenylate cyclase: Properties and function of the purified protein. *J. Biol. Chem.* 259:3568–77

28. Katada, T., Bokoch, G. M., Smigel, M. D., Ui, M., Gilman, A. G. 1984. The inhibitory guanine nucleotide-binding regulatory component of adenylate cyclase: Subunit dissociation and the inhibition of adenylate cyclase in S49 lymphoma cyc^- and wild type membranes. *J. Biol. Chem.* 259:3586–95

29. Katada, T., Northup, J. K., Bokoch, G. M., Ui, M., Gilman, A. G. 1984. The

inhibitory guanine nucleotide–binding regulatory component of adenylate cyclase: Subunit dissociation and guanine nucleotide-dependent hormonal inhibition. *J. Biol. Chem.* 259:3578–85

30. Harris, B. A., Robishaw, J. D., Mumby, S. M., Gilman, A. G. 1985. Molecular cloning of complementary DNA for the alpha subunit of the G protein that stimulates adenylate cyclase. *Science* 229:1274–77

31. Huff, R. M., Axton, J. M., Neer, E. J. 1985. Physical and immunological characterization of a guanine nucleotide–binding protein purified from bovine cerebral cortex. *J. Biol. Chem.* 260:10864–71

32. Florio, V. A., Sternweis, P. C. 1985. Reconstitution of resolved muscarinic cholinergic receptors with purified GTP-binding proteins. *J. Biol. Chem.* 260:3477–83

33. Stiles, G. L., Benovic, J. L., Caron, M. G., Lefkowitz, R. J. 1984. Mammalian β-adrenergic receptors: Distinct glycoprotein populations containing high mannose or complex type carbohydrate chains. *J. Biol. Chem.* 259:8655–63

34. Smigel, M. D. 1986. Purification of the catalyst of adenylate cyclase. *J. Biol. Chem.* 261:1976–82

35. Asano, T., Katada, T., Gilman, A. G., Ross, E. M. 1984. Activation of the inhibitory GTP-binding protein of adenylate cyclase, G_i, by β-adrenergic receptors in reconstituted phospholipid vesicles. *J. Biol. Chem.* 259:9351–54

36. Cerione, R. A., Codina, J., Benovic, J. L., Lefkowitz, R. J., Birnbaumer, L., Caron, M. G. 1984. The mammalian $β_2$-adrenergic receptor: Reconstitution of functional interactions between pure receptor and pure stimulatory nucleotide binding protein of the adenylate cyclase system. *Biochemistry* 23:4519–25

37. Stadel, J. M., Shorr, R. G. L., Limbird, L. E., Lefkowitz, R. J. 1981. Evidence that a β-adrenergic receptor–associated guanine nucleotide regulatory protein conveys guanosine 5'-O-(3-thiotriphosphate)-dependent adenylate cyclase activity. *J. Biol. Chem.* 256:8718–23

38. Asano, T., Pedersen, S. E., Scott, C. W., Ross, E. M. 1984. Reconstitution of catecholamine-stimulated binding of guanosine 5'-O-(3-thiotriphosphate) to the stimulatory GTP-binding protein of adenylate cyclase. *Biochemistry* 23:5460–67

39. Asano, T., Ross, E. M. 1984. Catecholamine-stimulated guanosine 5'-O-(3-

thiotriphosphate) binding to the stimulatory GTP-binding protein of adenylate cyclase: Kinetic analysis in reconstituted phospholipid vesicles. *Biochemistry* 23:5467–71

40. Cerione, R. A., Staniszewski, C., Benovic, J. L., Lefkowitz, R. J., Caron, M. G., et al. 1985. Specificity of the functional interactions of the β-adrenergic receptor and rhodopsin with guanine nucleotide regulatory proteins reconstituted in phospholipid vesicles. *J. Biol. Chem.* 260:1493–1500

41. Brandt, D. R., Asano, T., Pedersen, S. E., Ross, E. M. 1983. Reconstitution of catecholamine-stimulated guanosine triphosphatase activity. *Biochemistry* 22:4357–62

42. Cerione, R. A., Sibley, D. R., Codina, J., Benovic, J. L., Winslow, J., et al. 1984. Reconstitution of a hormone-sensitive adenylate cyclase system: The pure β-adrenergic receptor and guanine nucleotide regulatory protein confer hormone responsiveness on the resolved catalytic unit. *J. Biol. Chem.* 259:9979–82

43. Fung, B. K.-K., Hurley, J. B., Stryer, L. 1981. Flow of information in the light-triggered cyclic nucleotide cascade of vision. *Proc. Natl. Acad. Sci. USA* 78:152–56

44. Kuhn, H. 1980. Light- and GTP-regulated interaction of GTPase and other proteins with bovine photoreceptor membranes. *Nature* 283:587–89

45. Stryer, L. 1986. Cyclic GMP cascade of vision. *Ann. Rev. Neurosci.* 9:87–119

46. Abood, M. E., Hurley, J. B., Pappone, M.-C., Bourne, H. R., Stryer, L. 1982. Functional homology between signal-coupling proteins: Cholera toxin inactivates the GTPase activity of transducin. *J. Biol. Chem.* 257:10540–43

47. Navon, S. E., Fung, B. K.-K. 1984. Characterization of transducin from bovine retinal rod outer segments: Mechanism and effects of cholera toxin-catalyzed ADP-ribosylation. *J. Biol. Chem.* 259:6686–93

48. Cassel, D., Pfeuffer, T. 1978. Mechanism of cholera toxin action: Covalent modification of the guanyl nucleotide–binding protein of the adenylate cyclase system. *Proc. Natl. Acad. Sci. USA* 75:2669–73

49. Van Dop, C., Yamanaka, G., Steinberg, F., Sekura, R. D., Manclark, C. R., et al. 1984. ADP-ribosylation of transducin by pertussis toxin blocks the light-stimulated hydrolysis of GTP and cGMP

in retinal photoreceptors. *J. Biol. Chem.* 259:23–26

50. Watkins, P. A., Burns, D. L., Kanaho, Y., Liu, T. Y., Hewlett, E. L., Moss, J. 1985. ADP-ribosylation of transducin by pertussis toxin. *J. Biol. Chem.* 260:13478–82

51. Kanaho, Y., Tsai, S. C., Adamik, R., Hewlett, E. L., Moss, J., Vaughan, M. 1984. Rhodopsin-enhanced GTPase activity of the inhibitory GTP-binding protein of adenylate cyclase. *J. Biol. Chem.* 259:7378–81

52. Roof, D. J., Applebury, M. L., Sternweis, P. C. 1985. Relationships within the family of GTP-binding proteins isolated from bovine central nervous system. *J. Biol. Chem.* 260:16242–49

53. Gierschik, P., Codina, J., Simons, C., Birnbaumer, L., Spiegel, A. 1985. Antisera against a guanine nucleotide binding protein from retina cross-react with the β subunit of the adenylate cyclase-associated guanine nucleotide binding proteins, N_s and N_i. *Proc. Natl. Acad. Sci. USA* 82:727–31

54. Manning, D. R., Gilman, A. G. 1983. The regulatory components of adenylate cyclase and transducin: A family of structurally homologous guanine nucleotide binding proteins. *J. Biol. Chem.* 258:7059–63

55. Itoh, H., Kozasa, T., Nagata, S., Nakamura, S., Katada, T., et al. 1986. Molecular cloning and sequence determination of cDNAs coding for α subunits of G_s, G_i, and G_o proteins from rat brain. *Proc. Natl. Acad. Sci. USA* 83:3776–80

56. Lochrie, M. A., Hurley, J. B., Simon, M. I. 1985. Sequence of the alpha subunit of photoreceptor G protein: Homologies between transducin, *ras,* and elongation factors. *Science* 228:96–99

57. Medynski, D. C., Sullivan, K., Smith, D., Van Dop, C., Chang, F.-H., et al. 1985. Amino acid sequence of the α subunit of transducin deduced from the cDNA sequence. *Proc. Natl. Acad. Sci. USA* 82:4311–15

58. Robishaw, J. D., Russell, D. W., Harris, B. A., Smigel, M. D., Gilman, A. G. 1986. Deduced primary structure of the α subunit of the GTP-binding stimulatory protein of adenylate cyclase. *Proc. Natl. Acad. Sci. USA* 83:1251–55

59. Sullivan, K. A., Liao, Y.-C., Alborzi, A., Beiderman, B., Chang, F.-H., et al. 1986. The inhibitory and stimulatory G proteins of adenylate cyclase: cDNA and

amino acid sequences of the α chains. *Proc. Natl. Acad. Sci. USA* 83:6687–91

60. Tanabe, T., Nukada, T., Nishikawa, Y., Sugimoto, K., Suzuki, H., et al. 1985. Primary structure of the α subunit of transducin and its relationship to *ras* proteins. *Nature* 315:242–45

61. Yatsunami, K., Khorana, G. 1985. GTPase of bovine rod outer segments: The amino acid sequence of the α subunit as derived from the cDNA sequence. *Proc. Natl. Acad. Sci. USA* 82:4316–20

62. Halliday, K. 1984. Regional homology in GTP-binding proto-oncogene products and elongation factors. *J. Cyclic Nucleotide Res.* 9:435–48

63. Jurnak, F. 1985. Structure of the GDP domain of EF-Tu and location of the amino acids homologous to *ras* oncogene proteins. *Science* 230:32–36

64. Kaziro, Y. 1978. The role of guanosine 5'-triphosphate in polypeptide chain elongation. *Biochim. Biophys. Acta* 505:95–127

65. Fung, B. K.-K. 1983. Characterization of transducin from bovine retinal rod outer segments. I. Separation and reconstitution of the subunits. *J. Biol. Chem.* 258:10495–502

66. Wistow, G. J., Katial, A., Craft, C., Shinohara, T. 1986. Sequence analysis of bovine retinal S-antigen. Relationships with α transducin and G proteins. *FEBS Lett.* 196:23–28

67. Dixon, R. A. F., Kobilka, B. K., Strader, D. J., Benovic, J. L., Dohlman, H. G., et al. 1986. Cloning of the gene and cDNA for mammalian β-adrenergic receptor and homology with rhodopsin. *Nature* 321:75–79

68. Matsumoto, K., Uno, I., Ishikawa, T. 1985. Genetic analysis of the role of cAMP in yeast. *Yeast* 1:15–24

69. Matsumoto, K., Uno, I., Oshima, Y., Ishikawa, T. 1982. Isolation and characterization of yeast mutants deficient in adenylate cyclase and cAMP-dependent protein kinase. *Proc. Natl. Acad. Sci. USA* 79:2355–59

70. Casperson, G. F., Walker, N., Bourne, H. R. 1985. Isolation of the gene encoding adenylate cyclase in *Saccharomyces cerevisiae*. *Proc. Natl. Acad. Sci. USA* 82:5060–63

71. Matsumoto, K., Uno, I., Ishikawa, T. 1984. Identification of the structural gene and nonsense alleles for adenylate cyclase in *Saccharomyces cerevisiae*. *J. Bacteriol.* 157:277–82

72. Casperson, G. F., Walker, N., Brasier, A. R., Bourne, H. R. 1983. A guanine

nucleotide–sensitive adenylate cyclase in the yeast *Saccharomyces cerevisiae*. *J. Biol. Chem.* 258:7911–14

73. Masson, P., Jacquemin, J. M., Culot, M. 1984. Molecular cloning of the *tsm0185* gene responsible for adenylate cyclase activity in *Saccharomyces cerevisiae*. *Ann. Microbiol.* 135A:343–51

74. Kataoka, T., Broek, D., Wigler, M. 1985. DNA sequence and characterization of the *S. cerevisiae* gene encoding adenylate cyclase. *Cell* 43:493–505

75. DeFeo-Jones, D., Scolnick, E. M., Koller, R., Dhar, R. 1983. *ras*-Related gene sequences identified and isolated from *Saccharomyces cerevisiae*. *Nature* 306:707–9

76. Powers, S., Kataoka, T., Fasano, O., Goldfarb, M., Strathern, J., et al. 1984. Genes in *S. cerevisiae* encoding proteins with domains homologous to the mammalian *ras* proteins. *Cell* 36:607–12

77. Broek, D., Samiy, N., Fasano, O., Fujiyama, A., Tamanoi, F., et al. 1985. Differential activation of yeast adenylate cyclase by wild-type and mutant *RAS* proteins. *Cell* 41:763–69

78. Bourne, H. R. 1985. Transducing proteins. Yeast *RAS* and Tweedledee's logic. *Nature* 317:16–17

79. McGrath, J. P., Capon, D. J., Goeddel, D. V., Levinson, A. D. 1984. Comparative biochemical properties of normal and activated human *ras* p21 protein. *Nature* 310:644–49

80. Stryer, L., Bourne, H. R. 1986. G-proteins: A family of signal transducers. *Ann. Rev. Cell Biol.* 2:391–419

Ann. Rev. Pharmacol. Toxicol. 1987. 27:385–97

STATISTICAL METHODS AND APPLICATIONS OF BIOASSAY

Eugene M. Laska

Nathan S. Kline Institute for Psychiatric Research, Statistical Sciences and Epidemiology Division, Orangeburg, New York 10962

Morris J. Meisner

New York University Medical Center, Department of Psychiatry, New York, New York 10016

INTRODUCTION

A bioassay experiment is designed to estimate the relative potency of a test compound (T) to a standard compound (S). The relative potency of T to S is defined as the dose of T that produces the same biological response as does a unit dose of S (1).

Traditionally, relative potency has been estimated for a test compound that is a dilution of the standard. Currently, two different compounds that have parallel dose-response curves over some range of doses are rountinely assayed. This case is known as a comparative assay.

A bioassay experiment may be either quantal or quantitative, direct or indirect. If the response measure is binary, the assay is said to be quantal (2). Otherwise, it is quantitative. In a direct assay the threshold dose required for response is determined for each experimental unit. Thus, the observed data are dose units. In an indirect assay the experimental unit receives one or more specified doses of the preparation and the observed data may be either quantal or quantitative responses. Depending on the experimental design, several dose levels of T and S are given to the same or different experimental units. The former experiment is called a *crossover,* and the latter, a *parallel group* or *completely randomized design.*

In this chapter we discuss only indirect quantitative assays. We first review the elementary theory developed over the past forty years for the univariate

385

0362-1642/87/0415-0385$02.00

case. Next, we summarize recent work that extends the theory to the multivariate situation. This theory enables the computation of a single estimate of relative potency based on many measures of outcome. It also provides a method for pooling results across experiments. We then apply the theory to the problem of determining whether two preparations are bioequivalent and whether mixtures of compounds are synergistic, additive, or antagonistic.

UNIVARIATE BIOASSAY

The statistical analysis of a bioassay experiment requires a model that relates the average response to the dose of the preparations. If the average response is linearly related to the dose, and the line passes through the origin, the model is called a *slope-ratio assay*. However, a more commonly used model is the *parallel line assay*. In this assay response is linearly related to the log dose, and the line need not pass through the origin. The mathematical setup of the parallel line assay is as follows. Let the dose of the standard (test abbreviations in parentheses) preparation be denoted by z_S (z_T) and the log dose by $x_S = \log z_S$ ($x_T = \log z_T$). Let the response variable be denoted by Y_S for S and Y_T for T. The statistical model assumes that

$$Y_S = \alpha_S + \beta x_S + \epsilon_S \quad (Y_T = \alpha_T + \beta x_T + \epsilon_T), \qquad 1.$$

where ϵ_S (ϵ_T) is distributed normally with mean 0 and variance σ^2 for each value of x_S (x_T). In other words, $\alpha_S + \beta x_S$ is the average response due to the dose x_S of S, and $\alpha_T + \beta x_T$ is the average response due to the dose x_T of T. If T is a dilution of S, a proportion, ρz_T, of the test preparation will have an effect equal on the average to a dose, z_S of the standard preparation for every value of z_T in the range of doses for which the model holds. The relationships

$$z_S = \rho z_T$$

and

$$\alpha_S + \beta x_S = \alpha_T + \beta x_T$$

define the constant ρ, the relative potency of T to S. It follows that

$$\alpha_S + \beta \log \rho z_T = \alpha_T + \beta \log z_T$$

or

$$\log \rho = (\alpha_T - \alpha_S)/\beta. \qquad 2.$$

This expression defines the log of the relative potency in terms of the parameters α_T, α_S, and β of the *Parallel Line Model* 1. The geometric interpretation of the quantity, log ρ, is given in Figure 1.

To compute the point estimator of logρ, the point estimators, $\hat{\alpha}_S$, $\hat{\alpha}_T$, and $\hat{\beta}$ of the quantities α_S, α_T, and β are necessary. These numbers are obtained by using ordinary least squares regression and then substituting the results into *Equation 2*. These regression estimators are computed in a manner similar to the computation of slopes and intercepts in a straight-line regression problem, but in this case, because of parallelism, the slopes of the two lines are constrained to be equal.

Also, a confidence interval for logρ is useful. (A statistical procedure is said to produce a 95% confidence interval for a parameter when, if repeated many times, the true value of the parameter would be included 95% of the time. The values defining the interval depend on the observed responses in each repetition of the experiment.)

Fieller's Theorem (3, 4) provides a method used to obtain a confidence interval for a ratio of parameters when the estimators of both the numerator and the denominator are normally distributed random variables. Its application to bioassay derives from *Equation 2*, which expresses log relative potency as a ratio of the parameters $\alpha_T - \alpha_S$ to β from *Model 1*.

Let $\hat{d} = \hat{\alpha}_T - \hat{\alpha}_S$. From elementary regression theory it follows that $\hat{\delta}$ is a normal random variable with mean $\alpha_T - \alpha_S$, and $\hat{\beta}$ is a normal random variable with mean β. Then $E(\hat{\delta} - \mu\hat{\beta}) = 0$, where the notation E indicates the expected value of the random variable. In such a situation, Fieller's Theorem asserts that

$$(\hat{\delta} - \mu\hat{\beta})^2 \leq F_{1,\nu}(k_1\mu^2 - 2k_2\alpha3 + k_3)s^2$$

defines a confidence region for $\mu = \log\rho$. Here s^2 is the point estimator of σ^2 obtained from *Model 1*; k_1, k_2, and k_3 are constants that depend on the log doses and the number of test and standard observations; $\nu = N-3$, where N is the total number of observations, and $F_{1,\nu}$ is the 95th percentile of an F distribution with 1 and ν degrees of freedom. The confidence interval is determined by the roots, A and B, of the quadratic equation

$$a\mu^2 + b\mu + c = 0,$$

where $a = \hat{\beta}^2 - F_{1,\nu}k_1$, $b = -2\hat{\delta}\hat{\beta} + 2k_2F_{1,\nu}$ and $c = \hat{\delta}^2 - F_{1,\nu}k_3$. If $a > 0$ then the confidence region is the interval [B,A]. But if $a < 0$ and $b^2 - 4ac > 0$, then the confidence region is the exterior of the interval [B,A], i.e. the set log $\rho \leq B$ and log $\rho \geq A$. A third possibility is that the confidence region is the entire straight line. This uninformative consequence of Fieller's Theorem occurs when $a < 0$ and $b^2 - 4ac < 0$. No other cases are possible (5).

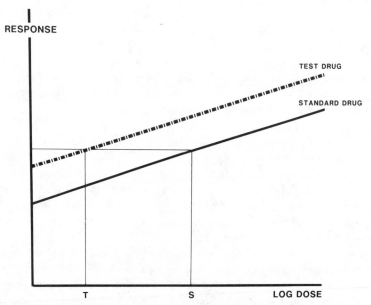

Figure 1   The length of the interval (T, S) is the log relative potency. The dose T of the test drug produces the same response as the dose S of the standard drug.

It is standard procedure to test the validity of the model of *Equation 1* via an analysis of variance (ANOVA) (1). In Table 1 the entry "Regression" tests the null hypothesis that the slope, β, is zero. This test is important for if β is zero, the concept of relative potency has no meaning because from *Equation 1* the relative potency parameter is undefined. "Parallelism" (Table 1) tests the assumption that the dose response lines for test and standard are indeed parallel. The model of *Equation 1* assumes that the average response of Y_S depends linearly on the log dose, x_S. The true relation between Y_S and x_S may be more complicated. They could be related by higher order terms, such as a quadratic involving the square of x_S. Also in Table 1, "Linearity" tests the possibility that a linear model is an inadequate representation of the dose-response relationship. The entry "Preparations" examines whether the same range of effectiveness is studied in the two treatments. It tests the null hypothesis that the weighted-population mean response of all doses of the standard equals that of all doses of the test used in the experiment. If so, the assay may still be valid. The magnitude of the difference indicates how great an extrapolation in the effect range is involved.

Although the ANOVA is traditionally used to test validity, it is somewhat inconsistent with the analogous tests based on the model of *Equation 1*. Using likelihood-ratio theory all tests can be based on *Equation* 1, thereby avoiding any possibility of inconsistencies. As an illustration, the estimator of σ^2

Table 1 Analysis of variance for parallel line
assay based on a completely randomized (parallel
groups) design

Source of variation	Degrees of freedom[a]
Between doses	$K_S + K_T - 1$
Regression	1
Parallelism	1
Preparations	1
Linearity	$K_S + K_T - 4$
Within doses	$N_S + N_T - K_S - K_T$
Total	$N_S + N_T - 1$

[a]N_S (N_T) is the number of experimental units receiving
the standard (test) preparation, and K_S (K_T) is the number
of different doses of the standard (test) preparation.

(required for instance by Fieller's Theorem) resulting from use of the AN-
OVA, is not the same as that resulting from the use of *Equation 1*. The
ANOVA method ignores, whereas the likelihood-ratio method incorporates,
the dose-response relationship (6).

COMBINATION OF UNIVARIATE ASSAYS

The problem of combining bioassays (1, 7–9) has received renewed attention
in recent years. Suppose that several independent bioassay experiments designed to estimate the relative potency of the same test and standard treatments are performed. Each one produces a point and 95% confidence interval
estimator of ρ. How could a single point and interval estimate of ρ be
produced on the basis of all of the data? Clearly, such combined estimates
should be more accurate than those produced by the individual experiments.
By application of the method of maximum-likelihood estimation, a combined
estimator can be obtained (7, 9). Two features of the combined estimator may
be mentioned: (*a*) the combined estimator of ρ depends not only on the
individual estimates of ρ but on the sample sizes, experimental design,
estimated residual error, and the statistics $\hat{\alpha}_T$, $\hat{\alpha}_S$, and $\hat{\beta}$ obtained in each of
the experiments; and (*b*) the estimator of log ρ is obtained from the solution to
a polynomial equation whose degree is greater than two. This latter situation
does not occur in the problems mentioned previously. For example, $\hat{\alpha}_T$ is
obtained from a linear equation. The Fieller confidence interval is obtained by
solving a quadratic equation. The new mathematical complication occurs
because estimation of the common relative potency is a nonlinear problem.
Such problems in mathematical statistics generally require the solution of
complicated nonlinear and nonquadratic equations.

Combining many bioassays involves first testing the validity assumptions in the individual studies. Even if a few such studies fail, they need not necessarily be excluded from the analysis. Complications arise when the slope of the regression lines of one or two of the studies has a sign that is opposite to those of the other studies. The additional hypothesis requiring investigation is whether the drugs share a common relative potency across experiments. This hypothesis can also be tested by the likelihood-ratio approach. Mathematical complications also arise here because such a hypothesis is not linear. In particular, instead of minimizing a sum of squares (as in straight-line regression theory), finding the likelihood-ratio test in this situation requires minimizing a function of the form

$$J(\mu) = \sum_{i=1}^{I} (\hat{\delta}_i - \mu\hat{\beta}_i)^2/(p_i\mu^2 + q_i\mu + r_i),$$

where p_i, q_i, and r_i are constants depending on the log doses in the ith experiment. I is the number of investigators and $\mu = \log\rho$. The value of μ that minimizes $J(\mu)$ is $\hat{\mu}$, the combined maximum-likelihood estimator of log relative potency. The solution can be found numerically. Various values of μ are systematically substituted into the above equation until the one that produces the minimum value of $J(\mu)$ is found. Another approach to finding the minimum is possible because $J(\mu)$ can be conveniently expressed as a ratio of two polynomials: $J(\mu)=P_1(\mu)/P_2(\mu)$. Standard techniques of differential calculus can then be used to obtain $\hat{\mu}$ as the root of a polynomial equation.

Finally, using likelihood-ratio methods, a Fieller-like confidence region (C) for $\log\rho$ may be obtained. In general, likelihood-ratio theory requires the specification of two hypotheses, H_0 and H_1. In the above case, H_0 is the hypothesis that, across all experiments, the log relative potency is equal to a specified value, $\mu_0 = \log\rho_0$. C is the acceptance region of H_0, i.e. the set of all μ_0 for which H_0 is not rejected. An exact method and an asymptotic method, both of which use the same H_0, have been developed. They differ in the choice of H_1, the "alternative hypothesis." If H_1 is the hypothesis that all experiments share an unknown common relative potency, then asymptotic or large-sample distribution theory must be used. If H_1 is the general linear model of *Equation 1*, a common relative potency across all experiments is not assumed, which results in the applicability of exact or small-sample distribution theory. The two approaches lead to different denominators in the likelihood ratio used to compute confidence regions. Nevertheless, the mathematical forms of the two confidence regions are very similar. Note that the word *region* rather than *interval* is used, for C may consist of one interval or many intervals. The possibility of many finite intervals in the confidence region does not occur when a confidence region for $\log\rho$ is computed for one bioassay. When the data is not pathological, however, C probably consists of one interval. If C is the asymptotic confidence region, then $\hat{\mu}$, the combined estimator of $\log\rho$, always belongs to C. If C is is the exact confidence region, it may be empty. This situation, too, does not occur with one bioassay. However, when the exact confidence region C is not empty, $\hat{\mu}$ always belongs to it.

SINGLE AND COMBINED MULTIVARIATE BIOASSAYS

Several papers have discussed multivariate bioassay (6, 10–13). Multivariate bioassay estimates relative potency when the observation of an experimental unit is not a single value but a vector of multiple responses representing different, but possibly correlated, outcomes. As in a univariate assay, each of the responses of the two drugs S and T are assumed to follow a linear model. For the ith response variable, we assume the model

$$Y_{S,i} = \alpha_{S,i} + \beta_i \log z_S + \epsilon_{S,i} \quad (Y_{T,i} = \alpha_{T,i} + \beta_i \log z_T + \epsilon_{T,i}), \quad 3.$$

where, as before, z_T and z_S are the log doses. For the ith response variable, *Model 3* is identical to *Model 1*, the model in the univariate situation. Here, however, if there are, for example, three responses, the covariances of the error terms $\epsilon_{T,1}$, $\epsilon_{T,2}$, and $\epsilon_{T,3}$ play a major role. The vector $\epsilon_T = (\epsilon_{T,1}, \epsilon_{T,2}, \epsilon_{T,3})$ is assumed to be multivariately normally distributed with mean vector $(0, 0, 0)$ and unknown variance-covariance matrix Σ. Note that, as in the univariate case, the standard and test formulations for each fixed i are assumed to have the same slope, β_i, although these slopes may be different for different response measures. If T is a dilution or new formulation of S, the relative potency should be the same, irrespective of the response measure used. The main goals of a multivariate bioassay are to (*a*) test the validity of the model of common slope; (*b*) test the hypothesis that there is a common relative potency for each variable; (*c*) estimate the scalar quantity, the common relative potency; and (*d*) determine a confidence interval for the common relative potency.

If two or more independent bioassay experiments are performed on T and S, as in the univariate case, each experiment separately yields a relative potency. In addition to the above points, another goal of combining multivariate bioassays (13–15) is (*e*) to analyze the data of all the experiments simultaneously to obtain a single point and interval estimator of relative potency.

The mathematics of these problems are more difficult than those of corresponding problems that arise in the univariate situation. Goal (*a*) is easiest to reach because it can be formulated as a linear hypothesis with respect to a multivariate model, at the same time being somewhat more general than the multivariate *Model 3*. The theory of tests of such linear hypotheses is well known. Thus, a test of (*a*) uses the F-test statistic. In short, (*a*) is treated as a special case of standard linear multivariate statistical theory. Hypothesis (*b*), on the other hand, does not arise univariately and is a nonstandard hypothesis testing situation because it is a nonlinear hypothesis. Asymptotic, i.e. large-sample, mathematical techniques are unavoidable. In the multivariate bioassay case, likelihood-ratio theory facilitates a large-sample test of the hypothesis of common relative potency. The same technique yields a maximum-likelihood estimator of the common relative potency and a corresponding 95% confidence interval. In a single multivariate bioassay experiment the methods that generate the tests and estimators described in (*a*)–(*d*) surprisingly turn out to require nothing more complicated than solving quadratic equations. However, analysis (*e*), combining several multivariate bioassays, involves solving higher order polynomial equations, as in the situation that arises from combining several univariate bioassays. A maximum-likelihood solution to the problem of combining multivariate bioassays has just recently appeared. The mathematical detail of the statistical analyses of these experiments is given in the references (13, 15) cited above. In the following sections we present some applications of these methods.

BIOEQUIVALENCE

There is considerable current interest in the interchangeability of generic and brand-name compounds (16–28). Suppose there is a standard drug S and a test drug T, which is a new formulation of the standard. The statistical problem is how to determine whether the two formulations are equivalent. The experimental procedure is accomplished in vivo, using a crossover or a completely randomized design. After either a single dose or multiple doses are administered to a pseudosteady state, blood samples are obtained to find the serum concentration over a single dose interval. All inferences about bioequivalence are made on the basis of this single dose.

The concentration curves are usually summarized by three measures: (*a*) the area under the curve *(AUC)*; (*b*) the peak concentration (C_{max}); and (*c*) the time to achieve the peak concentration (T_{max}). Usually each of the three measures (or a transformation such as their logarithms) is assumed to follow a normal distribution. The statistical hypothesis of interest is whether, for example, the expected values of the *AUC* given the standard drug S, *E[AUC|S]*, and the analogous quantity, *E[AUC|T]*, are equal. In practice, equality is not necessary, and if each of the three measures are similar, the formulations are said to be bioequivalent. Note that in the usual statistical situation the hoped for result is rejection of the null hypothesis, whereas in this case bioequivalence is concluded when the null hypothesis is not rejected. One must be sure, however, that the statistical power is adequate to reject if the drugs are not bioequivalent. Procedures for judging bioequivalence include classical statistical hypothesis testing, confidence intervals for the difference of, $E[AUC|S]-E[AUC|T]$, confidence intervals for the ratio $E[AUC|T]/E[AUC|S]$, and Bayesian methodology. Typically, the above methods are carried out univariately, that is, separately for each of the three measures.

One widely used rule accepts the proposition that two formulations are bioequivalent if the serum summary parameters of the test formulation are within 20% of those of the standard formulation. Let U_T and U_S denote the summary serum concentration parameters, and let $\Theta = U_T/U_S$. If with probability 0.95, $0.8 \leqslant 9\Theta \leqslant 1.2$, then the formulations are said to be bioequivalent under this rule.

Several different statistical approaches to obtaining confidence intervals have been suggested. Fieller's Theorem could be applied, and if the resulting interval falls within 0.8 to 1.2, then bioequivalence is accepted. Other authors have recommended methods for forming a confidence interval for Θ that is symmetric about 1. These approaches use the fact that there are many pairs of scalars for the t distribution with ν degrees of freedom that may be used to form a 95% confidence interval. In contrast to the usual scalars that are determined a priori, e.g. ± 1.96, these approaches choose limits that are data dependent to obtain a symmetric confidence interval.

Various post hoc statistical procedures are also used to perform power calculation to estimate the chance of detecting a difference, as a function of the true difference. These methods are post hoc in that the estimate of variability obtained from the results of the experiment is used in the power calculation.

The three measures usually used to summarize the serum concentration curves are obviously not three independent random variables but are rather components of a multivariate-response vector. It is clearly inappropriate to treat the responses univariately, since such a procedure results in several different measures of bioequivalence and ignores the covariance relationships between the components of the response vector. Therefore the appropriate approach is multivariate, in which a single measure of bioequivalence and a 95% confidence interval is obtained. In the case of measures that are ratios, a multivariate analogue of Fieller's Theorem can be applied. Also, rather than use the three summary measures of the concentration time curve, it may be more appropriate to use the actual observations of serum level at the times that they are obtained.

If the two formulations are found to be bioequivalent at one dose, the question of bioequivalence at a different dose is generally not tested in vivo. However, if there is therapeutic interest in a range of doses, it is logical to study the bioavailability over the full range. If the experimental design includes multiple doses of S and T, then the application of bioassay techniques is immediate and the scalar quantity relative potency is the natural indicator of bioequivalence. As mentioned above, if the confidence region for relative potency lies between 0.8 and 1.2, the two formulations may be said to be bioequivalent.

Finally, when there are several experiments it is important to have a single reply to the question of bioequivalence. Here the method of combining multivariate bioassays from two or more experiments provides a setting in which a single common relative potency and a corresponding 95% confidence region provide an unambiguous measure of bioequivalence.

MIXTURES

When two drugs, denoted by D_1 and D_2, are mixed in known quantities to produce a combination agent, its effectiveness is frequently compared to the effects of the constituent drugs acting separately. Suppose that the drugs are equipotent. If, for all doses x_1 and x_2, the effect of the mixture of dose x_1 of D_1 and dose x_2 of D_2 equals the effect of D_1 (or D_2) at dose $x_1 + x_2$, the mixture of the two drugs is said to be *additive*. Also, the two drugs are said to be *synergistic* or *antagonistic* according to whether the effect of the mixture is greater than or less than the effect of D_1 (or D_2) at dose $x_1 + x_2$. A curve of the doses (x_1, x_2) for which the effect of the mixture is constant is an *isobole*, and a collection of these curves, at different effect levels, is an *isobologram* (29). The type of joint action described by the additive model is *simple similar action*.

More generally, suppose the relative potency of D_1 to D_2 is $\mu = \log \rho$. Further, assume that the effect of the mixture is a random variable that is normally distributed. The null hypothesis H_0 states that the mixture is additive, i.e. the effect random variable has a mean equal to $\alpha + \beta \log(x_1 + \rho x_2)$. Notice that the model is statistical and makes no attempt to represent the biological action of the drugs (30–33). If the mixture is additive, point and interval estimators for the parameters may be obtained using maximum-likelihood theory, although numerical methods and asymptotic theory are required (34, 35).

The question of additivity versus synergism or antagonism may be tested as a statistical hypothesis using likelihood-ratio theory. Let the jth dose of the ith mixture be (x_{1ij}, x_{2ij}) where the ith mixture has the property that $x_{2ij} = \gamma_i x_{1ij}$. A common design is to have n_{ij} subjects receive the ith mixture at the jth dose level.

To perform the likelihood-ratio test, an alternative hypothesis, H_1, needs to be specified. One natural alternative is a model in which for each dose mixture of ratio γ_i, there is a separate constant $\mu_i = \log\rho_i$, such that the effects of the mixture of dose x_{1ij} of D_1 and dose x_{2ij} of D_2 is equivalent to the effect of dose $x_{1ij} + \mu_i x_{2ij}$ of D_1. For the ith mixture, the expected response is

$$\alpha + \beta\log(x_{1ij} + \mu_i x_{2ij}).$$

Substituting $x_{2ij} = \gamma_i x_{1ij}$, the expected response is equal to

$$c_i + \beta\log(x_{1ij} + x_{2ij}),$$

where

$$c_i = \alpha + \beta\log[(1 + \mu_i\gamma_i)/(1 + \gamma_i)].$$

The first step is checking that the dose-response lines of the mixture are parallel. This may be accomplished by fitting the model

$$E(\text{response}) = c_i + \beta_i\log(x_{1ij} + x_{2ij})$$

and testing the null hypothesis that the β_i are equal. If parallelism is rejected, the model of additivity is not possible and must be rejected. If parallelism is not rejected, the common slope β and c_i are estimated by least squares, and the quantities μ_i are determined from them in the same fashion as in the calculation in *Equation 2*.

Another alternative, H_1, assumes no structure other than that the responses are normally distributed. In either case the test of additivity proceeds first by independently maximizing the numerator likelihood under H_0 and the denominator likelihood under H_1 and computing their ratio Λ. To check significance $-2\log\Lambda$ is compared to the 95th percentile of a chi-square distribution.

The maximum-likelihood estimator, $\hat{\mu}$, is a by-product of the above calculation. In the computation of the numerator under the additivity model H_0, the value of μ for which the maximum of the likelihood-ratio statistic is achieved is the maximum-likelihood estimator.

To find a confidence interval first test that the relative potency of D_1 to D_2 is equal to a known constant, ρ_0. Under this H_0, the least-squares estimators of the remaining parameters α and β can then be obtained by standard regression theory because the resulting model is linear. The estimators depend, of course, on the particular value of ρ_0. Using either specification of H_1, the null hypothesis of additivity can be tested using the likelihood ratio. The resulting test statistic follows an F distribution, and rejection occurs when

396   LASKA & MEISNER

the statistic exceeds the 95th percentile. The 95% confidence interval then consists of all points ρ_0 for which this null hypothesis is not rejected.

ACKNOWLEDGMENTS

The authors would like to thank H. B. Kushner for his helpful comments and discussions.

Literature Cited

1. Finney, D. J. 1978. *Statistical Method in Biological Assay*. New York: Mac-Millan
2. Finney, D. J. 1947. *Probit Analysis. A Statistical Treatment of the Sigmoid Response Curve*. Cambridge: Cambridge Univ. Press
3. Fieller, E. C. 1940. The biological standardization of insulin. *J. R. Stat. Soc.* 137:1–53
4. Fieller, E. C. 1940. A fundamental formula in the statistics of biological assay, and some applications. 17:117–23
5. Buonaccorsi, J. 1979. Letter to the editor. *Am. Stat.* 33:162
6. Laska, E., Kushner, H. B., Meisner, M. 1985. Reader reaction: Multivariate bioassay. *Biometrics* 41:547–54
7. Bennett, B. M. 1962. On combining estimates of relative potency in bioassay. *J. Hyg.* 60:379–85
8. Armitage, P., Bennett, B. M., Finney, D. J. 1976. Point and interval estimation in the combination of bioassay results. *J. Hyg.* 76:147–62
9. Williams, D. A. 1978. An exact confidence region for a relative potency estimated from combined bioassays. *Biometrics* 34:659–61
10. Rao, C. R. 1954. Estimation of relative potency from multiple response data. *Biometrics* 10:208–20
11. Volund, A. 1980. Multivariate bioassay. *Biometrics* 36:225–36
12. Carter, E. M., Hubert, J. J. 1985. Analysis of parallel line assays with multivariate responses. *Biometrics* 41:703–10
13. Srivastava, M. S. 1986. Multivariate bioassay, combination of bioassays and Fieller's theorem. *Biometrics* 42:131–41
14. Volund, A. 1982. Combination of multivariate bioassay results. *Biometrics* 36:225–36
15. Meisner, M., Kushner, H. B., Laska, E. M. 1986. Combining multivariate bioassays. *Biometrics* 42:421–27
16. Westlake, W. J. 1972. Use of confidence intervals in analysis of comparative bioavailability trials. *J. Pharm. Sci.* 61:1340–41
17. Metzler, C. M. 1974. Bioavailability—a problem in equivalence. *Biometrics* 30:309–17
18. Westlake, W. J. 1976. Symmetric confidence intervals for bioequivalence trials. *Biometrics* 32:741–44
19. Westlake, W. J. 1979. Statistical aspects of comparative bioavailability trials. *Biometrics* 35:273–80
20. Rodda, B. E., Davis, R. L. 1980. Determining the probability of an important difference in bioavailability. *Clin. Pharmacol. Ther.* 28:247–52
21. Mandallaz, D., Mau, J. 1981. Comparison of different methods for decision-making in bioequivalence assessment. *Biometrics* 37:213–22
22. Selwyn, M. R., Dempster, A. P., Hall, N. R. 1981. A Bayesian approach to bioequivalence for the 2 × 2 changeover design. *Biometrics* 37:11–21
23. Fluehler, H., Grieve, A. P., Mandallaz, D., Mau, J., Moser, H. A. 1983. Bayesian approach to bioequivalence assessment: An example. *J. Pharm. Sci.* 72:1178–81
24. Metzler, C. M., Huang, D. C. 1983. Statistical methods for bioavailability. *Clin. Res. Pract. Drug. Reg. Affairs*, 1:109–32
25. Hauck, W. W., Anderson, S. 1984. A new statistical procedure for testing equivalence in two-group comparative bioavailability trials. *J. Pharmacokinet. Biopharm.* 12:83–91
26. Rocke, D. M. 1984. On testing for bioequivalence. *Biometrics* 40:225–30
27. Rocke, D. M. 1985. Correspondence. *Biometrics* 41:561–63
28. Selwyn, M. R., Hall, N. R. 1984. On Bayesian methods for bioequivalence. *Biometrics* 40:1103–8
29. Loewe, S. 1957. Antagonisms and antagonists. *Pharmacol. Rev.* 9:237–42
30. Ashford, J. R. 1958. Quantal responses to mixtures of poisons under conditions of similar action—the analysis of uncontrolled data. *Biometrika* 45:74–88
31. Plackett, R. L., Hewlett, P. S. 1963. A unified theory for quantal responses to

mixture of drugs: the fitting of data of certain models for two non-interactive drugs with complete positive correlation of tolerances. *Biometrics* 19:517–31

32. Ashford, J. R., Smith, C. S. 1964. General models for quantal response to the joint action of a mixture of drugs. *Biometrika* 51:413–28

33. Plackett, R. L., Hewlett, P. S. 1967. A comparison of two approaches to the construction of models for quantal responses to mixtures drugs. *Biometrics* 23:27–44

34. Scaf, A. H. 1974. Statistical analysis of isoboles. *Arch. Int. Pharmacodyn.* 208:138–65

35. Darby, S. C., Ellis, M. J. 1976. A test for synergism between two drugs. *Appl. Stat.* 25:296–99

Ann. Rev. Pharmacol. Toxicol. 1987. 27:399–427

SOLVENT TOXICOLOGY: RECENT ADVANCES IN THE TOXICOLOGY OF BENZENE, THE GLYCOL ETHERS, AND CARBON TETRACHLORIDE

George F. Kalf

Department of Biochemistry and Molecular Biology, Jefferson Medical College, Thomas Jefferson University, Philadelphia, Pennsylvania 19107

Gloria B. Post

Office of Science and Research, New Jersey Department of Environmental Protection, Trenton, New Jersey 08625

Robert Snyder

Joint Graduate Program in Toxicology, Rutgers College of Pharmacy, The State University of New Jersey, Rutgers, and The University of Medicine and Dentistry of New Jersey, Robert Wood Johnson Medical School, Piscataway, New Jersey 08854

INTRODUCTION

The field of solvent toxicology is quite broad and impossible to review fully in this format. We decided to stress benzene, the glycol ethers, and carbon tetrachloride. This review emphasizes the projected role of xenobiotic metabolism in hemopoietic toxicity caused by benzene, adverse effects on the male reproductive system caused by the glycol ethers, and hepatotoxicity caused by carbon tetrachloride.

399

0362-1642/87/0415-0399$02.00

BENZENE METABOLISM AND TOXICITY

Introduction

Benzene (Bz) is an important industrial chemical, a petroleum by-product, a component of unleaded gas, and thus a ubiquitous environmental pollutant [reviewed in (1)]. Bz is a myelotoxin; chronic exposure of humans and experimental animals to high concentrations results in blood dyscrasias including lymphocytopenia, thrombocytopenia, and pancytopenia or aplastic anemia (2, 3). Bz is also a carcinogen. It is associated with an increased incidence of acute myelogenous leukemia and some of its variants in humans (4–10), an increased incidence of several solid tumors (11, 12), and possibly leukemia/lymphoma (13) in rodents.

Since recent articles have reviewed the historical aspects of benzene toxicity (14), its genotoxicity (15), quinones as its toxic metabolites (16), and its developmental toxicity (17), we review recent findings on the metabolism of benzene and its hematotoxicity.

Metabolism

Benzene metabolism is required for toxicity. Possible pathways for the bioactivation of Bz in vivo are shown in Figure 1. In the liver, the major site of Bz metabolism (18), Bz is converted via a cytochrome P-450-mediated pathway (19) to benzene oxide, which is transformed by epoxide hydratase to the 1,2-dihydrodiol, which leads to catechol (C) formation (20) or rearranges nonenzymically to phenol (P), which is metabolized to hydroquinone (HQ) (21). The bone marrow is the target organ. It possesses a limited capacity to metabolize Bz, which cannot account for the amount of metabolites that accumulate in it (22–24). P is metabolized to HQ and C in the marrow by a myeloperoxidase-mediated pathway (25). The oxidation of HQ to p-benzoquinone (BQ) also probably occurs by a myeloperoxidase-mediated pathway, whereas C is presumably converted to 1,2,4-benzenetriol (BT) by the cytochrome P-450 system.

The quinones or semiquinones derived from HQ and/or C are generally considered to be the toxic metabolites, although an open-ring product such as *trans,trans*-mucondialdehyde is a possible toxic metabolite (26, 27). Ethanol consumption potentiates Bz toxicity in vivo by accelerating the hydroxylation of Bz and the conversion of P into toxic metabolites (28). Thus, it increases the hematotoxicity.

MICROSOMAL METABOLISM OF BENZENE   Bz induces the enzymes required for its metabolism. Post & Snyder (29) observed two benzene hydroxylase activities in rat liver microsomes from control, beta-naphthoflavone (BNF)-treated, and Bz-treated animals at all Bz concentrations and in pheno-

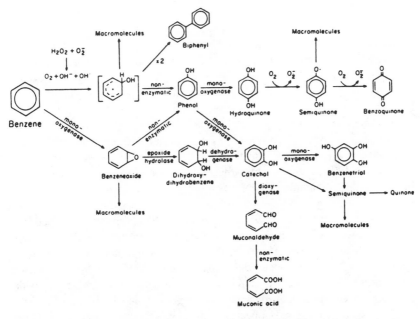

Figure 1 Metabolic pathways of benzene (taken from Ref. 45 with permission).

barbital (PB)-induced microsomes at concentrations of Bz up to 0.8 mM. Bz pretreatment increased activity without affecting total cytochrome P-450 content. This finding suggests the induction of a specific isozyme that was saturated at Bz concentrations > 0.4 mM, had a pH optimum of 6.6, and was stimulated by fluoride (30).

The inductive pattern of Bz hydroxylase is influenced by the addition of methyl groups to Bz (31). Toluene and xylene increased the metabolism of Bz, and consistent with the report by Post & Snyder (29), Bz induced benzene hydroxylase, but did not induce aniline hydroxylase or aminopyrine N-demethylase, whereas toluene and xylene did. Bz more readily induced the conjugating enzymes and increased the level of glutathione (GSH).

Cytochrome P-450 fractions from microsomes of benzene-induced rats have been compared to those obtained from untreated or PB-, BNF-, methylcholanthrene-, and ethanol-induced animals (32). Four distinct cytochromes P-450 were identified; isozyme A was induced by Bz and ethanol, and isozyme Bb was induced by all the inducers. The Bb isozyme induced by Bz appeared to differ from that induced by the classical inducers. The molecular activity of benzene hydroxylase of the microsomal fraction of rabbit bone marrow was about four times higher than that of liver microsomes (33). Pretreatment of the animals with Bz, but not PB, induced benzene monooxygenase activity, but did not affect the O-dealkylation activity in the marrow. Covalent binding of ^{14}C-labeled metabolites, but no free HQ or C, could be detected in incubations of Bz with bone marrow microsomes from Bz-induced animals (33).

Gilmour et al (34) found that Bz was converted to P by rat liver microsomes. They also observed that small amounts of HQ and C were produced from both Bz and P in a reaction mediated by cytochrome P-450 and stimulated by Bz pretreatment. The metabolism of Bz and P was competitively inhibited by toluene, and Bz and P reciprocally inhibited the metabolism of each other. Lunte & Kissinger (35) found that the rate of conversion of P to HQ by mouse liver microsomes was significantly higher than the rate of metabolism of Bz. P was converted to HQ, which was oxidized to p-BQ. Benzene hydroxylation in rabbit liver microsomes and reconstituted membrane vesicles containing cytochrome P-450 LM2 appeared to involve hydrogen peroxide, superoxide anion, and hydroxyl radical (36). Biphenyl was formed by the reconstituted system, indicating a cytochrome P-450-dependent formation of a hydroxycyclohexadienyl radical from the interaction of hydroxyl radical with Bz. These results would suggest that the microsomal cytochrome P-450-dependent oxidation of Bz requires hydroxyl radicals generated in a modified Haber–Weiss reaction between hydrogen peroxide and superoxide anion. However, these studies used only 17-μM Bz. Using a similar system with higher concentrations of Bz in alcohol, Gorsky & Coon (37) found a K_m for Bz of 18 mM with PB-induced rabbit liver microsomes and 105 mM with a cytochrome P-450 LM2 reconstituted system. When Bz concentrations were in the range of the K_m, superoxide dismutase, desferrioximine, or hydroxyl radical scavengers had no effect. The oxidation of Bz to P in a model hydroxyl radical–generating system consisting of xanthine, xanthine oxidase, and Fe-EDTA was not dependent on the substrate concentration. The rate of hydroxyl radical generation by the model system was regulated to be greater than the rate of product formation in the microsomal systems. Therefore, the lack of dependence on Bz concentration suggests that hydroxyl radicals are not involved in the metabolism of Bz to P when the concentration of Bz is near the K_m for cytochrome P-450 LM2. At concentrations of Bz below the K_m, the free-radical pathway of P formation becomes increasingly predominant.

It is commonly assumed that the microsomal cytochrome P-450 conversion of Bz to P occurs via an epoxide intermediate (38, 39), demonstrable by an NIH shift. Hinson et al (40) studied the role of the NIH shift in the formation of P from the deuterated benzene derivative, 1,3,5-[^{2}H$_3$]benzene, and found the expected products, 2,3,5-[^{2}H$_3$]phenol and 2,4-[^{2}H$_2$]phenol, which indicated that the shift had occurred. Analysis of the deuterium-isotope effect in the deuterated phenols suggests that the cyclohexadienone was formed either by the somerization of the epoxide or directly from the enzyme–substrate complex as a major intermediate in the hydroxylation of Bz.

Both epoxidation and free-radical insertion may be involved in the formation of P from Bz. Griffiths et al (41) reported on the production of P from Bz by a reconstituted microsomal system containing purified rat liver PB-induced cytochrome P-450. This production was inhibited by metyrapone and SKF 525A, but the conversion of P to secondary metabolites was not. The formation of the polyhydroxymetabolites from P was inhibited by radical-trapping agents and desferrioxamine. Interaction of Bz with cytochrome P-450 in the reconstituted microsomal system elicited a Type I spectral change, whereas interaction of P produced a Type II change indicative of an interaction of the substrate with the iron moiety. Also, an excess of unlabeled P did not dilute the labeled P derived from labeled Bz. These facts suggest that Bz interacts at the active site of cytochrome P-450 and undergoes epoxidation to benzene oxide, which rearranges to form P. This P is preferentially retained on the cytochrome P-450 but is shifted from the catalytic site to the iron moiety. There it can be attacked by hydroxyl radicals to form the polyhydroxy metabolites.

MITOCHONDRIAL METABOLISM OF BENZENE   Rat liver mitochondria, stripped of their outer membrane to avoid microsomal contamination (mitoplasts), metabolize Bz in an NADPH-dependent reaction to P and metabolites that covalently bind to mitochondrial (mt)DNA (42). A cytochrome P-450 that converts Bz to P has been solubilized from mitoplasts with 0.4% sodium cholate and purified 23-fold by polyethylene glycol (PEG) fractionation (43). The production of P from Bz by the 5–15% PEG fraction is completely dependent on NADPH and an exogenous bovine adrenodoxin/adrenodoxin reductase system that microsomal cytochrome P-450s do not use. This dependence provides evidence that the activity is indeed mediated by a cytochrome P-450 of mitochondrial origin.

THE EFFECT OF BENZENE AND ITS METABOLITES ON REPLICATION AND TRANSCRIPTION   Bz and its metabolites inhibit both nuclear and mitochondrial replication and transcription. DNA synthesis was inhibited in hemopoietic cells from mice exposed to a single dose of 3000-ppm Bz (44). It was also inhibited in mouse L5178YS lymphoma cells after their exposure to the metabolites, but not to Bz, which is not bioactivated in these cells (45). BQ was the most potent inhibitor, followed by HQ, BT, C, and P at concentrations that were not cytotoxic. Inhibition correlated with ease of oxidation. This correlation suggests that the oxidation of P or one of its metabolites produces   the   ultimate   reactive   compound   that   inhibits   DNA synthesis. Only BQ and BT induced single-strand (ss) DNA damage (46). BQ was about nine times more effective than BT in causing the damage. Ascorbic acid (47) protected against damage from BQ; superoxide dismutase did not protect against damage from BQ, but decreased the DNA damage from BT. Inhibition of intracellular superoxide dismutase increased the ssDNA damage. Such an increase suggests that ssDNA damage caused by BT results from superoxide anion radical generated during BT oxidation. Glutathione (GSH) also protected against DNA damage (48); BQ rapidly depleted the intracellular store of GSH. During BT treatment the GSH level dropped gradually, and only BQ affected the level of oxidized glutathione (GSSG). These observations imply that the two compounds act on GSH through different mechanisms and that GSH plays an important role in the detoxication mechanism (or mechanisms) for BQ and BT.

DNA replication in rat liver and rabbit bone marrow mitochondria in vitro is inhibited in a dose-dependent manner ky HQ, p-BQ, and BT (49). The activity of purified rat liver mitochondrial DNA polymerase-γ was inhibited by HQ and BQ by the metabolite's interaction with an active sulfhydryl group on the enzyme. The binding of [^{14}C]hydroquinone to the enzyme was prevented by N-ethyl maleimide as well as by unlabeled HQ or p-BQ, suggesting that both compounds bind to the same sulfhydryl (SH) group on the polymerase or that they are interconverted to the benzosemiquinone, which then binds.

Transcription in mouse lymphocytes (50) and macrophages (51) in vitro is inhibited in a dose-dependent manner by P, HQ, and p-BQ; the IC_{50} for BQ was 5×10^{-6} M for both cell types. Translation was also inhibited subsequent to the inhibition of RNA synthesis. Phenol was metabolized in macrophages by peroxidase to reactive species that inhibited RNA synthesis and covalently bound to macromolecules (51). Benzene was not metabolized. It inhibited RNA synthesis by infiltrating the plasma membrane and preventing the transport of labeled uridine into the cell, in a manner similar to that observed for lindane (52).

Rat and rabbit liver and cat and rabbit bone marrow mitoplasts are capable of bioactivating Bz in vitro to metabolites that inhibit mitochondrial transcription (53) and, consequently, translation. HQ, BQ, or P also caused a dose-dependent inhibition of transcription in rabbit bone marrow mitoplasts, with IC_{50} values ranging from 2×10^{-6} M for p-BQ to 2×10^{-3} M for C. Similar concentrations of p-BQ, HQ, and C inhibited mRNA synthesis in rabbit bone marrow nuclei incubated under conditions specific for RNA polymerase II (54).

COVALENT BINDING OF REACTIVE METABOLITES OF BENZENE WITH MACROMOLECULES   Bz and certain Bz metabolites are converted in nuclei and mitochondria to reactive species that covalently bind to macromolecules and that cause DNA damage in the form of strand breaks and covalently bound adducts in liver (55) and bone marrow (56). Reactive species from [^{14}C]benzene administered to rats and mice covalently bind to the macromolecules of various organs (57). Binding to RNA and protein is an order of magnitude greater than that to DNA. The level of DNA binding was low in several organs and highest in bone marrow. The covalent binding index (CBI) (cf 55) was 10, which approximately equals that of genotoxic carcinogens classed as weak initiators of carcinogenesis. The microsomal metabolism of Bz to reactive species capable of covalently binding to nucleic acids and proteins was induced by PB and inhibited by SKF 525A and GSH. This metabolism was selective. It was mediated by microsomes from liver but not from kidney, spleen, or lung (57). Ascorbate significantly reduced the ability of PB- and Bz-induced hepatic microsomes to metabolize labeled P or Bz to species capable of covalently binding to microsomal proteins (58). The metabolism of Bz to P was unaffected by GSH. However, GSH inhibited the covalent binding species observed from both substrates more than 95%. The metabolism of P to HQ was unaffected by either GSH or ascorbate. Bone marrow from guinea pigs with low dietary intakes of ascorbate showed a fourfold greater covalent binding of phenol equivalents in the presence of peroxide than did marrow from animals with high intakes. Myeloperoxidase appears to be responsible for the oxidation of P, as ascorbate blocks the oxidation of P, and H_2O_2 is for required the activation of P to covalently binding species. Partially purified guinea pig DT-diaphorase [NAD(P)H quinone oxidoreductase] inhibited the covalent binding from P by 70%. This effect was reversed by the diaphorase inhibitor, dicumeral (59). On the other hand, covalent binding was greatly enhanced by H_2O_2 and horseradish peroxidase or myeloperoxidase, and prevented by ascorbate. Quinone oxidoreductases reduce quinones to HQ or C via a two-electron transfer. This reduction suggests that covalent binding results from an electrophilic quinone species rather than from a semiquinone and the selective myelotoxicity of Bz may result from the high ratio of peroxidase activity to quinone reductase activity in the bone marrow (59). Lack of Bz toxicity in the liver may thus result from the conversion of quinone metabolites back to HQ and C by DT-diaphorase or by carbonyl reductase. Carbonyl reductase is very active on p-BQ and is the major NADPH quinone reductase of human liver (60).

Mitochondria can also activate Bz to intermediates that bind covalently to mtDNA. Rat liver mtDNA contains six deoxyguanosine adducts, and rabbit bone marrow mtDNA contains seven such adducts after incubation of mitoplasts with labeled Bz (61). A hydroxyl radical scavenger, mannitol, prevented the formation of four deoxyguanosine adducts. Two deoxyadenosine adducts were formed from [^{14}C]benzene in vitro. HQ, p-BQ, C, and Bz also formed adducts with deoxyguanosine when incubated with bone marrow mitoplasts in vitro (61).

Jowa et al (62) characterized the adducts formed when HQ or p-BQ reacts with deoxyguanosine (dG) in vitro. Two dG-adducts were formed with both HQ and p-BQ. Iron was required for the formation of the the adducts from HQ but not from p-BQ. This difference indicates the necessity for oxidation of HQ to BQ or the semiquinone. Similar adducts of dG were formed when p-BQ was allowed to react with single- or double-stranded DNA or with chromatin from rat liver nuclei. Adduct 2 was more stable. It was further characterized by NMR and mass spectra analysis to have the structure presented as Structure 1.

HEMOPOIETIC TOXICITY   Aplastic anemia from Bz poisoning could arise from toxic damage to one or more of the components of the hemopoietic system: stem cells, transit cells (progenitor cells in various degrees of differentiation), and/or bone marrow stroma or microenvironment (63).

Effects on stem cells   Several investigators have reported reductions in the number of multipotential stem cells (CFU-S) following exposure of mice to Bz (64, 65), whereas other workers have reported no change (66, 67). This discrepancy has been explained, in part, by a toxic effect of Bz on the transit cells, which signals stem-cell proliferation and differentiation, and thus depletes the stem-cell pool (68–70).

Effects on progenitor cells   Evidence that Bz acts primarily on committed progenitor cells was indicated by a decrease in the number of differentiating erythroid and myeloid progenitors in benzene-exposed rats, without an effect on the number of progenitor cells or mature cells in the bone marrow (71). Studies on the effects of Bz on the kinetics of ^{59}Fe uptake into maturing mouse erythrocytes indicated that the pronormoblast was the progenitor most sensitive to benzene, whereas stem cells and nondividing reticulocytes were relatively unaffected (72). The metabolites P, C, and HQ have also been reported to reduce ^{59}Fe incorporation into developing erythrocytes significantly, but not as much as Bz. The mixed-function oxidase inhibitor, 3-amino-1,2,4-triazole abolished the erythropoietic toxicity of Bz and P, but not of C or HQ (73). *Trans,trans*-mucondialdehyde, a six-carbon alpha, beta unsaturated aldehyde and an open-ring metabolite of Bz, is hemotoxic in CD-1 mice in a manner similar to benzene (26). It is also cytotoxic to human erythrocyte progenitor cells at micromolar concentrations (27). Other studies have shown that the number of erythroid (CFU-E) (74) and granulocyte/ macrophage (CFU-GM) (75) progenitor cells was depressed in benzene-exposed mice. However, low-level (10-ppm) exposure over a 54-day period did not decrease the number of CFU-E or CFU-GM unless hemopoiesis was stimulated by administration of a hemolytic dose of phenylhydrazine (76).

Effects on the stromal microenvironment   Hemopoiesis results from the interaction of stem cells with the supporting stroma. The stroma provides a favorable microenvironment for the regulated proliferation and differentiation of the stem cells (77). Reconstitution of the stroma and stem cells in vitro (78, 79), based on the growth of an adherent stromal layer from bone marrow cells in liquid culture, has stimulated new experimental approaches and provided important data about benzene toxicity to the bone marrow.

Several reports have indicated that Bz is toxic to the marrow microenvironment. Injection of normal bone marrow cells into benzene-exposed, lethally irradiated mice could not reconstitute normal hemopoiesis, as the number of granulocyte and macrophage colonies produced in vivo was decreased (66). However, incubation of normal bone marrow cells with Bz prior to administration to the animals did not reduce colony formation. This finding suggests that the microenvironment was deranged by benzene. Garnett et al (80) demonstrated that the marrow-adherent layer from benzene-treated mice did not differ in the number of CFU or in their ability to proliferate but was less able to support the differentiation of stem cells from unexposed mice. The development of an adherent layer in culture from the marrow cells of Bz-treated animals was altered; fat cells that normally appear during growth fail to develop, indicating that Bz affects marrow stromal cells. Gaido & Wierda (81) showed that HQ and p-BQ were most effective in decreasing the ability of stromal cells to support CFU-GM colony formation in a coculture system, whereas C and BT only inhibited at high concentrations. Adherent stromal cells from relatively Bz-resistant B6C3F1 mice support hemopoiesis better than stromal cells from sensitive DBA/2J mice (82). Marrow cellularity was reduced more in D2 than in B6 mice, but Bz had no effect on adherent stromal cell colonies or the number of granulocyte/macrophage precursors present. P, but not Bz, significantly decreased the ability of adherent stromal cells to support hemopoiesis of granulocyte and macrophage precursors, but no strain difference was evident. HQ, at levels that did not alter stromal cell number, inhibited granulocyte/macrophage colony formation and increased prostaglandin E_2 (PGE$_2$) levels (83). Pretreatment of the cultures with indomethacin decreased PGE$_2$ levels and protected against toxicity. Thus, the authors (84) suggested that HQ suppression of stromal cell–supported hemopoiesis is mediated by increased PGE$_2$ production and that this increase may be involved in myelosuppression by Bz. Taken together, these studies indicate that injury to bone marrow stromal cells may be an important factor in benzene-induced myelosuppression.

A possible target of Bz toxicity in the stroma is the macrophage. Macrophages are a major source of polypeptide growth factors required for the proliferation, development, and survival of progenitor cells of the various hemopoietic lineages (85). Post et al (51) demonstrated that P is metabolized in adherent mouse marrow macrophages by a peroxidase activity to one or more covalently binding species and that micromolar concentrations of HQ and p-BQ inhibit macrophage RNA synthesis. Adherent monocyte and macrophage cells from benzene-treated rabbits have been reported to inhibit the development of CFU-E and BFU-E colonies when cocultured with normal bone marrow (86). This finding suggests that Bz induces a CFU-E and BFU-E inhibiting activity in adherent blood cells.

Effect of benzene on lymphopoiesis   Peripheral lymphocytopenia is an early manifestation of Bz toxicity in both animals and humans (6, 16, 87), and is a distinctive feature of benzene-induced aplastic anemia (3). The ability of P, HQ, and C to suppress lymphocyte growth and function in vitro correlates with their capacity to undergo autooxidation and with their concentration in the bone marrow or lymphoid organs (88–91). HQ and its oxidation product, p-BQ, inhibit proliferation and differentiation in lectin-stimulated lymphocytes in culture (89, 90). These compounds also interfere with microtubule assembly (88, 91) at concentrations that are not cytotoxic and that can be achieved in vivo. P and C suppress lymphocyte activation only at cytotoxic concentrations. Suppression of lymphocyte blastogenesis by HQ has been postulated (88) to be mediated by the interaction of p-BQ with sulfhydryl groups on tubulin. This binding interferes with microtubular integrity, which is essential in cell division via spindle formation and in the regulation of surface receptor movement and signal transduction across the plasma membrane.

HQ and C are also immunotoxic in vivo. They are cytotoxic to spleen cells (92). HQ and C inhibit dextran sulfate– or lipopolysaccharide (LPS)-induced development of polyclonal plaque-forming cells (PC-PFC). These PC-PFC were obtained from progenitor cells from spleen and marrow of benzene-treated animals that were induced to differentiate by dextran sulfate or LPS. Both metabolites reduced the number of PC-PFC that developed from progenitors obtained from these organs. However, only C inhibited LPS-activated marrow progenitors from maturing to PC-PFC. HQ also inhibited pre-B cells (IgM⁻) from maturing to (IgM⁺) cells, and HQ reduced the ability of mitogens to stimulate the proliferation of IgM⁺ cells to CFU-B colonies (93). Thus, HQ and C, by a reduction of progenitor B-lymphocytes, are immunotoxic in vivo, and HQ inhibits marrow lymphopoiesis in vitro at a concentration of 10^{-7} M. This concentration can be achieved in vivo, suggesting that inhibition of precursor-cell maturation is important in the hemotoxicity from Bz (92). Proliferation and maturation of lymphocyte progenitor cells are regulated by polypeptide lymphokines, which are produced both in vivo and in vitro by T-lymphocytes. Bz, if metabolized in the lymphocyte to a reactive intermediate such as *p*-BQ, could inhibit the production of lymphokines. Post et al (50) demonstrated that HQ and *p*-BQ affected the dose–dependent inhibition of RNA synthesis in mouse spleen lymphocytes in vitro at micromolar concentrations that were not cytotoxic. They also demonstrated that exposure to *p*-BQ completely inhibits the proliferation and production of the T-cell lymphokine, interleukin-2, by concanavalin (conA)-stimulated T-lymphocytes.

A number of in vivo studies have been conducted by C. A. Snyder and his collaborators on the ability of Bz to affect lymphopoiesis and modulate the cell-mediated immune response. Protracted exposure of mice to a regimen known to cause thymic lymphomas decreased B-lymphocytes in bone marrow and spleen. It also decreased T-cells in thymus and spleen and the ability of T-cells to respond to mitogenic stimulation (94). Bone marrow cellularity was increased 3-fold and the numbers of thymic T-cells, 15-fold, whereas no compensatory response was seen in the spleen. This difference led to the speculation that a subpopulation of thymocytes may exist that are resistant to Bz and that proliferate in its presence (94). More importantly, short-term exposure of mice to Bz concentrations at or near the industrial standard-exposure level significantly depressed mitogen-induced blastogenesis of both B- and T-lymphocytes without reducing the total number of either type of cell (95).

Bz can modify both host resistance to a bacterial infectious agent (96) and T-cell-mediated tumor resistance (97). The immunosuppressive effects of Bz have been reported to be modulated by the prior administration of a fungal product, 6FMA, from *Aspergillus ochraceous* that has interferon-inducing properties (98). Ingestion of ethanol also increases immunosuppresion by Bz (28), as well as benzene-induced hematotoxicity (99) in experimental animals. If these findings can be extrapolated to humans, they might have considerable impact on workers who are exposed to Bz on a daily basis and who are moderate-to-heavy drinkers.

METABOLISM AND TOXICITY OF GLYCOL ETHERS

Introduction

The glycol ethers (GE; Table 1), often referred to as cellosolves, are an important class of industrial solvents that are miscible with both water and many organic solvents (100). Because of their low vapor pressure and high

Table 1 Names and structures of some important glycol ethers

Name	Abbreviation	Synonyms	Structure
Ethylene glycol monomethyl ether	EGME	2-methoxyethanol Methyl Cellosolve®	$CH_3OCH_2CH_2O$
Ethylene glycol monoethyl ether	EGEE	2-ethoxyethanol Cellosolve®	$CH_3CH_2OCH_2CH_2$
Ethylene glycol monobutyl ether	EGBE	2-butoxyethanol Butyl Cellosolve®	$CH_3(CH_2)_3OCH_2CH$
Propylene glycol monomethyl ether	PGME	1-methoxy-2- propanol	CH_3OCH_2CHOHO

rate of dermal absorption, significant exposure can occur through contact with the skin (101).

The older literature (101) and genotoxicity (102) of the GE have been reviewed recently. The genotoxic potential of these compounds, if any, is minimal. Occupational exposure to ethylene glycol methyl ether (EGME) has been associated with CNS, hematopoietic, and renal toxicity; few cases of illness from other GE have been reported.

Recently, attention has focused on the effects of the GE on the male reproductive system, on fetal and embryonic development, and on the hematopoietic system. We review these areas. Although testicular toxicity was first noted fifty years ago (see 103), the potential of the GE to cause this toxicity was not widely appreciated until much later. Reproductive effects were reviewed in 1983 (103); since then, much new information has become available.

Male Reproductive Effects

TESTICULAR TOXICITY OF GLYCOL ETHERS   Reports of testicular toxicity of EGME and EGEE (104–115) are summarized in Table 2. EGME and ethylene glycol ethyl ether (EGEE) cause testicular atrophy, decreased sperm counts, abnormal sperm motility and morphology, degeneration and atrophy of the seminiferous tubules, and impairment of fertility. EGME is more potent than EGEE (104, 107, 116). Their acetate derivatives are as potent testicular toxins as the parent compounds, presumably because the ether linkage is readily hydrolyzed (104). Other GE including ethylene glycol monobutyl ether (EGBE) (104, 111, 117–119), ethylene glycol phenyl ether (104), ethylene glycol isopropyl ether (112), ethylene glycol mono-*n*-propyl ether (120), propylene glycol monobutyl ether (PGME) (105, 111), and dipropylene glycol monomethyl ether (DPGME) (121) did not cause testicular damage.

Table 2 Testicular toxicity caused by EGME and EGEE[a]

Compound	Species	Exposure	Dose[b]	Reference
EGME	mouse	oral, 5 d/wk 5 wk	250 mg/kg	104
EGME	mouse B6C3F1	inhal, 6 h/d 9 d	1000 ppm	105
EGME	NZ rabbit	inhal, 6 h/d 5 d/wk, 13 wk	30 ppm	106
EGME	rat, SD	oral, 11 d[c]	100 mg/kg	107
EGME	rat, F344	oral, 5 d	150 mg/kg	108
EGME	rat, F344	inhal 6 h/d 9 d	1000 ppm	105
EGME	rat, SD	inhal, 6 h/d 5 d/wk, 13 wk	300 ppm	110
EGME	rat	inhal, 6 h/d 10 d	800 ppm	111
EGME	rat, alb	inhal, 4 h	625 ppm	112
EGEE	mouse, CD-1	H_2O, 14 wk	1% H_2O	113
EGEE	rat, SD	oral, 11 d[c] 11 d	500 mg/kg	107
EGEE	rat	sc, 4 wk oral, 13 wk	400 μl/kg 200 μl/kg	114
EGEE	rat, LE hooded	oral, 5 d	936 mg/kg	115
EGEE	dog	iv, 22 d oral, 13 wk	200 μl/kg	114

[a]Abbreviations: NZ, New Zealand; SD, Sprague–Dawley; alb, albino; LE, Long Evans; d, day; h, hour; wk, week; inhal, inhalation; iv, intravenous; sc, subcutaneous.
[b]Lowest dose at which treatment-related testicular effects were reported.
[c]Animals sacrificed at various times during the experiments.

TESTICULAR TARGET CELLS   In rats sacrificed at various times after exposure to EGME (108, 116) and EGEE (116), the meiotic spermatocytes in the pachytene stage were found to be most susceptible to the toxins, whereas cells in earlier (leptotene/zygotene) and later (early spermatid) stages were damaged only after exposure to higher doses or for a longer time period.

These findings were supported by studies in which male rats were mated at various times after exposure to EGME (115, 122, 123). Decreased fertility was observed at the postexposure time period during which the cells exposed at the meiotic spermatocyte stage would have matured to spermatozoa.

Recovery studies suggest that a high dose may cause irreversible damage (107, 110, 115). Effects on fertility or testicular morphology were seen at a postexposure time that would allow a full cycle of spermatogenic maturation, suggesting that the spermatogonia (stem cells) were affected.

GLYCOL ETHER METABOLISM AND ITS RELATIONSHIP TO TESTICULAR TOXICITY   The GE that are alkoxyethanols are primarily converted to the corresponding alkoxyacetic acids, which in some cases are conjugated with glycine (124–129). This conversion is thought to be mediated by alcohol dehydrogenase, presumably via the alkoxyacetaldehyde intermediate (127, 129, 130):

$$R–O–CH_2–CH_2–OH \rightarrow R–O–CH_2–CHO \rightarrow R–O–CH_2–COOH$$

[Alkoxyethanol→alkoxyacetaldehyde→alkoxyacetic acid R: CH_3 (EGME), $CH_3–CH_2$ (EGEE), $CH_3–(CH_2)_3$, (EGBE)].

Metabolites of EGME and EGEE (and their acetate derivatives) cause testicular toxicity. Methoxyacetic acid (MAA) (107, 130) and ethoxyacetic acid (EAA) (107) produce the same degree of toxicity as the parent compounds, and methoxyaldehyde, the postulated intermediate in the conversion of EGME to MAA, causes similar effects (131). Pyrazole, an alcohol dehydrogenase inhibitor, blocks conversion of EGME to MAA and protects against toxicity (127).

PGME causes none of the toxic effects of EGME, although it differs from EGME only by a single methyl group (105, 111). Unlike the alkoxyethanols, which are primary alcohols, PGME is a secondary alcohol and therefore a poor substrate for alcohol dehydrogenase (132). It is extensively metabolized to CO_2 (128). Metabolism of DPGME, which is also not a testicular toxin, is similar to that of PGME (133).

In primary mixed cultures of Sertoli and germ cells, MAA and EAA caused degeneration of pachytene and dividing spermatozoa (134); these cells are the targets of EGME and EGEE toxicity in vivo (108, 116). EGME and EGEE at much higher concentrations, and n-propoxy- and n-butoxyacetic acid, metabolites of GE that are not testicular toxins (104, 112, 117–120), had no effect. Furthermore, the ability of the four acids to induce testicular damage in vivo correlated with the in vitro results.

BIOCHEMICAL MECHANISM OF TESTICULAR TOXICITY   Exposure of Sertoli cells in culture to MAA, but not to EGME itself, decreased production of lactate but had no effect on protein synthesis or cell viability (135). Exposure to EGME decreased in vivo testicular lactate levels (136). These observations are significant because pachytene spermatocytes cannot utilize glucose and are dependent on lactate provided by Sertoli cells (137). Other results (134), however, do not support this hypothesis; addition of lactate to mixed Sertoli– germ cell cultures did not protect against MAA.

Hematological Effects

ETHYLENE GLYCOL MONOBUTYL ETHER   EGBE causes hemolytic anemia, as well as hemoglobinuria; decreased erythrocyte numbers, hemoglobin, and mean corpuscular volume; and increased mean cell volume, reticulocytes, and nucleated red blood cells; bone marrow and spleen hyperplasia; and increased extramedullary hemopoiesis (117–119). EGPE and its acetate cause similar changes (120).

EGBE may act by increasing the fragility of the erythrocyte membrane, and thus the susceptibility of the cells to hemolysis through its metabolite, butoxyacetic acid (138). However, increased erythrocyte osmotic fragility did not occur after exposure of rats to a concentration sufficient to decrease red cell number.

ETHYLENE GLYCOL MONOMETHYL ETHER   In contrast to EGBE, EGME and its acetate derivatives (104) decrease leukocyte numbers (lymphocytes and neutrophils), with less marked effects on erythrocytes (104–106, 111, 119).

EGME depletes the bone marrow of erythroid and myeloid cells (115, 119); abolishes normal extramedullary hemopoiesis (119); damages the endothelial cells of the marrow sinuses (119); and depletes lymphocytes from the thymus (105, 106, 111, 119), spleen (105), and lymph nodes (105). No changes were seen in various immune parameters after treatment with EGME or MAA (139). However, although the dose used produced thymic atrophy, it did not decrease bone marrow cellularity and leukocyte counts, as reported by others. As is the case for testicular toxicity, MAA produces the same hemopoietic toxicity as EGME (139), whereas the closely related PGME has no effect (105, 111).

The observations that EGME causes hematopoietic, lymphoid, and testicular damage might suggest that it acts by a similar mechanism in all of these rapidly dividing tissues. However, other sites of high cell turnover such as the intestinal epithelium and ovarian follicle are unaffected by EGME (105). Also, the most sensitive testicular cells are those undergoing meiosis rather than mitosis (see above).

Developmental Toxicity

A number of studies have shown that EGME, EGEE, and their acetate derivatives, as well as ethylene glycol dimethyl ether (140), can adversely affect embryonic and fetal development (111, 114, 141–148; Table 3). Effects observed include increased incidence of malformations and minor variations, increased embryo mortality, and decreased fetal growth at doses not maternally toxic. Rabbits were more sensitive than rats or mice (143–145). The types of defects caused by EGME are dependent on when in gestation it is given and on how many doses are administered (142).

EGME and EGEE also affect neurochemical and behavioral development in rats (149). Both behavior and neurotransmitter levels changed. Such

Table 3 Selected studies demonstrating the developmental toxicity of glycol ethers

Compound	Species	Exposure	Dose[a]	Reference
EGME	mouse	oral, d.g. 7–14	31.25 mg/kg	141
EGME	mouse	oral, d.g. 7–14[c]	500 mg/kg 1 dose, 300 mg/kg, 3 doses	142
EGME	rabbit	inhal, d.g. 6–18 6 h/d	50 ppm	143
EGME	rat	inhal, d.g. 6–17 6 h/d	100 ppm	111
EGME	rat	inhal, d.g. 7–15 7 h/d	500 ppm	144
EGEE	rabbit	inhal, d.g. 6–18 6 h/d	175 ppm	145
EGEE	rabbit	inhal, d.g. 1–18 7 h/d	160 ppm	146
EGEE	rat	inhal, d.g. 1–19 7 h/d	200 ppm	146
EGEE	rat	oral, d.g. 1–21	50 μl/kg	114
EGEE	rat	inhal, d.g. 6–15 6 h/d	50 ppm	145
EGEE	rat	dermal, d.g. 7–16 4x/d	233 mg	147
EGEEAc	rabbit	inhal, d.g. 6–18 6 h/d	100 ppm	145
EGEEAc	rat	inhal, d.g. 7–15 7 h/d	130 ppm	144
EGEEAc	rat	dermal, d.g. 7–16 4x/d	341 mg	148

[a]Lowest dose at which developmental toxicity was observed.
[b]Abbreviation: d.g., days of gestation.
[c]Multiple or single dose given during the period.

changes are also dependent on both the compound and the period of gestation during which exposure occurred.

Evaluations of teratogenic potential of PGME (111, 150), EGBE (144, 148, 151), and EGPE (152) have been negative. These compounds also do not produce testicular toxicity (see above), suggesting that metabolism may also be involved in teratogenicity. Significantly, ethylene glycol itself has recently been found teratogenic in both rats and mice (153, 154). A metabolite (or metabolites) of ethylene glycol, most likely glycolate, are responsible for its systemic toxicity (155, 156); the relationship between ethylene glycol metabolism and its developmental effects has not been examined.

Recent findings suggest a relationship between GE metabolism and teratogenicity. Addition of MAA or EAA blocked growth and development of rat embryos in culture (157). Propoxyacetic, butoxyacetic, and methoxypro-pionic acids, the analogous derivatives of the nonteratogenic GE (158), as well as EGME itself (157), showed much weaker toxicity in this system.

MAA is teratogenic in rats (159). EGME, MAA, and dimethoxyethyl phthalate were equally potent teratogens when administered to rats on day 12 of gestation (160). Metabolites of dimethoxyethyl phthalate include phthalate and EGME (161). The three compounds induced similar types of malforma-tions, including several unusual defects not induced by other teratogens.

MAA accumulates in the fetus after injection into pregnant rats (162), and radioactivity from 2-methoxy[1,2-^{14}C]ethanol injected into pregnant mice is incorporated into fetal macromolecules (163). The alcohol dehydrogenase inhibitor, 4-methyl pyrazole (160), or ethanol (164), which would be ex-pected to compete with EGME for metabolism, protects the fetus from teratogenic effects. However, fetal accumulation of MAA is not decreased by ethanol. This finding suggests that subsequent metabolism of MAA may be required for toxicity and that this metabolism may be blocked by ethanol (165). In support of this idea, coadministration of formate or acetate de-creased the incidence of paw malformations from EGME or MAA. Thus, competition of metabolites of MAA with endogenous carboxylic acids may contribute to the developmental toxicity of EGME (166).

MECHANISM OF CARBON TETRACHLORIDE–INDUCED HEPATOTOXICITY

Among toxic effects of CCl_4 in liver is a decrease in xenobiotic metabolism. Recent studies suggest that CCl_4 acts as a suicide substrate for cytochrome P-450 (167). The phenobarbital-induced form of the cytochrome P-450 is the most susceptible to attack. The trichloromethyl free radical, which results from the homolytic cleavage of CCl_4, may bind either at the heme group of cytochrome P-450 or at the active site of the enzyme near the heme group, thereby leading to inactivation (168, 169). Lipid peroxidation, which has been thought for many years to play a seminal role in CCl_4 toxicity, may relate directly to the decrease in cytochrome P-450 (170). In addition to the well-established route of lipid peroxidation (171), metabolism of [^{14}C]CCl_4 in rat liver microsomes was found to produce trichloromethyl free radicals, which were covalently bound to phospholipids (172). Isolation of phospha-tidylcholine from the phospholipid fraction and incubation with phospholi-pase A2 demonstrated that about half of the phospholipid had been rendered resistant to hydrolysis. Thus, it has been argued that whereas direct reaction of the radical with the heme moiety of cytochrome P-450 leads to destruction of the mixed-function oxidase, lipid peroxidation is more closely related to loss of microsomal enzymes such as glucose 6-phosphatase, UDP-glucuronyl-transferase, nucleoside diphosphatase, and perhaps other enzymes (173).

Hypoxia appears to potentiate CCl_4-induced hepatotoxicity (174). The production of ethane and pentane (thought to be indicators of lipid peroxidation in vivo, in an oxygen deficient atmosphere) from rats given CCl_4 reached a plateau at normal oxygen pressure (175) and reached a higher plateau at reduced oxygen levels. The initial phase of metabolism is thought to plateau because reactive metabolites of CCl_4 destroy cytochrome P-450. The reaction is more rapid anerobically. The metabolism of CCl_4 appeared to be accompanied by the destruction of a single, rather than a large number, of fatty acids. When oxygen tension was measured as a function of oxygen consumption and lipid peroxidation, as determined by malondialdehyde formation in rat liver microsomes during CCl_4 metabolism, both parameters were greatest in the range of 1–10 mm Hg (0.1–1.3 kPa) but were less at 80 mmHg (10.7 kPa) (173, 176).

Rechnagel & Glende (177) postulated that CCl_4 is metabolized via a homolytic splitting of the carbon–chlorine bond, which probably occurs anerobically following the reaction of CCl_4 with cytochrome P-450 (Fe^{2+}) (Figure 2) (178). The result is the formation of a complex composed of cytochrome P-450 (Fe^{3+}) and trichloromethyl free radical. This structure is analogous to the cytochrome P-450-oxy complex, which is probably involved in oxidative reactions. The trichloromethyl free radical may either be released from its complex in a manner similar to that by which the superoxide anion radical is released from cytochrome P-450 or it may undergo a one-electron reduction to yield $[Fe^{3+}\text{—}|CCl_3 \leftrightarrow Fe^{2+}\text{—}\cdot CCl_3]$. The trichloromethyl free radical can abstract a proton and form chloroform or, upon further reduction, yield a ferrodichlorocarbene complex (179), which can release HCl and CO in the presence of water. The mechanism of degradation of the carbene is probably analogous to that proposed by Kubic & Anders (180) for the thiol-stimulated conversion of dihalomethanes to CO (181). The residual cytochrome P-450 (Fe^{2+}) is free to react with CCl_4 again.

Slater (182) suggested that the trichloromethyl free radical may be less reactive than previously thought, but that it could react with oxygen to form a trichloromethyl peroxy free radical, which is a more reactive species (183, 184). "Unequivocal evidence" that trichloromethyl free radicals are formed during the metabolism of CCl_4 was provided in studies employing isolated rat hepatocytes and spin traps to identify the free radical species (185). Unsaturated lipid free radicals were also detected. There was no evidence that the trichloromethyl peroxy free radical was formed until the recent report of Connor et al (186). These investigators trapped a carbon dioxide anion radical resulting from CCl_4 metabolism in perfused liver using the spin trap N-t-butylnitrone. The authors concluded that the carbon dioxide anion radical

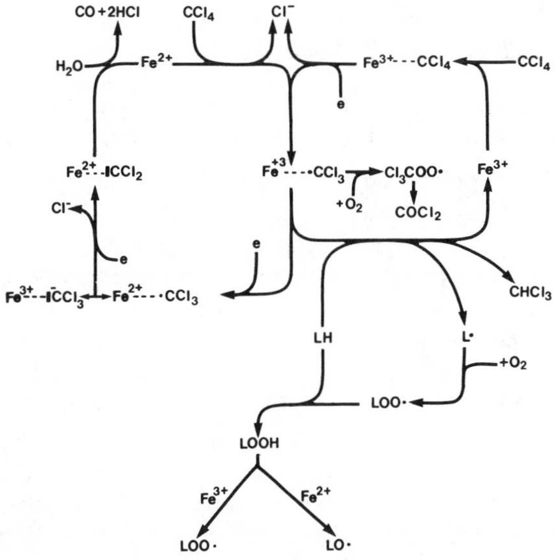

Figure 2 Formation of reactive metabolites from CCl_4.

arose from the trichloromethyl peroxy free radical. The trichloromethyl per-oxy free radical is thought to be a precursor to phosgene, which may also play a role in CCl_4-induced hepatotoxicity (187).

McCay et al (188) also used spin-trapping techniques to identify the trichloromethyl free radical in rat liver microsomes. They suggested that free radicals may be formed in a series of events initiated when a free radical reacts with a lipid moiety (LH; Figure 2). For example, during the homolytic cleavage of the C–Cl bond, radicals are formed that may react with lipid to yield L·, which can in turn react with O_2 to form the LOO· radical. LOOH may take either of two routes. Its action depends on the oxidation state of iron and results in the production of a highly complex series of reaction products (189). A similar series of reactions probably occurs in the liver.

The trichloromethyl radical can react directly with lipids or can be converted to the trichloromethyl peroxy radical; formation of the peroxy radical appears to depend on the availability of oxygen. The following series of events probably takes place in the hepatocyte: CCl_4 is reductively cleaved by cytochrome P-450 (190). This reduction yields trichloromethyl free radical in a region vicinal to unsaturated phospholipids. Thus, some radicals can add directly to double bonds to yield dienyl radicals. Others react with oxygen to form trichloromethyl peroxy radicals, which may also act in the initiation of lipid peroxidation. The lipid radicals resulting from the free-radical attack may react with oxygen as described above to initiate the process of lipid peroxidation, as Kappus (171) has suggested. Thus, oxidation of omega-3 unsaturated fatty acids yields ethane, whereas oxidation of omega-6 unsaturated fatty acids yields *n*-pentane.

Disturbances in Calcium Ion Homeostasis as a Final Common Pathway in Some Forms of Solvent Hepatotoxicity

Rechnagel (191), in attempting to relate CCl_4-induced lipid peroxidation to hepatic cell death and necrosis, recognized that lipid peroxidation occurred primarily in the region surrounding cytochrome P-450. He first attempted to invoke a useful concept, which he termed a "toxicological second messenger," to link events in the endoplasmic reticulum with general cell injury. The candidates he thought most likely to possess the required properties were 4-hydroxyalkenals, which are highly toxic products of lipid peroxidation. However, despite the attractiveness of this hypothesis, he recognized that 4-hydroxyalkenals react rapidly with cellular constituents in close proximity to their points of origin and would be unlikely to act as messengers to other loci in the cell. An alternative hypothesis developed by Rechnagel (191) and by Orrenius et al (192) suggests that alterations in Ca^{2+} homeostasis resulting from cell injury by CCl_4 or bromobenzene lead to cell death. Farber et al (193) had previously suggested that cell injury due to ischemia could be prevented if large increases in free intracellular Ca^{2+} could be prevented. They had argued that toxic liver cell death was associated with susceptibility of the cells to a large influx of extracellular Ca^{2+} (194). However, it was demonstrated that CCl_4, bromobenzene, and ethyl methane sulfonate were more toxic to liver cells in the absence of extracellular Ca^{2+} than in its presence. This finding suggested that redistribution of intracellular Ca^{2+} might be critical for cell death. CCl_4 inhibits the ability of microsomes to sequester Ca^{2+} but does not prevent the influx of extracellular Ca^{2+} either in vivo (195) or in vitro (196). Rechnagel (191, 197) argued that release of Ca^{2+} into the cytosol could result in a number of regulatory alterations. Such alterations could lead to triglyceride accumulation, a prominent feature of CCl_4-induced hepatotoxicity.

Bromobenzene caused a depletion of cellular GSH concomitant with the appearance of blebs on the surface of isolated hepatocytes (198). The blebs were postulated to be related to changes in membrane permeability associated with bromobenzene toxicity. Menadione, which also forms surface blebs, served as a model for hepatotoxicity induced by bromobenzene and other hepatotoxins. In this study Ca^{2+} accumulated in isolated perfused liver cells (199). Blebbing was also induced by the Ca^{2+} ionophore, A23187 (200), in a Ca^{2+}-free medium, suggesting redistribution of intracellular Ca^{2+}. Bellomo et al (201) also demonstrated impairment of calcium sequestration in mitochondria and the mobilization and loss of Ca^{2+} from both mitochondria and extramitochondrial spaces (199). Glutathione can prevent these effects. Orrenius et al (192), in agreement with Rechnagel (191), argued that these effects will cause the release of Ca^{2+} into the cytosol. They suggested that membrane-bound Ca^{2+}-ATPase, a sulfhydryl enzyme, is also inactivated by reactive intermediates and can no longer correct the imbalance of Ca^{2+} by promoting its secretion. The exact mechanism by which increased intracellular Ca^{2+} causes cell death is not yet completely understood. Further studies are needed to determine whether Ca^{2+} accumulation resulting from the cellular damage that reactive intermediates of solvent metabolism induce represents a final common pathway for cell death.

ACKNOWLEDGMENT

This research conducted in the laboratories of Drs. George F. Kalf and Robert Snyder was supported by grants ES02931 and ES03724 from NIEHS.

Literature Cited

1. Collegium Ramazzini Int. Conf. Benzene. 1985. *Am. J. Ind. Med.* 7:361–492
2. Laskin, S., Goldstein, B. D., eds. 1977. Benzene toxicity: A critical review. *J. Toxicol. Environ. Health Suppl.* Vol. 2
3. Goldstein, B. D. 1983. Clinical hematoxicity of benzene *Adv. Mod. Environ. Toxicol.* 4:51–61
4. Vigliani, E. C. 1976. Leukemia associated with benzene exposure. *Ann. N. Y. Acad. Sci.* 271:134–51
5. Infante, P. F., Wagoner, J. K., Rinsky, R. A., Young, R. J. 1977. Leukemia in benzene workers. *Lancet* 2:76–78
6. Infante, P. F., White, M. C. 1983. Benzene: Epidemiological observations of leukemia by cell type and adverse health effects associated with low-level exposure. *Environ. Health Perspect.* 52:75–82
7. Arp, E. W., Wolf, P. H., Checkoway, H. 1983. Lymphocytic leukemia and exposures to benzene and other solvents in the rubber industry. *J. Occup. Med.* 25:598–602
8. Decoufle, P., Blattner, W., Blair, A. 1983. Mortality among chemical workers exposed to benzene and other agents. *Environ. Res.* 30:16–25
9. Aksoy, M. 1985. Malignancies due to occupational exposure to benzene. *Am. J. Ind. Med.* 7:395–402
10. Aksoy, M. 1985. Benzene as a leukemogenic and carcinogenic agent. *Am. J. Ind. Med.* 8:9–20
11. Maltoni, C., Conti, B., Cotti, G. 1983. Benzene: A multipotential carcinogen. Result of long-term bioassays performed at the Bologna Institute of Oncology. *Am. J. Ind. Med.* 4:589–630
12. Maltoni, C., Conti, B., Cotti, G., Belpoggi, F. 1985. Experimental studies on benzene carcinogenicity at the Bologna Institute of Oncology: Current results and ongoing research. *Am. J. Ind. Med.* 7:415–46
13. Cronkite, E. P., Bullis, J. E., Inoue, T., Drew, R. T. 1984. Benzene inhalation produces leukemia in mice. *Toxicol. Appl. Pharmacol.* 75:358–61
14. Snyder, R. 1984. The benzene problem in historical perspective. *Fundam. Appl. Toxicol.* 4:692–99
15. Dean, B. J. 1985. Recent findings on the genetic toxicology of benzene, toluene, xylenes and phenols. *Mutat. Res.* 154:153–81
16. Irons, R. D. 1985. Quinones as toxic metabolites of benzene. *J. Toxicol. Environ. Health* 16:673–78
17. Schwetz, B. A. 1983. A review of the developmental toxicity of benzene. In *Carcinogenicity and Toxicity of Benzene*, ed. M. A. Mehlman, pp. 17–21. Princeton, NJ: Princeton Sci. Publ.
18. Sammett, D., Lee, E. W., Kocsis, J. J., Snyder, R. 1979. Partial hepatectomy

420   KALF, POST & SNYDER

reduces both metabolism and toxicity of benzene. *J. Toxicol. Environ. Health* 5:785–92

19. Gonasun, L. M., Witmer, C. M., Kocsis, J. J., Snyder, R. 1973. Benzene metabolism in mouse liver microsomes. *Toxicol. Appl. Pharmacol.* 26:398–406

20. Jerina, D., Daly, J., Witkop, B., Zaltzman-Nirenberg, P., Udenfriend, S. 1986. Role of the arene oxide-oxepin system in the metabolism of aromatic substrates. I. In vitro conversion of benzene oxide to a premercapturic acid and dihydrodiol. *Arch. Biochem. Biophys.* 128:176–83

21. Tunek, A., Platts, K. L., Przybylski, M., Oesch, F. 1980. Multi-step metabolic activation of benzene. Effect of superoxide dismutase on covalent binding to microsomal macromolecules, and identification of glutathione conjugates using high pressure liquid chromatography and field desorption mass spectrometry. *Chem. Biol. Interact.* 33:1–17

22. Andrews, L. S., Lee, E. W., Witmer, C. M., Kocsis, J. J., Snyder, R. 1977. Effects of toluene on metabolism, disposition and hemopoietic toxicity of [14C]benzene. *Biochem. Pharmacol.* 26:293–300

23. Andrews, L. S., Sasame, H. A., Gillette, J. R. 1979. 3H-Benzene metabolism in rabbit bone marrow. *Life Sci.* 25:567–72

24. Rickert, D. E., Baker, T. S., Bus, J. S., Barrow, C. S., Irons, R. D. 1979. Benzene disposition in the rat after exposure by inhalation. *Toxicol. Appl. Pharmacol.* 49:417–23

25. Sawahata, T., Rickert, D. E., Greenlee, W. F. 1985. Metabolism of benzene and its metabolites in bone marrow. In *Toxicology of the Blood and Bone Marrow*, ed. R. D. Irons, pp. 141–148. New York: Raven

26. Witz, G., Rao, G. S., Goldstein, B. D. 1985. Short-term toxicity of *trans, trans* mucondialdehyde. *Toxicol. Appl. Pharmacol.* 80:511–16

27. Goldstein, B. D., Witz, G., Jarid, J., Amoruso, M. A., Rossman, T., Wolder, B. 1982. Mucondialdehyde, a potential toxic intermediate of benzene metabolism. In *Biological Reactive Intermediates II. Chemical Mechanisms and Biological Effects*, ed. R. Snyder, D. V. Parke, J. J. Kocsis, J. Jollow, G. Gibson, C. M. Witmer, pp. 331–39. New York: Plenum

28. Nakajima, T., Okuyama, S., Yonekura I., Sato, A. 1985. Effects of ethanol and phenobarbital administration on the metabolism and toxicity of benzene. *Chem. Biol. Interact.* 55:23–38

29. Post, G. B., Snyder, R. 1983. Effects of enzyme induction on microsomal benzene metabolism. *J. Toxicol. Environ. Health* 11:811–25

30. Post, G. B., Snyder, R., 1983. Fluoride stimulation of microsomal benzene metabolism. *J. Toxicol. Environ. Health* 11:799–810

31. Pathiratne, A., Puyer, R. L., Brammer, J. D. 1986. A comparative study on the effects of benzene, toluene and xylene on their in vivo metabolism and drug metabolizing enzymes in rat liver. *Toxicol. Appl. Pharmacol.* 82:272–80

32. Baune, P., Flinois, J., LePrevost, E., Leroux, J. 1983. Influence of ethanol and benzene on cytochrome P-450 fractions in rat liver microsomes. *Drug Metab. Dispos.* 11:499–506

33. Gollmer, L., Graf, H., Ullrich, V. 1986. Characterization of the benzene monooxygenase system in rabbit bone marrow. *Biochem. Pharmacol.* 22:3597–602

34. Gilmour, S., Kalf, G., Snyder, R. 1986. Comparison of the metabolism of benzene and its metabolite phenol in rat liver microsomes. In *Biological Reactive Intermediates III. Molecules and Cellular Mechanisms of Action in Animal Models and Human Disease*, ed. J. J. Kocsis, D. J. Jollow, C. M. Witmer, J. O. Nelson, R. Snyder, pp. 223–35. New York: Plenum

35. Lunte, S., Kissinger, P. 1983. Detection and identification of sulfhydryl conjugates of p-benzoquinone in microsomal incubations of benzene and phenol. *Chem. Biol. Interact.* 47:195–212

36. Johansson, I., Ingelman-Sundberg, M. 1983. Hydroxyl radical–mediated cytochrome P-450 dependent metabolic activation of benzene in microsomes and reconstituted enzyme systems from rabbit liver. *J. Biol. Chem.* 258:7311–16

37. Gorsky, L. D., Coon, M. J. 1985. Evaluation of the role of free hydroxyl radicals in the cytochrome P-450 catalyzed oxidation of benzene and cyclohexanol. *Drug Metab. Dispos.* 13:169–74

38. Jerina, D. M., Yagi, H., Hernandez, O. 1977. Stereo selective synthesis and reactions of a diol-epoxide from benzo(a)pyrene. In *Biological Reactive Intermediates: Formation, Toxicity, and Inactivation*, ed. D. J. Jollow, J. J. Kocsis, R. Snyder, H. Vaino, pp. 371–78. New York: Plenum

39. Tunek, A., Platt, K. L., Bentley, P., Oesch, F. 1978. Microsomal metabo-

lism of benzene to species irreversibly binding to microsomal protein and effects of modifications of their mechanism. *Mol. Pharmacol.* 14:920–29

40. Hinson, J. A., Freeman, J. P., Potter, D. W., Mitchum, R. K., Evans, F. E. 1985. Mechanism of the microsomal metabolism of benzene to phenol. *Mol. Pharmacol.* 27:574–77

41. Griffiths, J., Kalf, G., Snyder, R. 1986. The metabolism of benzene and phenobarbital-induced liver mixed-function oxidase system. See Ref. 27, pp. 213–22

42. Kalf, G. F., Snyder, R., Rushmore, T. R. 1985. Inhibition of RNA synthesis by benzene metabolites and their covalent binding to DNA in rabbit bone marrow mitochondria in vitro. *Am. J. Ind. Med.* 7:485–92

43. Karaszkiewicz, J. W., Snyder, R., Kalf, G. F. 1986. Partial purification of benzene hydroxylase activity from rat liver mitoplasts. *Fed. Proc.* 45:1748

44. Lee, E. W. 1985. Effect of benzene on DNA synthesis in mouse hemopoietic cells following exposure by inhalation. *Toxicologist* 5:146

45. Pellack-Walker, P., Walker, J., Evans, H., Blumer, J. 1985. Relationship between the oxidation potential of benzene metabolites in their inhibitory effect on DNA synthesis in L5178YS cells. *Mol. Pharmacol.* 28:560–66

46. Pellack-Walker, P., Blumer, J. 1986. DNA damage in L5178YS cells following exposure to benzene metabolites. *Mol. Pharmacol.* 30:42–47

47. Pellack-Walker, P., Blumer, J. 1986. Multiple pathways for benzene-induced DNA damage: differences between benzoquinone and benzenetriol. *Proc. Am. Assoc. Cancer Res.* 27:106

48. Pellack-Walker, P., Frank, D., Blumer, J. 1986. The role of glutathione in 1,2,4-benzenetriol- and p-benzoquinone–induced DNA damage. *Proc. Am. Assoc. Cancer Res.* 27:81

49. Schwartz, C., Snyder, R., Kalf, G. 1986. The inhibition of mitochondrial DNA replication in vitro by the metabolites of benzene, hydroquinone and p-benzoquinone. *Chem. Biol. Interact.* 53:327–50

50. Post, G. B., Snyder, R., Kalf, G. F. 1985. Inhibition of RNA synthesis and interleukin-2 production in lymphocytes in vitro by benzene and its metabolites, hydroquinone and p-benzoquinone. *Toxicol. Lett.* 29:161–67

51. Post, G. B., Snyder, R., Kalf, G. F. 1986. Metabolism of benzene in macrophages in vitro and the inhibition of RNA synthesis by benzene metabolites. *Cell Biol. Toxicol.* 2:231–46

52. Roux, F., Puiseux-Dao, S., Treich, I., Fournier, E. 1978. Effect of linadane on mouse peritoneal macrophages. *Toxicology* 11:259–69

53. Kalf, G. F., Rushmore, T. R., Snyder, R. 1982. Benzene inhibits RNA synthesis in mitochondria from liver and bone marrow. *Chem. Biol. Interact.* 42:353–70

54. Post, G. B., Snyder, R., Kalf, G. F. 1984. Inhibition of RNA synthesis in rabbit bone marrow nuclei in vitro by quinone metabolites of benzene. *Chem. Biol. Interact.* 50:203–11

55. Lutz, W. K., Schlatter, C. H. 1977. Mechanism of carcinogenic action of benzene: irreversible binding to rat liver DNA. *Chem. Biol. Interact.* 18:241–45

56. Gill, D. P., Ahmed, A. 1981. Covalent binding of [^{14}C]benzene to cellular organelles and bone marrow nucleic acids. *Biochem. Pharmacol.* 30:1127–31

57. Artellinoi, G., Grilli, S., Calaeci, A., Mazzullo, M., Prodi, G. 1985. In vivo and in vitro binding of benzene to nucleic acids and proteins of various rat and mouse organs. *Cancer Lett.* 28:159–68

58. Smart, R. C., Zannoni, V. G. 1985. Effect of ascorbate on covalent binding of benzene and phenol metabolites to isolated tissue preparations. *Toxicol. Appl. Pharmacol.* 77:334–43

59. Smart, R. C, Zannoni, V. G. 1984. DT-Diaphorase and peroxidase influence the covalent binding of the metabolites of phenol, the major metabolite of benzene. *Mol. Pharmacol.* 26:105–11

60. Wermuth, B., Platts, K., Seidel, A., Oesch, F. 1986. Carbonyl reductase provides the enzymatic basis of quinone reduction in man. *Biochem. Pharmacol.* 35:1277–82

61. Rushmore, T. R., Snyder, R., Kalf, G. F. 1984. Covalent binding of benzene and its metabolites to DNA in rabbit bone marrow mitochondria in vitro. *Chem. Biol. Interact.* 49:133–54

62. Jowa, L., Winkle, S., Kalf, G., Witz, G., Snyder, R. 1986. Deoxyguanosine adducts formed from benzoquinone and hydroquinone See Ref. 34, pp. 825–32

63. Benestad, H. B. 1979. In *Aplastic Anemia*, ed. G. Gary, pp. 26–43. London: Baillierie Tindall

64. Uyeki, E. M., Elaskar, A., Shoeman, D. W., Bisel, T. U. 1977. Acute toxicity of benzene inhalation to hemopoietic

precursor cells. *Toxicol. Appl. Pharmacol.* 40:49–57

65. Green, J. D., Snyder, C. A., LoBue, J., Goldstein, B. D., Albert, R. E. 1981. Acute and chronic dose/response effects of inhaled benzene on multipotential hemopoietic stem (CFU-S) and granulocyte/macrophage progenitor (GM-CFU-C) cells in CD-1 mice. *Toxicol. Appl. Pharmacol.* 58:492–503

66. Frash, V. N., Yushkov, B. G., Karaulov, A. V., Skuratov, V. L. 1976. Mechanism of action of benzene on hematopoiesis. Investigation of hematopoietic stem cells. *Bull. Exp. Biol. Med.* 82:985–87

67. Speck, B., Cornu, P., Nissen, C., Groff, P., Weber, W., Jeannet, M. 1978. On the pathogenesis and treatment of aplastic anemia. In *Experimental Hematology Today*, ed. S. J. Baum, G. D. Ledney, pp. 43–48 New York: Springer-Verlag

68. Snyder, R., Lee, E. S., Kocsis, J. J., Witmer, C. M. 1977. Bone marrow depressant and leukemogenic actions of benzene. *Life Sci.* 21:1709–22

69. Gill, D. P., Jenkins, V. R., Kemper, R. R., Ellis, S. 1980. The importance of pluripotential stem cells in benzene toxicity. *Toxicology* 16:163–71

70. Cronkite, E. P., Inoue, T., Carsten, A. L., Miller, M. E., Bullis, J. E., et al. 1982. Effects of benzene inhalation on murine pleuripotential stem cells. *J. Toxicol. Environ. Health* 9:411–21

71. Irons, R., Heck, H. d'A., Moore, B. J., Muirhead, K. A. 1979. Effects of short-term benzene administration on bone marrow cell cycle kinetics in the rat. *Toxicol. Appl. Pharmacol.* 51:399–409

72. Lee, E. W., Kocsis, J. J., Snyder, R. 1974. Acute effect of benzene on ^{59}Fe incorporation into circulating erythrocytes. *Toxicol. Appl. Pharmacol.* 27: 431–36

73. Bolcsak, L. E., Nerland, D. E. 1983. Inhibition of erythropoiesis by benzene and benzene metabolites. *Toxicol. Appl. Pharmacol.* 69:363–68

74. Baarson, K. A., Snyder, C. A., Albert, R. E. 1984. Repeated exposure of C57B1 mice to inhaled benzene at 10 ppm markedly depressed erythropoietic colony formation. *Toxicol. Lett.* 20: 337–42

75. Tunek, A., Platts, K. L., Przybylski, M., Oesch, F. 1980. Multi-step metabolic activation of benzene. Effect of superoxide disimutase on covalent binding to microsomal macromolecules, and identification of glutathione conjugates using high pressure liquid

chromatography and field desorption mass spectrometry. *Chem. Biol. Interact.* 33:1–17

76. Dempster, A. M., Snyder, C. A. 1986. Effect of low-level benzene exposure on murine hemopoietic precursor cells. *Toxicologist* 6:285

77. Tavassoli, M., Friedenstein, A. 1983. Hemopoietic stromal microenvironment. *Am. J. Hematol.* 15:195–203

78. Dexter, T. M., Allen, T. D., Lajtha, L. G. 1977. Conditions controlling the proliferation of haemopoietic stem cells in vitro. *J. Cell. Physiol.* 91:335–44

79. Dexter, T. M. 1979. Hemopoiesis in long-term bone marrow cultures. *Acta Haematol.* 62:299–305

80. Garnett, H., Cronkite, E. P., Drew, R. T. 1983. Effect of in vivo exposure to benzene on the characteristics of bone marrow adherent cells. *Leukemia Res.* 7:803–10

81. Gaido, K., Wierda, D. 1984. In vitro effects of benzene metabolites on mouse bone marrow stromal cells. *Toxicol. Appl. Pharmacol.* 76:45–55

82. Gaido, K., Wierda, D. 1985. Modulation of stromal cell function in DBA/2 and B6C3F-11 mice exposed to benzene or phenol. *Toxicol. Appl. Pharmacol.* 81:469–75

83. Gaido, K., Wierda, D. 1986. Hydroquinone suppression of bone marrow stromal cell supported hemopoiesis in vitro is associated with prostaglandin E_2 production. *Toxicologist* 6:286

84. Wierda, D., Gaido, K. 1986. Indomethacin protects against in vivo benzene inhibition of stromal cell function. *Toxicologist* 6:286

85. Moore, M. A. S. 1978. Regulatory role of the macrophage in hemopoiesis. In *Stem Cells and Tissue Homeostasis*, ed. B. I. Lord, C. S. Potten, R. J. Cole, pp. 187–202. Cambridge: Cambridge Univ. Press

86. Haak, H. L., Speck, B. 1982. Inhibition of CFU-E and BFU-E by mononucuclear peripheral blood cells during chronic benzene treatment in rabbits. *Acta Haematol.* 67:27–33

87. Irons, R., Moore, B. J. 1980. Effect of short-term benzene administration on circulating lymphocyte subpopulations in the rabbit: Evidence of a selective B-lymphocyte sensitivity. *Res. Commun. Chem. Pathol. Pharmacol.* 27: 147–55

88. Irons, R. D., Neptun, D. A., Pfeifer, R. W. 1981. Inhibition of lymphocyte transformation and microtubule assembly by quinone metabolites of benzene:

Evidence for a common mechanism. *J. Reticuloendothel. Soc.* 30:359–72

89. Pfeifer, R. W., Irons, R. D. 1981. Inhibition of lectin-stimulated agglutination and mitosis by hydroquinone. Reactivity with intracellular sulfhydryl groups. *Exp. Mol. Pathol.* 35:189–98

90. Pfeifer, R. W., Irons, R. D. 1982. Effect of benzene metabolites on PHA-stimulated lymphopoiesis in rat bone marrow. *J. Reticuloendothel. Soc.* 31: 155–70

91. Pfeifer, R. W., Irons, R. D. 1983. Alteration of lymphocyte function by quinones through sulfhydryl-dependent disruption of microtubule assembly. *Int. J. Immunopharmacol.* 5:463–70

92. Wierda, D., Irons, R. 1982. Hydroquinone and catechol reduce the frequency of progenitor B lymphocytes in mouse spleen and bone marrow. *Immunopharmacology* 4:41–54

93. King, A. G., Landreth, K. S., Wierda, D. 1986. Hydroquinone inhibits bone marrow pre-B cell maturation in vitro. *Toxicologist* 6:169

94. Rozen, M. G., Snyder, C. A. 1985. Protracted exposure of C57B1/6 mice to 300 ppm benzene depresses B- and T-lymphocyte numbers and mitogen responses. Evidence for thymic and bone marrow proliferation in response to the exposures. *Toxicology* 37:13–26

95. Rozen, M. G., Snyder, C. A., Albert, R. E. 1984. Depressions in B- and T-lymphocyte mitogen-induced blastogenesis in mice exposed to low concentrations of benzene. *Toxicol. Lett.* 20:343–49

96. Rosenthal, G. J., Snyder, C. A. 1985. Modulation of the immune response to *Listeria monocytogenes* by benzene inhalation. *Toxicol. Appl. Pharmacol.* 80:502–10

97. Rosenthal, G. J., Snyder, C. A. 1986. Altered T-cell responses in C57B1/6J mice following sub-chronic benzene inhalation. *Toxicologist* 6:68

98. Pandya, K. P., Shanker, R., Gupta, A., Kahn, W. A., Ray, P. K. 1986. Modulation of benzene toxicity by an interferon inducer (6MFA). *Toxicology* 39:291–305

99. Baarson, K. A., Snyder, C. A., Green, J. D., Sellakumar, A., Goldstein, B. D., et al. 1982. The hematotoxic effects of inhaled benzene on peripheral blood, bone marrow and spleen cells are increased by ingested alcohol. *Toxicol. Appl. Pharmacol.* 64:393–404

100. National Institute for Occupational Safety and Health. 1983. *Current In-*

telligence Bulletin No. 39. Glycol Ethers, 2-Methoxyethynol and 2-Ethoxyethanol. US Dep. Health Human Serv. Publ. No. 83–112

101. Rowe, V. K., Wolfe, M. A. 1982. Derivatives of glycols. In *Patty's Industrial Hygiene and Toxicology*, ed. G. Clayton, F. Clayton, 2C:3911–4048. New York: Wiley. 3rd ed.

102. McGregor, D. B. 1984. Genotoxicity of glycol ethers. *Environ. Health Perspect.* 57:97–103

103. Hardin, B. D. 1983. Reproductive toxicity of the glycol ethers. *Toxicology* 27:91–102

104. Nagano, K., Nakayama, E., Koyano, M., Oobayashi, H., Adachi, H., et al 1979. Testicular atrophy of mice induced by ethylene glycol mono alkyl ethers. *Jpn. J. Ind. Health* 21:29–35

105. Miller, R. R., Ayres, J. A., Calhoun, L. L., Young, J. T., McKenna, M. J. 1981. Comparative short-term inhalation toxicity of ethylene glycol monomethyl ether and propylene glycol monomethyl ether in rats and mice. *Toxicol. Appl. Pharmacol.* 61:368–77

106. Miller, R. R., Ayres, J. A., Young, J. T., McKenna, M. J. 1983. Ethylene glycol monomethyl ether. I. Subchronic vapor study with rats and rabbits. *Fundam. Appl. Toxicol.* 3:49–54

107. Foster, P. M. D., Creasy, D. M., Foster, J. R., Thomas, L. V., Cook, M. W., et al. 1983. Testicular toxicity of ethylene glycol monomethyl and monoethyl ethers in the rat. *Toxicol. Appl. Pharmacol.* 69:385–99

108. Chapin, R. E., Dutton, S. L., Ross, M. D., Sumrell, B. M., Lamb, J. C. 1984. The effects of ethylene glycol monomethyl ether on testicular histology in F344 rats. *J. Androl.* 5:369–80

109. Chapin, R. E., Dutton, S. L., Ross, M. D., Swaisgood, R. R., Lamb, J. C. 1985. The recovery of the testis over 8 weeks after short-term dosing with ethylene glycol monomethyl ether: histology, cell-specific enzymes, and rete testis fluid protein. *Fundam. Appl. Toxicol.* 5:515–25

110. Rao, K. S., Cobel-Heard, S. R., Young, J. T., Hanley, T. R., Hayes, W. C., et al. 1983. Ethylene glycol monomethyl ether II. Reproductive and dominant lethal studies in rats. *Fundam. Appl. Toxicol.* 3:80–85

111. Doe, J. E., Samuels, D. M., Tinston, D. J., deSilva Wickramaratne, G. A. 1983. Comparative aspects of the reproductive toxicology by inhalation in rats of ethylene glycol monomethyl ether and

propylene glycol monomethyl ether. *Toxicol. Appl. Pharmacol.* 69:43–47

112. Samuels, D. M., Doe, J. E., Tinston, D. J. 1984. The effects on the rat testis of single inhalation exposures to ethylene glycol monoalkyl ethers, in particular ethylene glycol monomethyl ether. *Arch. Toxicol. Suppl.* 7:167–70

113. Lamb, J. C., Gulati, D. K., Russell, V. S., Hommel, L., Sabharwal, P. S. 1984. Reproductive toxicity of ethylene glycol monoethyl ether tested by continuous breeding of CD-1 mice. *Environ. Health Perspect.* 57:85–90

114. Stenger, E. G., Aeppli, L., Muller, D., Peheim, E., Thomann, P. 1971. Zur Toxikologie des Äthylenglykol-monoäthylathers. *Arzneim. Forsch.* 21:880–85

115. Oudiz, D. J., Zenick, H., Niewenhuis, R. J., McGinnis, P. M. 1984. Male reproductive toxicity and recovery associated with acute ethoxyethanol exposure in rats. *J. Toxicol. Environ. Health* 13:763–75

116. Creasy, D. M., Foster, P. M. D. 1984. The morphological development of glycol ether–induced testicular atrophy in the rat. *Fundam. Mol. Pathol.* 40:169–76

117. Dodd, D. E., Snellings, W. M., Maronpot, R. R., Ballantyne, B. 1983. Ethylene glycol monobutyl ether: acute, 9-day, and 90-day vapor inhalation studies in Fischer 344 rats. *Toxicol. Appl. Pharmacol.* 68:405–14

118. Tyler, T. R., 1984. Acute and subchronic toxicity of ethylene glycol monobutyl ether. *Environ. Health Perspect.* 57:185–91

119. Grant, D., Sulsh, S., Jones, H. B., Gangolli, S. D., Butler, W. H. 1985. Acute toxicity and recovery in the hemopoietic system of rats after treatment with ethylene glycol monomethyl and monobutyl ethers. *Toxicol. Appl. Pharmacol.* 77:187–200

120. Katz, G. V., Krasavage, W. J., Techaar, C. J. 1984. Comparative acute and subchronic toxicity of ethylene glycol monopropyl ether and ethylene glycol monopropyl ether acetate. *Environ. Health Perspect.* 57:166–75

121. Landry, T. D., Yano, B. L. 1984. Dipropylene glycol monomethyl ether: a 13-week inhalation toxicity study in rats and rabbits. *Fundam. Appl. Toxicol.* 4:612–17

122. McGregor, D. B., Willins, M. J., McDonald, P., Holmstrom, M., McDonald, D., et al. 1983. Genetic effects of 2-methoxy ethanol and bis(2-methoxyethyl) ether. *Toxicol. Appl. Pharmacol.* 70:303–16

123. Chapin, R. E., Dutton, S. L., Ross, M. D., Lamb, J. C. 1985. Effects of ethylene glycol monomethyl ether (EGME) on mating performance and epididymal sperm parameters in F344 rats. *Fundam. Appl. Toxicol.* 5:182–89

124. Hutson, D. H., Pickering, B. A. 1971. The metabolism of isopropyl oxitol in rat and dog. *Xenobiotica* 1:105–119

125. Jonsson, A. K., Pederson, J., Steen, G. 1982. Ethoxyacetic acid and N-ethoxyacetylglycine: metabolites of ethoxyethanol (ethylcellosolve) in rats. *Acta Pharmacol. Toxicol.* 50:358–62

126. Cheever, K. L., Plotnick, H. B., Richards, D. E., Weigel, W. W. 1984. Metabolism and excretion of 2-ethoxyethanol in the adult male rat. *Environ. Health Perspect.* 57:241–48

127. Moss, E. J., Thomas, L. V., Cook, M. W., Walters, D. G., Foster, P. M. D., et al. 1985. The role of metabolism in 2-methoxyethanol-induced testicular toxicity. *Toxicol. Appl. Pharmacol.* 79:480–89

128. Miller, R. R., Hermann, E. A., Langvardt, P. W., McKenna, M. J., Schwetz, B. A. 1983. Comparative metabolism and disposition of ethylene glycol monomethyl ether and propylene glycol monomethyl ether in male rats. *Toxicol. Appl. Pharmacol.* 67:229–37

129. Jonsson, A. K., Steen, G. 1978. n-Butoxyacetic acid, a urinary metabolite from inhaled n-butoxyethanol (butycellosolve). *Acta Pharmacol. Toxicol.* 42:354–56

130. Miller, R. R., Carrean, R. E., Young, J. T., McKenna, M. J. 1982. Toxicity of methoxyacetic acid in rats. *Fundam. Appl. Toxicol.* 2:158–60

131. Foster, P. M. D., Lloyd, S. C., Blackburn, D. M. 1985. Testicular toxicity of 2-methoxyacetaldehyde, a possible metabolite of ethylene glycol monomethyl ether, in the rat. *Toxicologist* 5:115

132. Von Wartburg, J. P., Bethuen, J. L., Vallee, B. L. 1964. Human liver alcohol dehydrogenase. Kinetic and physicochemical properties. *Biochemistry* 3:1775–82

133. Miller, R. R., Hermann, E. A., Calhoun, L. L., Kastl, P. E., Zakett, D. 1985. Metabolism and disposition of dipropylene glycol monomethyl ether (DPGME) in male rats. *Fundam. Appl. Toxicol.* 5:721–26

134. Gray, T. J. B., Moss, E. J., Creasy, D. M., Gangolli, S. D. 1985. Studies on

the toxicity of some glycol ethers and alkoxyacetic acids in primary testicular cell cultures. *Toxicol. Appl. Pharmacol.* 79:490–501

135. Beattie, P. J., Welsh, M. J., Brabec, M. J. 1984. The effect of 2-methoxyethanol and methoxyacetic acid on Sertoli cell lactate production and protein synthesis in vitro. *Toxicol. Appl. Pharmacol.* 76:56–61

136. Beattie, P. J., Brabec, M. J. 1985. 2-Methoxyethanol (ME) depletes testicular lactate. *Toxicologist* 5:463

137. Jutte, N. H. P. M., Jansen, R., Grootegoed, J. A., Rommerts, F. F. G., Clausen, O. P. F., et al. 1982. Regulation of survival of rat pachytene spermatocytes by lactate supply from Sertoli cells. *J. Reprod. Fertil.* 65:431–38

138. Carpenter, C. P., Pozzani, U. C., Weil, C. S., Nair, J. H., Keck, G. A., et al. 1956. The toxicity of butyl cellosolve solvent. *Am. Med. Assoc. Arch. Ind. Health* 14:114–31

139. House, R. V., Lauer, L. D., Murray, M. J., Ward, E. C., Dean, J. H. 1985. Immunological studies in B6C3F1 mice following exposure to ethylene glycol monomethyl ether and its principal metabolite methoxyacetic acid. *Toxicol. Appl. Pharmacol.* 77:358–62

140. Uemura, K. 1980. The teratogenic effects of ethylene glycol dimethylether on mouse. *Acta Obstet. Gynaecol. Jpn.* 32:113

141. Nagano, K., Nakayama, E., Oobayashi, H., Yamada, T., Adachi, H., et al. 1981. Embryotoxic effects of ethylene glycol monomethyl ether in mice. *Toxicology* 20:335–43

142. Horton, V. L., Sleet, R. B., John-Greene, J. A., Welsch, F. 1985. Developmental phase-specific and dose-related teratogenic effects of ethylene glycol monomethyl ether in CD-1 mice. *Toxicol. Appl. Pharmacol.* 80:108–18

143. Hanley, T. R., Yano, B. L., Nitschke, K. D., John, J. A. 1984. Comparison of the teratogenic potential of inhaled ethylene glycol monomethyl ether in rats, mice, and rabbits. *Toxicol. Appl. Pharmacol.* 75:409–22

144. Nelson, B. K., Setzer, J. V., Brightwell, W. S., Mathinos, P. R., Kuczuk, M. H., et al. 1984. Comparative inhalation teratogenicity of four glycol ether solvents and an amino derivative in rats. *Environ. Health Perspect.* 57:261–71

145. Doe, J. E. 1984. Ethylene glycol monoethyl ether and ethylene glycol monoethyl ether acetate teratology studies. *Environ. Health Perspect.* 57:33–41

146. Andrew, F. D., Hardin, B. D. 1984. Developmental effects after inhalation exposure of gravid rabbits and rats to ethylene glycol monoethyl ether. *Environ. Health Perspect.* 57:13–23

147. Hardin, B. D., Niemeier, R. W., Smith, R. J., Kuczuk, M. H., Mathinos, P. R., et al. 1982. Teratogenicity of 2-ethoxyethanol by dermal application. *Drug Chem. Toxicol.* 5:277–94

148. Hardin, B. D., Goad, P. T., Burg, J. R. 1984. Developmental toxicity of four glycol ethers applied cutaneously to rats. *Environ. Health Perspect.* 57:69–74

149. Nelson, B. K., Brightwell, W. S. 1984. Behavioral teratology of ethylene glycol monomethyl and monoethyl ethers. *Environ. Health Perspect.* 57:43–46

150. Hanley, T. R., Young, J. T., John, J. A., Rao, K. S. 1984. Ethylene glycol monomethyl ether (EGME) and propylene glycol monomethyl ether (PGME): Inhalation fertility and teratogenicity studies in rats, mice, and rabbits. *Environ. Health Perspect.* 57:7–12

151. Tyl, R. W., Millicovsky, G., Dodd, D. E., Pritts, I. M., France, K. A., et al. 1984. Teratologic evaluation of ethylene glycol monobutyl ether in Fischer 344 rats and New Zealand White rabbits following inhalation exposure. *Environ. Health Perspect.* 57:47–68

152. Krasavage, W. J., Katz, G. V. 1985. Developmental toxicity of ethylene glycol monopropyl ether in the rat. *Teratology* 32:93–102

153. Lamb, J. C., Maronpot, P. R., Gulati, D. R., Russell, V. S., Hammel-Barnes, L., et al. 1985. Reproductive and developmental toxicity of ethylene glycol in the mouse. *Toxicol. Appl. Pharmacol.* 81:100–12

154. Price, C. J., Kimmel, C. A., Tyl, R. W., Marr, R. W. 1985. The developmental toxicity of ethylene glycol in rats and mice. *Toxicol. Appl. Pharmacol.* 81:113–27

155. Clay, K. L., Murphy, R. C. 1977. On the metabolic acidosis of ethylene glycol intoxication. *Toxicol. Appl. Pharmacol.* 39:39–49

156. Chou, J. Y., Richardson, K. E. 1978. The effect of pyrazole on ethylene glycol toxicity and metabolism in the rat. *Toxicol. Appl. Pharmacol.* 43:33–34

157. Yonemoto, J., Brown, N. A., Webb, M. 1984. Effects of dimethoxyethyl phthalate, monomethoxyethyl phthalate, 2-methoxyethanol and methoxyacetic acid on post-implantation rat embryos in culture. *Toxicol. Lett.* 21:97–102

426   KALF, POST & SNYDER

158. Rawlings, S. J., Shuker, D. F. G.,
Webb, M., Brown, N. A. 1985. The
teratogenic potential of alkoxy acids in
post-implantation rat embryo culture:
structure-activity relationships. *Toxicol.
Lett.* 28:49–58
159. Brown, N. A., Holt, D., Webb, M.
1984. The teratogenicity of methoxyacetic acid in the rat. *Toxicol. Lett.* 21:97–
102
160. Ritter, E. J., Scott, W. J., Randall, J.
L., Ritter, J. M. 1985. Teratogenicity of
dimethoxyethyl phthalate and its
metabolites methoxyethanol and
methoxyacetic acid in the rat. *Teratology* 32:25–31
161. Campbell, J., Holt, D., Webb, M.
1984. Dimethoxyethylphthalate metabolism. Teratogenicity of the diester and
its metabolites in the pregnant rat. *J.
Appl. Toxicol.* 4:35–41
162. Scott, W. J., Nau, H. 1985. Weak acids
as human teratogens: Accumulation in
the young mammalian embryo. *Teratology* 31:25A
163. Sleet, R. B., John-Greene, J. A.,
Welsch, F. 1986. Localization of
radioactivity from 2-methoxy[1,2-
^{14}C]ethanol in maternal and conceptus
compartments of CD-1 mice. *Toxicol.
Appl. Pharmacol.* 84:25–35
164. Sleet, R. B., John-Greene, J. A.,
Welsch, F. 1985. Paw dysmorphogene-
sis in CD-1 mice treated with 2-
methoxyethanol and methoxyacetic acid
in combination with ethanol. *Teratology*
31:48A
165. Sleet, R. B., John-Greene, J. A.,
Welsch, F. 1986. Ethanol attenuation of
2-methoxyethanol (ME) teratogenicity
does not alter embryonal accumulation
of radioactivity from ME (1,2-^{14}C). *Toxicologist* 6:297
166. Sleet, R. B., Greene, J. A., Welsch, F.
1986. Reduction of methoxyethanol
(ME)-and methoxyacetic acid (MAA)-
induced paw malformations in CD-1
mice by small endogenous carboxylic
acids. *Teratology* 33:45C
167. De Groot, H., Haas, W. 1981. Self-
catalysed, O_2-independent inactivation
of NADPH- or dithionite-reduced microsomal cytochrome P-450 by carbon tetrachloride. *Biochem. Pharmacol.*
30:2343–47
168. Fernandez, G., Villarruel, M. C., De
Toranzo, E. G. D., Castro, J. A. 1982.
Covalent binding of carbon tetrachloride
metabolites to the heme moiety of
cytochrome P-450 and its degradation
products. *Res. Commun. Chem. Pathol.
Pharmacol.* 35:283–90
169. Yamazoe, Y., Sugiura, M., Kamataki,
T., Kato, R. 1979. The apparent loss of
cytochrome P-450 associated with
metabolic activation of carbon tetrachloride. *Jpn. J. Pharmacol.* 29:715–21
170. Masuda, Y. 1981. Carbon tetrachloride–
induced loss of microsomal glucose 6-
phosphatase and cytochrome P-450 in
vitro. *Jpn. J. Pharmacol.* 31:107–16
171. Kappus, H. 1985. Lipid peroxidation:
Mechanisms, analysis, enzymology and
biological relevance. In *Oxidative
Stress,* ed. H. Sies, pp. 273–310. New
York: Academic
172. Frank, H., Link, B. 1984. Anaerobic
metabolism of carbon tetrachloride and
formation of catabolically resistant phospholipids. *Biochem. Pharmacol.*
33:1127–30
173. De Groot, H., Noll, T. 1986. The crucial role of low steady state oxygen partial pressures in haloalkane free-radical-
mediated lipid peroxidation. Possible
implications in haloalkane liver injury.
Biochem. Pharmacol. 35:15–19
174. Shen, E. S., Garry, V. F., Anders, M.
W. 1982. Effect of hypoxia on carbon
tetrachloride hepatotoxicity. *Biochem.
Pharmacol.* 31:3787–93
175. Durk, H., Frank, H. 1984. Carbon tetrachloride metabolism in vivo and ex-
halation of volatile alkanes: Dependence
upon oxygen partial pressure. *Toxicology* 30:249–57
176. Noll, T., De Groot, H. 1984. The critical steady-state hypoxic conditions in
carbon tetrachloride-induced lipid peroxidation in rat liver microsomes.
Biochim. Biophys. Acta 795:356–62
177. Rechnagel, R. O., Glende, E. A. Jr.
1973. Carbon tetrachloride hepatotoxicity: An example of lethal cleavage. *CRC
Crit. Rev. Toxicol.* 2:263–67
178. Ahr, H. J., King, L. J., Nastainczyk,
W., Ullrich, V. 1980. The mechanism
of chloroform and carbon monoxide
formation from carbon tetrachloride by
microsomal cytochrome P-450.
Biochem. Pharmacol. 29:2855–61
179. Pohl, L., George, J. W. 1983.
Identification of dichloromethyl carbene
as a metabolite of carbon tetrachloride.
Biochem. Biophys. Res. Commun.
117:367–71
180. Kubic, V. L., Anders, M. W. 1978.
Metabolism of dihalomethanes to carbon
monoxide. III. Studies of the mechanism
of the reaction. *Biochem. Pharmacol.*
27:2349–55
181. Macdonald, T. L. 1982. Chemical
mechanisms of halocarbon metabolism.
CRC Crit. Rev. Toxicol. 11:85–120

182. Slater, T. 1982. Free radicals as reactive intermediates in tissue injury. See Ref. 27, pp. 575–89

183. Packer, J. E., Slater, T. F., Willson, R. L. 1978. Reactions of the carbon tetrachloride–related peroxy free radical ($CCl_3O_2\cdot$) with amino acids: Pulse radiolysis evidence. *Life Sci.* 23:2617–20

184. Mico, B. A., Pohl, L. R. 1983. Reductive oxygenation of carbon tetrachloride: Trichloromethylperoxyl radical as a possible intermediate in the conversion of carbon tetrachloride to electrophilic chlorine. *Arch. Biochem. Biophys.* 225:596–609

185. Albano, E., Lott, K. A. L., Slater, T. F., Stier, A., Symons, C. R., Tomas, A. 1982. Spin-trapping studies on the free-radical products formed by metabolic activation of carbon tetrachloride in rat liver microsomal fractions isolated hepatocytes and in vivo in the rat. *Biochem. J.* 204:593–603

186. Connor, H. D., Thurman, R. G., Galizi, M. D., Mason, R. P. 1986. The formation of a novel free radical metabolite from CCl_4 in the perfused rat liver and *in vivo*. *J. Biol. Chem.* 261:4542–48

187. Pohl, L. R., Schulick, R. D., Highet, R. J., George, J. W. 1984. Reductive-oxygenation mechanism of metabolism of carbon tetrachloride to phosgene by cytochrome P-450. *Mol. Pharmacol.* 25:318–21

188. McCay, P. B., Lai, E. K., Poyer, J. L. 1984. Oxygen- and carbon-centered free radical formation during carbon tetrachloride metabolism. *J. Biol. Chem.* 259:2135–43

189. Gardner, H. W., Kleiman, R., Weisleder, D. 1974. Homolytic decomposition of linoleic acid hydroperoxide: Identification of fatty acid products. *Lipids* 9:696–706

190. Noguchi, T., Fong, K. L., Lai, E. K., Alexander, S. S., King, M. M., et al. 1982. Specificity of a phenobarbital-induced cytochrome P-450 for metabolism of carbon tetrachloride to the trichloromethyl radical. *Biochem. Pharmacol.* 31:615–24

191. Rechnagel, R. O. 1983. A new direction in the study of carbon tetrachloride hepatotoxicity. *Life Sci.* 33:401–8

192. Orrenius, S., Thor, H., Di Monte, D., Bellomo, G., Nicotera, P., et al. 1985. Mechanisms of oxidative cell injury studied in intact cells. In *Microsomes and Drug Oxidations,* ed. A. R. Boobis, J. Caldwell, F. De Matteis, C. R. Elcombe, pp. 238–47. London: Taylor & Francis. 428 pp.

193. Farber, J. L., Chien, K. R., Mittnacht, S. 1981. The pathogenesis of irreversible cell injury in ischemia. *Am. J. Pathol.* 102:271–81

194. Schanne, F. A. X., Kane, A. B., Young, E. A., Farber, J. L. 1979. Calcium dependence of toxic cell death: A final common pathway. *Science* 206:700–2

195. Moore, L., Davenport, G. R., Landon, E. J. 1976. Calcium uptake of a rat liver microsomal fraction in response to in vivo administration of carbon tetrachloride. *J. Biol. Chem.* 251:1197–201

196. Lowery, K., Glende, E. A. Jr., Rechnagel, R. O. 1981. Rapid depression of rat liver microsomal calcium pump activity after administration of carbon tetrachloride or bromotrichloromethane and lack of effect after ethanol. *Toxicol. Appl. Pharmacol.* 59:389–94

197. Pencil, S. D., Glende, E. A. Jr., Rechnagel, R. O. 1982. Loss of calcium sequestration capacity in endoplasmic reticulum of isolated hepatocytes treated with carbon tetrachloride. *Res. Commun. Chem. Pathol. Pharmacol.* 36:413–28

198. Thor, H., Orrenius, S. 1980. The mechanism of bromobenzene-induced cytotoxicity studied with isolated hepatocytes. *Toxicology* 44:31–43

199. Mehendale, H. M., Svensson, S., Baldi, C., Orrenius, S. 1985. Accumulation of Ca^{2+} induced by cytotoxic levels of menadione in the isolated, perfused rat liver. *Eur. J. Biochem.* 149:201–6

200. Jewell, S. A., Bellomo, G., Thor, H., Orrenius, S., Smith, M. T. 1982. Bleb formation in hepatocytes during drug metabolism is caused by disturbances in thiol and calcium ion homeostasis. *Science* 217:1257–59

201. Bellomo, G., Jewell, S. A., Orrenius, S. 1982. The metabolism of menadione impairs the ability of rat liver mitochondria to take up and retain calcium. *J. Biol. Chem.* 257:11558–62

Ann. Rev. Pharmacol. Toxicol. 1987. 27:429–37

REVIEW OF REVIEWS

E. Leong Way

Departments of Pharmacology and Pharmaceutical Chemistry, Schools of Medicine and Pharmacy, University of California, San Francisco, California 94143

ANIMAL WELFARE AND RESEARCH

The right of scientists to conduct research on animals for the benefit of mankind is threatened today by animal activists. The need to justify the use of experimental animals for seeking the cause and treatment for diseases has become more than a nuisance; indeed, it has become an increasingly dangerous barrier to progress. These problems have necessitated that bioscientists leave their ivory towers to espouse their cause and to solicit allies in support of it. To this end, the Office of Public Affairs of the Federation of American Societies for Experimental Biology sponsored a special symposium "Government, Media, and the Animal Issue" at the 1986 Annual Meeting. This session drew a standing-room-only audience. The proceedings have appeared in the organization's official publication. They feature the comments of a panel of speakers including not only experts in federal and state relations, university public affairs, and city government but also representatives of the print and TV media (1).

The more militant animal activists create a climate of fear in the halls of scientific research and attract media attention by breaking into laboratories to steal valuable research animals. However, the major damage is done by more shrewd activists who have taken over the directorships of wealthy animal welfare organizations. Such activists have hampered research by lobbying for more and more legislation under the guise of promoting animal rights. Horton points out that in 1980 there were only six bills on animal research in state legislatures throughout the country, but by 1983 there were fifty bills. In 1985 eighty bills were pending in twenty-one states. Many of these bills are still active today. Although the biomedical community has been successful in staving off most of the bills, this merely preserves the status quo, whereas each victory for the animal activists represents a cumulative gain.

429

0362-1642/87/0415-0429$02.00

Illegal break-ins also serve the cause of animal activists because of the media exposure they receive. Morse details the happenings at his institution when animal activists vandalized a laboratory and stole videotapes documenting experiments on baboons. Officials at the University of Pennsylvania failed to react immediately and effectively because they thought that the animal-rights activists had no political base and would not challenge the validity of the research project. Moreover, the university officials believed that the National Institutes of Health would resist political pressure and support the beleaguered research project. They also felt that law enforcement would be galvanized into action by the illegal break-ins and destruction of property. However, the scientists and university administrators soon found that they had grossly underestimated the strength of the animal-rights activists and over-estimated the amount of support they would receive from NIH and law-enforcement officials.

Some very sage advice, flavored strongly with good common sense, on confronting animal-rights activists is provided by a politician and two media representatives. Mayor Moran of Alexandria points out that to protect one's profession, one must become known and involved in community affairs. Effective lobbying requires build-up of credibility before an issue is joined. If the issue is already joined do not give up but establish an agenda to continue the fight for another round. Nissenson, a news reporter, emphasizes the necessity of responding to a reporter. When you do not respond, the reporter assumes you have something to hide. It may not be possible to convert an antivivisectionist, but a responsible reporter can be persuaded by facts and logic. It is important, therefore, to find a way to communicate to the public that experimentation on cats, dogs, and other animals will benefit many people. The media are not the enemy, but ultimately are the most powerful ally for the truth. These views were echoed, but qualified, by Rensberger, a science writer. He notes that most people who write about science and medicine are extremely pro science and medicine. However, these writers also see themselves having watch-dog roles in journalism rather than as promoters of science.

DRUG DISCOVERIES

Sneader chronicles the background leading to the discovery of new drugs (2). This book is likely the most comprehensive book on the subject, although it makes some important omissions. Nearly all the drug groups that act on various organs and systems for the prevention, diagnosis, alleviation, and curing of diseases generally listed in older and current pharmacology text-books are discussed. Although both primary and secondary sources have been consulted, the citations could have been more precise. The primary references are more likely to refer to chemical aspects and the secondary ones to pharmacological and clinical facets. As a result, some interesting insights are given on the physical and chemical considerations in drug development and on the struggle between individuals and companies for patent rights. However, the discussion of pharmacological concepts leading to drug discoveries is unbalanced, and some misstatements are made with reference to pharmacologic or clinical matters.

Oxophenarsine (Mapharsen), naloxone (Narcan), and p-aminosalicylic acid are examples of notable omissions. Sneader devotes ten pages to arsenicals. In this section he emphasizes the efforts of Ehrlich and his colleagues that led to the discovery of compound 606, or arsphenamine, and later, to that of neoarsphenamine. He also relates the problems associated with the therapeutic application of these two agents because of solubility, stability, and irritant properties, but does not describe how these problems were finally solved. Tatum proposed the use of oxophenarsine, which circumvents these obstacles, and it became the drug of choice for treating syphilis for more than a decade, until it was supplanted by penicillin. Naloxone, because of its more selective effect as a pure opiate narcotic antagonist, has replaced nalorphine as the antidote of choice for opiate overdose. Moreover, naloxone has become the indispensable pharmacological tool for characterizing and identifying opiatelike action; Fishman & Blumgart deserve much credit for their innovation. p-Aminosalicylic acid was an important adjunct for the treatment of tuberculosis and was used in conjunction with streptomycin or isoniazid for at least two decades.

Examples of the lack of pharmacological balance are primarily the author's disregard for some highly important contributions by US investigators. The pioneering concepts of Ahlquist in proposing α- and β-adrenergic receptors, and those of Martin for μ, κ, and σ opiate receptors, opened new vistas and resulted in many new drugs. Yet, Sneader hardly discusses these works. Instead he devotes considerable space to the conceptualization of the H_2-histamine receptor, which was a subsequent event. No credit is given to Axelrod and Brodie, who provided the definitive information that the common active metabolite of acetanilid and acetophenetidin (phenacetin) is acetaminophen. This finding provided the pharmacologic rationale for the introduction of acetaminophen as a drug.

Sneader's book also contains some errors or misconceptions about drug action. The Straub tail effect of opiates is ascribed to the cat instead of the mouse. Diphenoxylate is stated to be nonaddicting because of its rapid metabolism by the liver. However, the chief reason diphenoxylate is nonaddicting is its poor solubility, which limits it absorption and intravenous usage. Buprenorphine is termed a κ agonist, but it is well-established to be a partial μ agonist. The main drawback to divinylether as an anesthetic is attributed to the inability of anesthetists to control its rapid action instead of to its proclivity to cause liver damage. In comparing the toxicity of aspirin and acetaminophen, Sneader appears to be unaware that prior to the introduction of safety caps, aspirin was a major cause of drug deaths among infants and children, and management of aspirin toxicity was complicated and difficult.

Some interesting and amusing anecdotes are provided with respect to the politics and human aspects of selecting generic names for drugs. Differences between the British and Americans in assigning generic names include such well-known examples as adrenaline/epinephrine, noradrenaline/norepinephrine, pethidine/meperidine, paracetamol/acetaminophen, mepacrine/quinacrine, ergometrine/ergonovine, etc. Sneader relates an amusing story about the latter drug that is likely true although he does not bother to substantiate it. The noted British pharmacologist, Sir Henry Dale, and collaborators had isolated an alkaloid from ergot, which they deemed new and named "ergometrine." However, three other laboratories reported the isolation of a substance from ergot with similar properties at about the same time. Because each of the four teams gave a different name to the new alkaloid, the American Medical Association found it necessary to adopt yet another name, ergonovine. This action so piqued Dale that he resigned as British correspondent of the AMA.

The value of the book lies in its more comprehensive treatment of drug discoveries than is generally covered in most pharmacology and medicinal chemistry textbooks or drug monographs. If there were an elementary course on drug discovery, the book would meet the need. However, historians would find it short of being a scholarly treatise. The errors within, although usually minor, are too much in evidence, and the impact of some major drug discoveries on the social and economic well-being of mankind, although mentioned in passing, could have been presented with better perspective. Despite these criticisms, I found the book useful and readable. There is much valuable information, coupled with interesting tidbits, for pharmacologsts, chemists, and medical historians.

RISK ASSESSMENT

In the introductory article of a new journal, intended as a vehicle for the presentation and critical analysis of recent developments in toxicology, Wilkinson discusses risk assessment and regulatory policy (3). He points out that although the development of many chemicals for the benefit of mankind ("and for profit") has immeasurably improved the quality of life, mistakes and miscalculations have been made due to insufficient consideration of the long-term consequences of releasing newly developed chemicals into the environment. As a result, the public, led by environmental activists, has demanded both more restrictive legislation and an assurance of the safety of chemicals. Balancing the demands of consumer advocates and industrial groups has become increasingly difficult for the federal government. Wilkinson addresses some problems inherent in regulating the potential human health risks of chemicals, in the current regulatory procedures, in attitudes for resolving these problems, and he describes some future approaches that might be considered.

The fundamental problem facing toxicologists and regulators is that chronic health effects of chemicals cannot be assessed by direct experimentation. Consequently, the investigator assessing risk must extrapolate data under laboratory conditions unlike those to be encountered in the field. Thus, as cited in a National Academy of Science report, regulatory processes need to be separated into two processes, risk assessment and risk management. Risk assessment is a scientific study. Alternatively, risk management is not; it involves a series of value judgments including benefits, costs, and political considerations (4). Thus, according to Wilkinson, the key elements to effective regulation are compromise and common sense. Compromise entails recognizing that every chemical cannot be tested for everything. Regulators should not demand from scientists more than they can provide. The public must be made fully aware of the fact that at the low levels of exposure usually encountered, the risks associated with the vast majority of chemicals are infinitesimal compared with the many other risks that are accepted as a part of everyday life.

NITROPLASTERS AND BIOAVAILABILITY

Woodcock and associates use a sexy introduction to introduce a pharmacokinetic analysis of the capacity of nitroplasters to deliver glyceryltrinitrate through the skin (5). The application of nitroplasters on the chest for prophylaxis of angina pectoris has gained considerable popularity, but so has its misuse for inducing erection by application on or near the penis. Nitroplasters incorporate a controlled drug-release system in which absorption of glyceryltrinitrate is a zero-order process and the amount of drug released per unit time is held below the transport capacity of the skin. The authors cite recent studies indicating that different nitroplasters, even when stated to have the same release rate, provide different plasma drug levels. Such findings suggest that the data were derived under different conditions or that the manufacturers' specifications are unreliable. For more definitive data, knowledge of the rate of release of nitrate from different plasters is essential. Also, bioavailability studies need to be held to a set of standard conditions in which the plaster application site and blood collection site are specified.

MAKING A SCIENTIFIC DYNASTY

Kanigel authors a fascinating account of the master-apprentice system underlying great discoveries in science (6). The lure to entice the reader is the description of the trials, tribulations, and triumphs of four generations of scientists. Each started as a student apprentice and then assumed the role of mentor. The scene is the house that James Shannon built, the National Institutes of Health, and the plot involves the love-hate relationships that develop between teachers and pupils working together. Worship and adulation turn into rage and resentment when recognition in terms of prizes and awards are doled to some, but not to the others, by third parties. The stories are true, and the characters are real. What makes the book particularly intriguing is that its leading characters are pharmacologists.

As a worker ploughing the same fields with a long-time, if not intimate, acquaintanceship with my four contemporaries, my interest could hardly not be titillated when the book became available. I was prepared at first to dislike the account because I was conditioned in part by a review that was not quite to my taste (7). As a friend of the family, I resented the intrusion into some private matters and the stirring-up of old controversies that might better have been brought up later. However, since the book has been published, there's no sense in trying to ignore its contents.

Upon reading the book, I had to concede that Kanigel, although he may have opened some old wounds and created a few new ones, had done a masterful job of reporting and writing. He has provided an absorbing and entertaining narration of the apprentiship system, which, clearly, he began only after digging deeply. His copious notes were gained not only by personal interviews with each of the four principals but with a strong supporting cast as well, including their superiors, pupils, colleagues, administrative underlings, and relatives. Thus, the views Kanigel presents are often a consensus rather than his own, and they reflect an attempt to be fair to the parties concerned. Particularly impressive is that the author also took the pains to understand the science. He succeeds admirably in translating the conceptualizations and experimental approaches of the pharmacologists into simple language for the lay public.

The head of the lineage is Bernard B. Brodie, or "Steve," who is described as brilliant, imaginative, demanding, and dictatorial. He brought American pharmacology to the forefront in the 1950s and 1960s with his innovations in drug metabolism and neuropharmacology. He was considered to be a maverick by some scientists because he appeared to be undisciplined in his approach and because he sometimes blatantly ignored some of the published literature and made conclusions not justified by the data. However, wins are based on hits and home runs, not strike-outs, and it is difficult to belittle Brodie's prodigious feats. In determining the physiological disposition of a drug, he was not content to determine just its biotransformation profile, as was the tendency of many chemists of his time, but he sought always to relate the therapeutic and toxic effects of a drug to its biotransformation products. In addition to biotransformation, rapid relocalization can be important in terminating drug action, and depletion of endogenous substrates can result in prolonged effects long after a drug has been metabolized. Altered disposition of bioamines can have genetic, evolutionary, or pathological bases, as well as be affected by drugs, and such changes might cause mental aberrations. These are the legacies of a highly fertile and inquiring mind.

His pupil, Julius Axelrod, is characterized as the ultimate efficient experimentalist. Axelrod's cohorts did not consider him demanding, but he was indirectly so by the excitement he showed for, and the close attention he paid to, their experiments. His intuitive insight permitted him to devise simple techniques to provide logical answers to complicated perplexing problems. Axelrod's first studies with Brodie on the biotransformation of acetanilid are classic. Acetaminophen was found to be the active metabolite of both acetanilid and acetophenetidin (or phenacetin), and when the latter compound was found to cause renal damage the sales of acetaminophen (Tylenol, Datril, etc) for headaches and menstrual pains were exceeded only by those of aspirin. Neither investigator benefitted financially from this basic discovery. Axelrod was not considered to be a conceptual theorist, but the conclusions he derived from his data are meaningful, logical, and difficult to refute. His experiments demonstrating termination of catecholamine action by neuronal reuptake processes and by catecholamine-O-methyl transferase biotransformation are the major reasons he shared the Nobel Prize, but he personally considers the discovery of the microsomal drug-metabolizing enzymes to be his best work. Conflict with respect to priority rights in this area caused the rift between him and his mentor.

Axelrod's student, Solomon Snyder, has no conflicts with his mentor. Snyder's respect and affection for his teacher have only grown with the years. As a scientist, Synder is a hybrid of his academic grandfather and father. Like Brodie, he concocts ideas at his desk, but although not a bench scientist, like Axelrod he uses intuitive insight and the tools at hand to solve complicated problems. He appears to be as demanding as his forebearers for data, but Snyder prefers psychological approaches, using the carrot more often than the stick to spur his students. His underlings usually meet his demands but do not feel threatened. They find him easy and exciting to work with. His laboratory was and is a production factory for the ideas he spews, generally along the lines of using biochemical, neuroanatomical, and neurophysiological data for correlating drug action on various types of receptors. Linking ornithine decarboxylase activity to tissue regeneration, correlation of antipsychotic activity to dopamine binding, catecholamine and histamine disposition mechanisms were some innovative contributions from his laboratory. However, the biggest splash he made (and the biggest headache he caused) resulted from the discovery of "the" opiate receptor with Candace Pert.

Candace Pert is hardly ever described as a mere scientist. The adjectives others used include smart, quick, imaginative, undisciplined, obsessed, and sloppy. The discovery of the opiate receptor gave her fame, but it also made her infamous because she sought greater recognition for her role on the project. The study also embroiled her and Snyder in a conflict with other laboratories that had initiated analogous experiments years earlier. Without minimizing the important contribution of these workers in facilitating the characterization of the opiate receptor, I accord major credit to Snyder and Pert for solving the problem in less than a year. Pert was a graduate student when these pioneering studies were performed, but any doubts of her independent capabilities can be met by subsequent work from her laboratory, which is concerned with the characterization of the bombesin receptor and the correlative studies on receptor sites and neuronal pathways using autographic imaging techniques.

Some interesting glimpses of the private lives and personalities of the characters are also provided. Although all four scientists evince sparks of genius, they did not always excel in the classroom. Snyder graduated *cum laude* but Brodie was a high-school dropout. Axelrod never received *A*'s in science courses, and all his applications to medical schools were rejected. There was discussion by Pert's teachers on whether to drum her out of graduate school because some thought her thinking and laboratory techniques sloppy. Brodie in his prime was a lady charmer, a skillful poker player, a writer of humorous articles on pseudoscientific topics, a practical joker, and an administrator torturer. One point not brought out by Kanigel is the affection and loyalty Brodie won from many of his former pupils, even though they were intimidated by him. Axelrod, although warm, kind, and affable in the laboratory, neatly comparmentalized his professional and private lives, and kept social interaction with his pupils to a minimum. He claims some of his best ideas came, not while in the laboratory, but when trying to go to sleep, listening to boring lectures, or shaving. Snyder, a gifted guitarist, has wide-ranging interests and is enjoyable company. However, he creates the most heat among his contemporaries. Most readily concede his creativeness, intellect, and instinct for important problems. However, debates about his ambitions, motivation, and means to achieve an end are often the topic of conversation in hallways, bars, and informal social gatherings. One famous pharamacologist told me flatly, "I will never cite Snyder." The adjectives used to portray Pert's personality are even more extreme than those used to describe her as a scientist, including impetuous, tempestuous, aggressive, earthy, candid, theatrical, intense, intimidating, and draining. She confides about her problems being a graduate student while also a wife and mother, and describes being mugged three times.

In sum, the genealogy of four academic generations points to an elite group that contributed major breakthroughs to biomedical science. Each member of the family in succession became renowned and, with the exception of Pert, has been the recipient of numerous major awards. Their common link appears to be an unbounded enthusiasm for science and an ability to impose unusual demands on their students, whether dictatorially, benevolently, psychologically, or exuberantly. All worshipped their mentors in the beginning and acknowledge deep debts to their predecessor. The masters, in turn, lavished much praise on their apprentices. However, being humans as well as scientists, they reflect strengths and weaknesses of a very peculiar animal species and became embroiled in priority conflicts. All are excited by good data, but the enthusiasm of each was tempered by his or her individual personality traits. All had the intuitive insight to solve major problems with the experimental tools at hand and asked the right question at the right time. Nonetheless, their approaches to projects were not always as systematic or rationalized in the manner demanded by peer-review committees for research grants. Indeed, Axelrod once told me, tongue in cheek, that one reason he never thought too seriously about any of the numerous academic offers he received was because he was afraid he would not be able to write grant proposals that would gain approval in time and amount. In truth, he had his cake and could eat it all at NIH.

The book makes great reading for the lay public as well as scientists. It is highly recommended for all and should be a must for graduate students and postdoctoral fellows embarking on a career in pharmacology.

Literature Cited

1. Kaganowich, G., O'Connor, K., Morse, D., Horton, H. 1986. Government, media and the animal issue. *Fed. Proc.* 45:7a–14a
2. Sneader, W. 1985. *Drug Discovery: The Evolution of Modern Medicines.* Chichester/New York: Wiley. 435 pp.
3. Wilkinson, C. F. 1986. Risk assessment and regulatory policy. *Comm. Toxicol.* 1:1–20
4. National Academy of Sciences. 1983. *Risk assessment in the federal government: Managing the process.* Natl. Res.

Coun. Natl. Acad. Sci. Washington, D.C.
5. Woodcock, B. G., Menke, G., Rietbrock, N. 1986. Nitroplasters and bioavailability. *Trends Pharmacol. Sci.* 7:338–40
6. Kanigel, R. 1986. *Apprentice to Genius: The Making of a Scientific Dynasty.* New York: MacMillan
7. Herron, C. R. Review of apprentice to genius. *New York Times,* October 5, 1986

SUBJECT INDEX

A

Abnormal involuntary movements
  levodopa therapy and, 116-17
Acephate
  immunotoxicity of, 37
Acetaminophen
  discovery of, 431
  extracorporeal removal of, 183-84
  overdose of, 169
Acetylcholine
  adenosine and, 326
  atonia and, 142-43
  calcium channels and, 352
  corelease of, 60
  cortical desynchronization and, 140
  cotransmission of, 53-57
  organization of, 138-39
  ponto-geniculo-occipital waves and, 141-42
  rapid eye movements and, 140-41
  REM sleep and, 139-46
Acetylcholine receptor
  kinetic analysis of, 219
  models for, 199
Acetylcholinesterase
  cholinergic neurons and, 138-39
Acetyl-CoA
  carnitine and, 258-60
N-Acetylcysteine
  acetaminophen overdose and, 183
  methylmercury poisoning and, 188
N-Acetylprocainamide
  extracorporeal removal of, 185
Achalasia
  calcium channel blockers and, 347
Acidemias
  organic
    carnitine and, 262-63
Acquired immune deficiency syndrome
  adenosine and, 333
Actinidin
  structure of, 195
Actinomycin D
  intercalation and, 195-96

Adenine nucleotides
  cell function and, 315-16
Adenocarcinoma
  diesel exhaust and, 286-87
Adenoma
  diesel exhaust and, 286
Adenosine
  bioavailability of, 322-24
  calcium channels and, 352
  cell function and, 315-16
  cellular energy and, 334
  gastrointestinal system and, 333
  immune system and, 333
  ion fluxes and, 325
  neurotransmitter release and, 325-26
  phosphatidylinositol and, 325
  pulmonary system and, 332-33
  respiration and, 334
  sedative effects of, 316
  uptake of, 334
Adenosine diphosphate
  metabolism regulation and, 261
Adenosine monophosphate
  extracellular adenosine and, 323
Adenosine receptors, 317-21
  cardiovascular system and, 331-32
  central nervous system and, 328-31
  cyclic AMP and, 324-25
  kidneys and, 332
  therapeutic targeting of, 335
Adenosine recognition sites, 327-28
Adenosine triphosphate
  extracellular adenosine and, 323
  sedative effects of, 316
Adenosine triphosphate receptors, 321-22
S-Adenosylhomocysteine
  cardiac adenosine and, 323
Adenylate cyclase
  adenosine and, 316-17
  adrenergic receptors and, 216, 225
  pertussis toxin and, 324
Adenylate kinase
  ATP-binding site of, 205

Adenylyl cyclase, 371-80
  adrenergic receptors and, 374-75
  G-proteins and, 372-74
  hormone-sensitive, 379-80
  yeast, 378-79
Adrenergic receptor
  adenylyl cyclase and, 374-75
  G-proteins and, 376-78
  subtypes of, 216
Adrenergic receptor metabolism, 215-31
  in vitro studies of, 221-26
  in vivo studies of, 226-30
  kinetic analysis of, 219-20
  measurement of, 217-18
Adriamycin
  cardiac toxicity of
    carnitine and, 271
Adult respiratory distress syndrome
  platelet-activating factor and, 246-47
Adverse drug reactions, 71-72, 76-78
Affective disorders
  muscarinic supersensitivity in, 148
Aflatoxin
  immunotoxicity of, 38-39
Alcohol
  dialyzability of, 177
  poisoning by, 169
Alcohol dehydrogenase
  chloral hydrate metabolism and, 182
  ethylene glycol metabolism and, 181
  glycol ethers and, 412
  structure of, 195
Alcoholism
  REM latency and, 147
Allergic reactions
  gold and, 32
  platinum complexes and, 32
Aluminum
  extracorporeal removal of, 186
Alveolar gas exchange
  diesel exhaust and, 288
Amanita phalloides
  poisoning by, 188
Amanita verna
  poisoning by, 188

439

CONTRIBUTING AUTHORS

CHAPTER TITLES, VOLUMES 23–27

Annual Reviews Inc.

A NONPROFIT SCIENTIFIC PUBLISHER

 4139 El Camino Way
P.O. Box 10139
Palo Alto, CA 94303-0897 • USA

ORDER FORM

Now you can order
TOLL FREE
1-800-523-8635
(except California)

Annual Reviews Inc. publications may be ordered directly from our office by mail or use our Toll Free Telephone line (for orders paid by credit card or purchase order, and customer service calls only); through booksellers and subscription agents, worldwide; and through participating professional societies. Prices subject to change without notice. ARI Federal I.D. #94-1156476

- **Individuals:** Prepayment required on new accounts by check or money order (in U.S. dollars, check drawn on U.S. bank) or charge to credit card — American Express, VISA, MasterCard.
- **Institutional buyers:** Please include purchase order number.
- **Students:** $10.00 discount from retail price, per volume. Prepayment required. Proof of student status must be provided (photocopy of student I.D. or signature of department secretary is acceptable). Students must send orders direct to Annual Reviews. Orders received through bookstores and institutions requesting student rates will be returned.
- **Professional Society Members:** Members of professional societies that have a contractual arrangement with Annual Reviews may order books through their society at a reduced rate. Check with your society for information.
- **Toll Free Telephone orders:** Call 1-800-523-8635 (except from California) for orders paid by credit card or purchase order and customer service calls only. California customers and all other business calls use 415-493-4400 (not toll free). Hours: 8:00 AM to 4:00 PM, Monday-Friday, Pacific Time.

Regular orders: Please list the volumes you wish to order by volume number.
Standing orders: New volume in the series will be sent to you automatically each year upon publication. Cancellation may be made at any time. Please indicate volume number to begin standing order.
Prepublication orders: Volumes not yet published will be shipped in month and year indicated.
California orders: Add applicable sales tax.
Postage paid (4th class bookrate/surface mail) by **Annual Reviews Inc.** Airmail postage or UPS, extra.

ANNUAL REVIEWS SERIES		Prices Postpaid per volume USA/elsewhere	Regular Order Please send:	Standing Order Begin with:
			Vol. number	Vol. number
Annual Review of ANTHROPOLOGY				
Vols. 1-14	(1972-1985)	$27.00/$30.00		
Vol. 15	(1986)	$31.00/$34.00		
Vol. 16	(avail. Oct. 1987)	$31.00/$34.00	Vol(s). _____	Vol. _____
Annual Review of ASTRONOMY AND ASTROPHYSICS				
Vols. 1-2, 4-20	(1963-1964; 1966-1982)	$27.00/$30.00		
Vols. 21-24	(1983-1986)	$44.00/$47.00		
Vol. 25	(avail. Sept. 1987)	$44.00/$47.00	Vol(s). _____	Vol. _____
Annual Review of BIOCHEMISTRY				
Vols. 30-34, 36-54	(1961-1965; 1967-1985)	$29.00/$32.00		
Vol. 55	(1986)	$33.00/$36.00		
Vol. 56	(avail. July 1987)	$33.00/$36.00	Vol(s). _____	Vol. _____
Annual Review of BIOPHYSICS AND BIOPHYSICAL CHEMISTRY				
Vols. 1-11	(1972-1982)	$27.00/$30.00		
Vols. 12-15	(1983-1986)	$47.00/$50.00		
Vol. 16	(avail. June 1987)	$47.00/$50.00	Vol(s). _____	Vol. _____
Annual Review of CELL BIOLOGY				
Vol. 1	(1985)	$27.00/$30.00		
Vol. 2	(1986)	$31.00/$34.00		
Vol. 3	(avail. Nov. 1987)	$31.00/$34.00	Vol(s). _____	Vol. _____

ANNUAL REVIEWS SERIES	Prices Postpaid per volume USA/elsewhere	Regular Order Please send:	Standing Order Begin with:
		Vol. number	Vol. number
Annual Review of COMPUTER SCIENCE			
Vol. 1 (1986)	$39.00/$42.00		
Vol. 2 (avail. Nov. 1987)	$39.00/$42.00	Vol(s). _____	Vol. _____
Annual Review of EARTH AND PLANETARY SCIENCES			
Vols. 1-10 (1973-1982)	$27.00/$30.00		
Vols. 11-14 (1983-1986)	$44.00/$47.00		
Vol. 15 (avail. May 1987)	$44.00/$47.00	Vol(s). _____	Vol. _____
Annual Review of ECOLOGY AND SYSTEMATICS			
Vols. 1-16 (1970-1985)	$27.00/$30.00		
Vol. 17 (1986)	$31.00/$34.00		
Vol. 18 (avail. Nov. 1987)	$31.00/$34.00	Vol(s). _____	Vol. _____
Annual Review of ENERGY			
Vols. 1-7 (1976-1982)	$27.00/$30.00		
Vols. 8-11 (1983-1986)	$56.00/$59.00		
Vol. 12 (avail. Oct. 1987)	$56.00/$59.00	Vol(s). _____	Vol. _____
Annual Review of ENTOMOLOGY			
Vols. 10-16, 18-30 (1965-1971, 1973-1985)	$27.00/$30.00		
Vol. 31 (1986)	$31.00/$34.00		
Vol. 32 (avail. Jan. 1987)	$31.00/$34.00	Vol(s). _____	Vol. _____
Annual Review of FLUID MECHANICS			
Vols. 1-4, 7-17 (1969-1972, 1975-1985)	$28.00/$31.00		
Vol. 18 (1986)	$32.00/$35.00		
Vol. 19 (avail. Jan. 1987)	$32.00/$35.00	Vol(s). _____	Vol. _____
Annual Review of GENETICS			
Vols. 1-19 (1967-1985)	$27.00/$30.00		
Vol. 20 (1986)	$31.00/$34.00		
Vol. 21 (avail. Dec. 1987)	$31.00/$34.00	Vol(s). _____	Vol. _____
Annual Review of IMMUNOLOGY			
Vols. 1-3 (1983-1985)	$27.00/$30.00		
Vol. 4 (1986)	$31.00/$34.00		
Vol. 5 (avail. April 1987)	$31.00/$34.00	Vol(s). _____	Vol. _____
Annual Review of MATERIALS SCIENCE			
Vols. 1, 3-12 (1971, 1973-1982)	$27.00/$30.00		
Vols. 13-16 (1983-1986)	$64.00/$67.00		
Vol. 17 (avail. August 1987)	$64.00/$67.00	Vol(s). _____	Vol. _____
Annual Review of MEDICINE			
Vols. 1-3, 6, 8-9 (1950-1952, 1955, 1957-1958) 11-15, 17-36 (1960-1964, 1966-1985)	$27.00/$30.00		
Vol. 37 (1986)	$31.00/$34.00		
Vol. 38 (avail. April 1987)	$31.00/$34.00	Vol(s). _____	Vol. _____
Annual Review of MICROBIOLOGY			
Vols. 18-39 (1964-1985)	$27.00/$30.00		
Vol. 40 (1986)	$31.00/$34.00		
Vol. 41 (avail. Oct. 1987)	$31.00/$34.00	Vol(s). _____	Vol. _____

ANNUAL REVIEWS SERIES	Prices Postpaid per volume USA/elsewhere	Regular Order Please send: Vol. number	Standing Order Begin with: Vol. number

Annual Review of **SOCIOLOGY**

Vols. 1-11	(1975-1985)	$27.00/$30.00		
Vol. 12	(1986)	$31.00/$34.00		
Vol. 13	(avail. Aug. 1987)	$31.00/$34.00	Vol(s). _____	Vol. _____

Note: Volumes not listed are out of print.

SPECIAL PUBLICATIONS	Prices Postpaid per volume USA/elsewhere	Regular Order Please Send:

Annual Reviews Reprints: **Cell Membranes, 1975-1977**

(published 1978)   Softcover .... $12.00/$12.50   _____ Copy(ies).

Annual Reviews Reprints: **Immunology, 1977-1979**

(published 1980)   Softcover .... $12.00/$12.50   _____ Copy(ies).

Intelligence and Affectivity:
Their Relationship During Child Development, by Jean Piaget

(published 1981)   Hardcover .... $8.00/$9.00   _____ Copy(ies).

Telescopes for the 1980s

(published 1982)   Hardcover .... $27.00/$28.00   _____ Copy(ies).

The Excitement and Fascination of Science, Volume 1

(published 1965)   Clothbound .... $6.50/$7.00   _____ Copy(ies).

The Excitement and Fascination of Science, Volume 2

(published 1978)   Hardcover .... $12.00/$12.50
                   Softcover .... $10.00/$10.50   _____ Copy(ies).

TO: **ANNUAL REVIEWS INC.,** a nonprofit scientific publisher
      4139 El Camino Way
      P.O. Box 10139
      Palo Alto, CALIFORNIA 94303-0897

Please enter my order for the publications listed above. California orders, add sales tax. Prices subject to change without notice.

Institutional purchase order No. _____

Amount of remittance enclosed $_____

Charge my account ☐ VISA

☐ MasterCard   ☐ American Express

INDIVIDUALS: Prepayment required in U.S. funds or charge to bank card below. Include card number, expiration date, and signature.

Acct. No. _____

Exp. Date _____   _____
                         Signature

Name _____
        (Please print)

Address _____
          (Please print)

_____ Zip Code _____

_____ Send free copy of current **Prospectus** ☐
Area(s) of Interest   Federal I.D.#94-1156476